# Echography of the Eye and Orbit

Olivier Bergès

Editor

# Echography of the Eye and Orbit

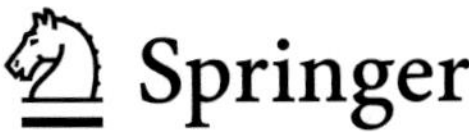 Springer

*Editor*
Olivier Bergès
Neuroradiology Department
Hôpital Fondation Adolphe de Rothschild
Paris, France

ISBN 978-3-031-41469-5          ISBN 978-3-031-41467-1   (eBook)
https://doi.org/10.1007/978-3-031-41467-1



This Springer imprint is published by the registered company Springer Nature Switzerland AG
The registered company address is: Gewerbestrasse 11, 6330 Cham, Switzerland

Paper in this product is recyclable.

*"I said one thing, you heard another, you
wrote a third."*
*Rabbi Israel Baal Shem-Tov*

*To you Monique, MEB, who deserve more
than a scherzo as Berlioz did, and far
more than the two chapters you wrote; for
you have always supported this project,
and allowed me to devote myself fully to it.
And to my friends, Dominique, Elisabeth, JB,
Mario, Michel, Patricia, Pierre...,
so close and so different, who have all helped
me from the start.*

# Foreword by Ronald H. Silverman

It is with great pleasure that I introduce this translation of *Echography of the Eye and Orbit*. Having spent much of my professional career immersed in the field of ophthalmic ultrasound, I have been witness to several decades of technological advances and broadening clinical application. This book, by world-renowned expert Olivier Bergès M.D. together with experts in transducer design, ocular biometry, ultrasound biomicroscopy, Doppler and clinical applications, offers a comprehensive and up-to-date guide to the theory and practice of ophthalmic echography.

The discipline of ophthalmic echography has a history of over a half-century, during which ultrasound technology and our clinical understanding of the eye and its diseases have evolved at an accelerating pace. *Echography of the Eye and Orbit* offers a timely and indispensable guide by the leaders in the field to the English-speaking world on the physical principles, latest technology, diagnostic applications and exam technique.

The chapters within this volume span a wide range of topics, expertly curated to provide a holistic understanding of diagnostic ophthalmic ultrasound. The volume begins with an exploration of the physics and technology behind ultrasound imaging, shedding light on the fundamental principles that underpin its use in ophthalmology. While this topic has been addressed before, the approach here is both wide-ranging and unique in expanding the discussion from the traditional single-element probes that have until recently dominated ophthalmic echography, to describe annular and linear array technologies, including probe design, imaging modes, artifacts and Doppler. Although Doppler has long been routinely used in virtually all other clinical specialities, Doppler technology and clinical use in ophthalmology may be new to many ophthalmologists and sonographers, making this an especially valuable contribution.

The book's scope extends from the cornea to the orbit. A chapter on ultrasound biomicroscopy covers anterior segment imaging and biometry with excellent and informative UBM images, sometimes supplemented by Doppler. Methods for measurement of the anterior chamber, the iridocorneal angle and retroiridal structures are described in considerable detail. The emphasis on quantitative methods offered on current instruments is critical for assessment of the angle in glaucoma.

The discussion proceeds from the anterior segment to cover imaging of pathologies of the vitreous, retina, choroid and orbit and the optimal techniques for conducting the exam in each case. The use of color-flow Doppler as a diagnostic tool, described in great detail, represents a leap in terms of diagnostic capability with respect to current B-scan systems that only offer structural imaging.

The publication of this volume in English is both welcome and timely, introducing the thinking and experience of French experts to a broader audience. The profound expertise of the authors will bring the reader, whether experienced professional or novice, valuable general knowledge and specific guidance on the latest technology and the practice of ocular echography. I am confident that this volume will become an indispensable guide and reference to all practitioners of ophthalmic echography.

Ronald H. Silverman, Ph.D.
Professor of Ophthalmic Science
Columbia University Irving Medical
Center
New York, USA

# Foreword to the French Edition by José-Alain Sahel

When Olivier Bergès wrote to me to ask me to write a preface to his forthcoming book on ultrasound, warning me that the deadlines would be short, I was surprised and flattered, then curious and finally happy to share my keen interest in the subject of this book and also some memories.

I have known Olivier Bergès for decades. Long before I returned to the Rothschild Foundation in 2001, I had followed his work, which was marked by a rigorous clinical diagnosis based on a methodical approach. Inspired by a great confidence in the power of this technology, he has accompanied its capacity to evolve and has never ceased to enrich the range of characteristics that he could detect and combine to describe a clinical picture. His approach is also marked by a concern to collaborate closely with clinicians to understand the context and the stakes of an investigation, which thus often becomes central and not only complementary. Integrated in a renowned radiology department, which deploys numerous imaging techniques, he has given ultrasound an inescapable status for all those who have benefited from his expertise. What is also remarkable is his willingness to share the knowledge he has acquired and built and to work with a large network of leading specialists who have participated in numerous training courses organized by Olivier and have contributed to the book presented today. The content of the book, which the reader will be able to consult very often, is rich in illustrations inserted in a didactic context that fully integrates the variety of tables to be explored and a broad perspective.

On a personal note, I would like to emphasize two elements of my experience. More than 30 years ago, following Prof. Brini in Strasbourg, I took charge of an ocular oncology consultation. He encouraged me to complete my training by taking ultrasound courses. With Prof. Flament, I had the opportunity to meet Dr. Poujol and Dr. Cantalloube at the XV–XX, great experts in B-mode ultrasound. I then attended

Karl Ossoinig's courses in Munich on standardized ultrasound, particularly in A-mode, an intense and demanding course. They made me aware of the complexity and power of ultrasound and at the same time of the fragmented nature of the expertise of an isolated clinician.

The work of Olivier Bergès, his lectures and courses were known to all. It is in a very particular context that they were able to develop: that of the Adolphe de Rothschild ophthalmological Foundation. This establishment has a particular charm for me, always renewed. I began my internship there more than 40 years ago and returned 20 years ago as the head of the department. Part of a little-known private non-profit sector, the Foundation welcomes a large number of patients who can benefit from the care of uncommon practitioners who are so exceptional that they have often not found their place or chosen to practice in the traditional academic world, but this has never prevented them from developing knowledge and skills that often make them international leaders. At the Foundation, there is a freedom of action, a simplicity, an almost family spirit and a collegiality that allows collaboration between departments in the service of patients. The Foundation has always welcomed unique personalities, whose names, such as Mawas, still resonate with many of us. I remember in the 1980s courses in strabology that were unique in the French landscape, the first intra-ocular implants, then orbital and pediatric surgery, not to mention neuro-imaging, interventional neuro-radiology and functional neurosurgery. The list of specialists who have practiced and still practice there is very impressive. Olivier Bergès is one of them. He has been able to take advantage of the diversity of clinical pictures that present themselves, of the particular attention paid by these clinicians to a precise diagnosis in order to decide on an effective and safe therapy, and above all of the willingness to collaborate to arrive at a decision that is, if not ideal, at least relevant.

This book therefore presents the expertise of the authors but also of all those who have entrusted them with patients and, in the end, it is to the patients themselves that it owes its richness, its complexity and its importance. As you will see, each chapter is preceded by a quotation that brings an element of variety, sometimes humor, often depth. In my turn, I will once again use an expression of Eugène Delacroix: "Accuracy is not the truth." Certainly, the concern of the right detail does not allow for apprehending the whole truth, but it is certain that the approximation, the lack of rigor, rhyme with the error.

After reading this book, it will be more difficult than ever to err in the analysis of clinical pictures for which ultrasound offers irreplaceable precision.

José-Alain Sahel<br>
Member of the Académie des Sciences<br>
and the Académie des Technologies<br>
Professor of Ophthalmology<br>
Sorbonne University<br>
Paris, France

Former Head of Ophthalmology<br>
department at the CHNO des<br>
Quinze-Vingts<br>
Rothschild Foundation Hospital<br>
Paris, France

Distinguished Professor and Chairman,<br>
Department of Ophthalmology<br>
University of Pittsburgh Medical<br>
Center<br>
Pittsburgh, USA

# Preface

Since its birth at the end of the 1950s, ultrasound of the eye and orbit has continued to grow, flourish and diversify, passing through its successive developments from the simple status of being useful to that of being envied. A-mode and B-mode ultrasound, once rivals, have been joined by color Doppler and (very) high-frequency ultrasound. This entire corpus continues to be perfected, refined and increased in specificity, thanks to ever-stimulating technological improvements, but also, by the same token, continues to become more complex.

The reader should not be surprised by the presentation of the images. I have decided to present them as they appear on the ultrasound screen: those obtained with a frequency of 10 MHz and a dedicated device have the anterior part of the eye on the left side of the image; those obtained with a frequency of 10–18 MHz and a multipurpose device, as well as the images obtained at 25 MHz (high frequency) or 50 MHz (very high frequency), have the anterior part of the eye at the top of the image. I hope that this "gymnastics of the mind" will not be a handicap.

Like any ultrasound, it is a dynamic examination "in real time" based of course on the clinical signs presented by the patient but which must be adapted "as we go along" to the first information obtained. It is therefore perilous to try to apply immutable protocols and rules of examination without exception. However, we have tried to take up this challenge and to study in this book not only the ultrasound semiology of the different ocular and orbital diseases but also to show the contribution of the different ultrasound techniques, but also the other medical imaging techniques, angiographies of the fundus, OCT, CT and MRI. In this way, the reader can deduce for himself the best way to conduct the examination and the diagnostic approach.

As will be reiterated throughout the book, it is not necessary to perform all the ultrasound techniques every time, but it is important to master their respective indications, especially as the problems of differential diagnosis become more acute. However, so that no one is lost, we have carefully detailed the technique of all the ultrasound techniques available today. A small caveat nevertheless: the technological evolution is so fast that some of the techniques exposed are still "works in progress," but one can wonder if, by the time the book is published, they will not render obsolete others that seem today clearly established. For this, we ask for the indulgence of our readers.

The constant improvement of ultrasound machines and the different ultrasound modes has made this ultrasound less operator-dependent, and not only because of the improvement of purely technical problems. An anecdote that will make the younger generation smile is that with the first machine, I used (the EO2), one had to take the image directly on the screen with a polaroid and an exposure time of the order of a second by pressing the trigger with the left hand, while with the right hand, one tried to obtain a demonstrative image without movement—nothing to do of course with the current image loops that allow one to choose very easily the image that shows the most characteristic sign.

You will note, especially when looking at the table of contents, that this is a collective work under the aegis of CTEREO, the French-speaking society of diagnostic ultrasound in ophthalmology. We also invite the readers to join CTEREO or SIDUO, the international society for diagnostic ophthalmic ultrasound as soon as they have finished reading the book. We wish a good and enriching reading to all. Thanks to all my co-authors for bringing their expertise to each of their favorite subjects, knowing that they could have written all the chapters. I would like to thank in particular Prof. de La Torre for having brought his mastery of standardized echography to the diagnosis of various ocular and orbital pathologies.

Finally, I would like to thank Prof. Sahel and Prof. Silverman for taking the time to write the forewords to this book.

Olivier Bergès<br>
Rothschild Foundation Hospital<br>
Paris, France

# Contents

# Editor and Contributors

## About the Editor

**Dr. Olivier Bergès, MD** Deputy Department Head, Neuroradiology Department, Rothschild Foundation Hospital, Paris, France. Founder member and president of French Society of Ophthalmic Ultrasound (CTEREO) and member of the executive board of Societas Internationalis Pro Diagnostica Ultrasonica in Ophthalmologia/International Society for Diagnostic Ophthalmic Ultrasound (SIDUO). e-mail: oberges@for.paris

## Contributors

**Jean Abascal** Ultrasound Project Manager, Biophysics Medical Clermont-Ferrand, France

**Prof. Philippe Arbeille, Ph.D., MD** Professor Emeritus of Biophysics (Clinical ultrasound), Director UMPS (Research unit Space Medicine/Physiology), School of Medicine, University of Tours, France. e-mail: arbeille@med.univ-tours.fr

**Alain Bectard** Engineer, Technical Support and After Sales Training for several ultrasound companies (CGR, ATL, Philips, SSI). e-mail: abectard51@gmail.com

**Dr. Violaine Caillaux, MD** Ophthalmologist, specialized in ocular imaging and in the diagnosis and treatment of retinal diseases. Member of CTEREO.

Explore Vision Ophthalmic Diagnostic Centers in Paris and in Rueil, France. e-mail: violainecaillaux@gmail.com

**The Late Prof. Michel Claudon MD, Ph.D.** Professor of Radiology, Nancy School of Medicine. Former Department Chair, Radiology Department, Brabois Hospital, CHRU Nancy, France; Former President of the CERF (French College of Radiology

Trainers); Former President of EFSUMB (European Federation of Societies for Ultrasound in Medicine and Biology) and of WFUMB (World Federation of Societies for Ultrasound in Medicine and Biology).

**Dr. Monique Elmaleh-Bergès, MD** Pediatric Neuroradiologist and Head/Neck Imaging, Robert Debré University Hospital, Paris, France. e-mail: monique.elmaleh@aphp.fr

**Dr. Audrey Feldman, MD** Ophthalmologist, Medical Retina and Ocular Imaging Hyperspecialist. Centre Lyon Est Ophtalmo, Saint-Priest, France. Member of CTEREO. e-mail: afeldman@lyonestophtalmo.fr

**Dr. Jean-Brice Gauthier, MD** Ophthalmologist, Department Chair of Ophthalmology, Laon Hospital, France. e-mail: jean-brice.gauthier@ch-laon.fr

**Dr. Patricia Koskas, MD** Neuroradiologist and specialist in ophthalmological imaging, Rothschild Foundation Hospital, Paris, France. Member of the Executive Board of French Society of Neuro-Ophthalmology (CNOF), Member of CTEREO. e-mail: pkoskas@for.paris

**Prof. Mario de La Torre, MD, Ph.D.** Head Professor and Chair of Ophthalmology, Universidad Nacional Mayor de San Marcos, Lima, Perú. Medical Director of DLT Ophthalmic Diagnostic Center, Former Chairman of the Ultrasound and Radiology of the Instituto Nacional de Oftalmología Lima, Perú. Secretary of SIDUO. Scientifical Director of Quantel Medical by Lumibird, Clermont-Ferrand, France. e-mail: mariodlt@gmail.com

**Dr. François Lafitte, MD** Neuroradiologist and specialist in ophtalmological imaging, Rothschild Foundation Hospital, Paris, France. Member of the Executive Board of French Society of Neuro-Ophthalmology (CNOF), Member of CTEREO. e-mail: flafitte@for.paris

**Dr. Jacques Laloum, MD** Ophthalmologist, Glaucoma specialist, Rothschild Foundation Hospital, Paris, France. e-mail: jlaloum@for.paris

**Prof. Pascal Laugier, Ph.D.** With a master's degree and Ph.D. in physical acoustics, plus medical training and postdoctoral training in biomedical ultrasound, all from the University of Paris, he held a full-time permanent position at National Center for Scientific Research (CNRS) as Research Director (Full-professor with the highest rank). He was the head of the Biomedical Imaging (2014–2018), a public laboratory affiliated with Sorbonne University of Paris, CNRS, and French National Institute of Health (INSERM). He was also a former director of the Parametric Imaging Lab (2001–2014). He co-authored some 220 articles in peer-reviewed journals, gave 120 invited talks and keynote speeches and co-edited two books entitled Bone Quantitative Ultrasound (Springer 2011, 2021). e-mail: pascal.laugier@upmc.fr

**Prof. Augustin Lecler, MD, Ph.D.** Neuroradiologist and specialist in ophthalmological imaging, Rothschild Foundation Hospital, Paris, France. Master of conferences, University of Paris. Member of CTEREO. e-mail: alecler@for.paris

**Dr. Elisabeth Nau, MD** Specialist in ophthalmologic imaging, Neuroradiology Department, Rothschild Foundation Hospital, Paris, France. Member of CTEREO. e-mail: enau@for.paris

**Dr. Pierre Pégourié, MD** Ophthalmologist, specialist in ophthalmic ultrasound since 1981. University Hospital of Grenoble, France. Member of the Board of the National Union of Ophthalmologists of France (SNOF). Founding Member and Past President of CTEREO. Member of SIDUO. e-mail: pegourie.pierre@club-internet.fr

**Dr. François Perrenoud, MD** Ophthalmologist, specialist in ophthalmic ultrasound. Former Practitioner of APHP Hospitals of Paris and CHIC Hospital of Créteil. Teaching Assistant in university degrees. Vice President of CTEREO

Explore Vision Ophthalmic Diagnostic Center Paris, France e-mail: fr.fraper@gmail.com

**Dr. Michel Puech, MD** Ophthalmologist, trained in ophthalmic ultrasound at Hôtel-Dieu Hospital, Paris. Founder and Medical Director of Explore Vision Ophthalmic Diagnostic Centers in Paris and in Rueil, France. Manager of VuExplorer Institute (a training organization in ocular imaging). Organizer of the annual conference "Ophthalmic Imaging from Theory to Current Practice." Teacher, Author or Co-author of several books and annual reports of the French Society of Ophthalmology. Former Treasurer of CTEREO. Member of SIDUO. e-mail: drmichelpuech@gmail.com

**Dr. Dominique Satger, MD** Ophthalmologist, Former Practitioner at Hôtel-Dieu and the Pitié Salpétrière Hospitals, Paris. Ophthalmic Ultrasound Specialist, University Hospital of Grenoble. France. Founding Member of CTEREO. e-mail: dsatger@gmail.com

**Dr. Mickaël Sellam, MD** Ophthalmologist, specialist in ocular imaging (echography, OCT, angiography), Member of CTEREO and SIDUO.

Explore Vision Ophthalmic Diagnostic Center Paris, France e-mail: drsellam@hotmail.fr

**Dr. Kamal Siahmed, MD** Ophthalmologist, specialist in ocular imaging, formerly practitioner at University Hospital Rouen, France. Ophthalmic center, Vernon, France Author and Co-author of several scientific articles and numerous oral presentations at international meetings on Imaging of the eye. Co-author of the annual report (2003) of the French Society of Ophthalmology on Vitreous Pathology (G. Brasseur *ed*). e-mail: dr.ksiahmed@gmail.com

**Dr. Maté Streho, MD, FEBO** Ophthalmologist, specialist in ocular imaging (echography, OCT and angiography), Member of CTEREO and SIDUO.

Explore Vision Ophthalmic Diagnostic Center Paris, France. e-mail: mstreho@ yahoo.fr

**Cédric Vénuat** Ultrasound Project Manager, Quantel Medical Clermont-Ferrand, France. e-mail: cvenuat@quantelmedical.fr

# Abbreviations

| | |
|---|---|
| A- | Amplitude |
| AA (AA amyloidosis) | Amyloid A, secondary amyloidosis |
| AAION | Arteritic anterior ischemic optic neuropathy |
| AC | Anterior Chamber |
| ACA | Anterior Chamber Angle |
| ACD | Anterior chamber depth |
| ACG | Angle-closure glaucoma |
| AION | Anterior ischemic optic neuropathy |
| AL (AL amyloidosis) | Light chain, primary amyloidosis |
| ALARA | As low as reasonably achievable |
| AMD | Age-related macular degeneration |
| AOD | Angle opening distance |
| ARA | Angle recess area |
| ASIC | Application-specific integrated circuit |
| AS-OCT | Anterior segment OCT |
| AVF | Arteriovenous fistula |
| AVI | Audio video interleave |
| B- | Brightness Here |
| BB | Bullet Ball, a small metallic ball projected by an airsoft gun (or a pellet gun) |
| BRVO | Branch Retinal Vein Occlusion |
| CD | Choroidal detachment |
| CDFI | Color Doppler flow imaging |
| CDI | Color Doppler imaging |
| CMUT | Capacitive micromachined ultrasonic transducer |
| CRA | Central retinal artery |
| CRAO | Central retinal artery occlusion |
| CRV | Central retinal vein |
| CRVO | Central retinal vein occlusion |
| CRVx | Central retinal vessels |
| CSF | Cerebrospinal fluid |

| | |
|---|---|
| CT | CT scan/CT scanner |
| DICOM | Digital imaging and communications in medicine |
| DIY | Do It Yourself, a cause of domestic accidents |
| ELP | Effective lens position |
| EMM | Epimacular membrane |
| EMR | Electronic medical record |
| ENT | Ear, Nose and Throat |
| FB | Foreign body |
| FDA | Food and drug administration |
| FEVR | Familial exudative vitreoretinopathy |
| FFT | Fast Fourier transform |
| FGPA | Field-programmable gate array |
| GA | General anesthesia |
| HDMI | High-definition multimedia interface |
| HFU | High-frequency ultrasound |
| HMI | Human machine interface |
| Hz | Hertz |
| ICA | Iridocorneal Angle |
| ICH | IntraCranial Hypertension |
| IICH | Idiopathic intracranial hypertension |
| IOFB | Intraocular foreign body |
| IOI | Idiopathic orbital inflammation |
| IOL | Intraocular lens implant |
| ION | Ischemic optic neuropathy |
| IOP | Intraocular Pressure |
| $I_{SPPA3}$ | Spatial-peak pulse-average acoustic intensity |
| $I_{SPTA3}$ | Spatial-peak temporal-average acoustic intensity |
| IT | Iris Thickness |
| IVH | Intravitreal hemorrhage |
| JPEG | Joint Photographic Experts Group |
| KILD | Kerato-irido-lenticular dysgenesis |
| LCD | Liquid crystal display |
| LED | Light-emitting diodes |
| LPI | Laser peripheral iridotomy |
| LV | Lens vault |
| M.I. | Muscle index |
| MGDA | Morning glory disc anomaly +++ |
| MH | Macular hole |
| MHz | Megahertz |
| MI | Mechanical index |
| MRI | Magnetic resonance imaging |
| NCO | Neonatal corneal opacity |
| NF | Neurofibromatosis |
| NFI | Neurofibromatosis type 1 |
| NF2 | Neurofibromatosis type 2 |

| | |
|---|---|
| OCT | Optical coherence tomography |
| OD | Oculus dexter |
| ON | Optic nerve |
| ONSD | Optic Nerve Sheath Diameter |
| Opht A | Ophthalmic artery |
| OS | Oculus sinister |
| PACG | Primary angle-closure glaucoma |
| PC | Personal computer |
| PDF | Portable document format |
| PFCL | Perfluorocarbon liquids |
| PFV | Persistent fetal vasculature |
| PHOMS | Peripapillary hyperreflective ovoid mass-like structures |
| PHPV | Persistent hyperplastic primary vitreous |
| PI | Peripheral iridotomy |
| pIOL | Phakic intraocular lens |
| PMMA | Polymethylmethacrylate |
| PRF | Pulse repetition frequency |
| PSV | Peak systolic velocity |
| PVD | Posterior vitreous detachment |
| PVR | Proliferative vitreoretinopathy |
| RB | Retinoblastoma |
| RD | Retinal detachment |
| RI | Resistive index |
| RMS | Rhabdomyosarcoma |
| SAS | Subarachnoidal Space |
| S.N.I. | Supero nasal index |
| SOV | Superior ophthalmic vein |
| sPCAs | Short posterior ciliary arteries |
| SRD | Serous retinal detachment |
| T | Tissue sensitivity |
| TAB | Temporal artery biopsy |
| TI | Thermal index |
| TIB | Thermal index for bone |
| TIC | Thermal index for the bones of the skull |
| TIS | Thermal index for soft tissue |
| TISA | Trabecular iris space area |
| UBM | Ultrasound biomicroscopy |
| US | Ultrasound/Medical diagnostic ultrasound |
| USB | Universal serial bus |
| USFDA | Food and Drug Administration in the US |
| VHFU | Very High-frequency ultrasound |
| VKH | Vogt-Koyanagi-Harada |
| VM | Vitreous membrane |
| VMT | Vitreous macular traction |

# Chapter 1
# Physical Principles of Ultrasound Propagation and Image Formation

Pascal Laugier

**Abstract** This chapter provides a comprehensive review of the physical principles of ultrasound propagation and image formation, with examples of the eye and orbit. Ultrasonic waves are first defined according to their speed, frequency and wavelength. The reflection and transmission of an ultrasonic wave, as well as scattering and the concept of attenuation, are subsequently outlined. The main steps of ultrasound image formation are then described, with a piezoelectric transducer acting as the ultrasound source and receiver, followed by an analysis of image resolution, and the conditions for its optimization at a given frequency. Finally, the principle of tissue characterization is discussed, based on the estimation of the backscatter coefficient as a function of frequency, and different applications to ophthalmology are presented.

## 1.1 Ultrasound Waves

An ultrasound wave is a pressure perturbation that travels through a medium at a well-defined speed. We can better understand this wave phenomenon by observing the waves on the surface of a pond that originate from the impact of a pebble thrown into the water. The wave originates from the initial disturbance of the water surface. The perturbation propagates and reproduces identically to itself at a distance from the point where it originated with a delay that depends on the speed at which the waves propagate. An object floating on the surface of the water undergoes an oscillatory movement as the wave passes and then, once the wave has passed, regains its initial position. In biological tissues, oscillations of very small amplitudes caused by a local variation in pressure propagate and thus allow for exploring the tissue depth-wise and generating an image of it from the echoes produced each time the pressure wave encounters an obstacle.

The pressure oscillations of an ultrasound wave are so fast and of such low amplitude that they are not perceived by humans. The frequency, which is expressed in Hertz (Hz), reflects the number of vibration cycles per second (1 Hz = 1 vibration

P. Laugier (✉)
Research Director at CNRS, and INSERM, Paris, France
e-mail: pascal.laugier@upmc.fr

© The Author(s), under exclusive license to Springer Nature Switzerland AG 2024

O. Bergès (ed.), *Echography of the Eye and Orbit*,
https://doi.org/10.1007/978-3-031-41467-1_1

Frequency range

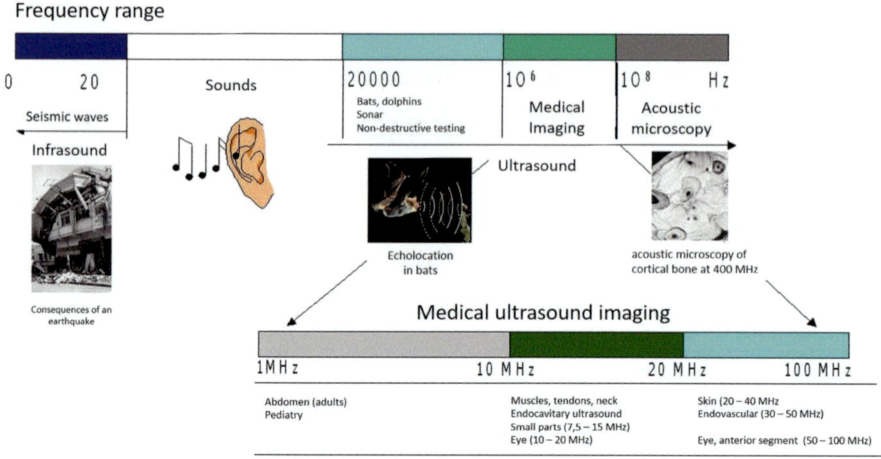


**Fig. 1.1  Scale of mechanical wave frequencies**. Ground tremors give rise to seismic waves. Their frequency is generally between 0.3 and 20 Hz, and they are referred to as infrasound. Ultrasound begins beyond the audible frequency band in humans, and it is a means of communication for some animals (e.g., dolphins). Bats are able to navigate in the dark by emitting ultrasound. Ultrasound in the 50-kHz to 1-MHz frequency range is used for exploring the seabed (sonar) or non-destructive testing of materials (nuclear, aeronautics, railway, automotive industry, etc.). Most medical applications are in the 2- to 20-MHz range, although higher frequency applications have recently been developed that are aimed at ultrasound of the skin, the anterior segment of the eye, or the endovascular wall. Frequencies greater than 100 MHz are referred to as acoustic microscopy

per second; 1 MHz = 1 megaHertz = 1 million vibrations per second). The frequencies of ultrasound waves in the field of medical imaging are mostly between 2 and 20 MHz, or even 50–100 MHz for the study of the cornea and the anterior segment of the eye. These frequencies are much higher than the frequency range of sound waves that the human ear can perceive (20–20,000 Hz) (Fig. 1.1).

## 1.2   Speed—Frequency—Wavelength

The speed of a wave is a characteristic of the propagation medium that reflects the distance traveled by the wave per unit of time (i.e., the speed at which the initial perturbation propagates through a medium). It is expressed in meters per second (m/s). The speed with which a perturbation is transmitted from one point to another in the medium depends on both the stiffness of the medium (or its inverse, compressibility) and its density (or inertia). Transmission of the wave increases with the stiffness of the medium, and it decreases as the density increases (greater inertia). The speed is represented as:

**Table 1.1** Propagation speeds in ocular and some other media [1–3]

| Medium | Speed of sound (m/s) |
| --- | --- |
| Air | 340 |
| Fat | 1462 |
| Water | 1524 |
| Vitreous body | 1513-1532 |
| Iris | 1542 |
| Ciliar body | 1554 |
| Liver | 1560 |
| Retina | 1576 |
| Optical nerve | 1615 |
| Lens of the eye | 1590-1640 |
| Subcapsular cataract | 1630-1641 |
| Sclera | 1597-1622 |
| Cortical bone | 3500-4000 |
| Metal (aluminum) | 6400 |

[a] Speed values in water and biological media are given at 37°

$$c = \sqrt{\frac{E}{\rho}} \tag{1.1}$$

where $E$ is the stiffness and $\rho$ the density. Because of the high-water content of biological soft tissues, ultrasound waves propagate in soft tissues substantially at the same speed, with a value close to the speed of propagation in water (the speed in water is 1524 m/s; the average speed in soft tissues is 1540 m/s). However, there are differences between tissues (Table 1.1). The speed of wave propagation in highly compressible gases (such as air) is much lower than the speed of wave propagation in water. The wave propagation speed in rigid media (bone, metal, glass, etc.) is higher than in water.

The wavelength is a measure of the spatial extent of a vibration cycle (i.e., the distance between two consecutive points in the medium in the same vibrational state: in the case of waves on the surface of the water, it is the distance between two adjacent crests or troughs). The wavelength is shorter the slower the wave propagates and the shorter the duration of a vibration cycle (high ultrasound frequency). The wavelength is thus a characteristic of both the wave and the propagation medium. It can be expressed mathematically as:

$$\lambda = \frac{c}{f} \tag{1.2}$$

where $f$ is the frequency. The wavelengths in a vitreous body at 10 and 20 MHz are 150 and 75 μm, respectively.

Wavelength is an important concept because it sets the resolution limit of the image. Image resolution is greater when the frequency of the ultrasound waves increases. However, ultrasound waves attenuate rapidly in biological tissues, and this occurs faster at higher frequencies. Ultrasound frequencies between 2 and 20 MHz are usually used in humans, which allows resolutions that are at best in the order of a few hundred microns. In the case of exploring small-sized (eye) or superficial (skin, anterior segment) organs, one can use higher frequencies and generate images with a resolution close to a few tens of microns [3].

## 1.3 Reflection and Transmission of an Ultrasound Wave

In biological tissues, ultrasound waves interact with the tissue structures encountered along their path. The waves can be reflected, scattered, or absorbed. Each of these interaction mechanisms results in a loss of energy from the incident wave and contributes to the total attenuation of the wave.

In terms of the image, reflection and scattering are the most important mechanisms because they give rise to the echoes from which the structures are identified on the ultrasound image.

Specular reflection refers to the change in direction of the wave when it encounters a large obstacle in relation to the wavelength. The incident beam is split in two: a reflected beam and a transmitted beam. In the case of an incidence perpendicular to the interface, the reflected beam leaves exactly in the direction from where the incident wave is coming from (an echo returns to the transducer), and the beam transmitted in the second medium continues in the initial direction (Fig. 1.2a). Otherwise, the angle of reflection $\theta_r$ is equal to the angle of the incidence $\theta_i$ and the transmitted beam is deflected (or refracted). The angle of refraction $\theta_t$ is governed by the following equation:

$$\frac{\sin\theta_i}{c_1} = \frac{\sin\theta_t}{c_2} \tag{1.3}$$

where $\theta_i$ and $\theta_t$ are the directions of the incident and transmitted beams, respectively, with respect to a right angle to the interface, and $c_1$ and $c_2$ are the propagation speeds in the first and second medium, respectively (Fig. 1.2b).

A representative morphological image of the explored medium is obtained on the basis of echoes from the reflection at the interfaces. During the examination, the operator always tries to position the ultrasound probe so as to orient the incident beam perpendicular to the structures examined in order to collect echoes of maximum amplitude. Refraction is not important in medical imaging, except when the mismatch between $c_1$ and $c_2$ is high. In this case, refraction can cause artifacts. The "Baum bump" is the most well known of these artifacts in ultrasound imaging of the eye. Two effects combine to explain this artifact: the biconvex shape of the lens and a higher propagation speed in the lens than in the vitreous body. These properties cause the ultrasound beam to be refracted to the edges of the lens, and the echoes from the

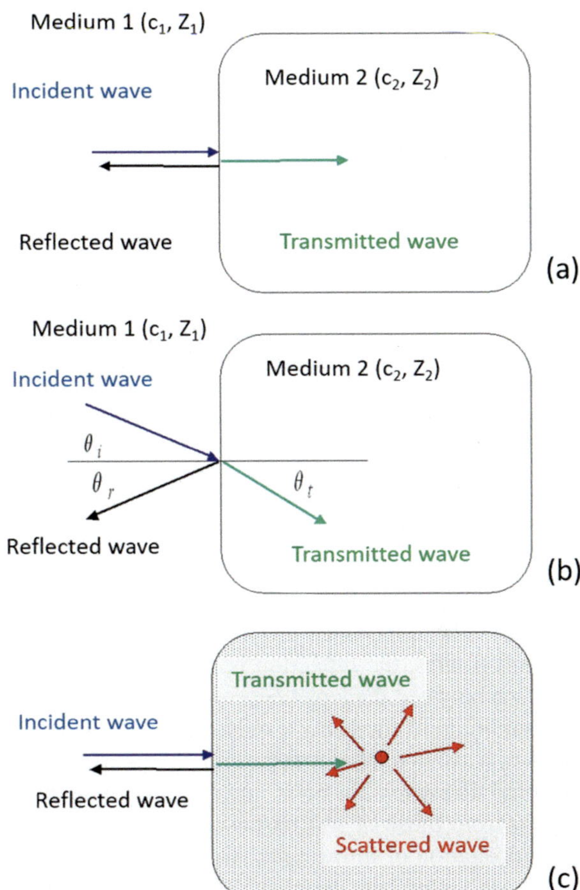



**Fig. 1.2  Interaction by specular reflection** in normal incidence (**a**), oblique incidence (**b**), and scattering (**c**)

posterior pole return faster to the transducer in the area swept through the lens. This results in a distortion of the image of the posterior pole (Fig. 1.3) (see Fig. 6.8).

To determine the amplitude of the echo, we define the acoustic impedance, a parameter related to the material characteristics of the medium. The acoustic impedance Z of tissues is defined by the product of the density $\rho$ and the propagation speed ($Z = \rho c$). The amplitude of the echo depends on the difference in the acoustic impedances of the two media and the direction of the incident beam with respect to the interface. In the case of a normal impact on the interface (i.e., the incident beam is perpendicular to the interface), the ratio of the amplitude of the echo ($A_r$) to the amplitude of the incident signal ($A_0$) is determined by:

$$R = \frac{A_r}{A_0} = \frac{Z_1 - Z_2}{Z_1 + Z_2} \tag{1.4}$$

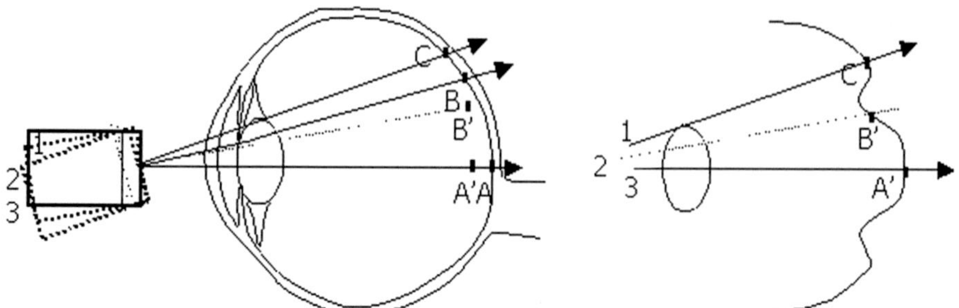

**Fig. 1.3 The "Baum bump" is explained by the change in speed and refraction across the lens.**
A beam that reaches the surface of the lens under non-normal incidence is refracted to the edges of
the lens. In addition, echoes from the posterior pole return faster to the transducer in the area swept
through the lens (where propagation is faster than in the vitreous). This results in a distortion of the
posterior pole because reflective area A is seen as being in A′ by the transducer in position 1, zone
B is seen as being in B′ by the transducer in position 2, etc., whereas zone C is seen as being in its
actual position by the transducer in position 3. This artifact is especially evident for myopic eyes
with a cataractous lens

This ratio defines the reflection coefficient *R*. The reflection at the interface is more
intense as the impedance difference $Z_1 - Z_2$ increases. At the interface between
two soft tissues, the reflection is generally of low amplitude. For example, for an
interface between the lens ($Z_{\text{lens}} = 1.73$) and the vitreous body ($Z_{\text{vitrous}} = 1.54$) [4],
the amplitude of the echo is only one-tenth of the incident amplitude. Most of the
incident wave is transmitted through the interface, and deeper structures can then be
explored. However, air, bone, and certain foreign bodies with impedances that differ
greatly from those of soft tissues are highly reflective and represent an obstacle to
the propagation of ultrasound. An acoustic shadow cone (an acoustic shadow area
where echoes are very attenuated or absent) then forms behind such highly reflective
structures (foreign body, calcified lens, some hyperechogenic tumors).

In other cases, highly reflective structures are responsible for a phenomenon of
reverberation. Such reverberation is caused by multiple reflections of the wave transmitted inside the structure (such as a foreign body); generates a series of close echoes,
the amplitude of which decreases rapidly; and gives rise to the characteristic presentation of a "comet tail" on the image. Reverberations can be seen in the presence of
a foreign body or intraocular gas.

## 1.4 Scattering

Scattering occurs due to the interaction of the wave with a small object at the scale
of the wavelength. The scattered wave is redistributed in all directions of space
(Fig. 1.2c). Although the contours of macroscopic structures (cornea, lens, eyeball,
tumor, etc.) are caused by reflection at interfaces, the echotexture (or internal image)

of tissues is due to echoes scattered by the multiple heterogeneities (or scatterers) of small size that are present in tissues such as blood capillaries, connective tissue, cell clusters, etc. On an ultrasound image, a solid tumor differs from a fluid mass by the presence of echo texture. A fluid area appears devoid of echoes.

The scattering power of a tissue is characterized by its backscatter coefficient. The laws of scattering are complex and beyond the scope of this book. One should simply note that the backscatter coefficient depends on the material characteristics (compressibility and density) of the scatterer, and it increases with the scatterer size and the number of scatterers per unit volume, as well as with the ultrasound frequency.

## 1.5   Attenuation

The wave amplitude and intensity (intensity is proportional to the square of the amplitude) attenuates when it propagates in tissues. The ultrasound intensity decreases exponentially with the depth z of penetration into tissues as follows:

$$I = I_0 e^{-\alpha z} \tag{1.5}$$

where $\alpha$ (expressed as $cm^{-1}$) is the attenuation coefficient and $I$ and $I_0$ are the intensities at depths z and z = 0, respectively. In soft tissues, $\alpha$ is proportional to the frequency. This is why the depth of penetration of ultrasound is less the higher the frequency.

The attenuation and heterogeneity of biological tissues are such that the dynamics of echoes (the ratio between the highest and lowest value of the echo intensity) can be substantial, ranging from $10^{10}$ to $10^{12}$. This is why quantities such as intensity or attenuation, and their dynamics, are generally expressed in decibels (dB), which is a more practical unit of measurement for comparing very different values. Of note, an attenuation of 10 dB corresponds to an intensity divided by 10. For example, an intensity ratio equal to $10^{10}$ corresponds to a difference of 100 dB, and an intensity ratio equal to $10^{12}$ corresponds to an attenuation of 120 dB, etc.

The attenuation coefficient depends on the nature of the tissue. For example, for the lens, the attenuation coefficient at 10 MHz is approximately 2 dB $mm^{-1}$, whereas it is negligible in the vitreous body. Because the attenuation coefficient is proportional to the frequency, its value at 50 MHz is close to 10 dB $mm^{-1}$ in the lens.

Reflection and scattering contribute to attenuation by redirecting some of the energy in different directions than that of the incident wave. Part of the wave is also absorbed by the tissues and converted into heat (Fig. 1.4). This loss of energy in the form of heat, when excessive, can lead to elevated temperatures that are damaging to cells and tissues. Diagnostic equipment is subject to standards that limit the power in order to avoid too much of an increase in temperature. However, the increase in temperature is used in certain therapeutic applications to cause necrosis and thus treat different pathologies such as glaucoma or melanoma [5, 6].

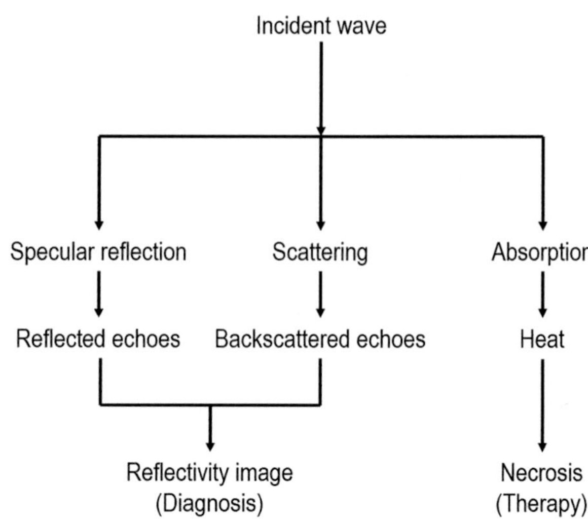



**Fig. 1.4 Diagram summarizing the interactions of ultrasound waves with tissues**. Wave attenuation results from loss by absorption, scattering, and specular reflection. Only scattered echoes and echoes reflected at an incidence close to normal can be used to generate an image

Attenuation results in rapid signal loss at depth. To compensate for this attenuation and ensure a satisfactory reading of echoes at all depths, most ultrasound scanners have a function to amplify the signal according to the depth. This function is set manually on some devices, although for others, an optimal gain curve is calculated and applied to the signal automatically.

## 1.6  Principle of Ultrasound Imaging

The main stages of ultrasound image generation are illustrated in Fig. 1.5. A piezo-electric transducer acts as an ultrasound source and receiver. Upon transmission, the transducer converts an excitatory electrical pulse into an ultrasound pressure wave. This ultrasound pulse propagates steadily in the biological environment. At a speed of 1540 m/s, ultrasound pulses travel 1 mm in 0.65 microseconds ($\mu$s).

The echoes from the reflection or scattering return to the transducer operating in reception mode immediately after the transmission phase. Each time an echo arrives at the surface of the piezoelectric sensor, the pressure wave is converted into a radio frequency electrical signal. The amplitude of the electrical signal is proportional to the amplitude of the echo. The envelope of the radio frequency signal is detected, stored, and then converted to gray scale. Once all the echoes have been received, the transducer is activated again in transmission mode to emit a new ultrasound pulse in an adjacent direction. Thus, each new transmission corresponds to a different line of the image. The image is generated by the set of lines that have swept the section (2D image) or the volume (3D image). There are currently different rapid scanning processes (mechanical or electronic). Mechanical scanning remains the most common scanning mode on devices dedicated to ophthalmology. The ultrasound

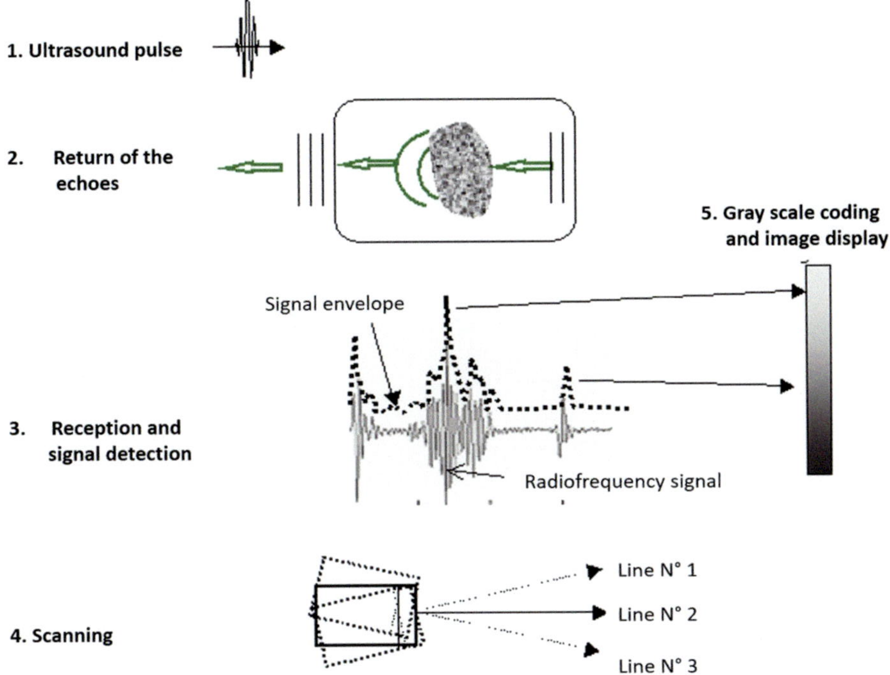



**Fig. 1.5** Illustration of the main steps in the construction of an ultrasound image

probe is controlled by a motor. The direction of the firing axis is given by the direction of the probe axis, which moves under the effect of the movement applied by the motor.

Ultrasound A-mode (A-scan) represents the amplitude of the signal as a function of time (Fig. 1.6). The time t that elapses between the transmission and reception of an echo (flight time) corresponds to the duration of a round trip of the ultrasound wave between the target and the sensor. The time of flight of an echo is determined by the following equation:

$$ct = 2z \tag{1.6}$$

Therefore, time indicates the depth z at which the reflecting (or scattering) structures are located. The amplitude of the echo provides information regarding the reflectivity of the target. A-mode is used to perform accurate distance measurements. Accurate knowledge of the speed c is essential to accurately convert the time of flight of echoes into distances on the image. For example, in the presence of silicone oil filling the posterior segment after intervention for retinal detachment with a much lower speed of propagation than that of the vitreous, the eye appears abnormally long on the ultrasound image.

B-mode (B-scan), which is the grayscale image representation of ultrasound data collected in a section plane, is the most commonly used mode.

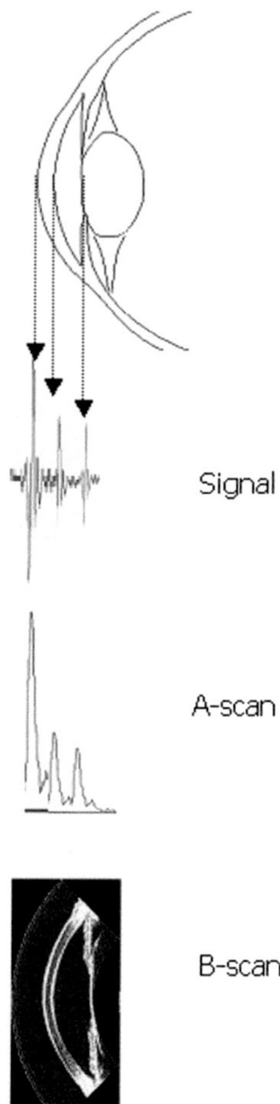

**Fig. 1.6** Illustration of an A-scan and B-scan for anterior segment exploration



## 1.7  Resolution

The level of detail of an image depends on the resolution capability of the imaging system. The resolution is defined by the minimum distance that must separate two targets for their images to be distinct. From a theoretical point of view, the resolution limit of an imaging system is determined by the wavelength. Because the wavelength decreases as the frequency increases, the resolution power increases with frequency. However, because attenuation also increases with frequency, the use of high-frequency probes is limited to the exploration of superficial or small-dimensional structures. A high resolution of approximately 30 μm is obtained when exploring the anterior segment at 80 MHz. To visualize the deeper posterior pole, the frequency must be reduced to 10 or 20 MHz, which results in lower resolution.

In ultrasound, three resolutions are usually defined according to the direction considered. A distinction is made between axial resolution (along the firing axis), lateral resolution (in the direction of the scanning), and azimuthal resolution (in elevation).

The axial resolution depends on the duration of the ultrasound pulse. It should be as brief as possible. The increase in frequency and mechanical damping of the vibrations of the probe contribute to optimizing the axial resolution. The axial resolution with a 10-MHz frequency probe is approximately 0.12 mm.

The lateral resolution depends on the beam width. Lateral resolution is improved by focusing. As in optics, a convergent lens can be placed in front of the piezoelectric transducer. Another solution has been to give the transducer a spherical cup shape, which allows for concentrating the ultrasound beam in the center of the radius of curvature.

The resolution is determined by the width of the focal spot. This is provided by:

$$d \propto \lambda \frac{F}{D} \tag{1.7}$$

where $\lambda$, $D$, and $F$ are the wavelength, transducer diameter, and focal length, respectively. The resolution is optimal at the focal length, but it degrades when moving away from the focal point. This variation in depth resolution with single-element fixed focal length sensors has led engineers to generate ultrasound probes from multi-element transducers for achieving a variable focus at depth. The optimal lateral resolution with a 10-MHz probe is approximately 150 $\mu$m.

Azimuthal resolution defines the thickness of the section. With a circular single-element transducer, the azimuth resolution and lateral resolution are identical.


## 1.8  Tissue Characterization

When a pathological process affects a tissue, biochemical or microarchitectural changes alter its acoustic properties. The practitioner usually evaluates the tissue echo pattern on the image to guide the diagnosis. However, grayscale ultrasound imaging (B-scan) uses only part of the information contained in the radio frequency signal. In particular, during the detection of the envelope of the radio frequency signal, the spectral content is lost. Digital processing of radio frequency signals allows for exploiting this spectral content and estimating quantitative parameters (attenuation coefficient and backscatter coefficient as a function of frequency). These tissue acoustic properties revealed by ultrasound tissue characterization methods allow for several aspects of tissues to be probed that are not usually represented (or poorly represented and subject to subjective interpretation) on the image. Ultrasound characterization using quantitative parameters completes the diagnostic arsenal by allowing for classification of tissues according to "ultrasound types" [7] or monitoring of tissue changes to follow a treatment [8].

From the beginning of the use of ultrasound by ophthalmologists, the potential for quantitative methods was recognized. Quantitative measurements of the reflectivity level of intratumoral echoes (signal amplitude), attenuation (decrease in echo amplitude as a function of depth), and echotexture (spatial distribution of echoes) have been performed in standardized A-mode [9, 10].

With the extensive use of personal computers and advances in digital signal processing, tissue characterization has advanced significantly over the past two decades. The main recent developments of these techniques in ophthalmology can be credited to a team at the Riverside Research Institute in New York.

Tissue characterization methods focus on estimating the backscatter coefficient as a function of frequency. Scattering theory allows the backscatter coefficient and its frequency variation to be related to tissue microstructural properties (mainly the size of the scattering structures) and its material properties, in particular the acoustic concentration of scattering entities. Acoustic concentration is defined as the product of the number of scattering entities per unit volume and the relative acoustic impedance difference between the scattering entities and the surrounding environment [11, 12]. By estimating these parameters locally, they can be mapped for the entire explored volume and represented as color-coded parametric images superimposed on the conventional grayscale ultrasound image [13]. Although this calculation function is currently not available on commercial devices, it has been implemented in a handful of research centers. The sensitivity of acoustic parameters to tissue microarchitecture and their diagnostic value have been demonstrated in several studies. Acoustic characteristics are correlated with the presence and characteristics of microvascularization zones of choroidal melanomas [14]. Hence, they may be used as prognostic indicators in patients with melanoma [15].

These tissue characterization methods, initially developed for 10-MHz ultrasound of the posterior pole, have since been adapted for high-frequency imaging of anterior segment structures [14]. In patients with melanoma localized to the iris, Ursea et al. showed a correlation between the acoustic parameters and melanocyte size and density [16].

Other methods of tissue characterization have been devised, combining several acoustic parameters (attenuation and backscatter coefficients) with texture parameters derived from statistical analysis of the amplitudes of echoes. Discriminant analysis using all these parameters has revealed excellent performance for differentiation of histological types of choroidal melanoma [17, 18]. However, this type of analysis has gradually been abandoned in favor of evaluating the backscatter coefficient alone.

# References


1. Goss SA, Johnston RL, Dunn F. Comprehensive compilation of empirical ultrasonic properties of mammalian tissues. J Acoust Soc Am. 1978;64:423–67.
2. de Korte CL, van der Steen AFW, Thijssen JM. Acoustic velocity and attenuation of eye tissues at 20 MHz. Ultrasound Med Biol. 1994;20:471–80.
3. Pavlin CJ, Foster FS. Ultrasound biomicroscopy of the eye. New York: Springer; 1995.

4. Thijssen JM, Mol MJ, Timer MR. Acoustic parameters of ocular tissues. Ultrasound Med Biol. 1983;11:157–61.

5. Coleman DJ, Silverman RH, Ursea R, Rondeau MJ, Lizzi FL. Ultrasonically induced hyperthermia for adjunctive treatment of intraocular malignant melanoma. Retina. 1997;17:109–17.

6. Silverman RH, Vogelsang B Rondeau MJ, Coleman DJ. Therapeutic ultrasound for the treatment of glaucoma: results of a multicenter clinical trial. Am J Opthalmol. 1991;111:327–37.

7. Coleman DJ, Lizzi FL, Silverman RH, Helson L, Torpey JH, Rondeau MJ. A model for acoustic characterization of intraocular tumors. Invest Ophthalmol Vis Sci. 1985;26:545–50.

8. Coleman DJ, Lizzi FL, Silverman RH, Ellsworth RM, Haik BG, Abramson DH, Smith ME, Rondeau MJ. Regression of uveal malignant melanomas following cobalt-60 plaque. Correlates between acoustic spectrum analysis and tumor regression. Retina 1985; 5:73–8.

9. Ossoining KC. Quantitative echography: the basis of tissue differentiation. J Clin Ultrasound. 1974;2:33–46.

10. Verbeek AM. Differential diagnosis of intraocular neoplasms with ulrasonography. Ultrasound Med Biol. 1985;11:163–70.

11. Feleppa EJ, Lizzi FL, Coleman DJ, Yaremko MM. Diagnostic spectrum analysis in ophthalmology: a physiscal perspective. Ultrasound Med Biol. 1986;12:623–31.

12. Lizzi FL, Ostromogilsky M, Feleppa EJ, Rorke MC, Yaremko MM. Relation of ultrasonic spectral parameters to features of tissue microstructure. IEEE trans Ultrason Ferreoelec Freq Contr. 1986;33:319–29.

13. Silverman RH, Rondeau MJ, Lizzi FL, Coleman DJ. Three-dimensional high-frequency ultrasonic parameter imaging of anterior segment pathology. Opthalmology. 1995;102:837–43.

14. Silverman RH, Folberg R, Boldt HC, Lloyd HO, Rondeau MJ, Mehaffey MG, Lizzi FL. Coleman DJ. Correlation of ultrasound parameter imaging with microcirculatory patterns in uveal melanomas. Ultrasound Med Biol 1997; 23:573–81.

15. Coleman DJ, Silverman RH, Rondeau MJ, Boldt HC, Lloyd HO, Lizzi FL, Weingeist TA, Chen X, Vangveeravong S, Folberg R. Noninvasive in vivo detection of pronostic indicators for high-risk uveal melanomas. Opthalmology. 2004;111:558–64.

16. Ursea R, Coleman DJ, Silverman RH, Lizzi FL, Daly SM. Harrison W. Correlation of high-frequency backscatter with tumor microstructure in iris melanoma. Ophthalmology 1998;105:906–12.

17. Thijssen JM, Verbeek AM, Romijn RL, de Wolff-Rouendaal D, Oosterhuis JA. Echographic differentiation of histologic types of intraocular melanomas. Ultrasound Med Biol. 1991;17:127–38.

18. Romijn RL, Thijssen JM, Oosterveld BJ, JA Verbeek AM. Ultrasonic differentiation of intraocular melanomas: parameters and estimation methods. Ultrasonic Imaging 1991;13:27–55.

# Chapter 2
# Ultrasound Devices and Probes


**Alain Bectard, Jean Abascal, Cédric Vénuat, Philippe Arbeille, Patricia Koskas, and Olivier Bergès**



**Abstract** In ophthalmology, ultrasound images are obtained using devices based on two technological principles: dedicated devices, for ophthalmology, and multipurpose devices. In this chapter, we review the various technical and technological aspects to understand how the information is generated by the transducer and then displayed as an image on the screen for both dedicated and multipurpose devices. For dedicated devices, we carefully review the transducer and the probe with all the characteristics essential for them to be optimal, but, being linked together, they must lead to an acceptable compromise; from the piezoelectric crystal to the motor/magnet/Hall effect sensor assembly allowing the movement (magnetic effect) and to the pre-amplification of the ultrasound signals in the probe, with special focus on high-frequency (50-MHz) probes and annular transducers. Then, we discuss the ultrasound system, the PC and the screen. The multipurpose ultrasound devices may be of two types: (1) a conventional multipurpose ultrasound device, with a beamformer and then processing boards, one per mode, and an integrated computer ensuring the presentation of the image for display, calculation, and transfer; and (2) a digital multipurpose ultrasound device, with acquisition boards digitizing the information from the probes; management of the beam is ensured by software in the computer terminal, separating the different modes for analysis. Here we analyze the technological evolution of transducers: piezocomposite assembly and capacitive micromachined ultrasonic transducer. Finally, we discuss fully digital imaging. Then, we review the biological effects and the safety of ultrasound scanners and probes,



A. Bectard
Several Ultrasound Companies (CGR, ATL, Philips, SSI), Paris, France

J. Abascal
Biophysic Medical Clermont-Ferrand, Clermont-Ferrand, France

C. Vénuat
Quantel Medical Clermont-Ferrand, Clermont-Ferrand, France

P. Arbeille
UMPS, University of Tours, School of Medicine, Tours, France

P. Koskas · O. Bergès (✉)
Rothschild Foundation Hospital, Paris, France
e-mail: oberges@for.paris

including the Food and Drug Administration's September 2008 recommendations, established to limit the acoustic power of ultrasound scanners. At last, we address the cleaning and decontamination of probes, insisting on the use of customized probe covers.

An ultrasound system provides an image, displayed on a screen, of the information captured by the probe in contact with the patient. Such systems comprise a probe equipped with an ultrasound transducer that emits and in return receives echoes due to the interfaces of the different media that the beam traverses.

In ophthalmology, ultrasound images are obtained using devices based on two technological principles:

- *Dedicated devices*, for ophthalmology, allowing exploration of the entire eyeball, equipped with a single-crystal 10 MHz (or more recently 15 MHz) B-mode probe, a 20-MHz long focal probe (or more recently, a 20 MHz B-mode probe with 5 ring annular technology); an A-mode diagnostic probe (at best 8 MHz, following the principles of standardized echography); an A-mode biometry probe (usually 10 to 12 MHz); a 50-MHz / or sometimes 35 MHz (and even 25-MHz) probe(s) for the study of the anterior segment; and sometimes a 3D module, $\pm$ tissue characterization. The advantages of these devices are their compactness, mobility, relatively low cost, and very good spatial resolution of B-images.
- Devices dedicated to exploring the anterior segment (ultrasound biomicroscopy) with an oscillating single crystal of 50 MHz (but sometimes only 35 MHz with a lower but nevertheless satisfactory resolution).
- *Multipurpose devices*, with a linear B-mode probe, a wide frequency band and a central frequency greater than 7.5 MHz (the maximum frequency able to go as high as 22 MHz), capable of also providing Doppler information (color, power, and spectral), sometimes with a 3D representation and an elastography module. The advantages of these devices are the excellent spatial resolution of the B-images obtained, the pre- and/or post-processing of the images, the excellent resolution in terms of density of the images, due to the excellent performance of the grayscale, the ability to better study the anterior superficial regions (eyelids, anterior segment),due to the focus and a less bothersome "dead zone", and by better studying the lateral para-equatorial regions of the eye and the lens. However, these devices are not very mobile, and they are expensive.

It is of course essential to understand how one's device "works" in order to get the best performance and in particular to customize the settings. However, also being aware of the technical specifications of other machines is useful. Therefore, in this chapter, we review the various technical and technological aspects to understand how the information is generated by the transducer and then displayed as an image on the screen for both dedicated and multipurpose devices.

## 2.1   Dedicated Ultrasound Devices

### 2.1.1   The Ultrasound Device and the Probes

- A-mode probes (Amplitude mode) are simple probes that operate only on a Transmit/Receive line.
- B-mode probes (Brightness mode) are mechanical scanning probes used to generate a 2D image defined by a large number of juxtaposed lines (e.g., 256 or 384 lines over 50 degrees with a 10-MHz sector probe).

Information from the probes is processed and then digitized for presentation and storage.

***An example in the Aviso ultrasound device from Quantel-Medical**

Sequences of images over several seconds can be stored. They are viewed in real time, delayed at normal speed, or viewed frame by frame. This makes it easier to select an image.

Different measurements are possible with B-imaging: distance; angle; surface; specific calculations for anterior chamber angle analysis: LV, AOD, IT, ARA, and TISA. Finally, display of an implant power calculation report is also possible.

**The device consists of the following:**

- different B-mode transducers (sector / linear scanning) and A-mode,
- an ultrasound scanner, allowing:

  - processing of data acquisition (transmitted by the transducers),
  - direct access to the necessary functions during acquisition,

- a computer, allowing display of the ultrasound image as well as the functions that allow:

  - insertion of patient information
  - insertion of post-exam information (including measurements, calculations, etc.),
  - recording of images or videos,
  - production of reports,
  - transfer of data in different formats (JPEG, AVI, PDF, DICOM, EMR, etc.).

### 2.1.2   Ultrasound and the Piezoelectric Effect

Natural or synthetic crystals that have piezoelectric properties are used in ultrasound transducers. They emit mechanical vibrations when stimulated electrically, and conversely, they provide electrical voltages proportional to the acoustic pressures detected.

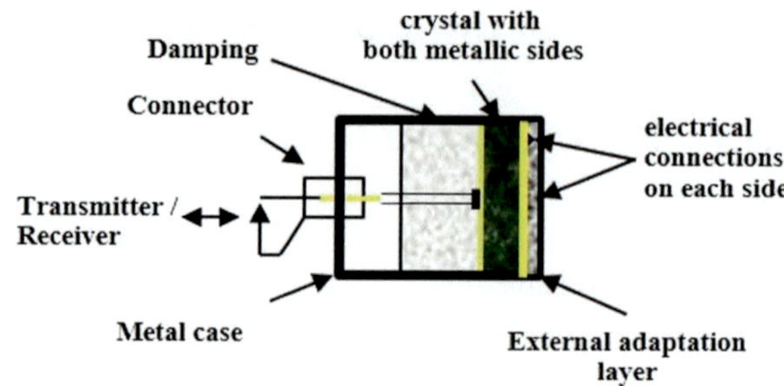


**Fig. 2.1** Diagram of a single crystal used in an ophthalmic dedicated ultrasound device

### 2.1.3 How are Transducers Made?

Transducers are composed of a piezoelectric crystal as well as different elements that determine their functioning (Fig. 2.1):

- An external adaptation layer on the front, to adapt to the surrounding environment
- A layer of absorbent material, at the back, which dampens the vibrations of the crystal
- An electrical link connecting the crystal to the emission and reception electronics, the front side being connected to the metal case (reference 0 V).

Various technologies are used for the crystal: natural, synthetic, or composite materials that combine the two.

The thickness of the crystal used determines the frequency range of the transducer. In the 20- to 50-MHz range, the thicknesses are less than 0.1 mm.

### 2.1.4 What Are the Characteristics of a "Good" Transducer

A transducer must be suitable for the intended exploration:

- The depth to be viewed and the desired resolution determine the frequency and sensitivity.
- The area to be prioritized determines the focal length and diameter of the crystal.

The characteristic features of transducers:

- Their opening, or useable diameter of the crystal
- Their focal length
- The depth of field is a result of the diameter of the crystal and the focal length
- Their central frequency of vibration
- Their bandwidth in frequency. It can be expressed as a percentage of the central frequency: 100% is a good value, equal to the central frequency, which is achieved with varying ease depending on the crystal technology. In practice, the central frequency may not be centered in relation to the frequency band.

- Their sensitivity.

All of these parameters are interrelated and must lead to an acceptable compromise.

## 2.1.5  How is a Probe Made?

**A-mode probes**: The transducer is simply mounted with a small support allowing agile and application-specific handling. A standardized A-probe has a narrow frequency band, which makes it easier to reproduce a central frequency value. In addition, it is not focused.

**B-mode probes**: They generate a two-dimensional section. The scan is usually mechanical, regulating the single transducer in a sectorial or linear movement.

## 2.1.6  How to Convert an Ultrasound Beam into an Image

The sequence by which a transducer works is as follows:

- Emission of a brief vibration that propagates in the medium to be explored (of the order of 1 $\mu$s or less):
  The necessary electrical impulse is very brief and can reach an amplitude of 100 V. It generates a very wide spectrum in which the transducer will draw the energy necessary to vibrate at its own frequency. This pulse is synchronized and triggers the pulse when the system is ready to record a line.
- Switch to reception mode to receive the feedback (much longer than the transmission time, in the order of 1 ms)

In reception mode, transducers are able to detect very weak signals as well as very strong signals:

> ***Example*** For a 10 MHz B-transducer: from 3 $\mu$V to 300 mV, a ratio of 100,000.
> 20 Log (100,000) = 20 $\times$ 5; or a dynamic range of 100 dB.

**Signal evaluation**

- **The transducer (Fig. 2.2)**:
  - Ultrasound signals are pre-amplified in the transducer, in order to make the transmission to the device (noise reduction) more reliable.

- There is also a complex integrated circuit (FGPA) in the probe, which controls the generation of the ultrasound emission (depending on the parameters of the device) and takes care of the functioning of the motor/Hall-effect sensor in order to generate the addressing indications for writing to memory.

**For example,** the emission rate varies from 2304 to 2720 Hz for a 10 MHz B-transducer and 3075 Hz for a 50 MHz linear transducer.

- **The ultrasound system** (Fig. 2.3):

  - An analog-to-digital converter in the device digitizes the ultrasound signals so that they can be stored in the memory.

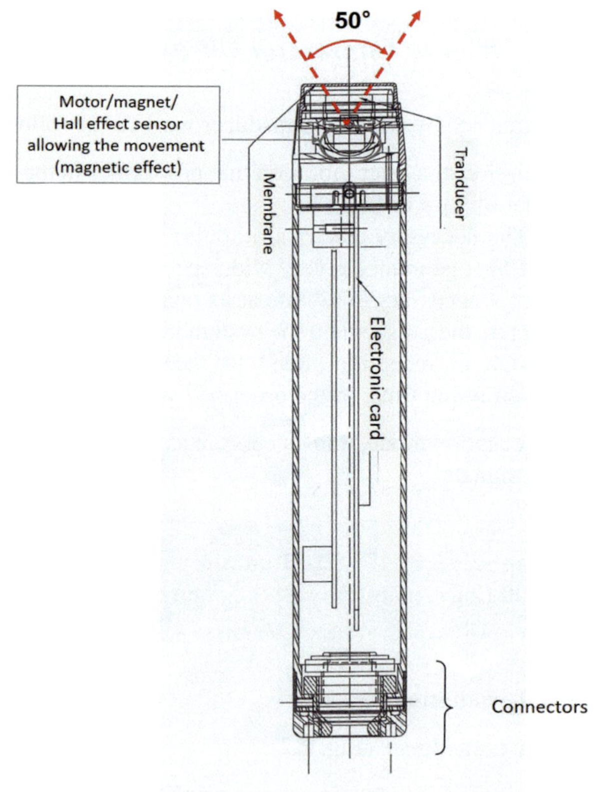


**Fig. 2.2** Diagram of a 10-MHz single-crystal probe of an ophthalmic dedicated ultrasound device

**Fig. 2.3** Diagram of an ophthalmic dedicated ultrasound scanner, showing the different steps between the probe and the display screen

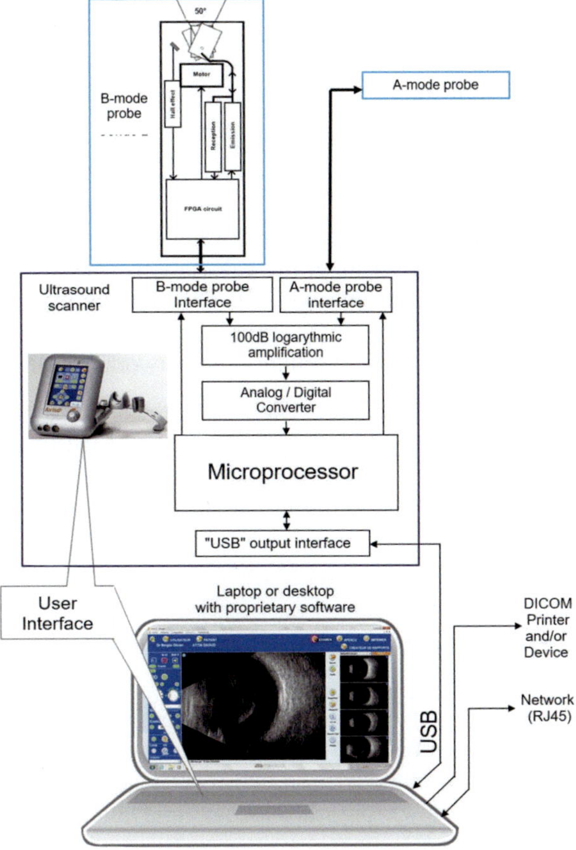


Note that in order to detect a signal, at least double the frequency must be used; for example, for a signal of 10 MHz, a frequency of 20 MHz is required, which provides a conversion/measurement every 50 ns.

- A microprocessor in the device manages the storage of the scanned ultrasound signals according to the addresses provided by the FGPA of the transducer and the presentation of the information for their visualization on a PC (based on an interface circuit by USB connection).
- The ultrasound device also provides the user interface for adjusting the acquisition parameters.

- **The PC:**

  - It provides the rest of the user interface and the presentation via a specific application:

    display of images (received from the ultrasound device) via Direct X (a set of application programming interfaces developed by Microsoft)
    integration of the Human Machine Interface (HMI) part, including the presentation of the software, entry of user data, patient, etc.
    management of the calculations (measurement of distances in biometric mode and B-mode, IOL calculations, etc.)
    formatting of the reports
    connection to printers and networks (EMR, DICOM).

  - The image matrix generated in the application depends on the graphics card, the screen resolution, and the size of the image allocated in the application. These settings are specified in Direct X.
  - The final result (resolution) depends directly on the quality of the PC's graphics card.

## 2.1.7  How Important is the Screen?

Regardless of the type of device, the settings and results will be assessed at the level of the image presented on the screen. There has been a succession of oscilloscopes with electrostatic deviation, which were very fast, then magnetic deflection tubes, which were slower but still adequate, and finally the first liquid crystal display (LCD) flat screens.

The current light-emitting diode (LED) screens (a matrix of tiny LED bulbs), which are part of the same category as the first LCD flat screens, are now essentially as fast as the older cathode ray tubes and as powerful in terms of contrast. The upper limit of cathode ray tubes is 1/3000 contrast, but the standard is 1/1500 to 1/2500. The current professional-quality LED screens generally have contrasts of 1/1000 to 1/2600. Finally, on recent ultrasound scanners, manufacturers use display corrections to make the best use of the dynamics of the type of screen used.

## 2.1.8  Is Full Digital Imaging Possible (Quality Computing) and, if so, How?

Fully digital imaging is desirable for all associated utilities (integration, miniaturization, stability, reliability, multiplicity of measurement, and calculation tools). As explained in #I.2.1.7, the results are analyzed on a screen. These screens are continuously being upgraded. The number of pixels has to increase for the image to have increased resolution. The pixel size must decrease, without a decrease in the brightness range. The image must be assessed according to its overall presentation. There are currently 15.4″ LED screens from $1320 \times 1080$ to $2880 \times 1800$ and 20″ from $1680 \times 1050$ with good contrast and display speeds compatible with the desired image quality/definition.

### 2.1.9  What Sets High-Frequency Transducers Apart?

High-frequency transducers are more difficult to manufacture because the thickness of the crystal decreases with frequency, and at 50 MHz, the reduced thickness is such that they become difficult to produce. Different synthetic materials provide very different performances in terms of sensitivities and frequency bands.

Attenuation in tissues increases rapidly with frequency. The same applies to oils or membranes that can be used as an intermediate in closed probes operating at 10 MHz. These materials, which already significantly attenuate at 20 MHz, become unusable at 50 MHz.

The only possible contact media for a 50-MHz probe are water-based ophthalmic gels or a layer of solidified gel. Therefore, all 35- and 50-MHz probes are open. A water bath is necessary, either in a scleral shell or in the probe itself using a very thin membrane, with an acoustic impedance equivalent to that of the medium being analyzed.

### 2.1.10  The Advent of Annular Transducers

Annular probes have been around for a long time, but their manufacture was technologically complex, especially for high-frequency probes. The focus of a transducer is achieved by its mechanical curvature (concave). However, this curvature has the disadvantage of de facto causing loss of resolution when the visualized target is not at the focal point. This problem is related to the fact that the reception of signals is not simultaneous on the surface of the transducer but creates a time lag for the reception of signals between the central and external part of the transducer, resulting in a phase shift of the signals.

The use of an annular transducer allows for processing and compensating for the delay in signals received on each ring, depending on the concave shape of the transducer, and thus improving the quality of the image. The second advantage of annular probes is that they improve the depth of field. Each signal received on each ring is analyzed and re-phased for each target point of the image (Fig. 2.4).

Processing of these signals is time-consuming but has become possible with the significant computing power of current computers, both in terms of the hardware of the circuit board controlling the probe and/or the computer configuration.

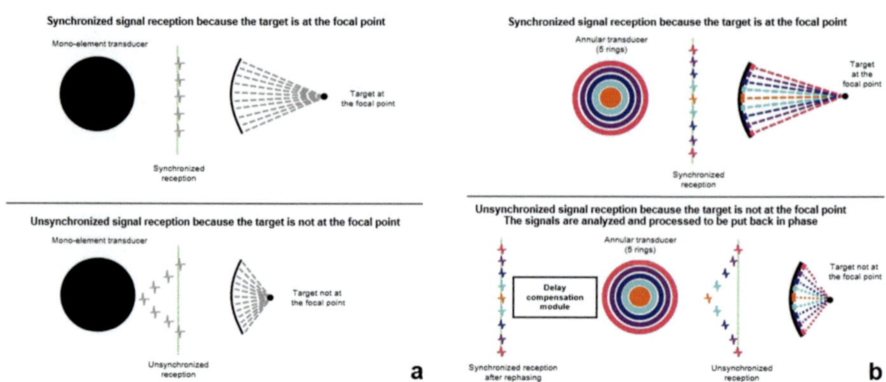



**Fig. 2.4** Comparison between a single-crystal transducer and an annular transducer (diagram): the latter allows for compensating for the delay of the received signals and thus increasing the focal area

## 2.2 Multipurpose Ultrasound Devices

### 2.2.1 The Ultrasound Device and the Probes

There are currently two types of multipurpose ultrasound devices, covering all price ranges, most often coupled to array transducers (linear or convex):

- either composed of a beam manager, commonly called a "beamformer" (a set of purely analog or mixed analog/digital acquisition boards connected to the transducers via a multiplexer used for transmission and reception, all coupled to a battery of specific analysis blocks (hybrid boards) or circuits, each providing imaging processing, 2D black and white, 2D coupled spectral Doppler, color Doppler, elastography and others), all connected to a computer providing presentation, storage, and a user interface (Fig. 2.5a).
- either composed of broadband analog/digital-capture boards (without specific processing) connected directly to the transducer elements; all connected (fast throughput) to a powerful computer that via the software provides all the treatments, both acquisition and analysis, for all types of mode (black and white 2D imaging, 2D coupled spectral Doppler, color Doppler, Elastography, and other modes), presentation, storage, and user interface (Fig. 2.5b).
- These systems are capable of generating measurements of distance, surface, and volume (2D); speed and quantity of flow (Doppler); tissue density (Elastography). The system and basic measurements can also be used to calculate specific values in relation to a protocol for acquiring precise values.

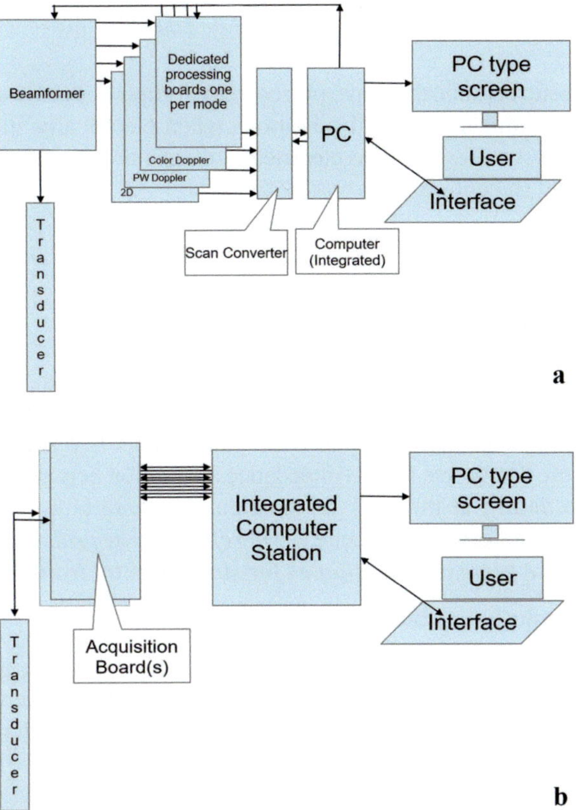



**Fig. 2.5** Diagram of a multipurpose ultrasound device. **a**: Conventional multipurpose ultrasound device: In this type of system, there is an analog or digital beamformer and then processing cards, one per mode; finally one or more cards ensure conversion (the acquired data arrive in the system at their own rate, depending on the type of acquisition, synchronous with ultrasonic emissions; they are written to image memory in a "random" way, then read and extracted from the image memory at a fixed rate depending on the associated software). An integrated computer ensures the presentation of the image for display, calculation, and transfer. The user interface allows for specific settings and annotations of the different selected obtained sections to be set (keyboard). **b**: Digital multipurpose ultrasound device: In this type of system, there is no longer a beam manager, but acquisition cards digitizing the information from the probes (RF signals—radio frequencies), management of the beam is ensured by software in the computer terminal, separating the different modes for analysis

- As for the transducers, they are most often array (a succession of piezoelectric elements, aligned), for which the scanning is electronic. They can be linear, convex, or mini-linear type arrangement with a "Phased-Array" sector scan (phase shift scanning); mechanical scanning transducers are rarely used because of the limited scanning speed.

### 2.2.2 Ultrasound and the Piezoelectric Effect

Natural or synthetic crystals that have piezoelectric properties are used in ultrasound transducers. They emit mechanical vibrations when electrically stimulated (emission), and conversely, they provide electrical voltages proportional to the acoustic pressures detected (reception).

### 2.2.3 How are Array Transducers Made?

These probes consist of a network of transducers with a thickness tailored to the desired frequency (a piezoelectric crystal, prepared from a large crystal or ceramic, cut into small elements); an impedance adaptation lens is placed in front of the elements to ensure transverse focus (impedance adaptation between the element and the analyzed medium); at the back of the elements there is a damper that limits vibrations to promote forward exchanges. *Therefore, array probes feature the same constraints and the same composition as for single-crystal transducers.*

**Technological evolution of the sensitive elements**

Progress in material machining techniques has made it possible to create a new entity called a Piezocomposite, allowing combination of small dimensions (essential for high-frequency elements) and resistance. Piezocomposite materials, by way of their production, are much more resistant to shocks than "piezoelectric materials". A polymer resin base supports small piezoelectric ceramic cylinders, which are electrically connected to each other to ensure the functions of the unitary element or a network of elements assembled into a linear or curved strip.

**For example,** to produce such a composite, a piezoelectric crystal is machined in two directions, in order to create a type of two-dimensional comb, cast in resin; then the stub is then removed leaving only the network of small elements, held by the resin (Fig. 2.6).

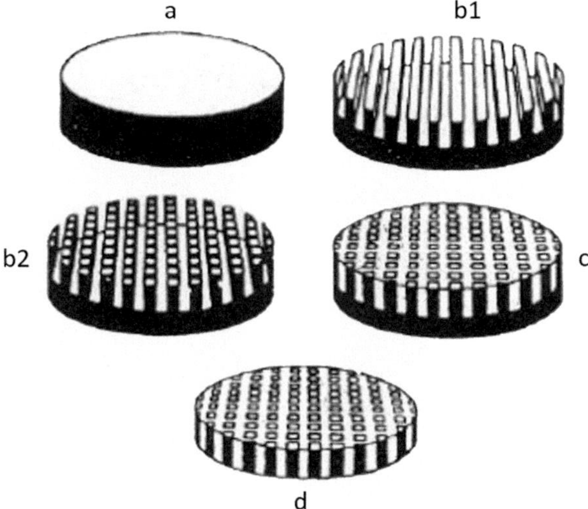


**Fig. 2.6** The process of piezocomposite assembly, more resistant than a single crystal. **a** Machining of a piezoelectric crystal; **b1**, **b2** creation of a type of 2D comb, then a network of small elements based on this crystal; **c** casting of the element in the resin; **d** removal of the stub, the small elements are held in place by the resin

## Images of probes

These images (Figs. 2.7, 2.8, and 2.9) show an example of a high-frequency probe, with exploded view drawings showing the stacking of the constituent elements of a linear strip type probe. This type of "sandwich" can be extended to micro-convex and phased arrays (mini-bars).

Frequency: 8–18 MHz.

A new electronic component will soon be able to assume the role of the elemental crystal, as promising research has allowed for producing active transmitter/receiver elements, capacitive micromachined ultrasonic transducer (CMUT), which will be able to replace piezoelectric elements in the near future. The characteristics of these non-resonant elements will allow these new probes to work at very wide frequency bands, from 1 to 200 MHz.

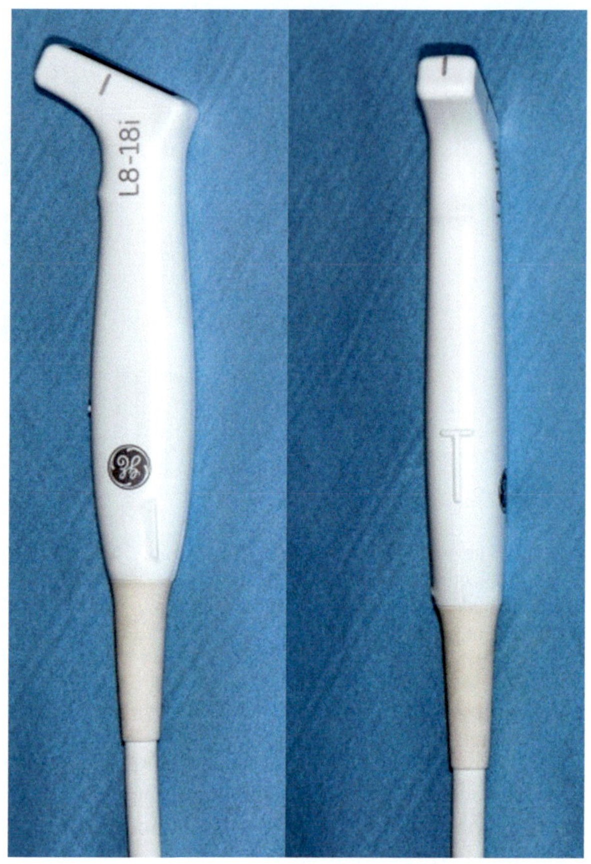


**Fig. 2.7 Front and side exterior views of an electronic probe** tailored to exploration of the eye and orbit, by its shape (golf club), its small size, its light weight, and its high frequency: 8–18 MHz

## 2.2.4 What Are the Characteristics of a "Good" Transducer

Ergonomics is paramount, the shape of the case as well as the flexibility of the cable and the weight of the assembly, to facilitate handling and access to the examination areas (Fig. 2.7).

For application-specific examinations, high frequencies are preferred because of the dimensions of the structures and the shallow depths analyzed. The proximal dead zone will be as small as possible (depending on the system's ability to control apodization). If required, one can install an interface (anechoic pocket) to shift this area out of the useful examination area, without attenuation of the signal.

**Fig. 2.8  Exploded view of an electronic probe,** showing the different components of the anterior part of this type of probe: the piezocomposite assembly, the support and connectors, the damper, the shielding, the housing, and the anterior membrane ensuring the impedance adaptation and focusing, perpendicular to the section plane

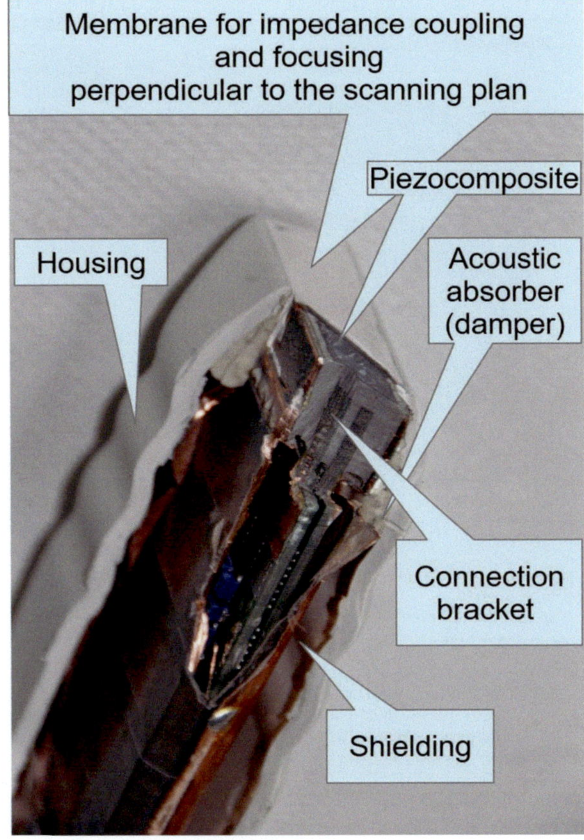


## *2.2.5   How to Convert an Ultrasound Beam into an Image*

There are two types of approaches: a system with hard-wired functions or an all-software-based digital system (detailed in paragraph Sect. 2.2.7.)

- **Systems with a wired interface and functions. All the functions of the ultrasound device, whether digital or analog, are ensured/supported by separate blocks:**

  - Creation of the emitted beam (with a characteristic dimension, direction, and focus), then, creation of the received beam (with a characteristic dimension, direction, and focus that can be dynamic); it is the Transducer/Ultrasound Interface, most often called a "Beamformer ".

  - Processing of the received beam information for each mode; most often there is a specific block per mode (2D, Doppler, Color, etc.) for adjustments of gain, filtering, autocorrelation, "FFT" (Fast Fourier Transformation), complex calculations to extract the Doppler signal, and others.

                                                                A. Bectard et al.

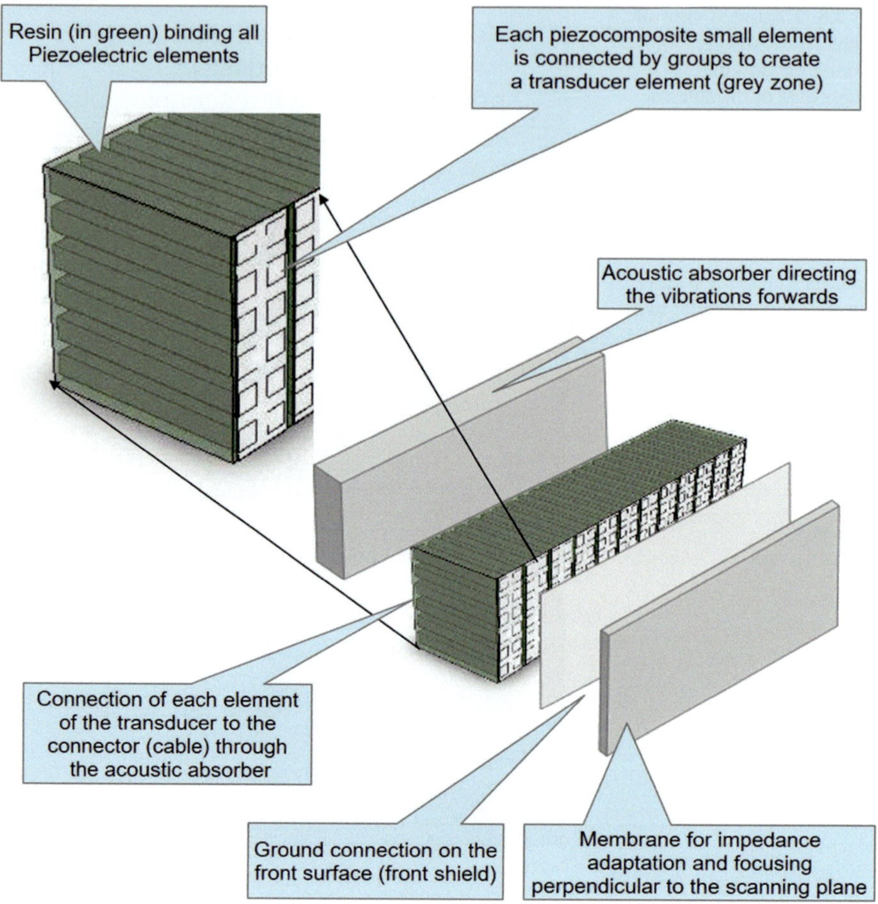


**Fig. 2.9** Diagram of the anterior piezocomposite assembly in front of an electronic probe and its adjacent entities ensuring correct generation of the ultrasonic beam
• Resin (green) linking all the piezoelectric elements
• Each small element of the piezocomposite is connected into groups to create an element of the probe (gray area)
• Damper, directs forward movements
• Connection to each element of the probe to the connector (cable) through the damper
• Connection to the ground on the front (shielding)
• Membrane ensuring impedance adaptation and focus perpendicular to the section plane

– Conversion for memory storage (tailored to the type of data acquired)
– Conversion for presentation on the screen(s), export(s), measurement(s), etc.
– User interface (keyboard, screen).

**As a result**, the same ultrasound beam from the probes is analyzed alternately by each block to ensure the functions by modes (bandwidth, shape, and direction are related to the original characteristics of this beam).

Of note, in this type of system, the processing of a mode is often linked to a specific module (board or set of boards), more or less software-oriented (use of application-specific integrated circuit), with the material restrictions allowing for possible improvements.


## *2.2.6  How Important is the Screen?*

Currently, computer screens using a standard (1680 × 1050) or HDMI (1920 × 1080) connection support high levels of definition that are widely compatible with the images to be presented. For multipurpose ultrasound scanners, image storage and presentation can be performed on DICOM servers and workstations.


## *2.2.7  Is Fully Digital Imaging Possible (Quality Computing) and, if so, How?*

Currently, the device can be almost exclusively digital; only the probe and input conversion are not.

- **Digital system. All the functions of the ultrasound device, after receiving the signals received by the probes, are provided by different software layers:**

  - The input/output interface, composed of electronic circuit boards ensuring digital/analog conversion to the probes (transmission) and analog/digital conversion (reception); the data from this block are native (RF) and non-organized, there is not yet the formation of a beam at this stage. These circuit boards have a large number of channels, with the widest possible bandwidth.
  - A computer station combining speed and power (professional motherboard with a large memory, microprocessor, and video game graphics processor) supporting a set of software applications ensuring all the functions of the ultrasound device:

    (a)  Management/creation of the transmitted signal
    (b)  Creation/management of the received signal
    (c)  Data processing (signal or beam) by mode or in parallel for compound modes (2D + Doppler, 2D + Doppler + color, 2D + elastography, etc.)
    (d)  Multiple conversions
    (e)  User interface management
    (f)  Presentation of the image
    (g)  Storage and transfer to other devices (DICOM and others).

**As a result**, the flow of data from the probes can be organized into a beam or a map of information, processed independently by each software layer (the bandwidth, shape, and direction of the transmitted or received signals have free access, simultaneously, by all software layers).

**Of note,** that in this type of system, signal processing at each stage is provided by software layers that can be controlled separately or in parallel to ensure the representation of diagnostic images of all modes, without hardware constraints; therefore, by simple software changes, the system can be altered or improved.

## 2.3  Biological Effects and the Safety of Ultrasound Scanners and Probes

As a preamble, no incidents due to the use of ultrasound in medicine have been reported to date, at least not when the ultrasound device is used for the applications intended by the manufacturer. This does not mean that no incidents have ever occurred but rather that for one reason or another they have not been formally documented [10].

However, one should note that when an ultrasound diagnosis energy is transmitted to the patient, the indication of the examination must always be relevant. Finally, the time spent probing, as well as the probe power, must follow the As Low As Reasonably Achievable principle throughout the examination. In practice, these criteria comprise capturing the information (B-Mode, Doppler, TM, etc.) in a minimum amount of time, avoiding the remaining several seconds in the same place without deriving additional information, and not redoing the scan 10 times the same section, etc. [11].

In approximately 1990–1995, estimation of the acoustic power of an ultrasound beam was generally based on the average energy of the beam: $I_{SPTA}$ (in mW/cm$^2$), or averaged intensity over a pulse cycle (the peak plus the interval between two peaks), with ultimately the $I_{SPPA}$, the intensity averaged only over the duration of the peak being defined. Currently, these $I_{SPTA}$ and $I_{SPPA}$ ultrasound power parameters are weighted by a theoretical absorption of biological tissues, in the form of a value of 0.3 dB/MHz/cm regardless of the tissue and the patient explored. These new parameters of ultrasound power are the $I_{SPTA3}$ and $I_{SPPA3}$.

It then became apparent that at low frequency (1.5 MHz), mechanical interaction of the beam with the tissue can be observed (with high energies not used in medicine) that can go as far as "tearing" the tissue (cavitation). This phenomenon reflects the mechanical index MI. Therefore, practitioners must be cognizant of the significance and the recommended upper limit, because **this index is displayed on the screens of all ultrasound scanners and for all modes**.

Additionally, to improve the **standard**, the thermal index (TI) has been defined, which measures the increase in temperature due to thermal agitation of the molecules of the tissue being traversed. The TI index accounts for this effect, which occurs more readily with high frequencies (the eye!). Again, it is necessary to know whether it is in the right range and to check its value on the ultrasound screen. An increase in one of these indexes beyond the recommended limits means that there is a malfunction of the device (they then appear in red or highlighted), which requires intervention by the manufacturer. The thermal index for bones (TIB), the thermal index for the bones of the skull (fetal ultrasound—TIC), and the thermal index for soft tissues (TIS) are also defined. That said, calculating the TI is not necessary if the output power divided by the area of the output beam at $-12$ dB is <20 mW/cm$^2$ and if the $I_{SPTA}$ is <100 mW [9].

Some tissues, such as those of embryos and fetuses and those of the eye, are particularly sensitive to the energy transmitted by medical imaging techniques (including ultrasound). Therefore, the acoustic power of the probes for these applications must be lower than with other applications. The physical (biological) effect produced on the tissues by acoustic radiation depends on the transmission power ($I_{SPTA3}$, $I_{SPPA3}$ mW/cm$^2$) as well as the frequency of repetition of the pulses and the ultrasound mode used (B-mode, color Doppler, pulsed, elastography, etc.)

In September of 2008, the US Food and Drug Administration (FDA) established recommendations to limit the acoustic power of ultrasound scanners (Table 2.1) [9].

The recommendations for the TI vary according to the application and depend on the duration of the exposure. A TI = 1 corresponds to a temperature increase limit of one degree. Currently, TI and MI parameters allow for evaluation of the biological effects (thermal and mechanical) of each radiation on tissues. In the case of litigation between the sonographer and the patient, these parameters allow confirmation of whether the sonographer carried out the examination in compliance with the standards for protection for patients or whether the examination carried out resulted in exposure of the patient to excessive risk.

To simplify things for sonographers, the devices are equipped with PRESET parameters that ensure optimum adjustment of the power, pulse rhythm, ultrasound frequency, and focus for each organ studied.

**Table 2.1** FDA recommendations for ultrasound power limits depending on the application (based on 9)

| Applications | $I_{SPTA3}$ (mW/cm$^2$) | $I_{SPPA3}$ (W/cm$^2$) | MI |
|---|---|---|---|
| Peripheral vessels | 720 | 190 | 1.9 |
| Cardiology | 430 | 190 | 1.9 |
| Other types of imaging[a] | 94 | 190 | 1.9 |
| Ophthalmology | 17 | 28 | 0.23 |

[a] Fetal, abdominal, pediatric, intraoperative, superficial organs (breast, thyroid, testicles, etc.), Transcranial (neonatal and adult)

## 2.4  Printers

Many printers are connectable:

- All standard printers for Windows PC (connected to a network or by USB, installed and following the Windows installer). However, attention should be paid to the quality of the support and image rendering.
- DICOM printers (connected to a network connection, require an Option and a suitable configuration in the AVISO PC interface, see user manual).

  These printers have no problems with image rendering, and they are intended to ensure a level of quality compatible with medical imaging. They require a DICOM configuration of the printer to accept the data from different ultrasound scanners.

## 2.5  Cleaning and Decontamination of Probes

The procedures for decontamination of probes can differ depending on the type of device used. However, ultrasound probes can be a vector for nosocomial infections and one must be very aware of this in ophthalmology.

Like endo-cavitary probes, ophthalmological ultrasound probes are classified as a semi-critical devices, requiring intermediate-level disinfection with bactericidal, mycobactericidal, virucidal, and fungicidal action.

### *2.5.1  The Use of Customized Probe Covers*

It is highly recommended, and it should be ubiquitous. They are single-use, made of latex material, individually packaged, and clean but not sterile. Such probe covers, which resembles a thimble, must be pulled over the probe (a dab of gel without any trapped bubbles at the end of the probe should be applied beforehand). Use of a probe cover allows for avoiding the standard decontamination protocol between each patient.

It is also essential to scrupulously follow the recommended procedures, both proper dilution of the products as well as the decontamination and disinfection times, use of personal protection equipment by the operator, to not forget to turn off the device before disconnecting the probes, and to avoid getting liquid on the connections and sockets of the cables.

## *2.5.2 Procedures*

It would be inappropriate to recommend a single procedure for decontamination of ophthalmic ultrasound probes. It took a particular significance during the COVID-19 pandemic.

The procedures described here are drawn from several sources:

- the recommendations for decontamination and disinfection given in the manufacturers' instructions for use [12, 13];
- the tailor-made procedures recommended by the hospital departments involved in the struggle against infections (committee for the control of the nosocomial infections - CLIN) [14, 15];
- the guidelines from national health authorities [16].

### A.  *Single-purpose ultrasound probe*

**Standard protocol**

1. Decontamination—pre-disinfection: Immerse the probe in a solution of alkazyme for 5 min or aniosyme for 5–15 min. Then clean the probe with a brush or a gauze swab for 1 min.
2. Rinse with distilled water.
3. Disinfection: Immerse the probe in a solution of alkacide for 5–20 min.
4. Rinse with distilled water and dry with a non-woven gauze swab.

**Protocol for patients at risk**

1. Decontamination – pre-disinfection: see above.
2. Rinse with distilled water.
3. Inactivation: the product used here is sodium hypochlorite at 9° (bleach) for 60 min.
4. Rinse with distilled water.
5. Disinfection: the probe is immersed in alkacide solution for 5–20 min.
6. Rinse with distilled water and dry with a non-woven gauze swab.

### B.  *Multipurpose ultrasound probe*

Because of the sophisticated electronics contained right behind the membrane covering the surface of the probe, bleach or disinfectants should never be used. Therefore, use of a probe cover in this case is particularly important. Two procedures are available.

**Procedure I**

1. Wipe the probe very thoroughly with a soft single-use paper tissue and remove any traces of gel.
2. Moisten a soft paper tissue with the disinfectant (Anios® detergent-disinfectant for elevated surfaces).
3. Coat the probe head with the moistened paper and leave it until it is used again.

**Procedure II**

1. Wipe the probe very carefully.
2. Arrange the probe heads on a clean paper tissue and spray them abundantly.
3. Before the examination, wipe the probes with a soft paper tissue.

For patients at risk, as for endo-cavitary probes, the probe can be soaked in a suitable container containing 2% glutaraldehyde for up to 30 min. However, this product is toxic and irritating and requires a well-ventilated room. It is better to use a probe cover and to not apply the probe directly to the cornea but rather to the closed eyelid.

## Abbreviations

| | |
|---|---|
| ALARA | As Low As Reasonably Achievable; |
| $I_{SPTA3}$ | average intensity over a pulse cycle (the peak plus the interval between two peaks) for a theoretical absorption of 0.3 dB/MHz/cm; |
| $I_{SPPA3}$ | average intensity only over the duration of the pulse (peak), for a theoretical absorption of 0.3 dB/MHz/cm; |
| MI | mechanical index; |
| TI | thermal index; |
| TIB | thermal index for bone; |
| TIC | thermal index for cranial bone; |
| TIS | thermal index for soft tissue. |

## References[1]


1. Courses available on the internet. http://www.ndt-ed.org/EducationResources/CommunityCol lege/Ultrasonics/cc_ut_index.htm
2. Manufacturers of ultrasound systems. http://www.quantel-medical.com/, "http://www.sup ersonicimagine.fr/, http://www.usa.philips.com/healthcare-solutions/ultrasound, http://www3. gehealthcare.com/en/products/categories/ultrasound", "http://www.hitachi-medical-systems. eu/products-and-services/ultrasound/platforms.html"
3. Manufacturers of piezocomposite crystals. http://www.neptune-sonar.co.uk/, "https://www. americanpiezo.com/products-services/composite-materials.html
4. Manufacturers of ultrasound probe. http://www.imasonic.fr/Company/Piezocomposite.php, http://www.vermon.com/vermon/
5. A reference. Research Center—Langevin Institute. http://www.espci.fr/fr/recherche/laboratoi res/institut-langevin/


---

[1] **For more information:**
Some references that are readily accessible on the internet.

6. Lexicon of acronyms used in this document. ASIC http://fr.wikipedia.org/wiki/Applic ation-specific_integrated_circuit, FPGA http://fr.wikipedia.org/wiki/Circuit_logique_progra mmable#FPGA, USB http://fr.wikipedia.org/wiki/Universal_Serial_Bus, RJ45 http://fr.wikipe dia.org/wiki/RJ45, CMUT https://tel.archives-ouvertes.fr/tel-01142993/file/Thèse_Audren_ BOULME.pdf
7. LCD screen. http://fr.wikipedia.org/wiki/%C3%89cran_%C3%A0_cristaux_liquides
8. Comparative screens. http://www.ybet.be/hard1ch16/hard1_ch16.php

## *For Biological Effects*

9. Information for manufacturers seeking marketing clearance of diagnostic ultrasound systems and transducers. Washington, DC: Guidance for Industry and FDA Staff US Department of Health and Human Services, Food and Drug Administration, Center for Devices and Radiological Health; 2008. http://www.fda.gov/cdrh/ode/guidance/560.pdf
10. Nelson TR, Fowlkes JB, Abramowicz JS, Church CC. Ultrasound biosafety considerations for the practicing sonographer and sonologist. J Ultrasound Med. 2009;28(2):139–50.
11. Arbeille, Ph. The biological effects of ultrasound. www.sfrnet.org/rc/org/sfrnet/htm/Article/ 2011/.../polyBasesPhysiques_14.pdf. May 24, 2011.

## *For Probe Decontamination*

12. Precautions to be taken to prevent the transmission of diseases, in particular Creutzfeld-Jacob disease, in the use of ocular ultrasound probes. Brochure published in January 2004 by Quantel Médical SA (Clermont-Ferrand).
13. Advice for the disinfection of probes with Anios detergent disinfectant high surfaces. Serge Vanneuville. Acuson Siemens, June 14, 2004.
14. Maintenance of the echo probe in ophthalmology. Dr. Chelly, Dr. Hammouten. CLIN of the Hyères Hospital Center; 2001 (Online editing (ch.hyeres.fr/CLIN)).
15. Disinfection of ultrasound probes. Gilles Heronneau. Le Manipulateur/AF PPE n° 156, March 2005.
16. Disinfection of medical devices—Guide to good practice. Ministry of Employment and Solidarity; 1998.

# Chapter 3
# Color Doppler Imaging

**Patricia Koskas, Olivier Bergès, and Augustin Lecler**

**Abstract** Being a core function of all modern multipurpose ultrasound devices, color Doppler imaging (CDI) has many indications in ophthalmology. In this chapter, we discuss the theory and the technique to obtain the best morphological and functional information. After describing the Doppler effect, this chapter presents the different Doppler modes, with an illustration for each. The first is the continuous Doppler, the oldest in vascular medicine, exploring vessels "blindly" without an associated imaging system, studying only the sounds and hence, not suitable for ophthalmological applications. For pulsed Doppler, with different representations, in the color mode, the images of the flows are superimposed on a B-image according to a color scale, translating the pulse repetition frequency, which must be adapted to the slow flows characteristic of ophthalmology and tailored when the settings are responsible of aliasing and blooming artifacts. In the spectral mode, which is the quantitative mode, the resistive index gives an idea of the flow for these vessels whose diameter is not known. Afterwards, we discuss the power Doppler, which is unfortunately sensitive to movements. Finally, we review micro-Doppler/B-flow/ smi/mvi which is a new method of vascular ultrasound independent of the Doppler effect, with no blooming or aliasing, which seems promising in ophthalmology.

The "Doppler" module is a core function of all modern multipurpose ultrasound devices. Ophthalmological pathology requires use of a high-end device equipped with a Doppler module of very good quality, given the small size of the vessels studied and their low velocities. Color Doppler and spectral Doppler allow the sonographer to collect information of a functional nature concerning the vascularization of the eye and orbit and, in the event of a circumscribed lesion, an approach to tissue characterization.

To obtain good-quality images and thus make the best diagnosis, the theory and technique of Doppler mode must be mastered.

P. Koskas · O. Bergès (✉) · A. Lecler
Rothschild Foundation Hospital, Paris, France
e-mail: oberges@for.paris



O. Bergès (ed.), *Echography of the Eye and Orbit*,
https://doi.org/10.1007/978-3-031-41467-1_3

## 3.1   The Doppler Effect

The Doppler effect is a physical phenomenon, generally applicable to propagated vibrations. First described by Christian Doppler in 1842 [1] (*On the colored light of double stars and some other celestial bodies in the sky*), initially applied to the analysis of the direction of movement of stars, this simple phenomenon can be verified on a daily basis in the visual and acoustic fields [2]. For example, the siren of an ambulance or the noise of a train traveling at a constant speed will be more acute (i.e., of higher frequency) when they are headed toward versus moving away from a fixed observer [2].

The Doppler effect ($\Delta F$) corresponds to the change in the apparent frequency of a periodic phenomenon following a displacement between the phenomenon and the observer [2, 3]. Regardless of the Doppler system (color, spectral, or power), a simple formula allows for calculating the Doppler frequency:

$$\mathbf{\Delta F = 2f_0 \cos \theta \frac{v}{c}}$$

where $f$ is transmission frequency, $v$ is velocity of flow from the blood column, $c$ is the speed of propagation of ultrasound in biological media, $\theta$ is the angle formed by the direction of flow of the blood column and the axis of the ultrasound beam.

Thus, the Doppler effect is proportional to $\cos\theta$ and therefore zero if the target moves perpendicular ($\theta = 90°$) to the Doppler pulse. Ideally, to achieve a maximum signal, the axis of the Doppler pulse must be placed parallel to the axis of the vessel being studied. However, the signal can be interpreted when the axis is at an angle provided it is less than 45°. Indeed, the greater the angle, the larger the error in the velocity measurement. With an angle greater than 60°, the measurement fluctuates at least 20%, which is unacceptable in terms of reproducibility.

### 1.   Continuous Doppler

Initially, the Doppler phenomenon was applied in vascular medicine in the form of continuous Doppler: a system for exploring vessels "blindly" without an associated imaging system, studying only the sounds, and the representation in the form of curves of the signals collected in a vessel identified only by anatomical means. This type of Doppler, widely used to assess large vessels, is not suitable for ophthalmological applications.

### 2.   Pulsed Doppler

Pulsed Doppler has the advantage of "visually" selecting the vessel for which a Doppler signal is to be recorded. With the duplex system combining B-mode imaging of the vessel with manifestation of the pulsed Doppler axis, one can ensure that the intended vessel is being imaged and therefore identified anatomically.

Currently, the probes used for vascular studies are no longer mechanical but rather electronic. For ophthalmological applications, electronic probes are small-sized and usually linear, with parallel crystals that are excited successively by group to obtain the scan and the reconstructed image on the screen. The Doppler signal is obtained by assigning a group of crystals to the signal acquisition, with the other crystals participating in the acquisition of the image in B-mode.

### 3.a.  Color mode (Fig. 3.1)

Color Doppler mode is a pulsed emission Doppler. A color image is produced on the screen that corresponds to the overlay of an image acquired in B-mode (2D) and a 2D Doppler image in color. The colors correspond to a color scale, reflecting different speeds, which are generally presented alongside the image [4].

By convention, a flow toward the probe is assigned the color at the top of the color scale and a flow away from the probe is assigned the color from the bottom of the color scale. This color scale is often symmetrical on either side of 0, between pre-established speeds. For ophthalmological studies, a scale tailored to low velocity flows (+5/9 cm/s or −5/9 cm/s) is chosen to obtain accurate representation of the vascularization of the posterior part of the eyeball and the orbit. Out of habit, in ophthalmology, vessels with flows heading toward the probe are coded in red. They often correspond to arteries. Vessels moving away from the probe are coded in blue, and they often correspond to veins.

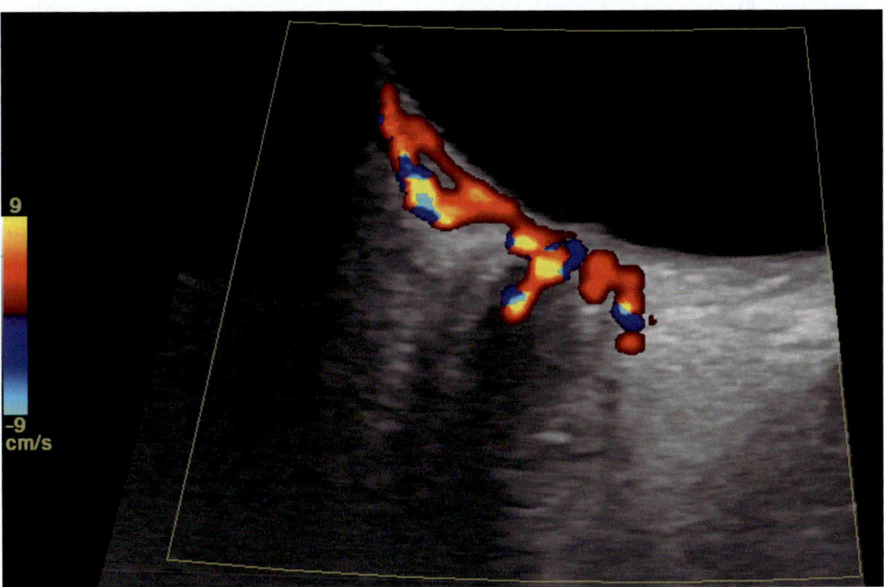


**Fig. 3.1  Vessels of the optic nerve head in color mode**: the central retinal artery (CRA) can clearly be seen, depicted in red, and the central retinal vein, depicted in blue in the center of the anterior part of the optic nerve, and the posterior short ciliary arteries on either side of this anterior part of the optic nerve. Note that even with a speed scale ranging from −9 to + 9 cm/s, small blue/green dots are discernible on the CRA and the medial posterior short ciliary arteries corresponding to an aliasing phenomenon

This speed scale reflects the concept of pulse repetition frequency (PRF): It needs to be carefully adjusted and tailored to the velocity of the vessels being studied. It avoids the phenomenon of aliasing, which arises when the PRF is set at a value too low for fast-flow vessels, located depth in the orbit (see Chap. 4: artifacts).

Outside the orbit, in larger vessels, this aliasing phenomenon related to a failure of adjustment should not be confused with eddies or turbulence related to the presence of stenosis. With turbulence, color inversion takes place, but by black and not white.

In ophthalmology, in color mode, this aliasing phenomenon is useful for recognizing a vessel with a flow that is faster than the maximum of the fixed velocity scale, such as the ophthalmic artery, for which the maximum speed is close to 50 cm/s. By comparison, the velocity scale set for the vessels of the optic nerve head ranges from +6 to −6 cm/s. The aliasing artifact does not occur in power Doppler mode. In spectral mode, the color scale must be carefully tailored to each vessel being studied.

Care must also be taken to avoid blooming artifacts (*see* Chap. 4—artifacts), which correspond to oversampling of the Doppler signal, resulting in a vessel appearing wider than it really is. This artifact depends on the Doppler gain.

To obtain a good color Doppler image, one must choose a window that is not too wide, that is well oriented (in practice, for the eye, the window remains straight), a suitable field of view (adapted zoom) for B-mode, a 2D gain (B-mode) that is quite low, a color-adapted gain (with no colored pixel artifacts outside the vessels), medium color persistence to retain the impression of real time and, finally, application of the above notions of the PRF settings.

Currently, most devices allow a triplex mode combining a B-mode image, a color Doppler image, and the recording of a pulsed Doppler spectrum of the selected vessel. However, in ophthalmology, the frame rate obtained with this mode is too low (because it takes several pulses, between 8 and 16, to obtain a color line, and the competition of the three systems slows down the electronic calculations for the generation of the image). Therefore, this triplex mode is rarely used to explore the eye and the orbit.

### 3.b.  Spectral mode (Fig. 3.2)

This is a quantitative mode. Spectral analysis in pulsed Doppler mode allows intravascular flow to be assessed along two axes: time on the x-axis and the Doppler frequency on the y-axis. Access to the actual velocity is possible via angular correction of the Doppler pulse in relation to the axis of the vessel and knowledge of the Doppler frequency. On modern devices, this velocity is provided in real time. The systolic and diastolic parameters can readily be assessed. The size of the pulsed Doppler gate should be tailored to the size of the vessel.

The formula for the flow rate as a function of velocity is:

$$Q = \pi\, v\, \frac{D^2}{4}$$

where Q is flow, v is the average velocity, and D is the vessel diameter.

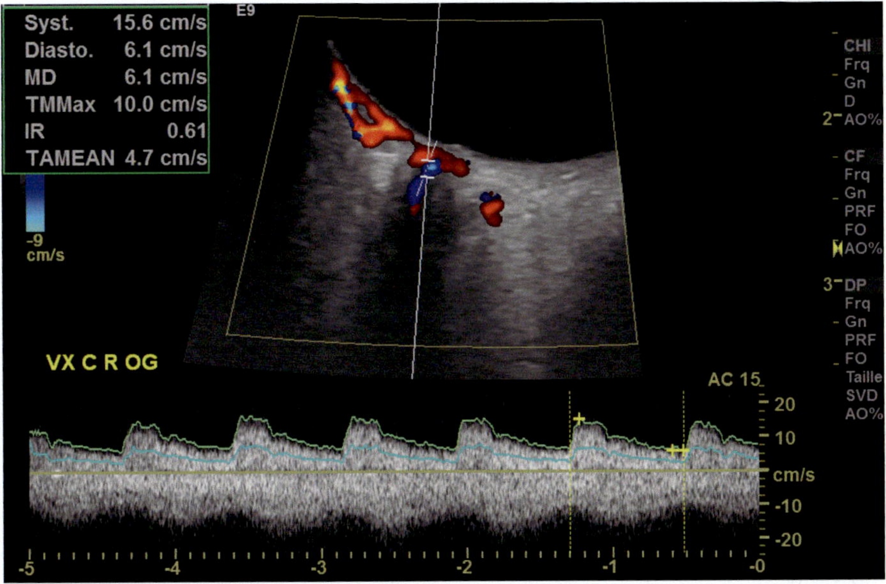


**Fig. 3.2  Vessels of the optic nerve head in spectral mode**: In this person, on the spectral analysis curve, the flow of the central retinal artery is positive and well defined, whereas that of the vein, which is also substantial, has a blurred outline. The velocimetric constants used to characterize the flow of these small vessels are the peak systolic velocity (PSV), the telediastolic velocity (end diastolic velocity [EDV]), and the resistive index (RI). The pulsatility index is generally not used for these small vessels. As shown in Table 3.1, RI A Oph > RI CRA > RI SPCA

However, obtaining a reliable and reproducible measurement of the diameter of ophthalmic vessels is difficult because of their small size and sinuosity as well as technical errors. Of note, an error, even a small one, will be squared in the formula. Therefore, flow rate measurement of orbital vessels is not currently feasible.

To compare velocities and not flows, semiological analysis is required. However, this analysis remains reliable.

The resistive index (RI) (from Pourcelot) reflects the resistance to the flow of red blood cells in a vessel. It allows for obtaining a useful qualitative equivalent of the flow rate.

$$RI = \frac{S - D}{S}$$

where S is the Peak Systolic Velocity and D is the End Diastolic Velocity.

In ophthalmological pathologies, the peak (maximum) systolic velocities (PSVs) and RIs of the arteries are systematically assessed: the central retinal artery (CRA), the posterior short ciliary arteries (PSCAs), and the ophthalmic artery (Oph A). The systolic upstroke or acceleration time is also assessed. For veins, the central retinal vein (CRV), the superior ophthalmic vein (SOV), and the inferior ophthalmic vein (IOV), their direction of circulation and their spectrum type are observed. The maximum velocity (Vmax) and the average velocity (Vm) can also be assessed. In practice, the inferior ophthalmic vein is rarely visible except in children examined under general anesthesia with halogenated anesthetics (*see* Fig. 8.11).

As is the case for brain damages, the flow of ophthalmic vessels (especially those of the eyeball) is systolic-diastolic.

Calculation of the RI is important in ophthalmological pathologies; it is independent of the Doppler angle of the pulse (Table 3.1). Oph A RI > CRA RI > sPCA RI is usually observed. If this is not the case, the recordings must be redone while making sure that no pressure is exerted on or even no contact is made with the orbit/eyelids (*see* Figs. 7.21 and 8.7) that could alter the velocimetric constants and lead to the belief, although erroneous, of a pathology.

As far as velocities are concerned, there is a great deal of inter-individual variability. However, in the same individual, in the absence of ocular pathology, the hemodynamic parameters are almost always symmetrical, especially for the CRA.

### 3.c. **Power Doppler (Fig. 3.3)**

Power Doppler is a mode that uses quantification of the number of intravascular red blood cells to encode the signal strength [5]. Therefore, it does not allow for determining the direction of the flow, although it is very sensitive in terms of detecting flows with very low velocities. It is independent of the angle of insonation, allowing for exploration of vessels that are perpendicular to the ultrasound beam and not very accessible. However, it is also very sensitive to movement (artifacts) because of the low PRF and is therefore not useful in ophthalmology apart from examinations performed under general anesthesia. With the latest generation of ultrasound scanners, this advantage of power Doppler with slow flows is no longer relevant because color mode has also become sensitive to very slow flows. All that is required is that the Doppler gain is set to the limit to reduce motion artifacts.

### 4. **Micro-Doppler/B-flow/superb microvascular imaging (SMI) or microvascular flow imaging (MVI/MV-flow) (Fig. 3.4)**

This new method of vascular ultrasound is another mode of representation of circulating red blood cells, independent of the Doppler effect, and is superposable on B-images [4–6].

**Table 3.1 Peak Systolic Velocity (PSV) and Resistivity Index (RI) values for the different orbital arteries**: Ophthalmic Artery (Oph A), Central Retinal Artery (CRA), lateral and medial short Posterior Ciliary Arteries (sPCA), according to our personal experience

|  | PSV (cm/s) | RI |
| --- | --- | --- |
| Oph A | 45 ± 10 | 0.75 ± 0.05 |
| CRA | 15 ± 3 | 0.62 ± 0.05 |
| Lat sPCA | 13 ± 3 | 0.55 ± 0.07 |
| Med sPCA | 12 ± 3 | 0.53 ± 0.08 |

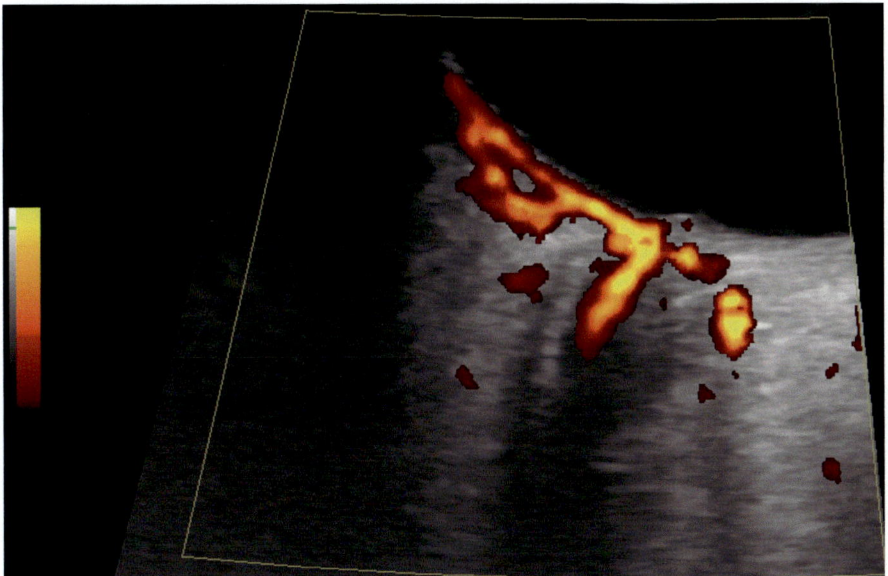

**Fig. 3.3  Vessels of the optic nerve head in power Doppler**: The central retinal vessels are discerned over a distance that is just slightly longer than in color mode but with no information on their direction

- It provides real-time visualization of blood flow by encoding circulating red blood cells on a grayscale.
- The advantages are no "blooming"; the signal concerns only red blood cells and therefore the lumen, better spectral and spatial resolution, and absence of disadvantages related to Doppler (angle, aliasing).
- The main disadvantages are that there is no quantitative approach.

3D visualization of vessels is currently possible because of specific software. Contrast medium can also be injected to increase visualization of vessels with very low velocities.

However, in ophthalmological pathologies, the phenomenon of blooming is a significant issue and hinders performance of the examination in current practice and interpretation of the hemodynamic data obtained. Therefore, the main indication for injecting ultrasound contrast medium is to assess the vascularization of a tissue process, mainly if there is little vascularity by standard examination.

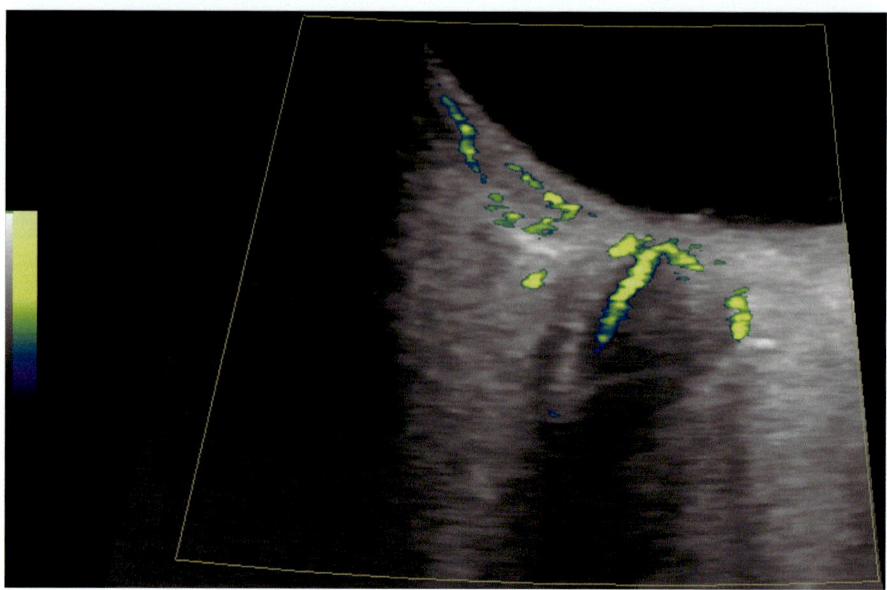

**Fig. 3.4 Vessels of the optic nerve head in B-flow mode**: As in energy mode, this is not a mode to discern the direction of flow, but because of no 'blooming' artifacts, the vessels are represented with their actual caliber

# References


1. Doppler CA. Über das farbige Licht der Doppelsterne und einiger anderer Gerstirne des Himmels. (On the colored light of double stars and a few other stars in the sky.) Abh Konigl-Böhm Ges. 1843;2:465–82.
2. Sadik J-C, Doppler E. Principes physiques—Doppler. In: Sadik J-C, editor. Echographie Doppler des vaisseaux du cou et de l'encéphale. Paris: Médecine Sciences Flammarion; 1995. p. 5–15.
3. Tranquart F, Bergès O, Koskas P, Arsene S, Rossazza C et al. Color Doppler imaging of orbital vessels: personal experience and literature review. J Clin Ultrasound. 2003; 31(5):258–73.
4. Berger M, Adams Q. B-flow technology. https://www.logiqclub.net/club/files/news
5. Tola M, Yurdakul M, Cumhur T. Combined use of color duplex ultrasonography and B-flow imaging for evaluation of patients with carotid artery stenosis. AJNR Am J Neuroradiol. 2004;25(10):1856–860.
6. Yurdakul M, Tola M, Cumhur T. B-flow imaging for assessment of 70–99% internal carotid artery stenosis based on residual lumen diameter. J Ultrasound Med. 2006;25(2):211–5.

# Chapter 4
# (Very) High-Frequency Ultrasound

**Olivier Bergès and François Lafitte**

**Abstract** This chapter is an overview of (very) high-frequency ultrasound, especially the technological advances made since the invention of ophthalmic ultrasound biomicroscopy by Charles Pavlin: the very high-frequency ultrasound "Artemis", high-frequency ultrasound with 20-MHz long and short focus probes, very high-frequency Doppler, as well as its applications for the anterior segment of the eye (cornea, iris, anterior chamber angle, ciliary body tumors) but also the posterior segment (the optic disc, the study of maculopathies and the periphery, in particular the sclera). The indications and results are reviewed in detail in Chap. 11 for the anterior segment and in Chap. 12 for the posterior segment.

## 4.1 History

Ophthalmology is one of the oldest applications of ultrasound for medical diagnoses: in 1956, Mundt and Hughes [1] published the first study on the use of ultrasound for the diagnosis of ocular tumors. In 1957, Oksala and Lehtinen [2] described the various ultrasound aspects in amplitude mode (A-mode) of most eye diseases, and in 1958, Baum and Greenwood produced the first ultrasound images in brightness mode (B-mode) with a device they constructed using a combined scan, a 15-MHz probe and an immersion technique [3, 4].

For purely technological reasons, for more than 10 years, only the A-mode was used in ophthalmology. As early as 1963, Ossoinig developed the concept of standardized echography [5, 6], which he advanced over the next 40 years. Back then, it was accepted that, given their superficial location, the eye and the orbit had to be examined with a high-frequency probe of 8–12 MHz. The work of Purnell, Bronson, and Coleman [7–9] developing B-mode has lent credence to this notion.

O. Bergès (✉) · F. Lafitte
Rothschild Foundation Hospital, Paris, France
e-mail: oberges@for.paris

     47
O. Bergès (ed.), *Echography of the Eye and Orbit*,
https://doi.org/10.1007/978-3-031-41467-1_4

### 4.1.1 Ultrasound Biomicroscopy

In 1990, Pavlin, Sherar, and Foster published their first study on high-frequency ultrasound (HFU) of the eye, using a 100-MHz probe [10, 11]. Ultrasound biomicroscopy (UBM) was conceived in 1991 and rapidly became popular around the world. The device, marketed by Humphrey-Zeiss, ultimately used a 50-MHz probe with a single oscillating crystal allowing for exploration of a cell of 5 mm × 5 mm. Dedicated to the study of the anterior segment, UBM required an immersion technique, with the crystal oscillating in a small bath of methylcellulose or serum held in place by a small cup inserted between the eyelids [12] (see Fig. 7.14a). Humphrey's device was widely distributed throughout the world [13, 14]. In France, because of certification issues, the device was not available until 2000, when it was marketed by the company Paradigm (Fig. 4.1).

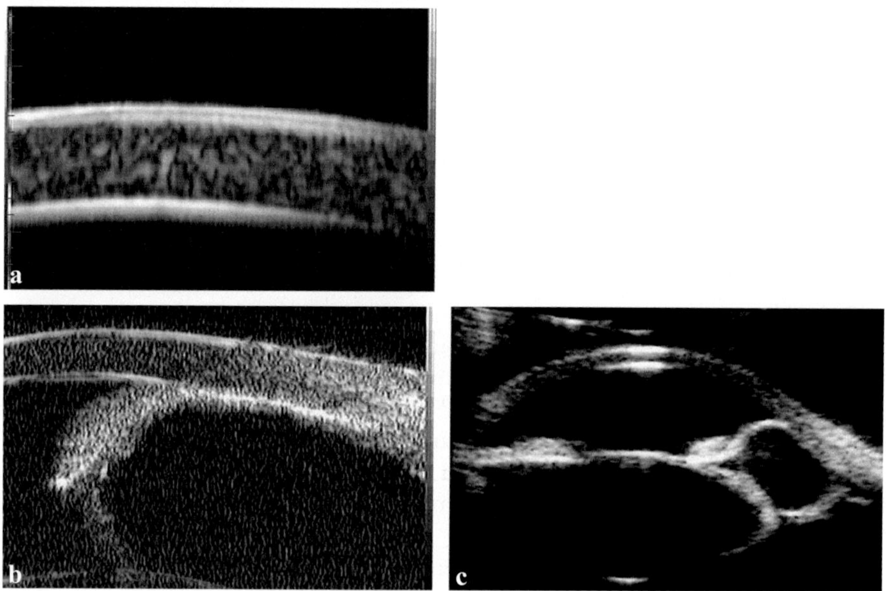

**Fig. 4.1 Ultrasound biomicroscopy (UBM) at 50 MHz: advantages and limitations. a**: Axial section of the center of the cornea at high resolution, providing very precise details of the epithelium, Bowman's membrane, and the stroma. **b**: Iris stromal cyst. The examination confirms that it is a cyst, fully anechoic, but because of its large size, it cannot be measured, nor can its deep part be visualized. **c**: The same iris stromal cyst seen with a 20-MHz probe. It measures 3.2 mm × 4.1 mm in diameter × 2.8 mm thick; it does not exceed the equator of the lens

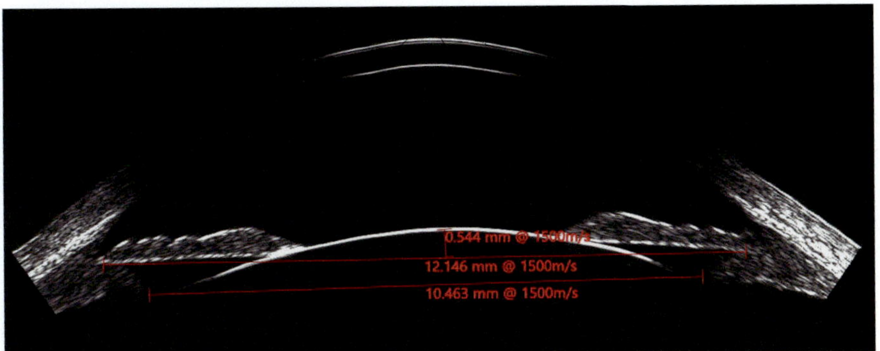


**Fig. 4.2  Anterior Segment B-Scan with ultra high resolution**—Artemis Insight very high-frequency digital ultrasound B-scan (ArcScan, Inc). Red caliper lines are shown measuring the sulcus-to-sulcus diameter, crystalline lens rise from the sulcus plane, and ciliary body inner diameter. The arciform scan parallel to the anterior side of the cornea provides a nice image of the entire anterior segment with high spatial resolution, less than 10 μm. *Reprinted with permission from Reinstein DZ, Archer TJ, Vida RS, Piparia V, Potter JG. New Sizing Parameters and Model for Predicting Postoperative Vault for the Implantable Collamer Lens Posterior Chamber Phakic Intraocular Lens. J Refract Surg. 2022 May;38(5):272–279*

## *4.1.2  VHFU—Artemis*

A few years after the development of UBM, in New York, another very HFU (VHFU) device, called Artemis, was conceived, with a scan that was no longer sectorial but rather arciform, parallel to the theoretical curvature of the cornea [15, 16], thereby generating an image of the entire anterior chamber and no longer only 5-mm wide. More specifically designed to assess the anterior segment after refractive surgery, the axial resolution could reach 4 μm at the level of the cornea. Combined with specific measurement software, this device allows for precise analyses of the different layers of the cornea (Fig. 4.2). Marketed by the company UltraLink, the distribution of this device has been limited because of its high price.

## *4.1.3  HFU (Quantel Medical): 20 MHz Short and Long Focal Length Probes*

At the end of the 1990s, in France, at the instigation of Michel Puech [17], the Quantel Medical company developed a 20-MHz short focal length probe to assess the anterior segment and a 20 MHz long focal length probe to assess the posterior pole (optic disc and macula), which has proven useful also for assessing the ocular wall, especially the sclera, even on the periphery. For the anterior segment, despite a lower spatial resolution than with a 50 MHz probe, the visibility of the entire anterior segment, including the lens, and the significantly higher resolution than with a 10 MHz probe

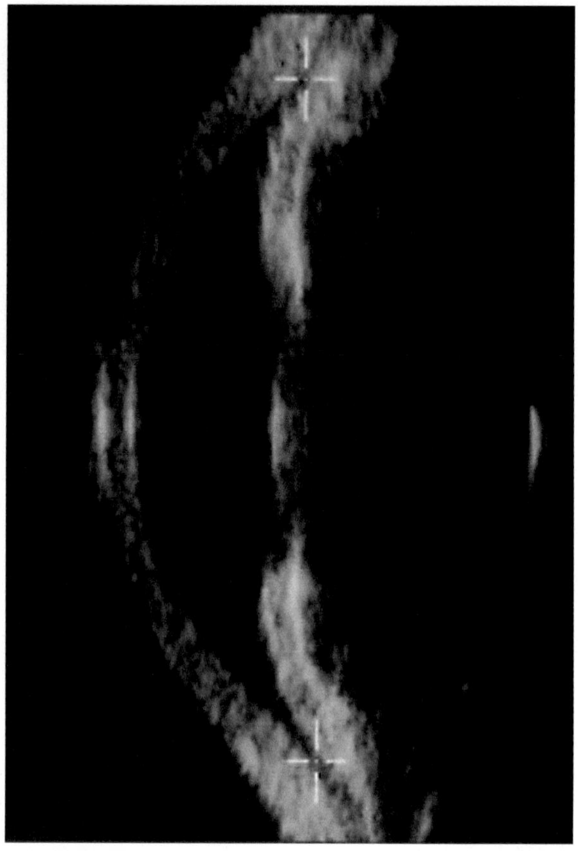

**Fig. 4.3 Axial section of the anterior segment with a 20-MHz probe with a long focal length requiring a 25-mm high cup filled with gel**. Satisfactory presentation of the various structures and in particular the posterior capsule of the lens. Good resolution of the chamber angles allowing angle-to-angle diameter measurement according to 3 to 9 o'clock.

provides well-codified indications for this probe (Fig. 4.3), in particular assessment of tumors of the ciliary body, which are often not fully visible with a 50 MHz probe because their size often exceeds 4 mm in thickness [18].

## *4.1.4 High Frequency Doppler*

At the end of the 2nd millennium, the teams of Pavlin in Toronto [19] and Coleman in New York [20] performed research on the detection of microflux of the arterial circle of the iris with VHFU, which did not lead to a commercialized device, however. Fujifilm Healthcare should present such a device quite soon.

### 4.1.5	*Ophthalmic Dedicated Device*

More recently, at the beginning of 2006, Quantel Medical again developed a new ultrasound device dedicated to ophthalmology, with 10 MHz, 25 MHz short focal-length and 20 MHz long focal-length probes and a new 50 MHz linear scan probe, allowing, as for Artemis, visualization of the entire anterior chamber (Fig. 4.4).

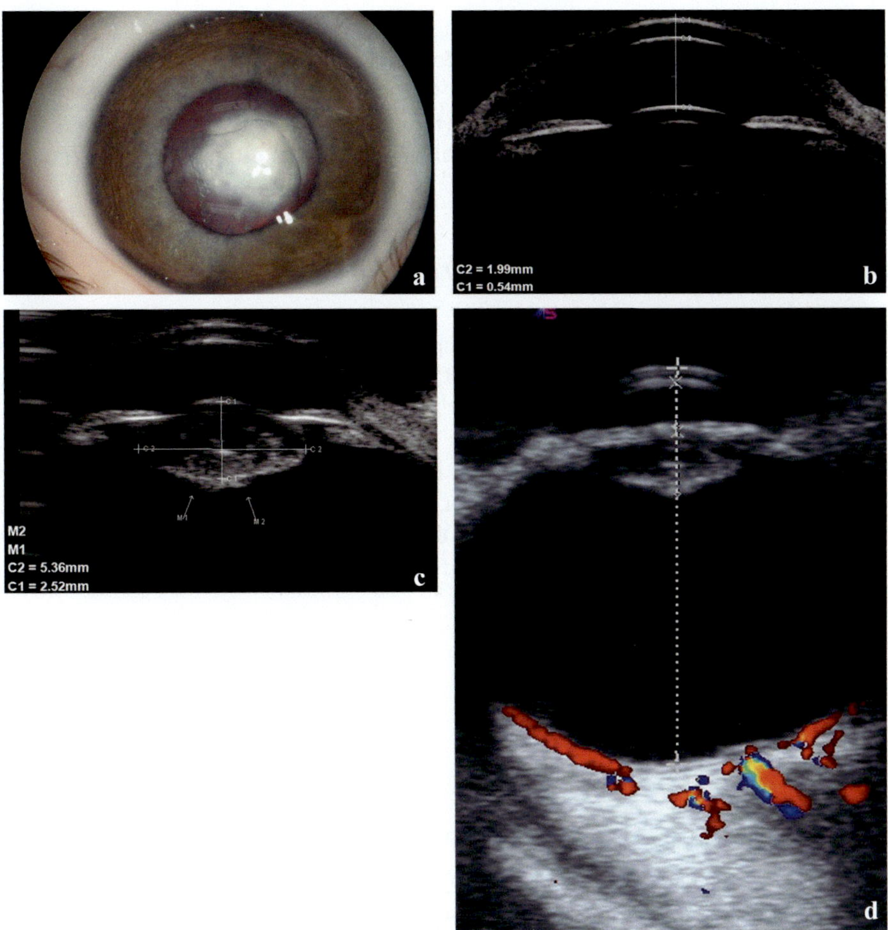


**Fig. 4.4  Leukocoria related to persistent fetal vasculature (PFV) in a 2-month-old child.** Comparison of different imaging. **a**: Clinical presentation; **b**: axial section of the anterior segment at 50 MHz; **c**: sagittal section of the anterior segment with a short focal length 25 MHz probe showing the anterior PFV behind the posterior lens capsule (→); **d**: axial section in CDI with a 5–12 MHz probe. The cornea, normal, and the anterior chamber are best assessed at 50 MHz. Cataract and perilental echoes (→) are best discerned with a 25 MHz probe. Although the resolution is lower, CDI allows for excluding an associated posterior form of PFV

This proved to be very efficient and rapidly became popular in many centers, replacing the device designed by Pavlin. Even though this device has been upgraded, and the P60 Ultrasound BioMicroscope is still sold by Paradigm Medical Industries Inc.

### 4.1.6   UBM Versus (V)HFU

By convention and to pay tribute to Charles Pavlin, who passed away in November 2014, the acronym UBM is reserved in this book for images generated with an ultrasound biomicroscope, whereas HFU (HFU if F = 20 MHz to 50 MHz) or VHFU (VHFU if F $\geq$ 50 MHz) will be used for all other types of ultrasound scanners.

### 4.1.7   Tendency to Use Higher Frequencies

For multipurpose devices also, there is a tendency to use higher frequencies: in ophthalmology, they were originally 7–15 MHz for the B-mode and 5 MHz for Doppler.

For the program "eye", the frequency is now centered around 16 MHz for the B-mode and 6.3 MHz for Doppler, and for the program "anterior segment", the frequency is centered around 16 MHz for the B-mode and 10.5 MHz for Doppler. Although it is not really high frequency, this is of course a great help for studying anteriorly located lesions and in particular ciliary body tumors.

## 4.2   Applications

### 4.2.1   The Anterior Segment

For more than 15 years, the pathologies studied using HFU have been well codified.

**4.2.1.1.** The cornea is assessed at 50 MHz. If it is a check-up after refractive surgery, the Artemis ultrasound from UltraLink, especially because of its various programs, provides slightly better information [15, 16, 21, 22].

**4.2.1.2.** The iris is assessed at 50 MHz. Cysts of the posterior epithelium of the iris are common, especially in young people [23]. Although often only one eye is symptomatic, systematic analysis of all the quadrants of both eyes shows that it is most often a bona fide iridociliary polycystic dysplasia [24, 25], which is difficult to treat when it results in plateau iris and glaucoma [26]. These are readily differentiated from rarer cysts of the iris stroma [27] and solid lesions [28, 29], mainly nevi and melanomas. Benign nevi, when they are large, frequently have a hypoechoic surface plaque. Melanomas are typically larger, multilobulated, attenuating (see Chap. 13), heterogeneous with anechoic structures, with necrosis, large vessels, or authentic microcysts inside or around the lesion [30, 31]. Although HFU is well suited for assessing the morphology of these solid lesions, most often it cannot differentiate such melanocytic lesions from other solid lesions [32, 33].

**4.2.1.3.** The chamber angle should be assessed at 50 MHz by horizontal and vertical sections to explore the 3, 6, 9, and 12 o'clock meridians or even by sections assessing the intermediate meridians. Each section must have biometric measurements of the chamber angle in order to classify it as normal ($> 15°$), borderline ($10°$ to $15°$), narrow ($5°$ to $10°$), very narrow/filiform, or closed ($< 5°$). Because of anatomical variations and to ensure greater reproducibility (both inter- and intra examiner), to measure the angle in degrees, the angle opening distance (AOD) between the iris and the trabeculum is preferentially measured at 500 $\mu$m from the scleral spur; the angle is considered normal if the AOD is $> 250$ $\mu$m, borderline when $= 150$ $\mu$m to 250 $\mu$m, narrow if AOD $= 100$ $\mu$m to 150 $\mu$m, and very narrow or filiform when $< 100$ $\mu$m. These figures should be compared in an illuminated environment (myosis) and in the dark (mydriasis) [34, 35]. Other values are used to quantify the aperture of the angle, such as surfaces: the angle recession area (ARA) and trabecular-iris space area (TISA) at 500 $\mu$m or 750 $\mu$m from the scleral spur. These surfaces have been extensively studied by optical coherence imaging (OCT) of the anterior segment [36–39], but with ultrasound, even with semi-automatic calculation software, determination of these surfaces is often time-consuming, so they are not so frequently used in daily practice. In any case, the shape of the iris needs to be considered, distinctly concave in case of pigmentary glaucoma [40, 41], as well as the position of the ciliary body in relation to the scleral spur to detect plateau iris [42–44], which requires specific treatment.

HFU is also useful for check-ups after filtration surgery [45, 46], to assess the filtration "bleb" and flap.

**4.2.1.4.** Ciliary body tumors (Fig. 4.5) are often relatively large at the time of diagnosis, and although 50-MHz ultrasound is preferable for small lesions that are less than 4 mm thick [47, 48], other tumors should be analyzed with a 25-MHz probe. However, VHFU at 50 MHz remains useful in the following cases [45]:

- to measure the thickness of the sclera next to the tumor and to detect scleromalacia
- to measure the distance between the tumor and the scleral spur.

Ultrasound can sometimes reveal characteristic signs that allow for an accurate diagnosis [23, 49], and in combination with clinical evaluation, it allows for appropriate therapeutic management of such lesions.

**4.2.1.5.** Analysis of the anterior segment behind a corneal opacity, regardless of the cause, entails use of a 50 MHz probe to assess the cornea (Fig. 4.6), the anterior chamber, the iris, and the ciliary body and a 25 MHz probe to assess the condition of the lens (Fig. 4.4).

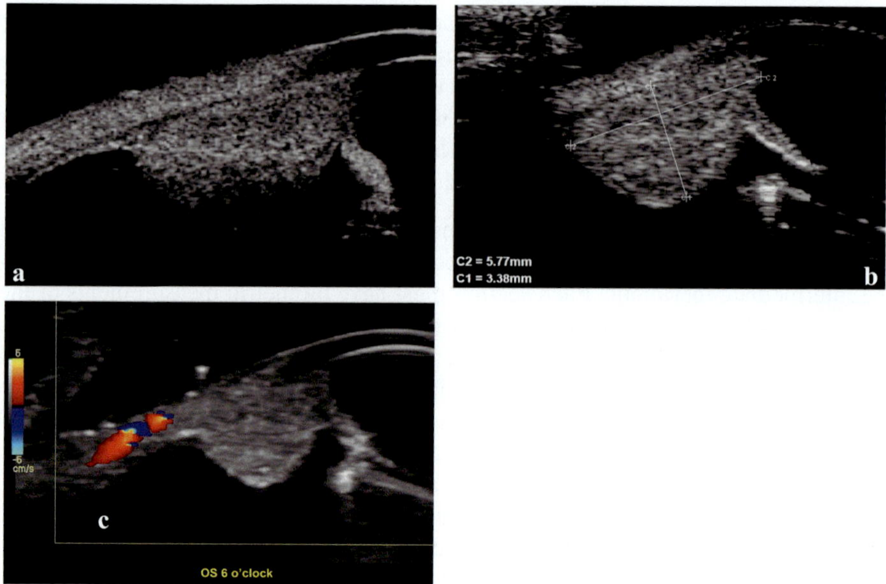



**Fig. 4.5 Anterior segment, 25 MHz probe contribution**. Inferior iridociliary melanoma treated with proton beam therapy 8 years ago. **a**: Section of the ciliary body mass according to the 6 o'clock meridian at 50 MHz; **b**: section of the ciliary body mass according to the 6 o'clock meridian at 25 MHz; **c**: section of the ciliary body mass according to the 6 o'clock meridian by color Doppler imaging with an 8–18 MHz probe. At 50 MHz, the mass in question can be seen, highly attenuating, but it cannot be measured, in particular its thickness. Small synechia can be discerned between the tumor scar and the cornea. At 25 MHz, the resolution is much less good, as is the analysis of the echotexture (the difference between the iris and the less echogenic lesion is less obvious), but the lower attenuation allows for measurement of its diameters and thickness. In color Doppler imaging, with an 8–18 MHz probe, there is good penetration of the ultrasound beam, but the echotexture of the lesion can also be clearly appreciated. Finally, the color mode confirms the avascular character of the mass, which much later became a scar

## 4.2.2 The Posterior Pole

Long focal length 20-MHz probes greatly improve the resolution of the structures of the posterior pole, optic disc, and macula [50]. This is also the case for the new 20 MHz 5 rings annular array probe. Admittedly, this resolution is lower than that of OCT obtained with a laser beam at 820 nm. The advantage of ultrasound remains being able to assess the entire posterior segment and thereby accurately analyze the entire vitreoretinal interface.

**4.2.2.1.** The optic disc is best assessed at 20 MHz, whereas 10 MHz is still better for assessment of the retrobulbar optic nerve (see Figs. 7.6 and 7.18).

**4.2.2.2.** A macular hole or vitreomacular traction (and all other maculopathies) are best evaluated with a 20-MHz probe [51, 52] (see Chaps. 7 and 12).

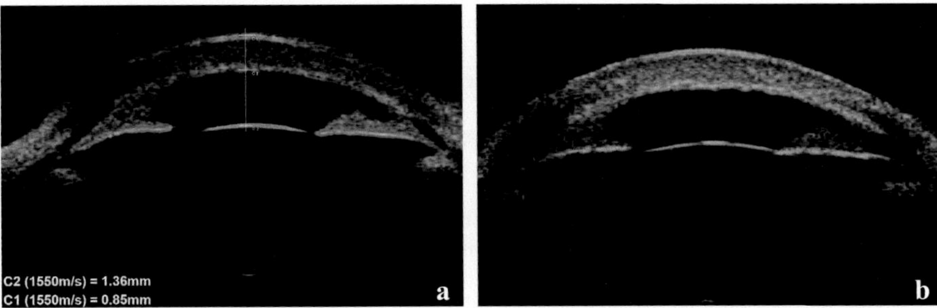


**Fig. 4.6  Anterior segment at 50 MHz—Peters syndrome a**: Axial section, the focal area being centered on the anterior chamber; **b**: axial section, the focal area being centered on the cornea. On both sections, one can clearly see the substantial thickening of the cornea. However, its hyperechoic echotexture and the irregular defect of the endothelium and Descemet membrane are only properly discerned on the section focused on the cornea. Irido-lenticular synechiae are already visible (a little better on the section focused on the anterior chamber) but require centered sections for an exhaustive study

**4.2.2.3.** A 20-MHz probe is also useful for assessing the peripheral wall, not only for the masses [50, 53], but especially the sclera [54].

# References


1. Mundt GH, Hugues WE. Ultrasonics in ocular diagnosis. Am J Ophthalmol. 1956;41:488–98.
2. Oksala A, Lehtinen A. Diagnostic value of ultrasonics in ophthalmology. Ophthalmologica. 1957;134:387–95.
3. Baum G, Greenwood I. The application of ultrasonic locating techniques to ophthalmology: theoretic considerations and acoustic properties of ocular media: part 1. Reflective properties Am J Ophthalmol. 1958;46:319–29.
4. Baum G, Greenwood I. The application of ultrasonic locating techniques to ophthalmology. II : Ultrasonic slit lamp in the ultrasonic visualization of soft tissues. Arch. Ophthalmol, Chicago 1958;60:263–79
5. Ossoinig KC and Steiner H. Standardization in Ultrasonic Diagnosis—a tissue model for the diagnosis of intraocular tumors [German] in: Diagnostica Ultrasonica in Ophthalmologia (Proceedings of SIDUO I, Berlin 1964, Buschmann W and Hildebrandt I, editors.) pp. 129–133, Math. Naturwiss. Reihe XIV der Humboldt-Universität Berlin, 1965
6. Ossoinig KC. Acoustic diagnosis of ocular tumors—experimental and clinical examinations with the A-scan method [German] Klin. Monatsbl Augenheilk. 1965;146:321–37.
7. Dakters JG, Yashon D, Purnell EW, Volk M, White RJ. Ultrasonography for diagnosis of orbital tumors. JAMA. 1968;203(9):803–5.
8. Bronson NR. Development of a simple B-scan ultrasonoscope. Trans Am Ophthalmol Soc. 1972;70:365–408.
9. Coleman DJ, Lizzi FL, Jack RL. Ultrasonography of the eye and orbit. Philadelphia: Lea & Febiger; 1977.
10. Sherar MD, Starkoski BG, Taylor WB, Foster FS. A 100 MHz B-scan ultrasound backscatter microscope. Ultrason Imaging. 1989;11(2):95–105.
11. Pavlin CJ, Sherar MD, Foster FS. Subsurface ultrasound microscopic imaging of the intact eye. Ophthalmology. 1990;97(2):244–50.

12. Pavlin CJ, Harasiewicz K, Foster FS. Eye cup for ultrasound biomicroscopy. Ophthalmic Surg. 1994;25(2):131–2.
13. Pavlin CJ, Harasiewicz K, Sherar MD, Foster FS. Clinical use of ultrasound biomicroscopy. Ophthalmology. 1991;98(3):287–95.
14. Pavlin CJ, Foster FS. Ultrasound biomicroscopy imaging of the eye. New York: Springer–Verlag; 1995.
15. Reinstein DZ, Silverman RH, Raevsky T, Simoni GJ, Lloyd HO, Najafi DJ, Rondeau MJ, Coleman DJ. Arc-scanning very high-frequency digital ultrasound for 3D pachymetric mapping of the corneal epithelium and stroma in laser in situ keratomileusis. J Refract Surg. 2000;16(4):414–30.
16. Reinstein DZ, Sutton HF, Srivannaboon S, Silverman RH, Archer TJ, Coleman DJ. Evaluating microkeratome efficacy by 3D corneal lamellar flap thickness accuracy and reproducibility using Artemis VHF digital ultrasound arc-scanning. J Refract Surg. 2006;22(5):431–40.
17. Puech M. High resolution ultrasound imaging of the macula communication. ASOU. 1998.
18. Siahmed K, Bergès O, Desjardins L, Lumbroso L, Brasseur G. Imagerie des tumeurs du segment antérieur : Avantages de l'échographie (10,20 et 50 MHz) et de la tomographie en cohérence optique (OCT) J Fr Ophtalmol. 2004;27(2):169–73.
19. Pavlin CJ, Christopher DA, Burns PN, Foster FS. High-frequency Doppler ultrasound examination of blood flow in the anterior segment of the eye. Am J Ophthalmol. 1998;126(4):597–600.
20. Silverman RH, Kruse DE, Coleman DJ, Ferrara KW. High-resolution ultrasonic imaging of blood flow in the anterior segment of the eye. Invest Ophthalmol Vis Sci. 1999;40(7):1373–81.
21. Cusumano A, Coleman DJ, Silverman RH, Reinstein DZ, Rondeau MJ, Ursea R, Daly SM, Lloyd HO. Three-dimensional ultrasound imaging. Clin Appl Ophthalmol. 1998;105(2):300–6.
22. Reinstein DZ, Ameline B, Puech M, Montefiore G, Laroche L. VHF digital ultrasound three-dimensional scanning in the diagnosis of myopic regression after corneal refractive surgery. J Refract Surg. 2005;21(5):480–4.
23. Lois N, Shields CL, Shields JA, Mercado G. Primary cysts of the iris pigment epithelium. Clinical features and natural course in 234 patients. Ophthalmology. 1998;105(10):1879–85.
24. Kunimatsu S, Araie M, Ohara K, Hamada C. Ultrasound biomicroscopy of ciliary body cysts. Am J Ophthalmol. 1999;127(1):48–55.
25. Fine N, Pavlin CJ. Primary cysts in the iridociliary sulcus: ultrasound biomicroscopic features of 210 cases. Can J Ophthalmol. 1999;34(6):325–9.
26. Crowston JG, Medeiros FA, Mosaed S, Weinreb RN. Argon laser iridoplasty in the treatment of plateau-like iris configuration as result of numerous ciliary body cysts. Am J Ophthalmol. 2005;139(2):381–3.
27. Rosenthal G, Klemperer I, Zirkin H, Lifshitz T, Pe'er J. Congenital cysts of the iris stroma. Arch Ophthalmol. 1998;116(12):1696.
28. Marigo FA, Esaki K, Finger PT, Ishikawa H, Greenfield DS, Liebmann JM, Ritch R. Differential diagnosis of anterior segment cysts by ultrasound biomicroscopy. Ophthalmology. 1999;106(11):2131–5.
29. Augsburger JJ, Affel LL, Benarosh DA. Ultrasound biomicroscopy of cystic lesions of the iris and ciliary body. Trans Am Ophthalmol Soc. 1996;94:259–71; discussion 271–4.
30. Giuliari GP, Krema H, Mc Gowan HD, Pavlin CJ, Simpson ER. Clinical and ultrasound biomicroscopy features associated with growth in iris melanocytic lesions. Am J Ophthalmol. 2012;153(6):1043–9.
31. Marigo FA, Finger PT, McCormick SA, Iezzi R, Esaki K, Ishikawa H, Liebmann JM, Ritch R. Iris and ciliary body melanomas: ultrasound biomicroscopy with histopathologic correlation. Arch Ophthalmol. 2000;118(11):1515–21.
32. Nordlund JR, Robertson DM, Herman DC. Ultrasound biomicroscopy in management of malignant iris melanoma. Arch Ophthalmol. 2003;121(5):725–7.
33. Shields JA, Shields CL, Mercado G, Gunduz K, Eagle RC Jr. Adenoma of the iris pigment epithelium: a report of 20 cases: the 1998 Pan-American Lecture. Arch Ophthalmol. 1999;117(6):736–41.

34. Conway RM, Chew T, Golchet P, Desai K, Lin S, O'Brien J. Ultrasound biomicroscopy: role in diagnosis and management in 130 consecutive patients evaluated for anterior segment tumours. Br J Ophthalmol. 2005;89(8):950–5.

35. Pavlin CJ, Harasiewicz K, Foster FS. An ultrasound biomicroscopic dark-room provocative test. Ophthalmic Surg. 1995;26(3):253–5.

36. Woo EK, Pavlin CJ, Slomovic A, Taback N, Buys YM. Ultrasound biomicroscopic quantitative analysis of light-dark changes associated with pupillary block. Am J Ophthalmol. 1999;127(1):43–7.

37. Friedman DS, He M. Anterior chamber angle assessment techniques Surv Ophthalmol. 2008;53(3):250–73.

38. Radhakrishnan S, See J, Smith SD, Nolan WP, Ce Z, Friedman DS & al. Reproducibility of anterior chamber angle measurements obtained with anterior segment optical coherence tomography. Invest Ophthalmol Vis Sci. 2007;48(8):3683–8.

39. Leung CK, Li H, Weinreb RN, Liu J, Cheung CY, Lai RY, & al. Anterior chamber angle measurement with anterior segment optical coherence tomography: a comparison between slit lamp OCT and Visante OCT. Invest Ophthalmol Vis Sci. 2008 ;49(8):3469–74.

40. Kim DY, Sung KR, Kang SY, Cho JW, Lee KS, & al. Characteristics and reproducibility of anterior chamber angle assessment by anterior-segment optical coherence tomography. Acta Ophthalmol. 2011;89(5):435–41.

41. Pavlin CJ. Ultrasound biomicroscopy in pigment dispersion syndrome. Ophthalmology. 1994;101(9):1475–7.

42. Adam RS, Pavlin CJ, Ulanski LJ. Ultrasound biomicroscopic analysis of iris profile changes with accommodation in pigmentary glaucoma and relationship to age. Am J Ophthalmol. 2004;138(4):652–4.

43. Wang N, Wu H, Fan Z. Primary angle closure glaucoma in Chinese and Western populations. Chin Med J (Engl). 2002;115(11):1706–15.

44. Mandell MA, Pavlin CJ, Weisbrod DJ, Simpson ER. Anterior chamber depth in plateau iris syndrome and pupillary block as measured by ultrasound biomicroscopy. Am J Ophthalmol. 2003;136(5):900–3.

45. Sihota R, Dada T, Gupta R, Lakshminarayan P, Pandey RM. Ultrasound biomicroscopy in the subtypes of primary angle closure glaucoma. J Glaucoma. 2005;14(5):387–91.

46. McWhae JA, Crichton AC. The use of ultrasound biomicroscopy following trabeculectomy. Can J Ophthalmol. 1996;31(4):187–91.

47. Khairy HA, Atta HR, Green FD, van der Hoek J, Azuara-Blanco A. Ultrasound biomicroscopy in deep sclerectomy. Eye. 2005;19(5):555–60.

48. Pavlin CJ, McWhae JA, McGowan HD, Foster FS. Ultrasound biomicroscopy of anterior segment tumors. Ophthalmology. 1992;99(8):1220–8.

49. Weisbrod DJ, Pavlin CJ, Emara K, Mandell MA, McWhae J, Simpson ER. Small ciliary body tumors: ultrasound biomicroscopic assessment and follow-up of 42 patients.

50. Maberly DA, Pavlin CJ, McGowan HD, Foster FS, Simpson ER. Ultrasound biomicroscopic imaging of the anterior aspect of peripheral choroidal. Am J Ophthalmol. 1997;123(4):506–14.

51. Foster RE, Murray TG, Byrne SF, Hughes JR, Gendron BK, Ehlies FJ, Nicholson DH. Echographic features of medulloepithelioma. Am J Ophthalmol. 2000;130(3):364–6.

52. Siahmed K, Bergès O, Brasseur G. Comparaison de l'échographie à 10, 20 MHz et de la tomographie en cohérence optique dans l'évaluation des trous maculaires. J Fr Ophtalmol. 2005;28(7):733–6.

53. Simonini VM, Lodi L. Encephalofacial angiomatosis (Sturge-Weber syndrome): report of three cases. Acta Clin Croat. 2012;51(Suppl 1):91–8.

54. Good P. Usefulness of 20 MHz probe for the evaluation of the sclera. Presentation at the XXVI SIDUO meeting (Naples, 2016).

# Chapter 5
# Ultrasound Settings

**Olivier Bergès and Michel Claudon**

**Abstract** Even if customized programs are used to allow reproducibility, settings are important to improve image quality. They are essential to understand and master to obtain an informative image, both in B-mode and in Doppler; however, they are even more crucial in Doppler, to avoid artifacts. Successively, the following settings are reviewed in this chapter:

**For the B-mode**

- The size of the image and area of interest and the adjustment of the frequency
- The adjustment of the focal length(s) to the area of interest
- The gain
- The contrast
- The time gain compensation curve

**For the Doppler**

- The Doppler frequency
- The Doppler beam angulation
- The angular correction
- The size of the Doppler window and gate
- The pulse repetition frequency
- The wall filters
- The acoustic power

O. Bergès (✉)
Rothschild Foundation Hospital, Paris, France
e-mail: oberges@for.paris

M. Claudon
Brabois Hospital, CHRU Nancy, Nancy, France

© The Author(s), under exclusive license to Springer Nature Switzerland AG 2024
O. Bergès (ed.), *Echography of the Eye and Orbit*,
https://doi.org/10.1007/978-3-031-41467-1_5

We only cover the ultrasound settings that allow for improving the image quality and provide for greater quality in terms of esthetics, exchange, and communication. Of note, multipurpose ultrasound devices have settings that ensure a customized program that is reproducible and that takes into account the following:

**For B-mode**

1. General gain
2. Exploration depth ≠ zoom
3. Focal lengths (number, position) in the axial plane
4. Acoustic power (see Chap. 1)
5. Dynamic = bandwidth = contrast
6. Grayscale = γamma
7. Frequency
8. Harmonic imaging: Possible with a broad-frequency band probe; it is set by default in the programs for exploring the eye and orbit with multipurpose ultrasound devices, allowing for improvement in lateral resolution, enhanced contrast by increasing the useable dynamic range, and improvement of the axial spatial resolution without an increase in the acoustic intensity emitted at the expense of a slight loss of penetration at depth.
9. Cross beam
10. Speckle reduction (after the beamformer / beam manager)
11. Noise levels: relatively low, so as to remove twinkling, without reducing the signal
12. Line density

Contrast with the I/S number

The juxtaposition of parallel exploration lines allows for generating a section in the plane of the displacement of the transmitter. The number of exploration lines determines the density of the information on the screen (this is the lateral resolution of the image) but compromised with frame rate ++.

**For Doppler**

1. Line density
2. Frequency (compromise penetration/resolution)
3. Sample volume
4. Wall filters (decreasing background noise) + + +
5. Averaging, providing an indication of the persistence
6. Pulse repetition frequency (PRF) if increased, slow flow, aliasing
7. Number and sample size
8. Spectrum compression = γamma

## 5.1 In B-mode

### 5.1.1 Size of the Image and Area of Interest and Adjustment of the Frequency

This is fairly obvious, but it is the first thing to try. There is a trade-off between the higher the frequency, the better the resolution, but at the cost of lower penetration. Thus, for broad exploration of the eyeball or orbit, the most suitable frequency is 10–15 MHz. This is already high frequency as compared with the frequencies used for abdominal or transcranial exploration. For better resolution, especially of the eye wall, optic disc, macula, or even the periphery, a 20 MHz probe with a long focal length should be used (see below). However, for exploring the anterior segment, a high-frequency probe (25 MHz or close to this value) or very-high-frequency probe (50 MHz) is used.

**5.1.1a Anterior segment:** The size of the explored cell is small, at 16 mm in diameter × 9 mm deep for an axial section at 50 MHz or 25 MHz. The attenuation, intimately linked with the possible resolution, will dictate the choice between these two probes. The best resolution (35 μm) is obtained at 50 MHz but with significant attenuation, thus not allowing routine visualization of the posterior lens capsule or study of large tumors of the ciliary body (> 6 mm thick). The attenuation is lower at 25 MHz, allowing these two applications, but at the cost of lower resolution: 70 μm. These axial resolutions are significantly higher than those of a 10-MHz probe: 0.15 mm. With recent multipurpose ultrasound devices, a high-frequency probe (18 to 22 MHz) can be used as well as a program devised for exploring the anterior segment of the eye, eyelids, and anterior orbit. The depth of exploration with very good spatial resolution (very close to that obtained at 25 MHz) is even greater, reaching 15 to 20 mm (Fig. 5.1).

**5.1.1b Posterior segment, transocular**

**5.1.1c Orbit, transocular or paraocular**

Whether for the eye or the orbit, recent dedicated ophthalmic ultrasound devices allow for adjusting the size of the image, which allows visualization (and especially measurement) of very myopic globes, for which the axial length is close to or even greater than 40 mm (Fig. 5.2).

With multipurpose ultrasound scanners, an exploration area adapted to the area to be studied is selected and must not be too localized. One can also select the frequency within the broad band of the probe (higher for surface structures and lower for deep structures).

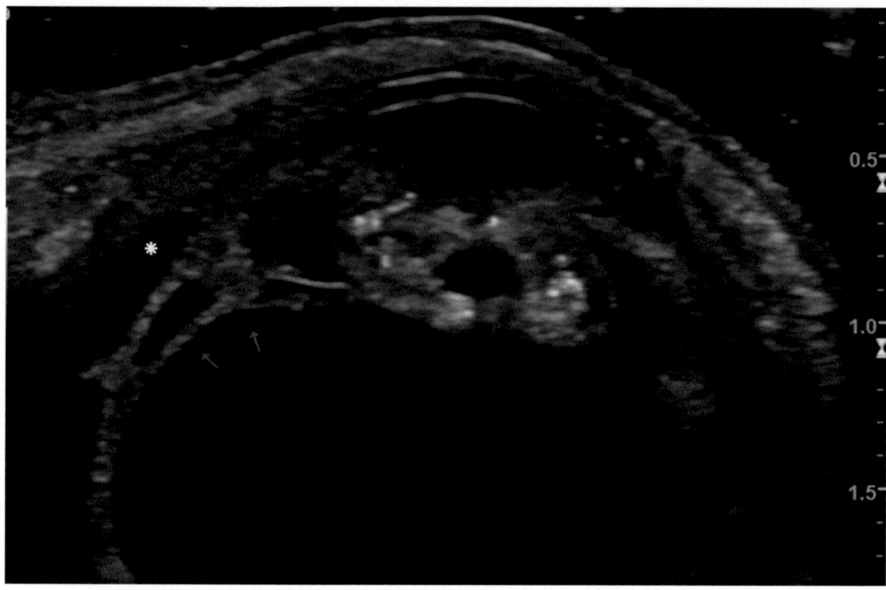

**Fig. 5.1 Compromise between the area of interest, image size, resolution, penetration, and frequency.** Ultrasound of the anterior part of the right eye according to the 3 o'clock meridian with a multipurpose ultrasound device and an 8–18-MHz probe. Persistence of a choroidal detachment after drainage on Day 30 of a voluminous choroidal hematoma after expulsive hemorrhage and posterior dislocation of the nucleus. The peripheral anechogenic choroidal detachment going up to the ciliary body (*) can clearly be seen as well as vitreous membranes (→) connecting the detached choroid to the very echogenic residual lenticular masses. Note the good penetration of the ultrasound beam up to 1.8 cm, with focal zones placed at 6 mm and 11 mm

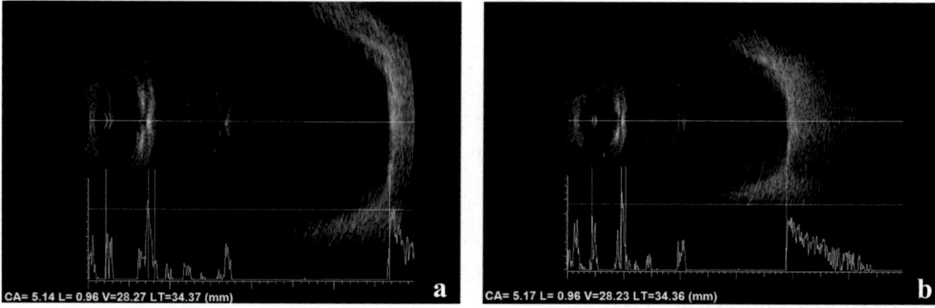


**Fig. 5.2 Contribution of an exploration depth of 60 mm for measuring very myopic globes,** B-mode guided biometry. **a**: With a standard depth of 40 mm, this globe measured at 34.7 mm barely fits into the cell, and most of the orbit is cut off. **b**: With an exploration depth of 60 mm, the globe and orbit are well visualized. Note the excellent reproducibility of the B-mode-guided biometry technique, with minimal standard deviation for these two sections

For 10- and long focal length 20 MHz probes, the scanning angle is fixed at 50°; and for 25- and 50 MHz probes, the width of the exploration cell is stable: 16 mm. The scan speed (frame rate) can also be varied. For the posterior segment, it can be set from 9 to 16 Hz. For the anterior segment, the frame rate is approximately 8 Hz. With a multipurpose ultrasound device, because it uses an electronic scanning probe, it is faster, varying according to depth, number of focal lengths, and line density: on average, 50 Hz, ranging from 5 to 330 Hz.

Aside from the initially selected area of interest, one should also be aware that a zoom function can be used (25 mm with a 10 MHz probe and 30 mm with a long focal length 20 MHz probe) similar to an optical zoom, allowing for better resolution of the image due to an increased number of lines and points. The same zoom function is possible with multipurpose ultrasound devices. Of note, by increasing the number of lines and number of points per line, there is a new compromise and a need to reduce the frame rate.

## 5.1.2   Adjustment of the Focal Length(s) to the Area of Interest (Fig. 5.3)

**5.1.2a With dedicated ophthalmic ultrasound devices,** each probe has a characteristic focal area.

- From 21 to 25 mm for a 10 MHz B-probe (it is immediately clear that the resolution is optimal for the ocular wall but will be less for the anterior and para-equatorial vitreous and for the orbit, especially at the apex)
- 24–26 mm for a long focal-length 20 MHz probe (for the posterior pole), and 11–13 mm for a 25 MHz high-frequency probe
- From 9 to 11 mm for a very-high-frequency probe of 50 MHz

In addition, for exploring the anterior segment, as long as the image is not frozen, the manifestation of the focal area can be perceived on the screen in the form of two thin green dotted lines, allowing verification that the structures to be studied are indeed within this focal zone. However, it is smaller than the entire anterior segment: For an axial section of the entire anterior segment, a section is made with the iris plane and the anterior lens capsule located at the deep part of this focal zone (appearing very clear); however, the cornea, far in front of the focal area, may appear slightly blurred. Of note, one can/must distinguish the two interfaces corresponding to the epithelium and the Bowman membrane. This section is mainly used for measurements: thickness of the cornea, depth of the anterior chamber, and diameters: from angle to angle and from sulcus to sulcus. However, if a fine analysis of the cornea is desired, the probe must be moved a little further, so as to place the cornea within the focal area (Fig. 5.4).

**5.1.2b With multipurpose ultrasound devices,** there are usually two focal zones (sometimes three or four, but be careful: the more the number is increased, the more

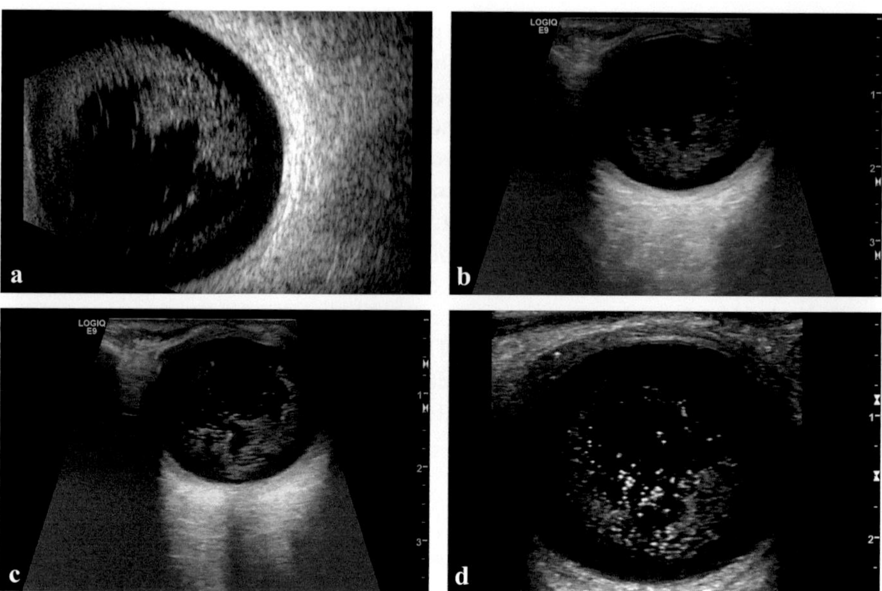

**Fig. 5.3** Asteroid hyalosis The calcium phosphate deposits of the vitreous collagen matrix characteristic of asteroid hyalosis only appear punctiform at the level of the focal zone(s): at the posterior part (a and b) and the anterior part of the eye (c). However, these same points are wide and blurred at a distance from these focal areas. Also, the small dots are best defined with a high-frequency probe (d)

the frame rate is reduced!) adjustable, which must be positioned carefully, to optimize the spatial resolution; they allow for an axial resolution of less than 400 $\mu$m to be achieved with the 8–18 MHz probe of the Logiq E9 and less than 300 $\mu$m with the 12–22 MHz probe of the Logiq *e* (from General Electric).

All this concerns the axial resolution of the probe. One must also consider the lateral resolution of the probe, which, at the focal point of the probe of dedicated ophthalmic ultrasound devices is 300 $\mu$m for a 10 MHz probe, 250 $\mu$m for a long focal-length 20 MHz probe, 120 $\mu$m for a 25 MHz high-frequency probe, and 60 $\mu$m for a 50 MHz very-high-frequency probe. With multipurpose ultrasound devices, this lateral resolution is less than 700 $\mu$m with the 8–18 MHz probe of the Logiq E9 and less than 500 $\mu$m with the 12–22 MHz probe of the Logiq *e*.

When the transducer is rectangular, the final azimuthal resolution, or the thickness of the section, also depends on the probe. It is of the same order as the lateral resolution.

When the transducer is circular (the various probes of dedicated ophthalmic ultrasound devices), this azimuthal resolution corresponds to the lateral resolution.

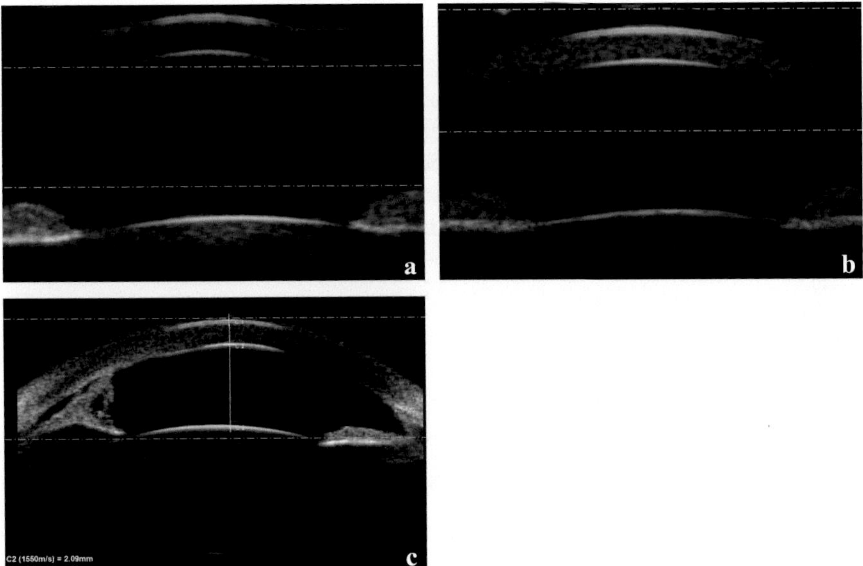

**Fig. 5.4 Importance of the position of the focal zone on the appearance of the cornea. a**: Axial section of the central part of the anterior segment, the focal area, represented by the dotted green lines, is located between the cornea and the anterior lens capsule **b**: Axial section of the central part of the anterior segment, the focal zone, represented by the dotted green lines, is located on either side of the cornea, clearly showing the two lines corresponding to the epithelium and Bowman membrane as well as the homogeneous hypoechogenicity of the stroma. **c**: Peters syndrome, axial section of the anterior segment. Because the eye is small, the cornea and the temporal iridocorneal synechia are located within the focal area, with high resolution: in particular, note the temporal sectorial hyperechogenicity of the cornea corresponding to clinical opacity as well as the defect of the endothelium/Descemet membrane at the corneal extremity of the synechia related to the cleavage syndrome

## *5.1.3 The Gain (or Sensitivity Setting)*

It is the equivalent of the potentiometer on an amplifier, corresponding to the amplification of the reflected echoes, and is very different from the acoustic power of the system. This is the most frequently used setting. It is expressed in decibels (dB), which is a relative scale that differs from one ultrasound device to another.

**5.1.3a standardized A-mode:** it allows for quantification and reproducibility, after calibration of the probe with a silicone tissue model (when the attenuation is regular, 45°, separating the space into two identical triangles—(see Fig. 7.13) which defines the standard gain or tissue sensitivity setting: T. Images with high T + 9 and low T-9 gain should also be acquired. Tissue gain acquisition allows for quantifying the reflectivity of a lesion (as a percentage of the scleral peak, taken as a reference). To obtain the attenuation of the lesion, simply press the K key, which provides an average height of the peaks of 50%. The attenuation is given in decibels per millimeter and in a more understandable manner by the angle kappa that the slope of decay of the echoes makes with the horizontal plane.

**5.1.3b B-mode** does not allow for a perfectly reproducible standard gain value. Rather, the gain for the study of the ocular wall and the orbit must be defined intuitively: a relatively low gain, whereby the different layers of the ocular wall and particularly the meninges around the optic nerve can be clearly seen. Out of habit, the vitreous is generally assessed with a maximal gain. However, reducing the gain by a few decibels is sometimes useful to avoid oversaturating the image with random echoes.

### 5.1.4  Contrast

This setting, which is subjective, depends on a number of parameters, such as the following:

- The user's preferences (in the United States, the entire dynamic range is usually used, with a setting at 90 dB, and the white tends to become gray)
- The quality of the probe
- The quality of the screen

It is also directly related to the printer setting.

For 10 MHz probes, the most appropriate setting to obtain a clear and unsaturated retina but with sufficient display of pathologies in the vitreous or near retina is approximately 70 dB.

If the dynamic range is set too low, the small signals in the vitreous will be able to be displayed, at the cost of saturation of the retina. If the dynamic range setting is at the maximum (90 dB), the weak signals of the vitreous may disappear (Fig. 5.5).

Therefore, the dynamic range needs to be adjusted according to the area explored, but this adjustment is tedious and rarely used.

"*Sync. Contrast*" can also be used to automatically synchronize the dynamic range setting with that of the gain.

For other probes, the dynamic range adjustment is less critical.

### 5.1.5  Time Gain Compensation (TGC)

The energy of the ultrasound beam is slowly depleted as it moves through tissues. This effect can be counterbalanced by amplifying distant echoes more than proximal echoes. This is called the TGC (see Fig. 7.10).

On the dedicated ophthalmic Aviso ultrasound device, the TGC is not set over the entire image, but it is possible to set the TGC from 0 to −30 dB on the first 18 mm of the image, which reduces echoes from the membrane and the gel, resulting in better

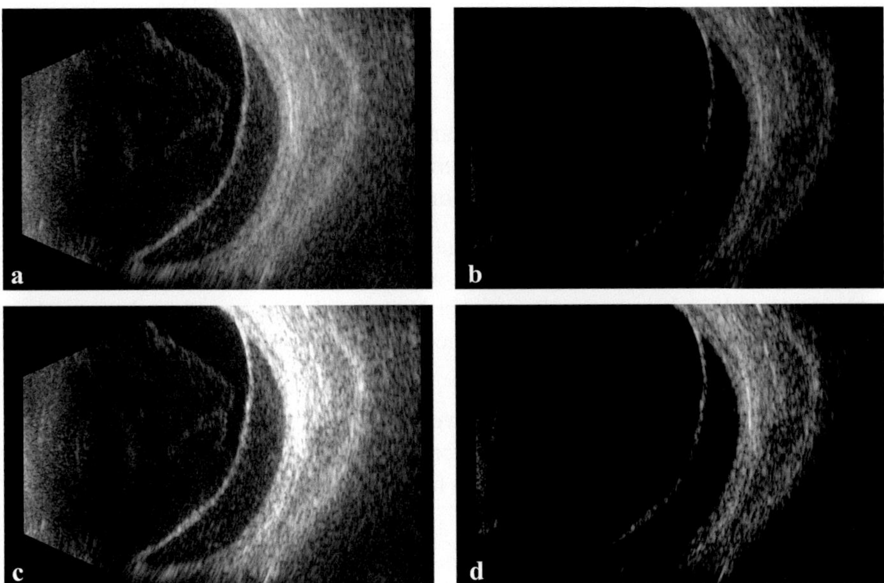

**Fig. 5.5  Effect of gain and dynamic range on visualization of eye structures.** Same section with intravitreal hemorrhage and retinal detachment. **a**: Gain = 110 dB – dynamic range = 90 dB **b**: Gain = 81 dB – dynamic range = 90 dB **c**: Gain = 110 dB – dynamic range = 60 dB **d**: Gain = 81 dB – dynamic range = 60 dB At a high gain, one can readily see the intravitreal hemorrhage restricted by the detached posterior hyaloid membrane and the hemorrhagic retinal detachment, but the reflectivity of these membranes cannot be fully assessed. By viewing them with a relatively low gain, only the detached retina remains visible, and the hemorrhagic echoes are no longer visible. Clearly, the dynamic range is a matter of personal choice, especially at a high gain

images. This also avoids "saturation" of corneal echoes when immersion technique is used (especially for B-mode guided biometry). With multipurpose ultrasound devices, a series of small push buttons allow the TGC to modify the amplification of echoes according to their depth.

## 5.2  In Doppler

Many settings are already determined by the programs, but one should be aware of how to adjust them to obtain the maximum information.

**5.2.1 The Doppler frequency:** By default, it is set to 8 MHz, which allows visualization of the arteries of the optic nerve head and the ophthalmic artery if it is located at the anterior part of the orbit, along the medial rectus muscle. When the ophthalmic artery is deeper, the Doppler frequency can be decreased (to 5 MHz) to highlight it.

**5.2.2 Doppler beam angulation:** Given the direction of the vessels in the orbit and their small size, the angle of the Doppler pulse remains in the axis of the probe and is not angled.

**5.2.3 Angular correction:** In spectral mode, angular correction is applied for the ophthalmic artery and the central retinal artery but not for the short posterior ciliary arteries because their actual direction around the optic nerve head is not known.

**5.2.4 Size of the Doppler window and gate:** Because these are small vessels, with slow flows, the size of the Doppler window should be as small as possible. To have the best possible color signal, the gain in B-mode should be reduced as much as possible. Similarly, in spectral Doppler, the size of the Doppler gate must be as small as possible: 1 mm.

**5.2.5 PRF:** The velocities of the different vessels are rather slow, from a few centimeters per second for veins to 40 to 60 cm/s for the ophthalmic artery. The arteries of the optic nerve head and other orbital arteries have intermediate velocities: 10 to 20 cm/s.

- In color mode, a speed scale of $\pm 5$ to 6 cm/s is chosen, with red colors at the top and blue colors at the bottom. With this setting, in color mode, the arteries of the optic nerve head are encoded in red (sometimes yellow in connection with a discrete aliasing artifact). The ophthalmic artery, which has a much faster circulation, is readily recognized because of the aliasing artifact, which often gives it a yellow appearance centered by a blue line. Loops of varying tightness are often seen for this vessel and therefore a broad range of features are possible.
- In spectral mode, the velocity scale is usually adapted to the central retinal vessels, from $-10$ to $+20$ cm/s; a scale also valid for the posterior short ciliary arteries. For the ophthalmic artery, which has a much faster flow, one must modify the setting on demand: ranging from $-10$ cm/s to more than $+50$ cm/s after angular correction.

**5.2.6 Wall Filters:** They should be decreased to reduce background noise, especially for the very small vessels of the eyelids and lesions of the anterior segment, iris, and ciliary body (Fig. 5.6).

**5.2.7** Acoustic Power: MI and TIs Must Be Less Than 0.2 (see Chap. 2).

*Knowing how to adjust the settings is essential to obtaining an informative image, both in B-mode and Doppler. However, in Doppler, this is even more crucial to avoid artifacts (see Chap. 6).*

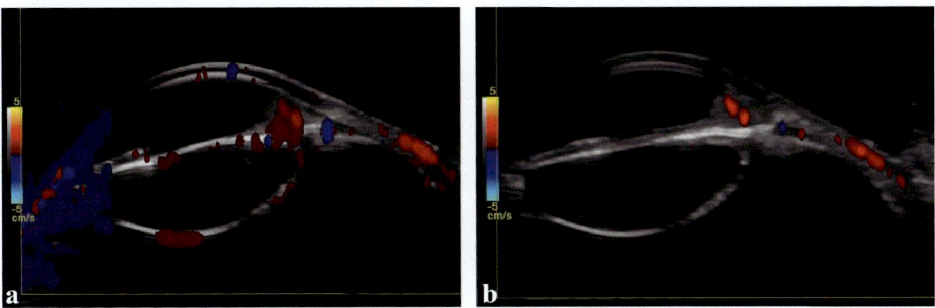

**Fig. 5.6 Importance of wall filters**: Color Doppler imaging of an iridociliary melanoma. **a**: With the standard program for assessing choroidal melanomas **b**: After reducing the wall filters. In **a** there are colored spots everywhere, masking the small lesion for the most part and preventing the appreciation of its vascularization, which is clearly visible in **b**. This helps to confirm the presumed diagnosis. The correction of the wall filters allows for preventing the micromovements (the examiner's hand and the patient's eye), which are the source of these artifacts

# Chapter 6
# Artifacts in Ultrasound

**Michel Claudon and Olivier Bergès**

**Abstract** With various causes, artifacts are nearly constant, both in B-mode and in Doppler. These phenomena of artificial origin are readily recognizable, although sometimes difficult to detect. Knowing how to recognize them is important to avoid diagnostic errors. They can sometimes be a diagnostic help, but more often it is useful to know how to minimize them. We first review the artifacts in B-mode. The different artifacts are classified, described and illustrated according to whether they are related to (1) the physics of ultrasound and acoustics: reverberation echoes, comet tail/dirty shadowing, mirror image, posterior (acoustic) enhancement, acoustic shadowing, edge shadow (oblique reflection, refraction), velocity artifacts (Baum bump), scattering artifacts - dispersion (speckle); (2) the ultrasound technique and sensors: side-lobe artifacts and partial volume artifacts; (3) ultrasound and sensor malfunctions and environmental artifacts; and (4) complex artifacts (intraocular gas). Then artifacts encountered in Doppler are studied, in relation to unsuitable velocity scale settings (absence of flow if pulse repetition frequency is too high, aliasing if pulse repetition frequency is too low), spectrum broadening (turbulence), and color coding outside of vessels (perivascular blooming artifact, twinkling artifact, and artifacts related to movements).

## 6.1 Introduction: Definition and Proposal of a Classification

Generally, an artifact is an entity or phenomenon of artificial origin, encountered during an observation or experiment on a natural phenomenon. In ultrasound, the ultrasound image is generated from the information (position and intensity of the echo) collected by the probe and transmitted to the device. Random echoes are

M. Claudon
Brabois Hospital, CHRU Nancy, Nancy, France

O. Bergès (✉)
Rothschild Foundation Hospital, Paris, France
e-mail: oberges@for.paris



O. Bergès (ed.), *Echography of the Eye and Orbit*,
https://doi.org/10.1007/978-3-031-41467-1_6

*echoes that do not correspond to a real entity* and appear on the reconstructed image as artifacts.

Artifacts [1–4] can be classified according to whether they are related to:

- physical and acoustic phenomena,
- the technology and malfunctions of the ultrasound apparatus or sensors,
- the environment (interactions between devices), which have become a rarity nowadays.

Such artifacts can hinder interpretation or lead to errors, but they can sometimes also be useful and help with the recognition of tissues or lesions and thus can be useful for diagnosis. There is a need to know what strategy to adopt to eliminate or minimize them.

## 6.2 Artifacts in B-mode

### 6.2.1 Artifacts Related to the Physics of Ultrasound and Acoustics

#### 6.2.1.1 Reverberation

Reverberation Echoes

Also called delayed echoes, these are random echoes, delayed, spaced regularly, generated by an orthogonal incidence between two or more media interfaces with very different acoustic impedances. Such artifacts are frequently encountered in daily practice (Fig. 6.1), and they can come from the posterior side of the iris plane, the lens, an intraocular implant, or the cornea.

Comet Tail, Dirty Shadowing

These occur at the level of very reflective entities: calcifications, large foreign bodies, and tissue–gas or liquid–air interfaces (Fig. 6.2). These are successive repetitions of echoes between the surface of the structure and a more proximal plane.

Intraocular foreign bodies (IOFBs), made of aluminum or glass, produce comet-tail artifacts, whereas those made of wood produce shadowing. The presence of an artifact allows for the identification of unknown IOFBs. And, the type of artifact allows for characterizing its nature [5, 6]. Tantalum markers used for proton therapy are frequently encountered IOFBs (Fig. 6.3).

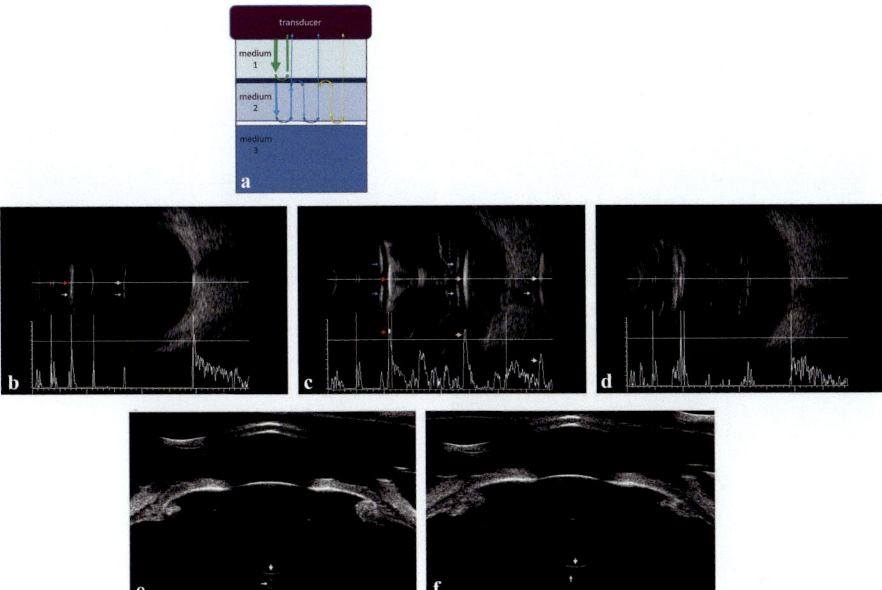

**Fig. 6.1  Reverberation echoes. a: Diagram explaining the formation of reverberation echoes**:
the ultrasound beam can be transmitted or reflected at the interface between two media with different
acoustic impedance, with extension of the time of flight; **b: axial section (B-mode guided biometry).** The anterior lens capsule (➤red arrow) and the iris (→ white arrow) give rise to para-
equatorial repetitions for the lens (➤ pink arrow) and the iris (→grey thin arrow) **c: axial section
(B-mode guided biometry)** of an eye with a posterior chamber intraocular lens (IOL), made of polymethylmethacrylate (PMMA). The optics of the implant (➤ red arrow), hyperechoic, are clearly
visible both in B-mode and in reconstructed A-mode. The first repetition (➤ pink arrow) is behind
the equator of the globe and the second (➤ white arrow) in the anterior intraconal orbital space.
Because of the marked difference in acoustic impedance between PMMA and the vitreous, the
second repetition is almost as echogenic as the structure at the origin of the artifact, but in B-mode,
the artificial image is more diffuse, less sharp. The second repetition is not very echogenic, both in
B-mode and A-mode. The appearance of the artifacts immediately behind (and outside) the optics
of the implant and the very echogenic repetition of the implant behind the equator are characteristic
of this type of implant (of this material). Also note the repetitions of the iris (→ and → and →
dense to light blue thin arrows). **d: Acrylic IOL.** The echogenicity of the implant and the reverberation artifact are less than for a PMMA IOL, in B-mode and reconstructed A-mode, and there is
no second repetition. Here again, the appearance of the implant optics and its artifact behind the
equator are characteristic of this type of implant (of this material). **e:** Reverberation artifacts in the
cornea (epithelium and endothelium), axial section at 50 MHz. This repetition (→) (epithelium and
endothelium) projects behind the posterior capsule of the lens (➤ white arrow), weakly echogenic
(or most often even non-visible) at 50 MHz because of the significant attenuation at this frequency.
**f:** The same section at 50 MHz, the probe being discreetly deeper in the gel than in **e**. In **f**, the
repetition of the epithelium, invisible, is now projected on the posterior capsule of the lens (➤
white arrow), and that of the endothelium discreetly behind it (→ white thin arrow)

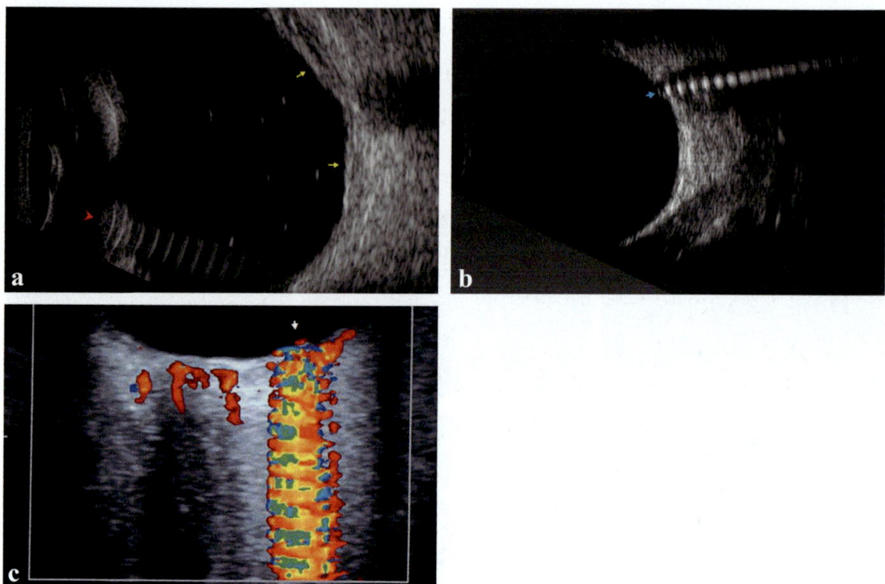

**Fig. 6.2 Comet tail artifact. a**: Behind a residual silicone mini bubble lodged behind the iris against the temporal ciliary body (▶ red arrowhead); recurrent retinal detachment and gliosis are seen in the nasal and temporal areas of the optic disc. (→ yellow arrows). **b**: Behind a residual micro bubble of perfluorocarbon liquid (PFCL) at the posterior pole (➡ blue arrow). Care should be taken to not zoom the image too much; otherwise, the artifact may not be obvious, because it is, in this case, very long in a characteristic way, all the more obvious here because it projects itself on the shadow of the optic nerve. **c**: Behind a micro bubble of residual PFCL at the posterior pole (➡ white arrow), with the retina being reattached – color Doppler imaging. The artifact may not be evident in B-mode within the highly echogenic retrobulbar fat, but it becomes so in CDI

### 6.2.1.2 Mirror Image

These are representations on the image of an entity on both sides of a concave or oblique interface (Fig. 6.4). For example, the subclavian artery examined by the supraclavicular route gives rise to a mirror image, visible in B-mode and in color Doppler, owing to reflection of ultrasound by the pleural dome. They are only rarely observed at the level of the eye or orbit.

### 6.2.1.3 The Posterior Enhancement Artifact (Acoustic)

Acoustic enhancement is generated at the level of a structure with less attenuation than the surrounding environment, with the overall amplification of the signal applied to the image enhancing the echoes behind this structure. The intensity of a posterior acoustic enhancement is proportional to the anteroposterior diameter of the less attenuating entity. In ophthalmology, the eyeball can be considered an ultrasound

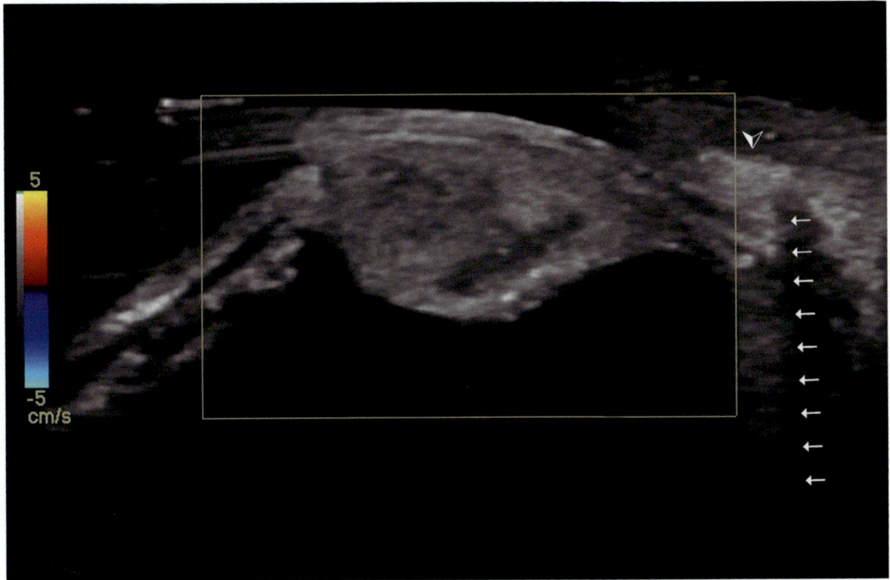

**Fig. 6.3  Comet tail artifact**. Comet tail artifact (⇐ white arrows) behind a tantalum marker (▷white arrowhead) for proton beam therapy of a melanoma of the ciliary body—color Doppler imaging. Examination performed 2 years after the treatment, which was effective: absence of visible intratumoral vessel, and heterogeneous echotexture indicating areas of necrosis

cyst, with non-visibility of its side walls and posterior enhancement of the retrobulbar fat (relative to the periocular fat). It is used as a "water pouch" for studying retrobulbar orbital structures (fat, vessels, muscles, and optic nerve).

Harmonic imaging accentuates the acoustic enhancement behind a fluid structure. It is a major semiological element, accentuating the liquid nature of a structure, like a small cyst (Fig. 6.5). However, this acoustic enhancement is also encountered in other lesions with low ultrasound attenuation, such as, lymphomas, or cysts containing cholesterol crystals.

### 6.2.1.4  Acoustic Shadowing

These are formed by the absence of transmission of the ultrasound beam behind a highly reflected or absorbent interface, with structures that are:

- highly mineralized (bone, urinary stones, calcified atheroma plaque, voluminous dense foreign bodies)
- gaseous (digestive, lung, aerobilia, intraocular gas bubble)
- metallic.

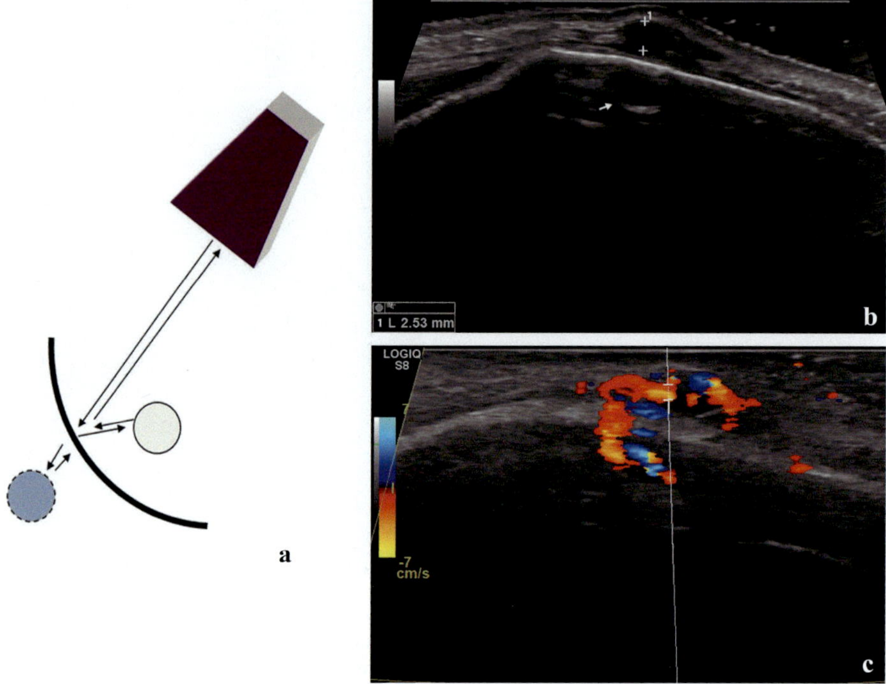

**Fig. 6.4 Mirror image artifact. a**: Diagram explaining the formation of the artifact image. The artifact image (blue) is a mirror image of the actual image (beige) due to reflections on the concave interface. This artifact is rarely observed in ocular ultrasound because, for example, the image of the nucleus of a dislocated lens in front of the ocular wall would project onto the hyperechoic retrobulbar fat and would, therefore, be invisible. **b**: B-mode and **c**: color Doppler imaging of a small false aneurysm of a small arteriovenous malformation of the right frontal region with a low flow rate, measured at 4.53 mm diameter × 2.53 mm thick and responsible for a mirror image (→ white arrow) in relation to the frontal bone. This artifact is also visible in color Doppler imaging, with the malformation naturally not crossing the bony wall

The phenomenon is amplified with high-frequency probes and harmonic mode. It is minimized by multi-scan probes. In some cases, the presence of a posterior shadowing (especially if it is large) prevents visualization of the structures behind it (e.g., it is often very difficult to visualize the optic nerve and orbit behind a large retinoblastoma containing macro-calcifications). However, sometimes it helps with the diagnosis, such as choroidal osteoma, a foreign body, and macro-calcifications in retinoblastoma (Fig. 6.6).

### 6.2.1.5   Edge Shadow (Oblique Reflection, Refraction)

Edge shadows are due to refraction of the ultrasound beam approaching a round structure tangentially. This type of artifact is well known in ocular ultrasound, especially

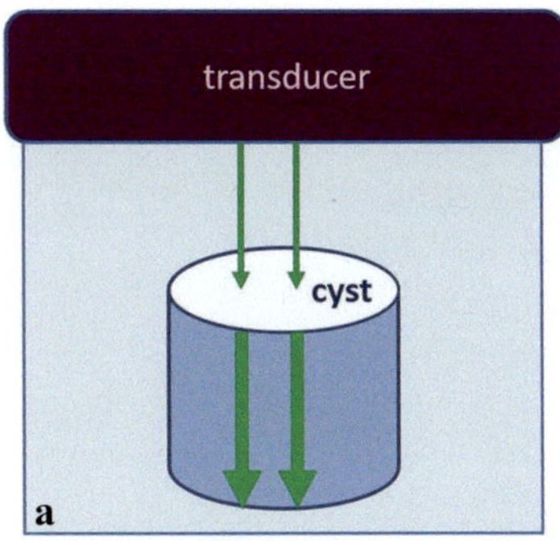
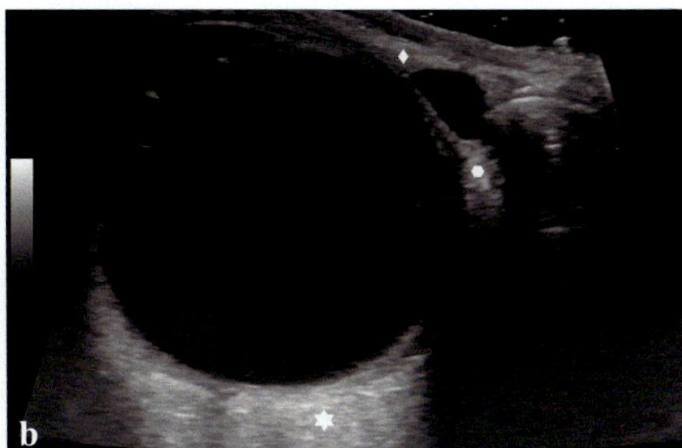



**Fig. 6.5  Posterior (acoustic) enhancement. a**: Diagram demonstrating posterior or acoustic enhancement: fluid structures such as cystic lesions lead to an increase in transmission, with increased visibility of deep structures. **b**: Clearly visible (⬢ white hexagon) behind and in the largest axis of this small cyst of the lacrimal gland (dacryops). However, the most perfect cyst remains the eyeball itself, with the non-visibility of its side walls and enhanced retrobulbar orbital fat (✹ white star) that is more echogenic than the extra-conal peribulbar fat (◆ white rhombus)

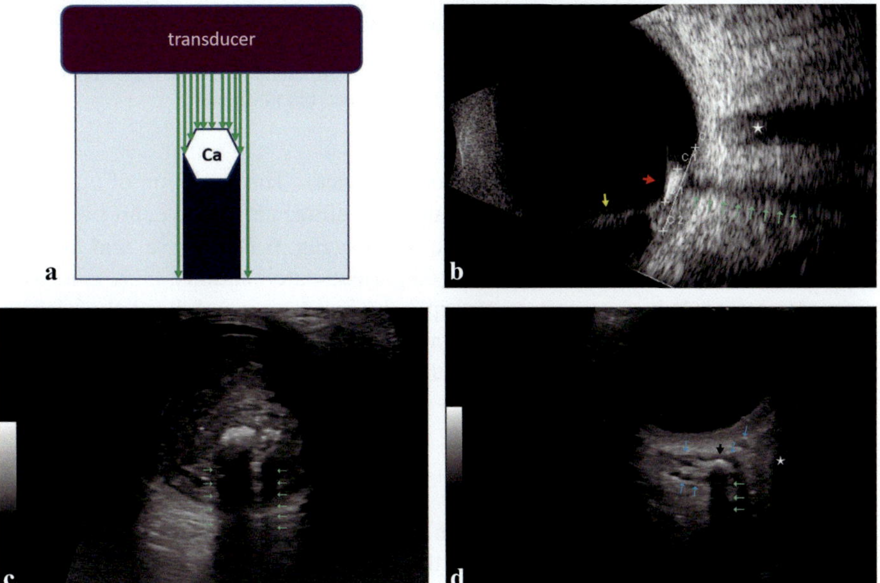



**Fig. 6.6  Posterior acoustic shadowing. a: Diagram explaining the formation of the artifact** that typically appears behind calcium-rich structures. **b**: Behind a metallic foreign body (c1 ➡ red arrow) with fibrosis (c2) and detachment of retina (→ yellow arrow) **c**: In a large stage E retinoblastoma with macro-calcifications **d**: Behind a phlebolith (➤ arrow) indicating an orbital varix, empty in the supine position, but nevertheless one can discern some serpiginous (→blue arrows) vascular structures around the calcification. In all cases, the posterior shadowing (⇉ green arrows) on the retrobulbar orbital fat is obvious, and it helps guide the diagnosis, not to be confused with the optic nerve (★ white star)

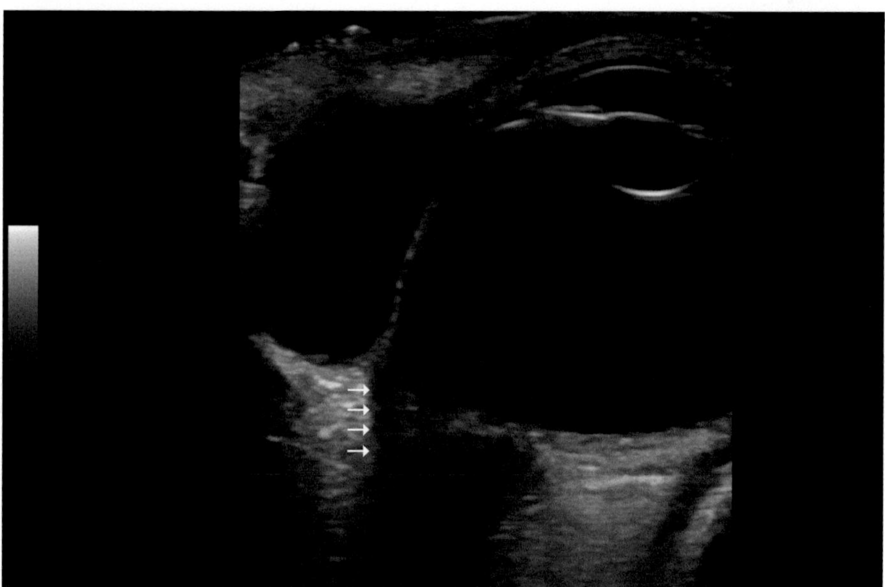

**Fig. 6.7 Edge shadowing**. Clearly visible (⇉ white arrows), lateral to the acoustic enhancement due to a dermoid cyst of the lacrimal fossa, very hyperechoic, but not liquid

with linear probes of multipurpose ultrasound devices. The deviation of ultrasound is responsible for a loss of sonification and, therefore, an empty echo band. This phenomenon occurs at the edges of cystic lesions (Fig. 6.7), the eye, and the sides of vessels (carotid). In case of unrecognized parietal calcifications, there is a risk of misinterpretation. It is necessary to multiply the incidences and move the probe as far as possible, because the refractive artifact always remains in the axis of the beam, unlike posterior shadowing due to (parietal) calcification.

### 6.2.1.6　Velocity Artifacts

In case of different media, with different propagation velocities, deformation of the image occurs. In ophthalmology, the best known is the Baum bump [7], which creates a false deformation of the posterior pole driven by the lens, with the velocity of ultrasound faster than in other ocular media, and by the refraction of echoes as soon as the incidence of the ultrasound beam is not fully orthogonal to the capsules (see Chap. 1) (Fig. 6.8). A more or less similar appearance is observed in the case of a silicone posterior chamber IOL (see Chap. 8).

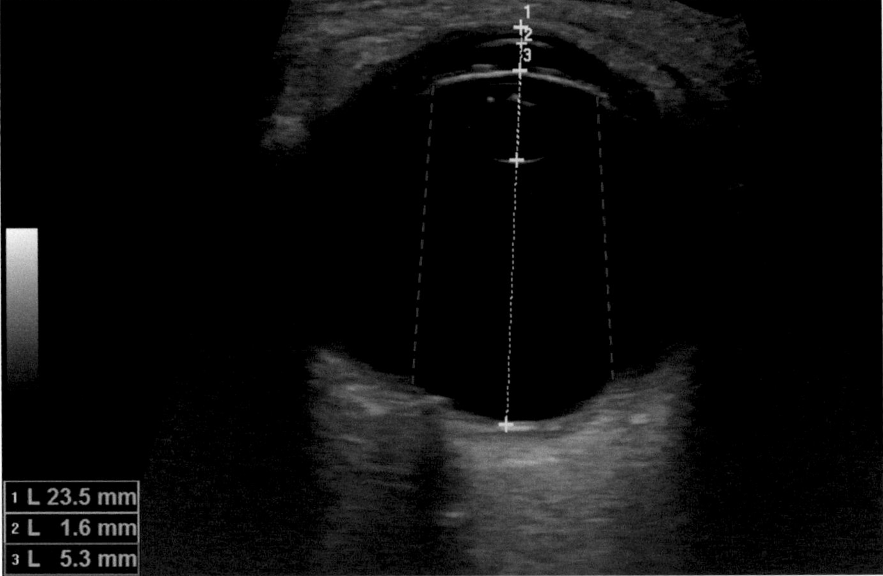


**Fig. 6.8 Baum bump artifact**. The lens causes an apparent deformation of the ocular wall (•••••••• dotted red lines). However, the biometric values are perfectly reliable on the line of the visual axis, orthogonal to the lens. The artifact is even more marked when the lens is echogenic (dense cataract) and the eyeball is myopic

### 6.2.1.7 Scattering Artifacts—Dispersion (Speckle)

Most ultrasound images are formed by reflection echoes from scattering on an irregular surface (Fig. 6.9a) and by dispersion echoes in a heterogeneous medium. The echogenicity of parenchyma is essentially generated by dispersion echoes for which the intensity depends on the tissue homogeneity. The parenchyma of each organ has a characteristic echogenicity. The image of the tissue in the analysis area depends on the setting of the ultrasound, the ultrasound sensor, and the handling of the sensor during acquisition (Fig. 6.9b).

## 6.2.2 Artifacts Related to the Ultrasound Technique and Sensors

### 6.2.2.1 Side-Lobe Artifacts

These artifacts are related to the emission, not of a single ultrasound beam, but the main beam and several side beams [8] (Fig. 6.10). Encountered with all probes, this artifact is minimized by harmonic mode.

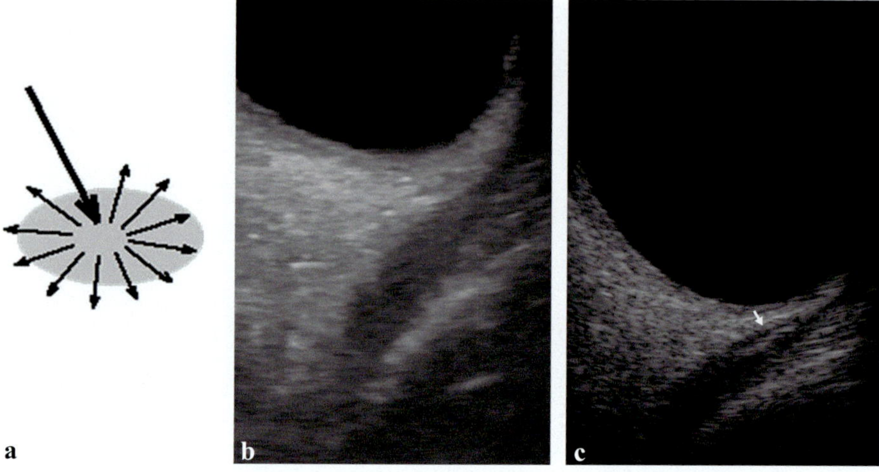

**Fig. 6.9 Scattering-dispersion artifacts—(speckle). a**: Diagram explaining the speckle phenomenon **b** and **c**: image of the same medial rectus muscle **b**: with a multipurpose ultrasound scanner and an 8–18 MHz broadband probe **c**: with an ophthalmic dedicated ultrasound device and a 10 MHz probe When the ultrasound beam is perpendicular, the heterogeneous muscle fibrils appear hyperechoic in **c** (➜ white arrow) but give rise to a blurred appearance in **b** in relation to the speckle

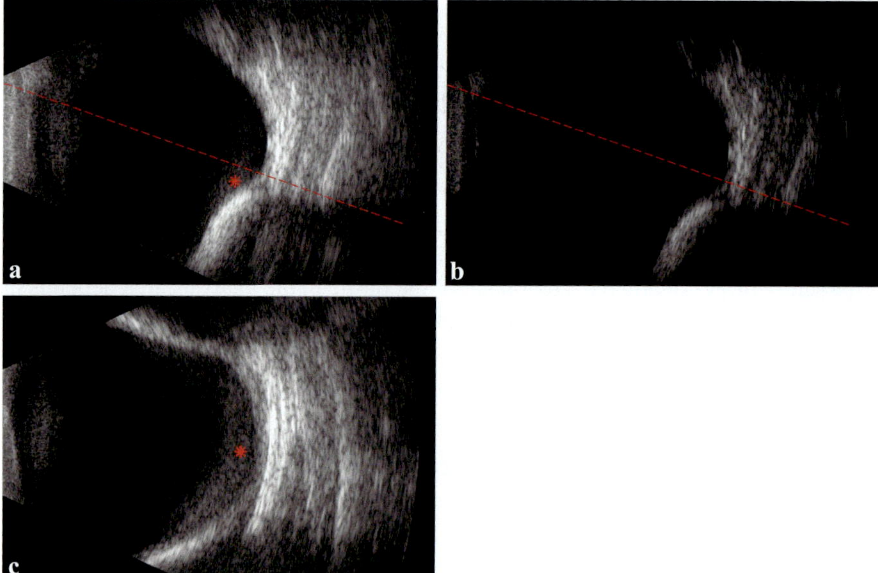

**Fig. 6.10 Side-lobe artifact. a** and **b**: sections exploring a meridian **c**: section exploring a quadrant according to the axis outlined in **a** and **b** (•••••••••• red dotted line) **a and c**: sections at high sensitivity setting **b**: reduced sensitivity setting section At high sensitivity setting, fog artifact (✳ red star) is caused by hyperechoic indentation with posterior shadowing

### 6.2.2.2 Partial Volume Artifacts

These are related to the width of the section. Resolution of the width is related to the width of the slice of the ultrasound beam. It is lower than the lateral resolution of an electronic scanning device. Thus, two contiguous entities can be non-dissociable on the reconstruction of the image. For example, in B-mode, visualizing the subarachnoid spaces surrounding optical fibers is rare if they are not dilated (Fig. 6.11).

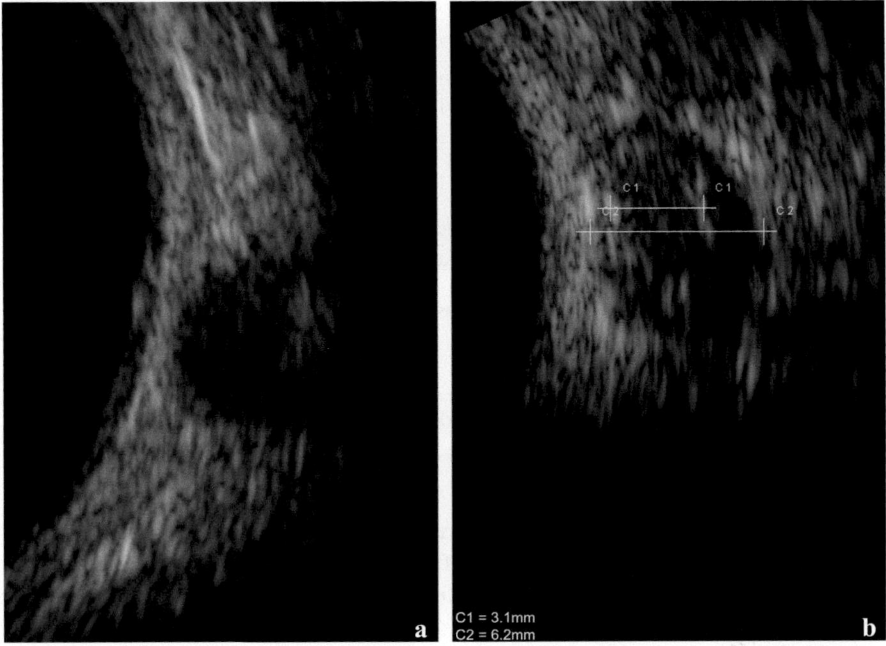


**Fig. 6.11 Partial volume artifact. a**: normal optic nerve, coronal section **b**: dilation of the subarachnoid spaces due to idiopathic intracranial hypertension; optic nerve, coronal section In **a**, the meninges are non-dissociable and appear as a rather echogenic crown around the hypo-echogenic optical fibers. It is even difficult to measure the diameter of the optical fibers and that of the optic complex. In **b**, in relation to the dilation of the subarachnoid spaces, the arachnoid and the dura mater are better integrated; the dilation of the subarachnoid spaces is clearly visible. The diameter of the optical fibers (C1) is measured at 3.1 mm and the diameter of the optical complex (C2) at 6.2 mm

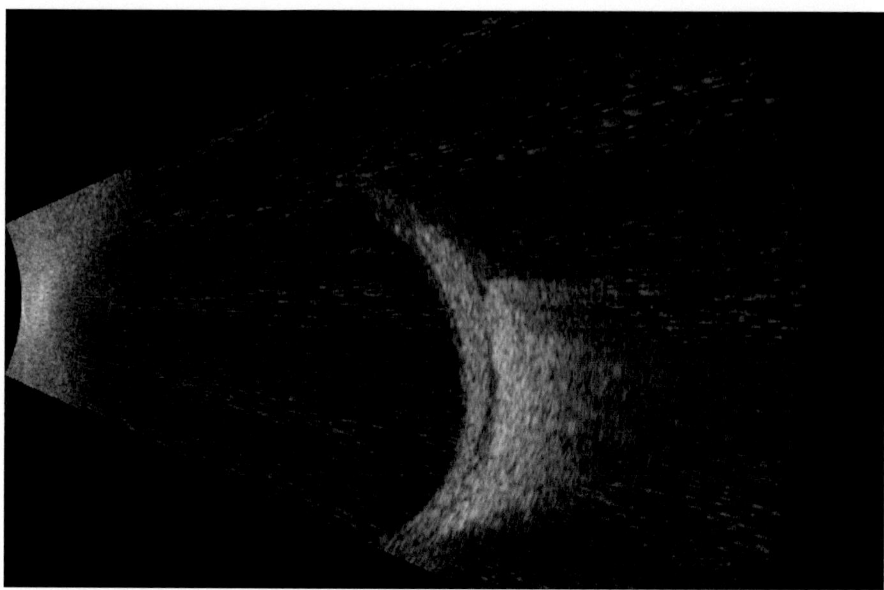

**Fig. 6.12 Artifacts (superimposed echoes) caused by a faulty cable**. The cable (or its shielding) needs to be repaired

### 6.2.3 Artifacts Related to Ultrasound Machine and Sensor Malfunctions

These malfunctions can involve the hardware (the device, probe, or cable) but also the image reconstruction software. These malfunctions give rise to very diverse artifacts: added echoes, absent echoes, or deformation of the analyzed area. They can be due to detachment of the probe membrane; degradation of the cable or its shielding (Fig. 6.12); a short circuit between ceramic components of the sensor; or failure, of varying intermittence, of the electronic circuit board of the probe (Fig. 6.13).

Faced with such problems, which are readily recognizable, one should contact the manufacturer's after-sales service.

### 6.2.4 Environmental Artifacts

Equipment in the environment close to the ultrasound system can cause adverse effects related to interference (Fig. 6.14). Such artifacts tend to result in superimposed echoes. They have become extremely rare with the much more effective shielding of probes, which are now only rarely sensitive to the various devices used in hospitals, especially anesthesia equipment.

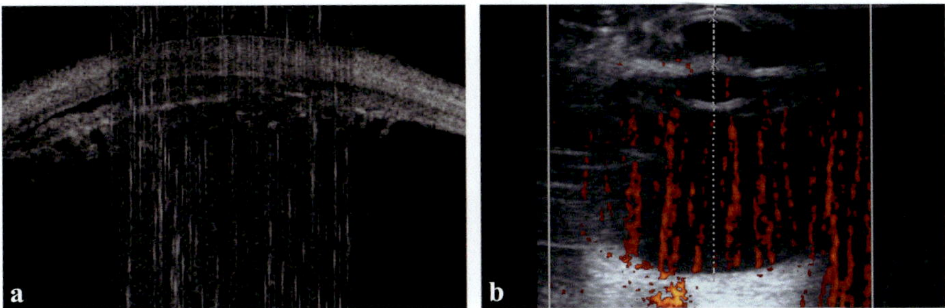

**Fig. 6.13 Artifacts created by a failure of the probe's electronic circuit board. a:** 50 MHz probe, ophthalmic dedicated ultrasound device **b:** power Doppler with 5–10 MHz probe of a multipurpose ultrasound device more obvious in power Doppler but also an issue in B-mode. In both cases, there is no other solution than to call the manufacturer (after-sales service)

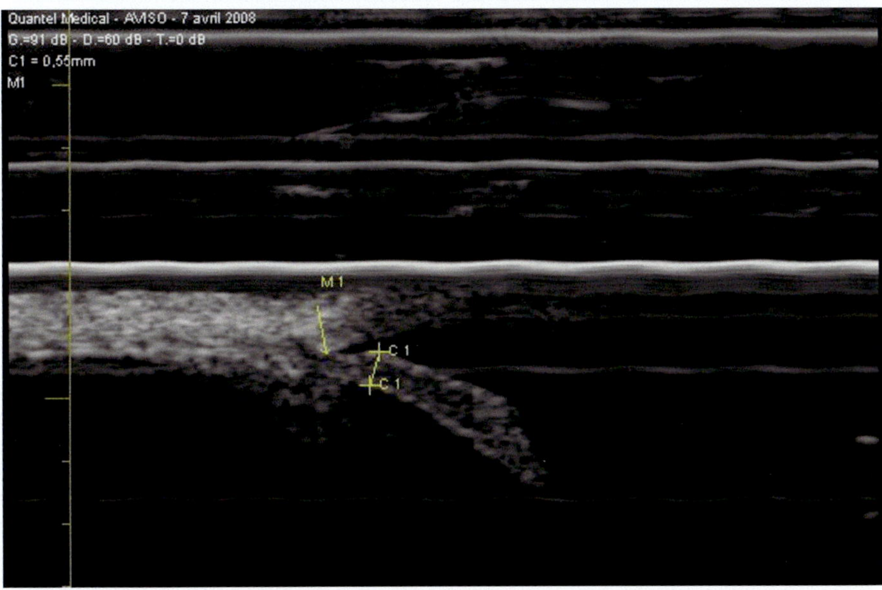



**Fig. 6.14 Artifacts (superimposed echoes) related to the environment, caused by a nearby device (OCT).** These types of artifacts have become rare

## 6.2.5 Complex Artifacts

Intraocular gas has a characteristic appearance in B-mode [9]. Gas–vitreous liquid and gas–tissue interfaces are so reflective that no structure behind a gas bubble can be evaluated. However, B-mode ultrasound can be performed to identify the presence of intraocular gas, determine the percentage of filling of the vitreous cavity, and, by mobilizing the gas bubble(s), assess the existence of recurrent retinal detachment

(Fig. 6.15). Silicone oil also greatly impairs assessment of the posterior segment and can sometimes pass into the anterior segment. It does not prevent performing very-high-frequency ultrasound [10]. This tamponade preclude any ultrasonic biometry (see Chap. 10).

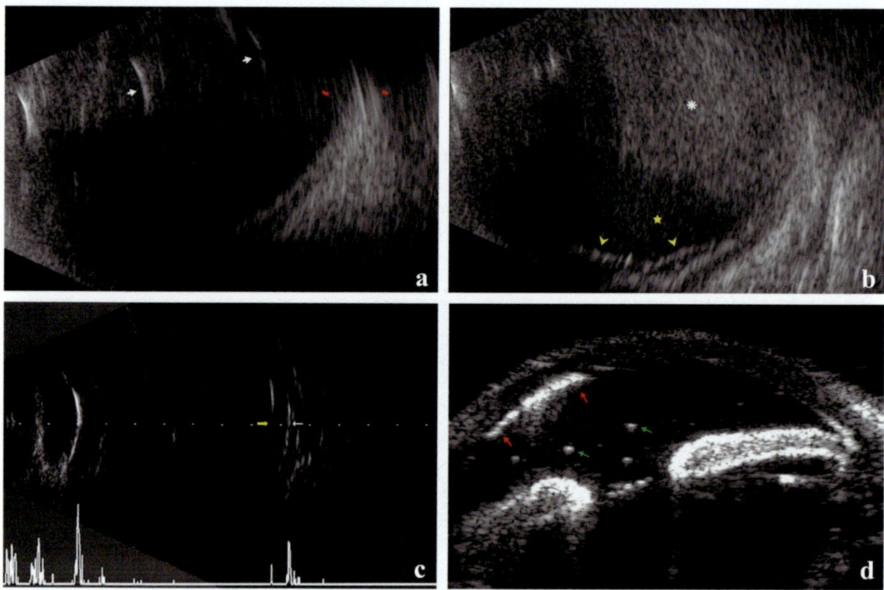

**Fig. 6.15 Combined artifacts. a** and **b**: artifacts of different types in relation to the presence of an intraocular, partially resorbed, SF6 bubble, the intervention having taken place only 15 days prior, in particular preventing analysis of the ocular wall behind the gas. Of note, reverberations (➡ white arrows) and posterior acoustic shadows (➡ red arrows) are seen, as is a poorly outlined moderately echogenic zone (✳ white star). The residual volume of the bubble is approximately 35% of the globe. However, by moving the patient's head, one can discern a localized inferior temporal recurrent retinal detachment (▷ yellow arrowheads). The fundus is not accessible in this patient because of post-operative hemorrhage after vitrectomy (★ yellow star). **c** and **d**: artifacts in relation to an intraocular silicone bubble after intervention for retinal detachment. **c**: axial section at 10 MHz; **d**: para-axial section of the anterior segment at 40 MHz. The velocity of ultrasound in silicone oil is 980 m/s, which gives the impression that the eye is nearsighted. In addition, there is dispersion of the ultrasound beam, which prevents ready recognition of the interface of the silicone bubble (➡ yellow arrow) and the vitreoretinal interface (⬅ white arrow). Hence, accurate biometry is neither easy nor reproducible under these conditions. In addition, there is passage of micro-silicone bubbles to the anterior chamber, some floating in the anterior chamber (➡ green arrows), and others grouped behind the cornea (➡ red arrows) because they are lighter than the aqueous humor, which only moderately hinder assessment of this anterior segment. Finally, others are attached to the different structures of the anterior segment, iris, anterior lens capsule, and zonule, thus contributing to a very contrasted image, with few grey levels

## 6.3  Artifacts in Doppler Mode

As in B-mode, the settings are important for Doppler, in both color and spectral modes, and especially for low-velocity, ocular, and orbital vessels, for which the gain, focal length, and filters must be controlled as well as the velocity scale. As in B-mode, various artifacts occur [11], and diagnostic errors can be avoided if the sonographer is aware of these pitfalls.

### 6.3.1  In Relation to Unsuitable Velocity Scale Settings

- **If the pulse repetition frequency (PRF) is too high**, a slow flow may not be visualized (Fig. 6.16)
- **If the PRF is too low**, there is insufficient coding and **aliasing**. Because CDI uses a pulsed beam, this artifact is observed if the recorded Doppler frequency exceeds half of the PRF (Nyquist–Shannon sampling theorem). There is a color inversion of flows that are too fast in color mode, switching from red to blue by desaturated (clear) colors (Fig. 6.17) and aliasing in spectral mode (Fig. 6.18). At the usual settings, an aliasing artifact occurs on orbital vessels with rapid flows, such as the ophthalmic artery, which allows it to be recognized very quickly in color mode and to record its flows in spectral mode. In practice, the correction of aliasing is straightforward: an increase of the PRF or velocity scale is associated with a readjustment of the baseline.

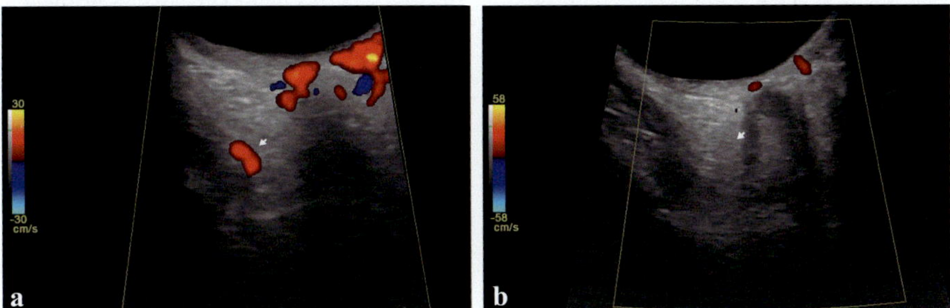

**Fig. 6.16** **Effect of the pulse repetition frequency (PRF) setting (velocity scale) on correct visualization of the ophthalmic artery a**: with a velocity scale from − 30 to + 30 cm/s **b**: with a velocity scale from − 56 to + 56 cm/s. The ophthalmic artery (➡ white arrow) is clearly visible in **a** next to the medial rectus muscle. In **b**, with a PRF that is too high, the vessel has "disappeared"

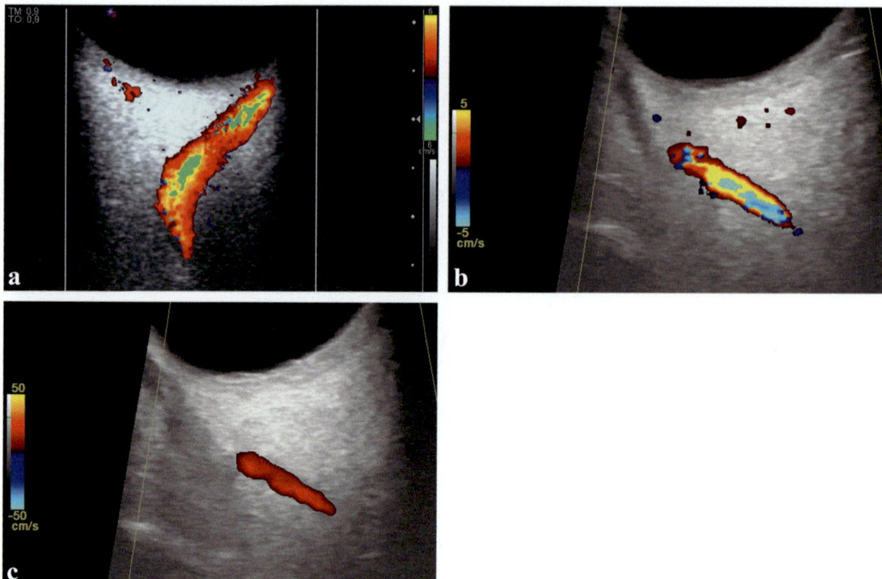

**Fig. 6.17** **Aliasing or directional ambiguity—color mode. a**: dural fistula of the cavernous sinus: the superior ophthalmic vein is inverted, coded in red, and arterialized. However, in the center, the maximum systolic speed, measured at 12.7 cm/s, is faster than the maximum speed of the velocity scale (6 cm/s) and therefore is coded in green/blue at places of greater velocity, passing through light colors. **b and c**: Normal ophthalmic artery. **b**: With a velocity scale from − 5 to + 5 cm/s **c**: with a velocity scale from − 50 to + 50 cm/s. The peak systolic velocity of the ophthalmic artery is from 30 cm/s to 50 cm/s. In **c**, it is, therefore, coded in red in color mode. However, in **b**, at the usual setting adapted to the vessels of the optic nerve head, there are many colored blue *artifactual dots* in the center of the vessel. This artifact helps to recognize this vessel in relation to other orbital arteries in simple color mode

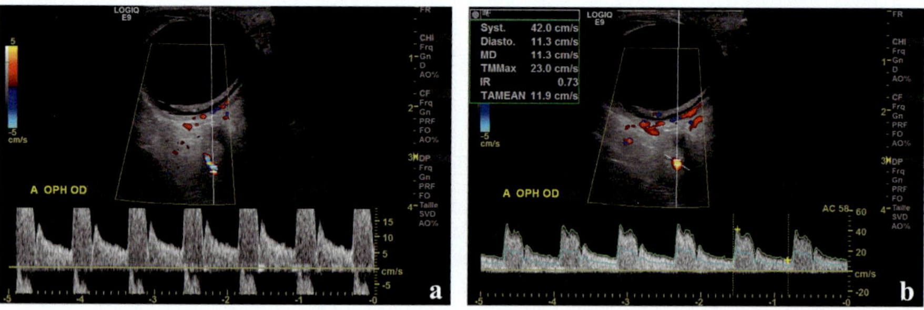

**Fig. 6.18** **Aliasing or spectral ambiguity: normal ophthalmic artery—spectral mode. a**: with a velocity scale from − 10 to + 20 cm/s. **b**: with a velocity scale from − 20 to + 60 cm/s. The ophthalmic artery usually has a flow of approximately 50 cm/s. In **a**, the systolic flow circulates much faster than 20 cm/s; therefore, its spectrum appears as partially negative. In **b**, the velocity scale is a perfect fit and the ophthalmic artery has resumed a purely positive normal spectrum. Note also the total retinal detachment

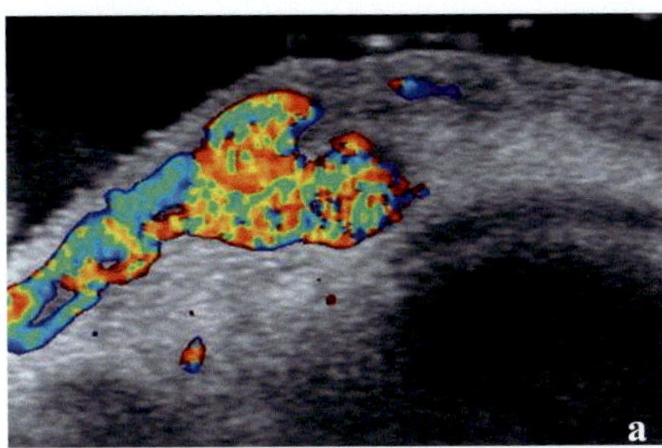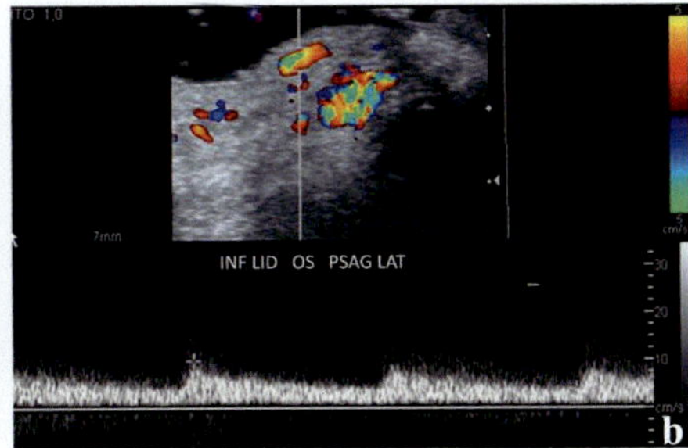


**Fig. 6.19  Spectrum broadening artifact**. Post-traumatic aneurysm of the lower left eyelid, in a 28-year-old man. **a** Color mode, showing a hypervascular lesion with a lot of turbulence. **b** Spectral mode at the level of the feeder vessel; turbulence and the change in direction of flow within the Doppler gate are responsible for the broadening of the spectrum in spectral mode. See the complete iconography of this aneurysm in Chap. 20: Vascular Lesions (Fig. 20.21)

### 6.3.2   Spectrum Enlargement Turbulence

Care must be taken not to confuse the phenomenon of aliasing related to an incorrect setting and the eddies or turbulence within a vessel related to the presence of stenosis, or within arteriovenous malformations or aneurysms. Color inversion takes place with turbulence, but through black and not white, with turbulence at the level of the affected vessel. Thus, artificial Doppler frequencies are noted around the original Doppler frequency (Fig. 6.19), thereby widening the spectral analysis curve.

### 6.3.3   Color Coding Outside of Vessels

The classical clinical circumstances represented by arteriovenous fistula or tight stenosis are not usually found in ophthalmology; however, one should consider the following:

- **Perivascular blooming artifact** (Fig. 6.20).

This is a phenomenon whereby the color overflows the vascular wall, making the vessel appear wider than it actually is. It depends on the gain, and this artifact is reduced by decreasing the gain. However, care must be taken not to remove important velocimetric information.

- **Twinkling artifact**

These are multiple echoes with phase-shift in color Doppler. This artifact is observed behind calcifications of irregular surfaces (urinary stones, atheroma plaques, etc.) [12]. In ophthalmology, this artifact is readily visible behind calcifications of the lens (calcified cataract) (Fig. 6.21a), calcified tumors (especially retinoblastoma)

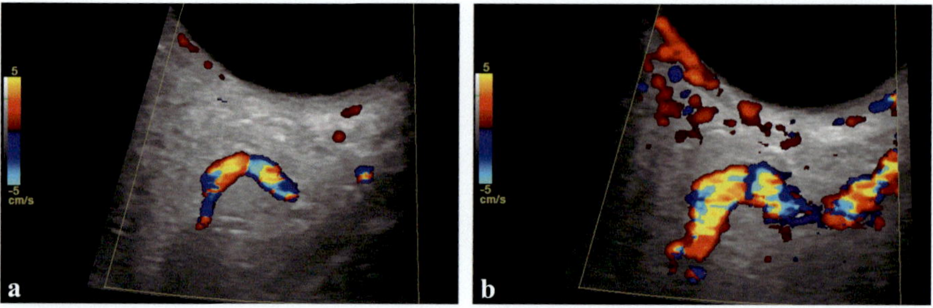

**Fig. 6.20 Blooming artifact. a**: Color Doppler with low gain. The artery, which is curved, explaining the color changes of the vessel, has a normal caliber. **b**: Color Doppler with high gain. The ophthalmic artery appears to have a caliber that is twice as large, by color coding outside the vessel wall

(see Fig. 14.4), calcified optic disc drusen, or even foreign bodies or calcifications on atrophic globes [13]. In case of drusen, it may complicate exploration of the central retinal vessels, in color as in spectral modes (Fig. 6.21b).

- **Artifacts related to movements**

These can be observed because of movements of the probe or movements of adjacent tissues (especially vessels) (Fig. 6.22).

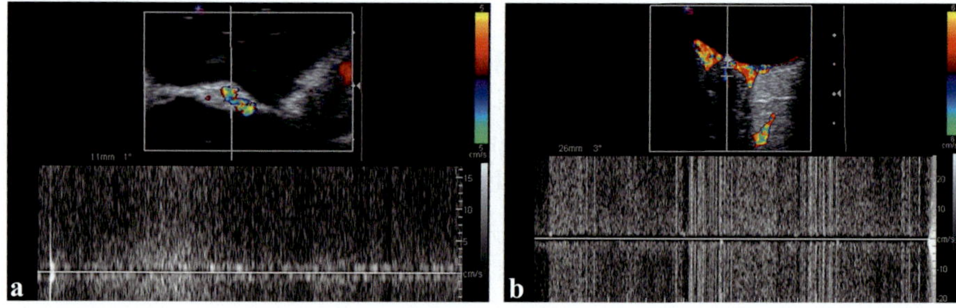

**Fig. 6.21 Twinkling artifact. a**: In connection with a calcified congenital cataract **b**: In relation to large calcified optic disc drusen. In spectral Doppler, there is no recognizable flow but only random background noise, and in **a**, in color mode, two colored spots can be seen that are too bright as compared with vessels of identical size. In **b**, to study the flows of the central retinal vessels, simply move the probe or the Doppler gate (see Figs. 19.11 and 14.4)

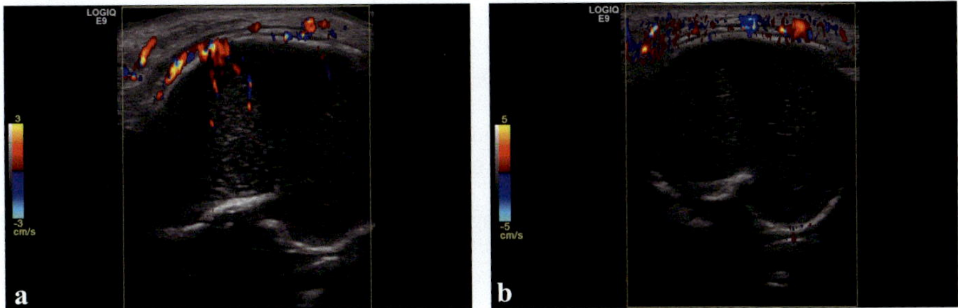

**Fig. 6.22 Artifactual colored dots from "motion"**: Low-grade sarcoma with fibro-myxoid component of the lacrimal sac in a 6-month-old baby, the examination carried out without anesthesia. **a**: Spontaneous section in which numerous artifactual colored dots are seen at the periphery of the lesion owing to uncontrolled movements of the baby. **b**: Section performed after having taken care that there is no uncontrolled movement. The small peripheral flows of this large lesion are not in keeping with a simple dacryocystocele (see Fig. 26.3)

## 6.4   Conclusion

With various causes, artifacts are nearly constant, both in B-mode and in Doppler. These anomalies are readily recognizable, although sometimes difficult to detect. Knowing how to recognize them is important to avoid diagnostic errors. Sometimes artifacts can be minimized by simple actions (change of the position of the probe, etc.) or by adjusting the settings (harmonic mode, gain, etc.).

## References


1. Hedrick WR, Hykes, DL, Starchman DE. Ultrasound physics and instrumentation, 4th Edition Mosby; 2005.
2. Prabhu SJ, Kanal K, Bhargava P, Vaidya S, Dighe MK. Ultrasound artifacts: classification, applied physics with illustrations, and imaging appearances. Ultrasound Q. 2014;30(2):145–57.
3. Feldman MK, Katyal S, Blackwood MS. US artifacts. Radiographics. 2009;29(4):1179–89.
4. Scanlan KA. Sonographic artifacts and their origins. AJR Am J Roentgenol. 1991;156(6):1267–72.
5. Laroche D, Ishikawa H, Greenfield D, Liebmann JM, Ritch R. Ultrasound biomicroscopy localization and evaluation of intraocular foreign bodies. Acta Ophthalmol Scand. 1998;76(4)/491–5.
6. Modjtahedi BS, Rong A, Bobinski M, McGahan J, Morse LS. Imaging characteristics of intraocular foreign bodies: a comparative study of plain film X-ray, computed tomography, ultrasound, and magnetic resonance imaging. Retina. 2015;35(1):95–104.
7. Baum G. A discussion of acoustic artifacts in ophthalmic ultrasonography. Am J Ophthalmol. 1965;60(3):493–8.
8. Laing FC, Kurtz AB. The importance of ultrasonic side-lobe artifacts. Radiology. 1982;145(3):763–8.
9. Whitacre MM. B-scan ultrasonography of eyes containing intravitreal gas. Am J Ophthalmol. 1991;112(3):272–7.

10. Grigera DE, Zambrano A, Cazon GP, Cavanagh E, Girado SG. Ultrasound biomicroscopy in silicone oil-filled eyes. Retina. 2000;20(5):524–31.
11. Pozniak MA, Zagzebski JA, Scanlan KA. Spectral and color Doppler artifacts. Radiographics. 1992;12(1):35–44.
12. Chelfouh N, Grenier N, Higueret D, Trillaud H, Levantal O, Pariente JL, Ballanger P. Characterization of urinary calculi: in vitro study of "twinkling artifact" revealed by color-flow sonography. AJR Am J Roentgenol. 1998;171(4):1055–60.
13. Ustymowicz A, Kreja J, Mariak Z. Twinkling artifact in color Doppler imaging of the orbit. J Ultrasound Med. 2002;21(5):559–63.

# Chapter 7
# Indications and Examination Techniques

Olivier Bergès

**Abstract** This chapter deals with the indications and examination techniques of ophthalmic ultrasound. First, the axial section at 10 MHz in "simple immersion", which allows for immediate evaluation of the emmetropia and ametropias, is reviewed. Then the transocular sections at 10 MHz along the meridians or along the quadrants are covered, as are the para-ocular sections. The choice of gain (sensitivity setting) and the time gain compensation curve are then discussed. Then correct measurement is presented. Second, the indications and examination techniques of the anterior segment are covered, with high-frequency and very-high-frequency ultrasound, in terms of axial sections, meridian sections and quadrant sections. Then, color Doppler imaging of the eye and its anterior segment is discussed, again regarding the indications and the examination techniques, with the three representation modes. Finally, 3D and tissue characterization are mentioned.

## 7.1 Indications and Examination Techniques

Modern ocular and orbital ultrasound relies on a large number of different techniques: 10 MHz B-mode, (standardized) A-mode, (long focal length) 20 MHz B-mode, immersion B-mode (20/25 MHz short focal length, sometimes 35 MHz and 50 MHz), and color Doppler imaging (CDI). Each can answer a specific question and must be tailored to the clinical condition of the patient. Naturally, systematically performing all these techniques every time is out of the question, and the examination should only be undertaken after a careful and discriminative analysis of the clinical signs presented by the patient, which must remain the motivation for and guide of the examination.

O. Bergès (✉)
Rothschild Foundation Hospital, Paris, France
e-mail: oberges@for.paris


O. Bergès (ed.), *Echography of the Eye and Orbit*,
https://doi.org/10.1007/978-3-031-41467-1_7

### *7.1.1   10 MHz B-Mode*

The eyeball is usually examined first with B-mode, with a probe of approximately 10 MHz. At this frequency, both the different ocular structures and the orbital structures can be visualized with an acceptable level of resolution.

Various devices can be used (see Chap. 2).

- These are most often *ophthalmic dedicated ultrasound devices*, using a mechanically oscillating single crystal, with a narrow frequency band B-mode probe, usually close to 10 MHz (or 15 MHz), and a fixed focusing distance, usually between 21 and 25 mm, often also possessing an A-mode probe, a biometric module, and sometimes a 3D module and a tissue characterization module. The devices are characterized mainly by excellent spatial resolution. Recent devices use an annular probe, resulting in better and more equal spatial resolution over the entire image.
- *Multipurpose ultrasound devices* can also be used, with multicrystal and multi-channel electronic probes that have a wide frequency band centered on 10 MHz or more, with several variable focal areas. They are characterized by excellent spatial representation (especially on the anterior and lateral parts of the image) but above all by excellent density resolution. They usually have the capacity for Doppler imaging (color, power, and spectral, and sometimes B-flow /m-SMI), and sometimes 3D imaging.

The examination is performed on a relaxed patient in a supine position, after corneal anesthesia. As a coupling agent, use of ophthalmic gel is advised: carbomer 0.2% (Lacrygel®, Europhta, or Lacrynorm® Chauvin).

#### 7.1.1.1   Orientation of the Probe

Traditionally, the anterior part of the eye is located on the left of images with ophthalmic dedicated devices and at the top of images with multipurpose devices. Also, traditionally, the right (temporal side of the right eye and nasal side of the left eye) is located at the top of images with ophthalmic dedicated devices and on the right of images obtained with the multipurpose devices. To achieve this, one must correctly orientate a mark placed on the probe (see Figs. 7.3, 7.6, and 7.7).

The following are performed in succession:

#### 7.1.1.2   Axial Section of the Eye and Orbit

Always acquiring an axial section first allows for, among other things, biometric evaluation of the eyeballs. This section must be acquired in "simple immersion" [1], (see Chap. 10) (Fig. 7.1). Otherwise, through the eyelids, discerning the anterior side of the cornea is difficult. One can immediately determine whether it is an emmetropic,

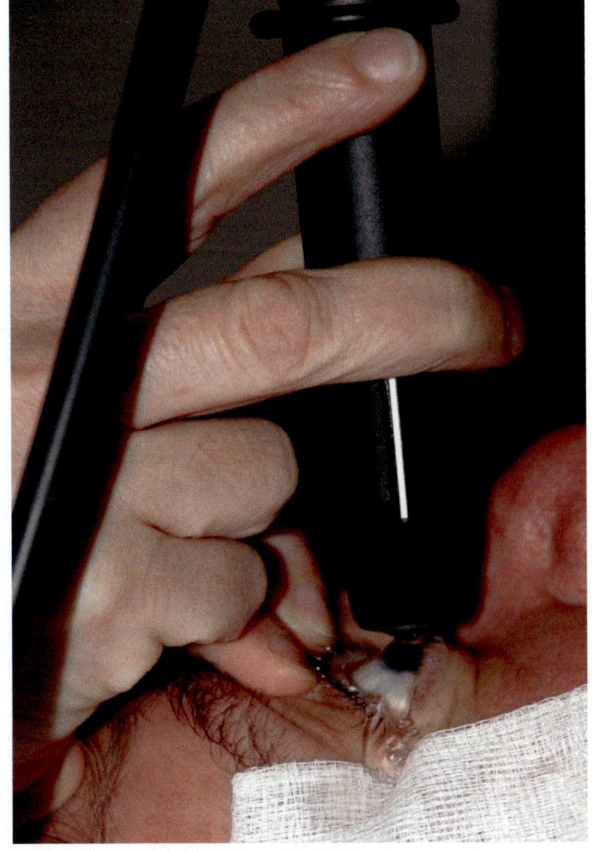

**Fig. 7.1 Axial section by a "simple immersion" technique**. The tip of the probe is placed in contact with the gel, positioned on the cornea between the two eyelids. To ensure a primary gaze, the patient is asked to look at a point on the ceiling with the other eye

hyperopic, or myopic eyeball (Fig. 7.2). One should acquire an axial section of both eyes. This will confirm or refute, for example, pseudoexophthalmos in connection with unilateral myopia with anisometropia ($\pm$ amblyopia), atrophy of one of the two globes, or buphthalmia.

### 7.1.1.3 Transocular Multidirectional Assessment Exploring the Various Meridians and Quadrants

The assessment must be exhaustive: the operator must assess the entire volume of the globe and the orbit. For this, at least four sections need to be acquired according to the 3, 6, 9, and 12 o'clock meridians. Then, rotating the probe by 90°, the four corresponding quadrant sections, nasal, inferior, temporal, and superior are imaged (Figs. 7.3, 7.4, and 7.5).

The intermediate meridians (1:30, 4:30, 7:30, and 10:30 o'clock) and their corresponding quadrants can also be systematically recorded. The first rule of ultrasound

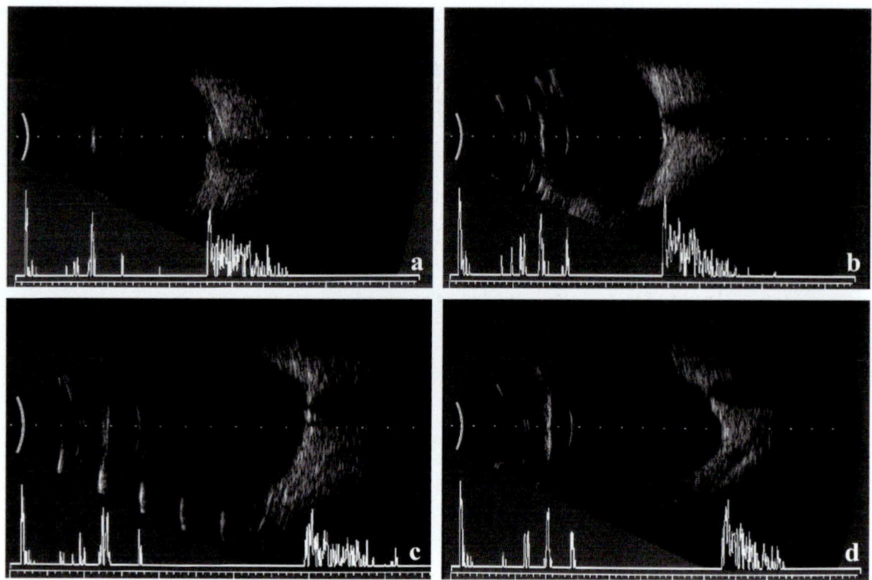

**Fig. 7.2 Axial section of the eyeball by "simple immersion" technique: results**. **a**: Hyperopic eye (AL = 21.6 mm); **b**: emmetropic eye (AL = 22.8 mm); **c**: highly myopic eye (AL = 29.7 mm) with staphyloma located nasal to the optic disc, the macular plane being oblique to the visual axis; **d**: very highly myopic eye (AL = 31 mm) with temporal peripapillary staphyloma including the macula

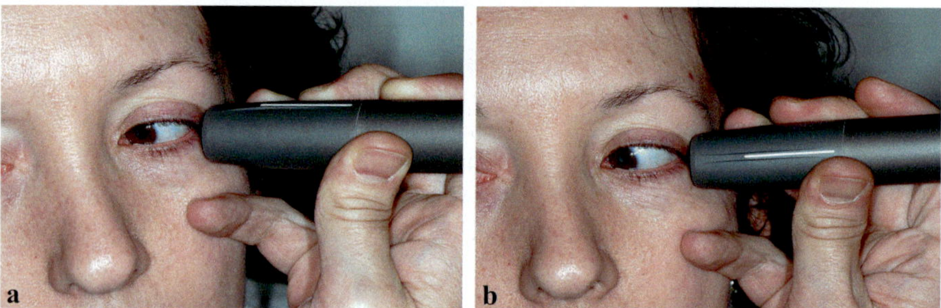

**Fig. 7.3 Transocular section: technique**. a: Nasal quadrant OS; b: 9 o'clock OS. The probe is rotated by π/2 to explore a corresponding quadrant or meridian. Note the position of the marker, by convention always positioned to the right or upwards

imaging must be followed: **be as perpendicular as possible to the structure (or lesion) to be assessed**. For example, to examine the optic disc and the optic nerve, the probe is tilted only slightly with a primary gaze, whereas for examining the tendon of an extraocular muscle, it must be tilted maximally by asking the patient to look in the opposite direction to which the probe is placed (Fig. 7.6). An integrated performance of meridian sections and quadrant sections helps comply with the rule that

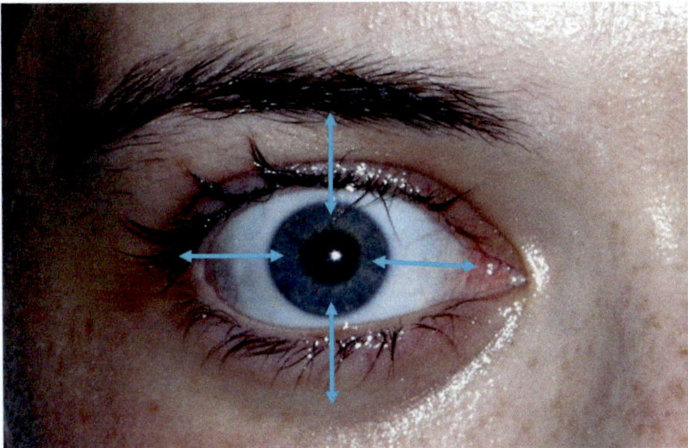

**Fig. 7.4 Technique for exploring the four main meridians in B-mode, by transocular approach**. The probe must be placed beyond the limbus on the meridian opposite to (across from) the one to be studied and tilted back and forth to explore the entire meridian, from the optic disc to the ocular periphery, keeping the opposite rectus muscle visualized in its largest axis, in the center of the screen

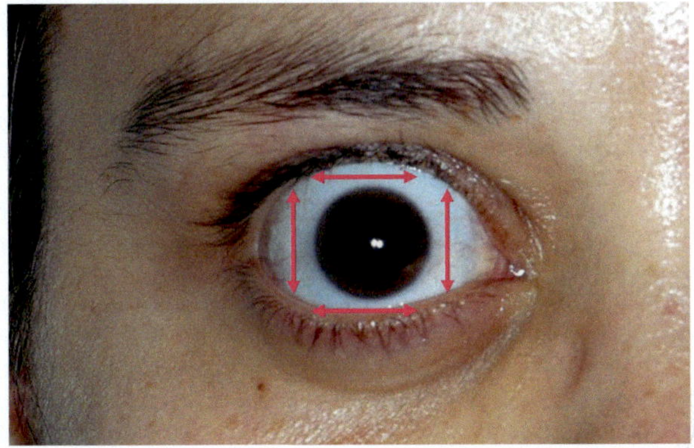

**Fig. 7.5 Technique for exploring the four main quadrants in B-mode, by transocular approach**. The probe must be placed beyond the limbus opposite to (across from) the quadrant to be explored. The opposite rectus muscle, seen in a cross-section, must be located in the center of the screen. To visualize the tendon, the probe has to be tilted more than for visualizing the muscle belly

applies to any cross-sectional imaging: **examining a lesion or a structure in at least two orthogonal sections**. Even with B-probes becoming very compact and easy to handle, exploring the periphery of the temporal field is sometimes difficult because of the nasal bridge. For these transocular sections, the probe is placed directly on the conjunctiva, which provides the best spatial resolution, or on the gently closed eyelids (Fig. 7.7).

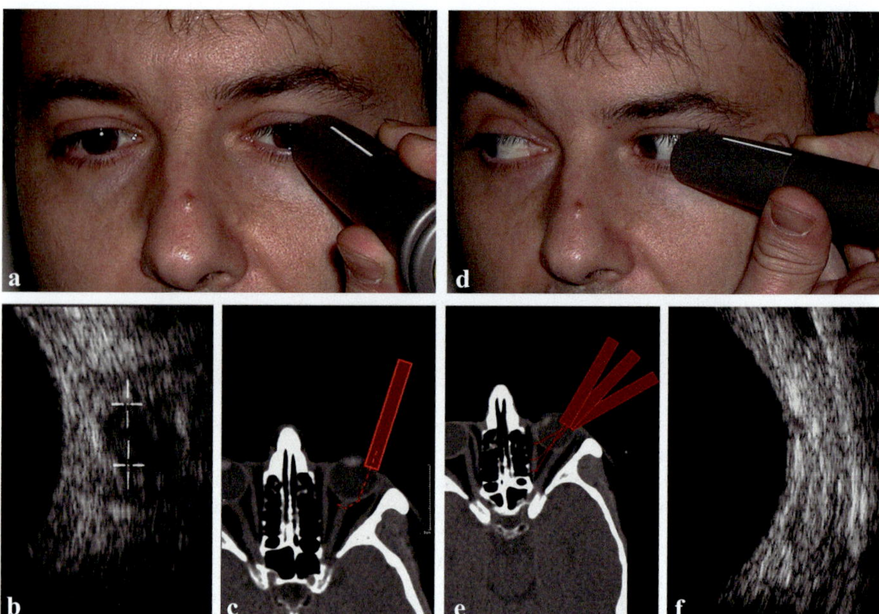

**Fig. 7.6 Perpendicularity to what is being visualized. a**: Technique for exploring the posterior pole of the left eye: the eye is in primary gaze, with the probe placed near the limbus and tilted only slightly toward the posterior pole. **b**: Schematic outline of exploration of the posterior pole of the left eye and the retrobulbar optic nerve on a CT axial section. The path of the ultrasound beam is not linear because it is slightly deflected each time it encounters an angle, a medium of different acoustic impedance. This way, it can approach the retrobulbar optic nerve orthogonally. **c**: Result of such a section showing the retrobulbar optic nerve in cross-section. **d**: Technique for exploring the medial periphery of the left eye: the eyes look far to the right, with the probe placed at a distance from the limbus and greatly angled toward the ocular periphery. **e**: Schematic outline of exploration of the left medial rectus muscle on a CT axial section, with the patient looking to the right. Note the double movement of angulation of the probe and slight translation of the end of the probe on the eyelid, so as to remain as perpendicular as possible to the muscle to be studied, from its tendon to its posterior part. **f**: Result of such a section exploring the tendon of the medial rectus muscle "in cross-section"

### 7.1.1.4 Para-Ocular Sections

To complete the orbital assessment, placing the probe on the eyelids with a large amount of gel, and rotating, again systematically and exhaustively around the eye (Fig. 7.8). These sections are especially useful in case of pathology of the eyelids and superficial anterior structures such as the lacrimal gland and the tear ducts, which are sometimes visible even when normal with a multipurpose device.

Once all the sections have been acquired, the operator must mentally reconstruct the entire explored volume.

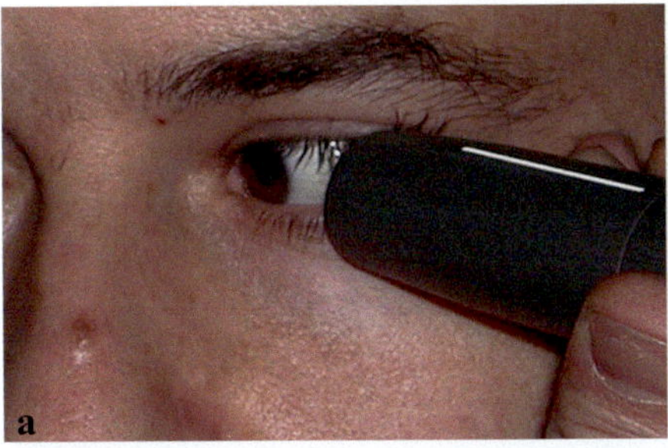 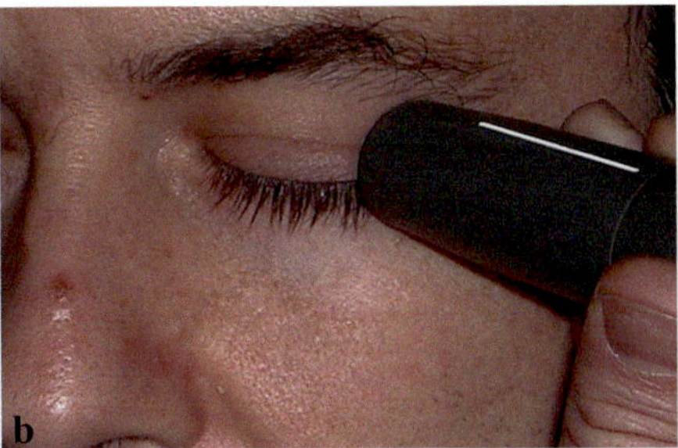

**Fig. 7.7  Transocular section of the medial quadrant of the left eye. a**: By transconjunctival approach; **b**: by trans-palpebral approach. With a 10 MHz probe, a transconjunctival (**a**) or transpalpebral (**b**) approach can be used. With a long focal length 20 MHz probe, only a transconjunctival approach can be used, because at this frequency the eyelids attenuate the ultrasound beam too much

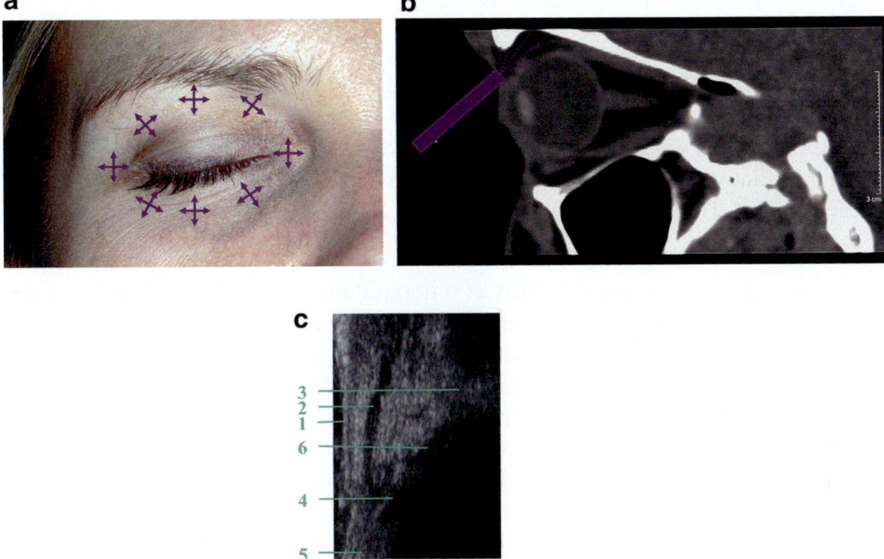

**Fig. 7.8  Technique for exploring the anterior para-ocular segment. a**: Technique for exploring the anterior para-ocular segment: This compartment must be assessed in different directions; **b**: transverse view of the superior quadrant. Diagram of the angulations to be carried out (on a CT sagittal section along the main axis of the orbit); **c**: result of such a vertical section of the upper eyelid and superior extraconal peribulbar space with a 15-MHz probe. 1: skin—2: orbicular muscle—3: septum—4: Müller muscle—5: tarsus—6: levator palpebrae superioris muscle

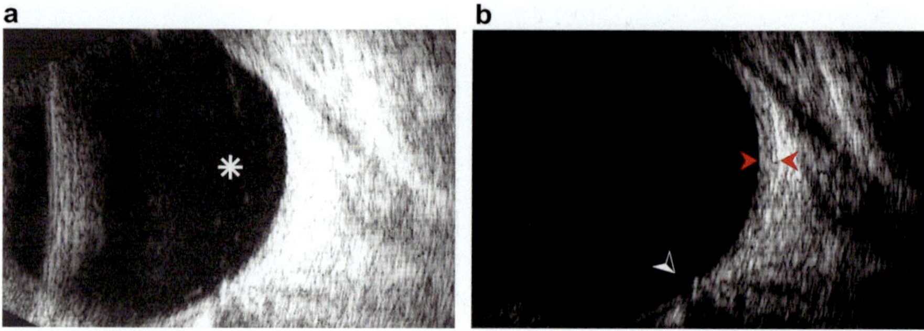

**Fig. 7.9 Section exploring the 9 o'clock meridian of the left eye. a**: At maximum gain; **b**: at reduced gain. Maximum gain is used to analyze the echotexture of the vitreous body (✳ white star), in this case with simple floaters and without detachment of the posterior hyaloid membrane. The optic disc and the medial rectus muscle can be discerned. However, a reduced gain is necessary to visualize the retino-choroid layer, which is moderately echogenic (▶◀ red arrowheads), the optic disc (➤ white arrowhead), the optic nerve, and the extraocular muscle(s)

### 7.1.1.5 Choice of Sensitivity Setting (Gain)

This represents the amplification of the reflected echoes and is expressed in decibels, which is a relative scale. Therefore, obtaining a similar image with different devices can be difficult. The sensitivity setting must be adjusted according to the structure to be examined:

- For the eyeball, one usually starts at a maximum gain, which allows for seeing small low-reflective vitreal floaters and detachment of the posterior hyaloid membrane. However, when an ocular pathology is detected (membrane or parietal mass), it is necessary to approach the degree of reflectivity with reduced gain, a gain that allows for examining the ocular wall and the retrobulbar optic nerve, derived from the tissue sensitivity setting in standardized A-mode (Fig. 7.9). It can also be useful to know at what setting a structure is no longer visible, by gradually lowering the gain (see Chap. 12).
- This reduced gain is usually used for procedures for the orbit as well as for the wall of the globe. However, as in standardized A-mode, when an anechoic or very hypoechoic orbital process is detected, gradually increasing the gain is useful to better discern the internal echotexture of the lesion. As a corollary, in case of a very echogenic lesion, gradually decreasing the gain is useful.

### 7.1.1.6 Time Gain Compensation (TGC) Setting

This setting for the TGC curve is intended to compensate for the attenuation of the ultrasound beam in depth. Superficial structures are better assessed with multicrystal electronic probes of multipurpose devices. However, in all cases, the gain must be reduced at the level of these anterior superficial structures, then the slope must occupy

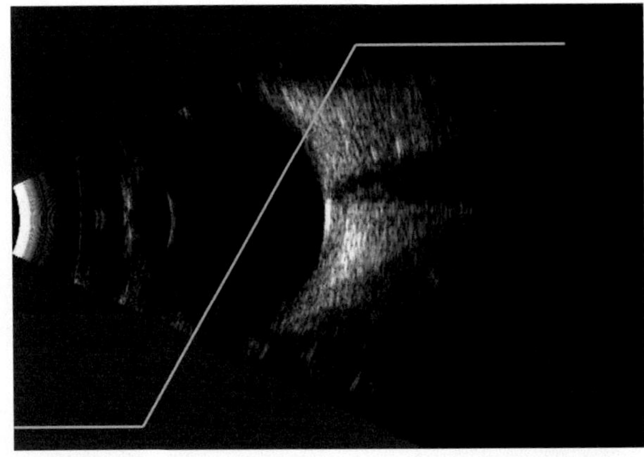

**Fig. 7.10 Time gain compensation (TGC) setting**: The anterior gain is reduced because there is very little attenuation of the visualized structures at this level. Then, the attenuation slope is regular throughout the eyeball. And the gain is maximal after the sclera

the entire ocular space, the gain being maximum at the level of the orbit, behind the episclera (Fig. 7.10).

#### 7.1.1.7 Measurements

The first rule for obtaining correct measurements is to be as perpendicular to the lesion to be measured as possible. Once a lesion has been detected by systematic sections (meridians and quadrants), the operator must position the probe as perpendicular to it as possible and to make two sweeps according to the meridian and according to the quadrant considered. In addition, as noted previously, when using ultrasound, a lesion needs to be analyzed in at least two orthogonal planes, which allows for measuring two diameters and one thickness. For intraocular lesions, the thickness should be measured on a meridian section and not on a quadrant section (Fig. 7.11). Although the maximum value is the most significant, it is useful, such as for biometry, to obtain at least three concordant measurements in the three planes of space and to average them, along with the standard deviation (which must be less than 0.10). Very often, this orthogonality to the lesion allows for more precise measurement than with CT or MRI.

### 7.1.2 A-Mode

Quantitative analysis of the echotexture of a lesion (reflectivity, attenuation of the ultrasound beam by the lesion, and homogeneity or heterogeneity of the lesion) is much easier and more accurate than with B-mode (Fig. 7.12). The best way to perform this examination is by following the rules of standardized echography [2, 3]. An unfocused 8-MHz pencil probe is placed on the bulbar conjunctiva beyond the limbus and oriented successively toward the 9:00 o'clock, … 10:30, 12:00, 1:30,

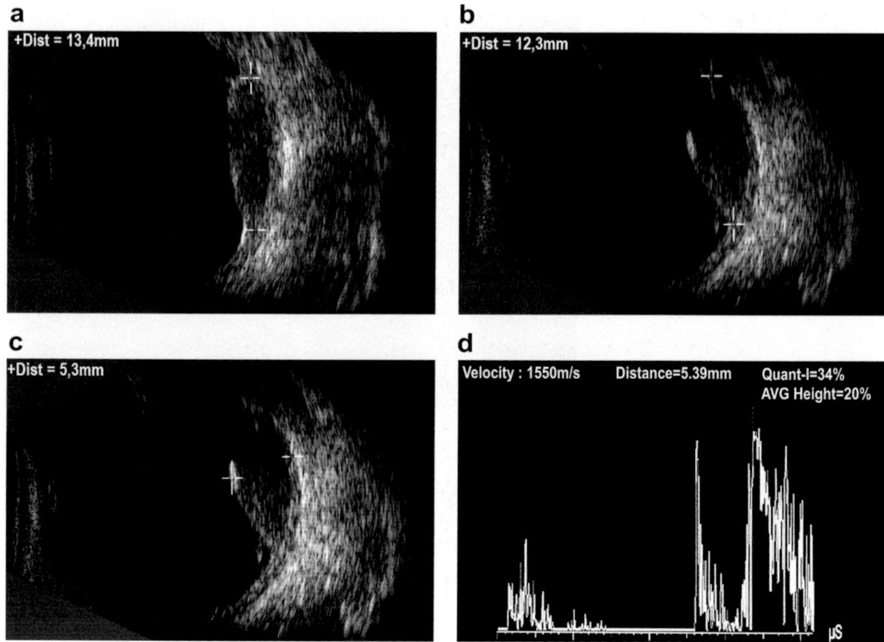

Fig. 7.11 **Measurements of a lesion: choroidal melanoma of the superior quadrant**. a: Section of the superior quadrant, providing the horizontal (transverse) diameter of the tumor: 13.4 mm; **b**: Section exploring the 12 o'clock meridian, providing the sagittal (vertical) diameter of the tumor: 12.3 mm; **c**: The same section exploring the 12 o'clock meridian, providing the thickness of the tumor: 5.3 mm. Note the position of the calipers: perpendicular to the axis of the tumor; **d**: A-mode, also providing the thickness of the tumor. When care is taken to be fully perpendicular to the two surfaces of the tumor, this measurement is more accurate: 5.39 mm. However, at the periphery, one is easily oblique, with a resulting higher value

3:00, 4:30, 6:00, and 7:30 o'clock meridians to perform an exhaustive multidirectional assessment, followed by focusing on the lesion in question, taking care to be perpendicular to the structure/lesion to be assessed, from the posterior pole to the ocular periphery. A silicone tissue model is used to determine the standard gain. This standardized technique alone allows for quantifying results, such as the reflectivity and attenuation of a lesion or characterization of a structure (see Chap. 12). Echo amplification follows an $S$-shaped curve, amplifying weak echoes more than strong echoes. Then, acquisitions according to the different meridians and especially of a pathological lesion are made at standard or tissular (T), high (T + 9), and reduced (T−9) sensitivity settings. This standard gain, which varies for each probe/ultrasound device, is fundamental and is determined regularly, at least once a month, using a silicone tissue model (Fig. 7.13) [4].

On an axial section, in immersion, at standard or tissue (T) sensitivity (see Chap. 10), one can discern the two peaks of the cornea and the two peaks of the anterior and posterior capsules of the lens, with the vitreous appearing anechoic or

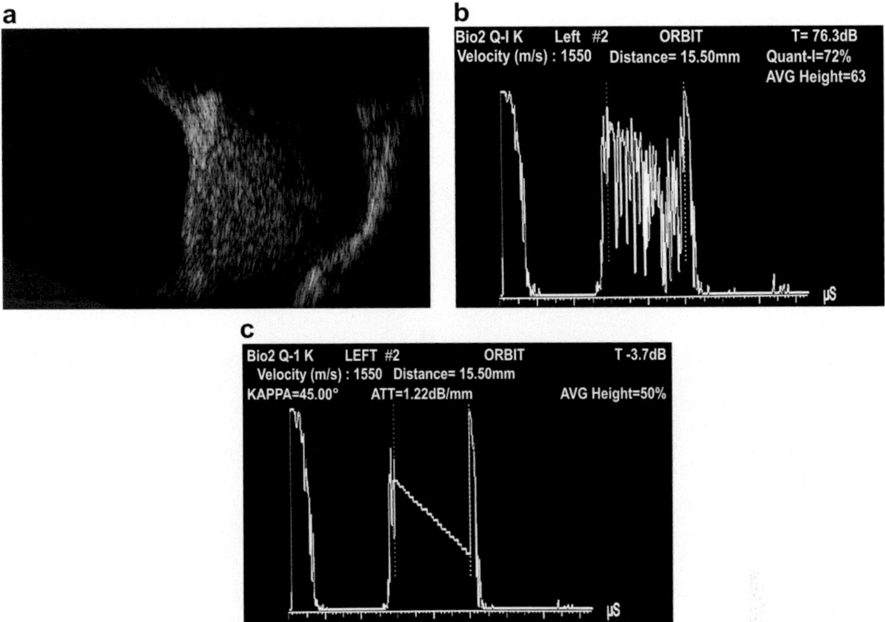

**Fig. 7.12  Benign mixed tumor of the left lacrimal gland, transocular approach. a**: B-mode; **b**: standardized A-mode at tissue sensitivity (T = 76.3 dB) for assessing the reflectivity of the lesion, revealing a fairly reflective lesion (Quant I = 72%), very homogeneous and regular; **c**: standardized A-mode at T -3.7 dB, resulting in an average peak height of 50% to determine the attenuation of the ultrasound beam by the lesion. Its attenuation is regular, with a kappa angle = 45°

containing minor echoes (floaters). The vitreoretinal interface is represented by a very large peak (> 90% of the scleral peak), with less than three deflections. The choroid is discreetly less echogenic than the retina, and the sclera has the highest peak (100%), so it serves as a reference for the other structures. The orbital fat then results in regular and strong attenuation of the ultrasound beam.

### 7.1.3   Ultrasound of the Anterior Segment

Quality cross-sectional imaging of the anterior segment has been possible only since the work of Charles Pavlin in the early 1990s [5] and the development of a new technique that he called ultrasound biomicroscopy, which very quickly became highly popular because of its multitude of applications but also because of its easy-to-remember acronym: UBM. Since this "pioneering" time, ultrasound devices dedicated to ophthalmology most often associate the exploration of the eyeball at 10 MHz and exploration of its anterior segment with a 50-MHz probe (very-high-frequency ultrasound [VHFU]) or with a probe of lower frequency although greater than or

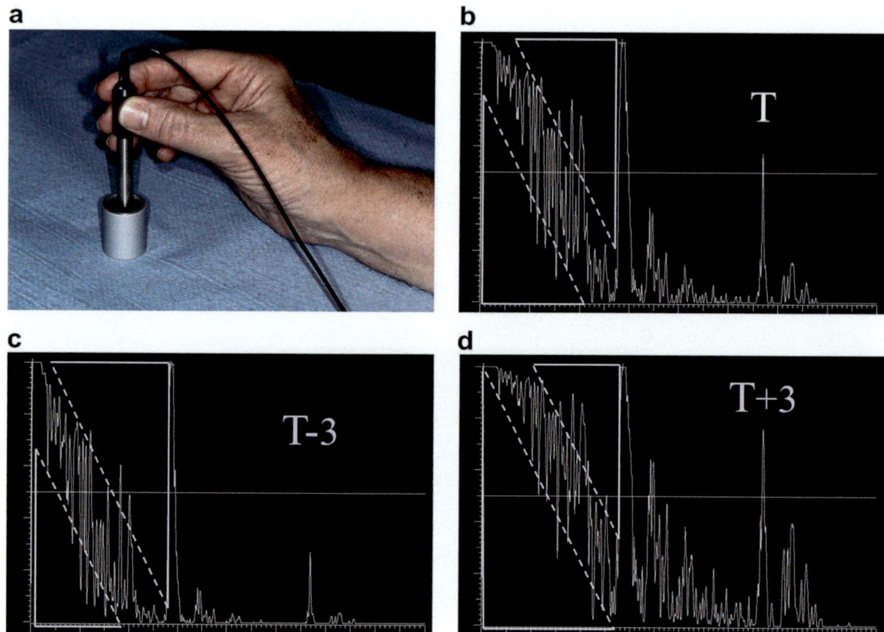


**Fig. 7.13 Calibration of the standardized A-probe: determining tissue sensitivity. a**: Technique: the probe is placed on a silicone tissue model, coupled with a drop of saline or gel; **b**: result when tissue sensitivity (T) is obtained: the two triangles on either side of the echo decay curve have equal areas; **c**: result if the gain is too low: the lower triangle is too small; **d**: result if the gain is too high: the upper triangle is too small

equal to 20 MHz (high-frequency ultrasound [HFU]). The exploration cell of this probe is wide (16 mm), thus allowing imaging of the entire anterior segment from one angle to another, which could not be done with UBM, for which the width of the exploration cell was only 5 mm. At the time, a section of the entire previous segment was required: a reconstruction would have to be performed with Adobe Photoshop based on three images acquired separately.

Although recent ultrasound devices have become very popular, the UBM ultrasound device by the company Paradigm is still commercially available, and we discuss both equipments in this chapter.

UBM involves a complementary examination with high spatial resolution, the axial resolution being about 70 $\mu$m with a 20-MHz probe and 35 $\mu$m with a 50-MHz probe (much higher than the 0.15 mm resolution of a 10-MHz probe). Ultrasound of the anterior segment is performed with an immersion technique, regardless of the frequency used. Some ultrasound devices also have 35/40-MHz probes, but the technique is identical. The exploration cells of 50-MHz and 25-MHz probes are identical: the width is approximately 16 mm, but the depth is related to the attenuation of the ultrasound beam, which is much higher at 50 MHz than 25 MHz. For an axial section at 50 MHz, the posterior capsule of the lens (located approximately 12 mm from the crystal) is not visualized or only seen inconsistently, partially, and very attenuated.

The most frequent indications are as follows:

- Exploration of tumors of the anterior segment, essentially those of the iris (see Chap. 13), thus exploration of localized bulging of the iris, to allow for detecting the difference between a cyst and a solid tumor but also tumors of the ciliary body: when they are small, they can be seen completely with a 50-MHz probe, but when they are voluminous (e > 5 mm), a high-frequency probe ($\approx$ 20 MHz) allows for seeing them entirely and measuring them. The 50-MHz probe analyzes fine semiological criteria such as the thickness of the sclera (to look for scleral effraction or scleromalacia) and the distance of this ciliary mass to the angle (see Chaps. 4 and 13).
- Exploration of glaucoma, especially narrow-angle glaucoma, and follow-up of glaucoma after surgery,
- Assessment of the cornea and anterior segment in case of opacity and after refractive surgery,
- Traumatic pathology of the anterior segment,
- Assessment of the peripheral anterior vitreous (anterior proliferative vitreo-retinopathy [PVR], uveitis, etc.).

### 7.1.3.1 Choice of Frequency

A 50-MHz probe is selected for such imaging of the anterior segment, in particular for the cornea, iris, glaucoma, conjunctiva and superficial sclera, and small tumors of the ciliary body, less than 4 mm in diameter.

However, an exploration at 25 MHz is indicated, in addition to or directly for:

- assessment of more voluminous tumors of the ciliary body (or cilio-choroidal) because their thickness often exceeds 5 mm with consequent attenuation of the ultrasound beam.

but also for:

- fine study of the lens and intraocular implants,
- assessment of the anterior segment and ocular periphery behind a corneal opacity, especially after eye trauma.

Initially, high-frequency probes at 25 MHz with a short focal length (9 to 11 mm from the crystal), designed to study the anterior segment, did not exist and 20-MHz probes were used with a long focal length (24 to 26 mm), designed for study of the posterior pole. Also, an immersion cup of at least 25 mm tall was used, which made handling tricky. However, the results obtained were comparable (see Fig. 4.3).

50-MHz Probes

Several devices use 50-MHz probes, with sector scanning or linear scanning. With sector-scanning probes, in particular with the UBM device still marketed by Paradigm, these devices are based on UBM; the exploration cell is small (5 mm × 5 mm) and, therefore, does not allow for visualizing the entire anterior segment on a single section.

With recent linear-scan probes, the exploration cell is wider (16 mm) and, therefore, allows for visualizing the entire anterior segment from one angle to another, except sometimes in the case of very large buphthalmia, with a white-to-white distance greater than 15 mm. However, at this very high frequency, in relation to attenuation, the posterior lens capsule is seen rarely or inconsistently, and therefore, the effective exploration cell is 16 mm × 5 mm.

Regardless of the frequency, the examination is performed with the patient in a supine position after thorough topical anesthesia. With open probes involving sectorial scanning, the crystal oscillates freely in a methylcellulose/serum bath, a few millimeters from the structures to be assessed, with the help of a small plastic cup placed on the eye between the eyelids (Fig. 7.14a). With closed probes (25- and 50-MHz linear scanning), one can only place thicker gel (carbomer) on the cornea between the eyelids, which can be kept open with a small lid speculum (Fig. 7.14b), or a water bag tip can be used (Fig. 7.14c). The eyelids can also simply be held open with the operator's fingers. This technique is also applicable to examining the anterior segment with a multipurpose device with a high-frequency probe (Fig. 7.14d). As it is usually the case for ultrasound, the operator must be perpendicular to the structure (or lesion) to be studied. For example, the angulation of the probe will be different for visualizing the peripheral eye wall, ciliary body, iris, or cornea.

### 7.1.3.2    Focal Length

To optimize spatial resolution, the structures (or lesions) to be studied must be in the immediate vicinity of the focal point of the probe. The higher the frequency, the more this rule needs to be followed (see Fig. 5.4). Moreover, the higher the frequency, the narrower the focal length is around the focal point.

With a 50-MHz linear-scan probe, the focal area is represented during acquisition by two dotted green lines, and the area of interest should be located in the center or immediately below this area. These indicator lines disappear when the image is "frozen". For a cross-section of the entire anterior segment, the compromise consists in locating this focal zone in front of the anterior capsule of the lens (Fig. 7.15a and b). However, if a thin section of the cornea is desired (especially if the latter is opaque), another section locating the cornea in the center of the focal area should be acquired (Fig. 7.15c).

With a UBM device from Paradigm, the choice of "delay" determines the optimal focus area of the probe. During the acquisition of images, it is represented on the screen as a thin yellow line that must be located immediately below the structure to

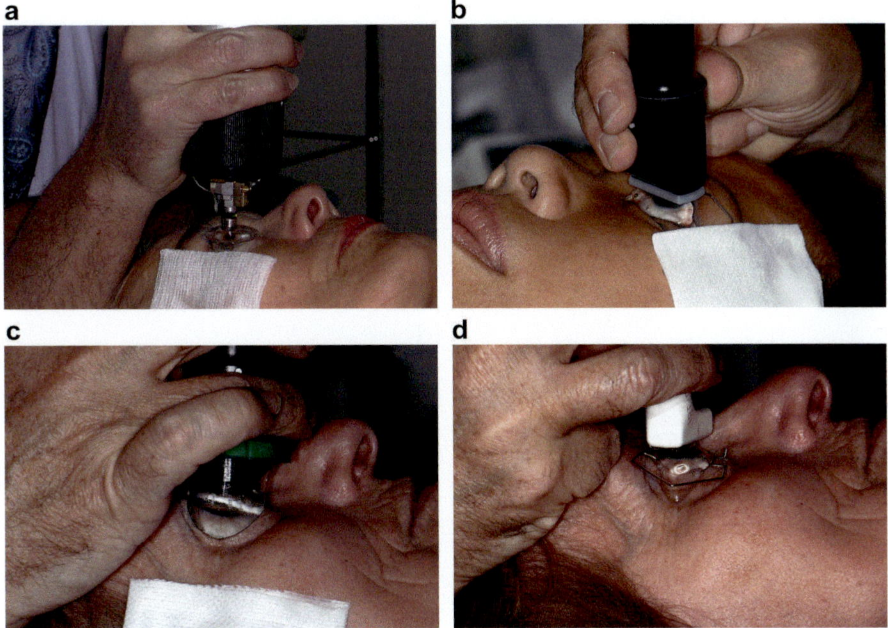

**Fig. 7.14  Ultrasound of the anterior segment: practical realization**. **a**: Ultrasound biomicroscopy. The crystal, without protection, oscillates freely in a bath of methylcellulose contained by a small cup slipped between the eyelids, in the conjunctival fornix. **b**: Very high frequency ultrasound (VHFU) using a dedicated ophthalmic ultrasound device, gel, and a lid speculum. The probe is closed by thick, solidified gel, with minimal attenuation (compared to the plastic protection of a probe, such as that of a 25 MHz probe). The tube of gel should be gently pushed against the cornea to avoid an emulsion of micro air bubbles that would lead to a high level of artifact in the images obtained. **c**: VHFU using a modern ultrasound device, a water bag (Clearscan™), without a lid speculum. The preparation can take a little longer at first, but it prevents issues due to micro air bubbles, and use of a lid speculum is not essential. **d**: HFU using a multipurpose ultrasound device with immersion involving a thick layer of carbomer gel, a lid speculum, and an 8–18 MHz probe

be studied, but it disappears as soon as the image is frozen (Fig. 7.15d and e). For an average resolution, which is most often chosen, this delay is 2.24 mm. For high resolution, used for detailed evaluation of the cornea, it is 3.54 mm. Thus, the spatial resolution is optimal, while the crystal oscillates in the gel at a distance from the cornea without risk of erosion.

### 7.1.3.3  Selection of the Sensitivity Setting

At very high frequencies, the dynamic range is much smaller than at 10 MHz. More so than at 10 MHz, at very high frequencies, the sensitivity setting values (entirely relative) depend on the device used. A high-sensitivity setting is useful, provided that it does not lead to random background noise. The cornea is assessed at a slightly lower

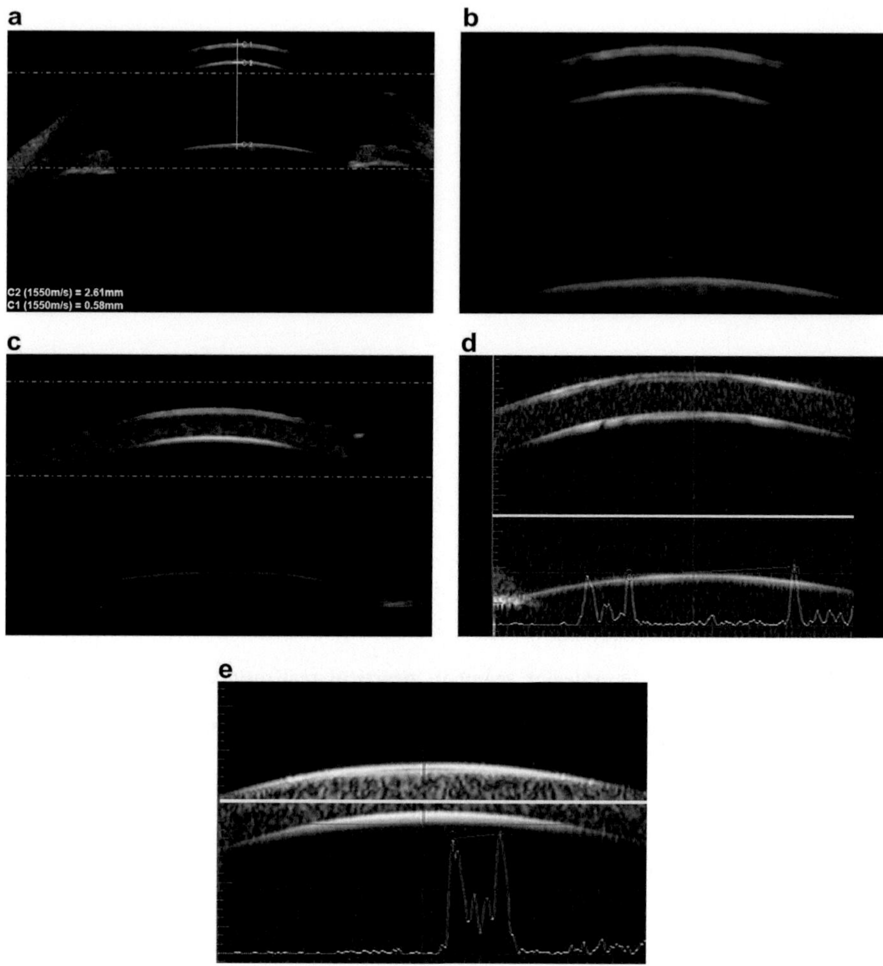

**Fig. 7.15 VHFU at 50 MHz, axial sections** in a patient with a plateau iris configuration. **a:** Horizontal axial section of the entire anterior segment from angle-to-angle according to 3–9 o'clock, with the focal area represented by the two green dotted lines. **b:** The same section, zoomed, showing the two anterior interfaces of the cornea corresponding to the epithelium and Bowman's membrane (even though the cornea is not centered in the focal area). Hence, it can readily be verified that the imaging is perpendicular and at the center of the cornea and that the various measurements will be reliable. **c:** Axial section of the cornea in the center of the focal area: The stroma appears discreetly more echogenic, and the resolution is optimal. **d:** Ultrasound biomicroscopy (UBM) section centered on the anterior chamber, the focal area represented by the yellow line located at the junction of the middle one-third and posterior one-third of the anterior chamber. **e:** UBM section centered on the cornea, the focal area represented by the yellow line located just in front of and at the center of the endothelium. Note the thin hyporeflective line and the small dropout on the reconstructed A-mode line showing the epithelium and Bowman's membrane. The thickness of the cornea in the center is measured at 514 μm (at a velocity of 1620 m/s). Note the difference in appearance of the cornea (resolution, reflectivity) between the two sections, simply due to the proximity or distance of it from the optimal focal line

sensitivity setting than for the anterior chamber and the structures of the chamber angle.

### 7.1.3.4 Technique

The following are usually carried out in succession:

- **7.1.3.4.1.** One or two axial sections of the anterior segment are acquired.

With a 50-MHz probe of a current ultrasound device, a section can be acquired according to 3–9 o'clock, one in light and another in the dark, or two sections in light, one according to 3–9 o'clock and another according to 6–12 o'clock. Checking that the incidence is correct is easy: after zooming the image, one must individualize the two interfaces corresponding to the epithelium and Bowman's membrane (Fig. 7.15b). These sections allow for obtaining biometric measurements: the thickness of the cornea, depth of the anterior chamber, diameter from angle-to-angle, diameter from sulcus-to-sulcus, and lens vault (Fig. 7.16). The diameters are slightly larger on the vertical section than the horizontal section: the report must specify the section used to obtain these values. The thickness of the cornea and the depth of the anterior chamber would ideally be measured from peak to peak on reconstructed A-mode (Fig. 7.15d and e), but the accuracy with calipers is acceptable. However, these values are obtained with ultrasound velocity of 1550 m/s. To obtain the actual value, a correction must be added to account for the velocity of ultrasound in the cornea of 1620 m/s (actual thickness = the value recorded × 1620/1550) and in the anterior chamber of 1532 m/s (actual depth = the value recorded × 1532/1550). In addition to these biometric values, these sections also serve to provide an idea of the morphology and situation of the iris. The thickness of the lens often cannot be measured at 50 MHz, so this value, as well as the total axial length, is obtained by a biometric assessment performed immediately beforehand, which is a mandatory prerequisite for all ultrasound explorations of the anterior segment.

With a UBM device (from Paradigm), two axial sections should be acquired: one showing the center of the cornea, the central part of the anterior chamber (AC), and the pupil, with the focal line located in the middle of the anterior chamber, and the other centered on the cornea, with the focal line located right in front of the center of the corneal endothelium. The first one allows for measuring the depth of the anterior chamber, preferably on a reconstructed A-mode, perpendicular to the interfaces of the cornea and the anterior lens capsule, whereas the second one allows for measuring the thickness of the center of the cornea, again on a reconstructed A-mode, perpendicular to the center of the cornea (Fig. 7.15d and e). Again, the device yields measurements with an average ultrasound velocity in tissues equal to 1550 m/s. Naturally, the actual values must be stated in the report, especially in case of glaucoma. This device also allows for acquiring an axial section of the cornea at very high resolution, which is especially useful in case of opacity or edema of the cornea and after refractive surgery.

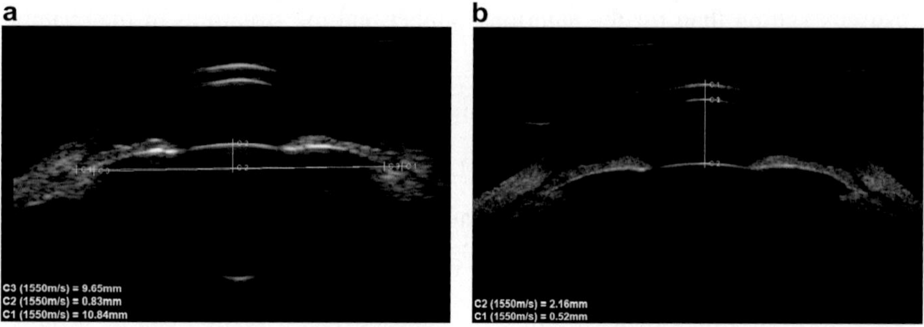

**Fig. 7.16** Axial sections of the anterior segment in a highly hyperopic patient (AL = 21.3 mm). **a:** With a 25-MHz probe allowing satisfactory measurement of angular diameters: the angle-to-angle diameter (C1) of 10.8 mm, the sulcus-to-sulcus diameter (C3) of 9.6 mm, and the lens vault of 879 μm (increased). **b:** With a linear scanning 50 MHz probe: angular markers are more obvious; therefore, diameters are usually measured at this frequency. The thickness of the cornea (543 μm) and the depth of the anterior chamber (2.13 mm) are also measured on this section

- **7.1.3.4.2.** Sections exploring the region of the anterior chamber angle and adjacent structures according to eight systematic meridians (9:00 o'clock, … 10:30, 12:00, 1:30, 3:00, 4:30, 6:00, and 7:30 o'clock), then by focusing the assessment on a known or discovered anomaly (Fig. 7.17a and b), with the scleral spur as a reference point, appearing as a small hyperechogenic point at the junction of the two curves representing the corneal endothelium and the outer limit of the uvea. This section allows for various biometric measurements for the chamber angle (see Chap. 11) [5]. To allow for good reproducibility of these measurements, the criteria for proper performance of these sections must be checked so that the two hyperechoic lines (epithelium and endothelium) limiting the cornea in the periphery are clearly seen and the iris is as short as possible. The resolution is insufficient at high frequency (Fig. 7.17c) to allow for these measurements and assessment of the angle, and therefore VHFU is mandatory.
- **7.1.3.4.3.** Orthogonal sections to these meridian sections successively assess the ocular periphery, the pars plicata of the ciliary body (Fig. 7.17d) and the iris, from its root to the pupil, taking care to be fully perpendicular to the structures to be assessed.

### 7.1.4   20-MHz BMode Study (for the Posterior Pole)

This is a complementary exploration that is undergoing rapid development. The probe is placed on the conjunctiva at the limbus in a temporal and then a nasal position. Cross-sections and vertical sections of the optic disc, macula, and intermaculo papillary region are generated (Fig. 7.18). One can acquire more peripheral sections, as long as the region studied is close to the focal point of the probe (approximately 25 mm), so for assessment of the ocular wall, and mainly the sclera. Because of

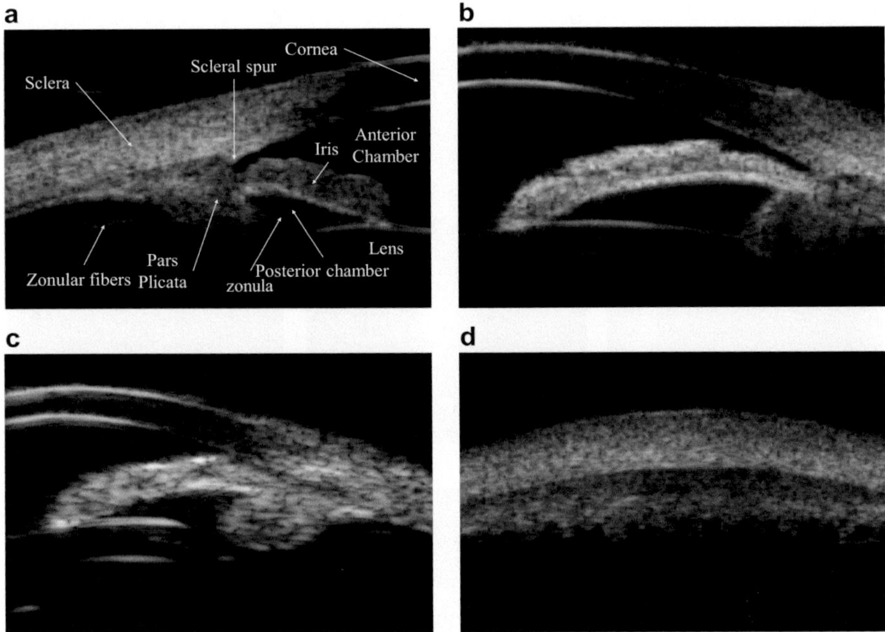



**Fig. 7.17** Appearance of the ciliary body at 20 MHz and 50 MHz. **a**: Section at 50 MHz of the chamber angle at 3 o'clock. The region stands out around the scleral spur, which must absolutely be identified before evaluating this anterior chamber angle. **b**: Section at 50 MHz of the chamber angle at 9 o'clock in a different patient. The angle is narrower but fully analyzable. **c**: Section at 25 MHz of the chamber angle at 9 o'clock (the same patient as in b). When the angle is narrow, the resolution is insufficient to recognize the scleral spur and thus to study the anterior chamber angle. **d**: Orthogonal section at 50 MHz passing through the pars plicata, clearly showing the ciliary processes and valleys

the greater attenuation and background noise, the variation of gain is limited, and the posterior hyaloid membrane appears significantly less reflective than at 10 MHz, often even being undetectable.

### 7.1.5 Color Doppler Imaging (CDI) (See Chap. 3)

This is a technique that has been applied in ophthalmology since the early 1990s, when technological advances allowed for studying slow flows [6]. The ocular and orbital vessels visualized by the Doppler effect are superimposed on a B-mode image. The results can be expressed in three modes:

- **Color mode**. The ocular and orbital vessels appear in gradients of red and blue depending on the direction and speed of the blood flow. Arbitrarily, for the orbit, the vessels heading towards the probe, mainly arteries, are coded in red, and

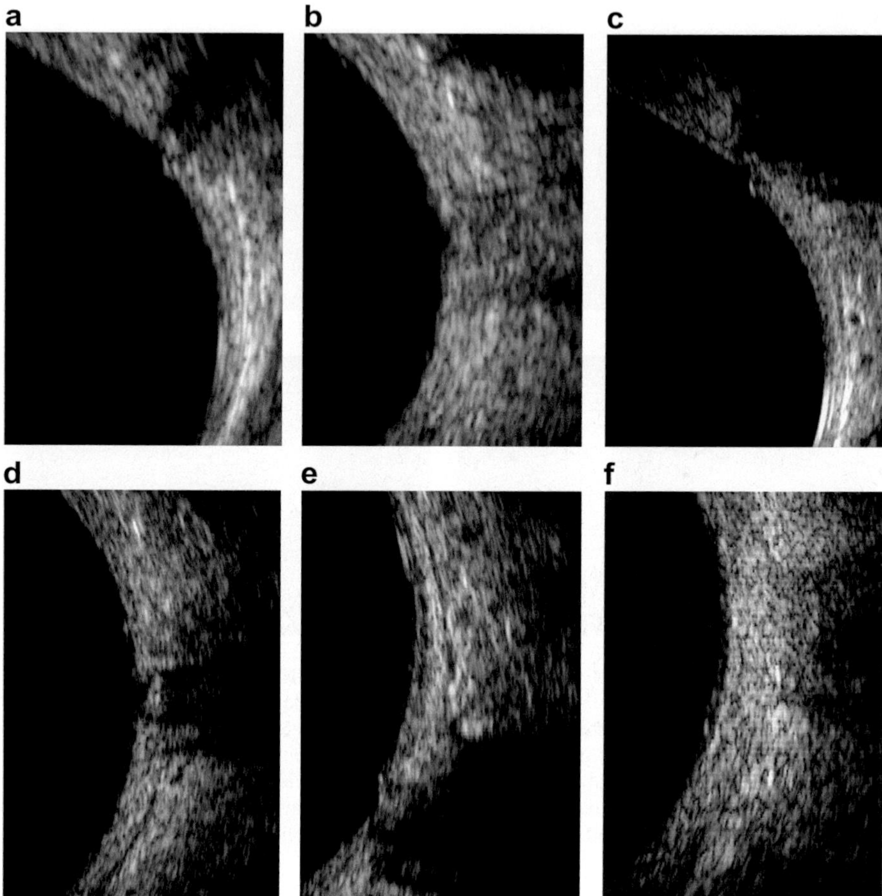

**Fig. 7.18 Examination of the optic disc and macula: superiority of 20 MHz. a**: Para-axial section of the posterior pole at 10 MHz; because it is a right eye, the macula is located above the optic disc; **b**: vertical section of the optic disc at 10 MHz; **c**: para-axial section of the posterior pole at 10 MHz; **d**: vertical section of the optic disc at 10 MHz; the physiological cupping and the peripapillary neural bulge can readily be analyzed; **e**: horizontal section of the posterior pole of the left eye at 20 MHz. The resolution is excellent, and the three parietal layers can be clearly discerned and can even be measured, albeit with less accuracy than with OCT: at 4.31 mm from the center of the optic disc, the echogenic retina is measured as 310 $\mu$m, the less echogenic choroid as 420 $\mu$m, and the very echogenic sclera as 460 $\mu$m. The hypoechoic normal thin episcleral border can readily be visualized; **f**: vertical section of the macula. In addition to the normal virtual episcleral space, there is a thin partial PVD at the posterior pole

the vessels that move away from the probe, most often veins, are coded in blue. Each color is lighter and brighter the faster the flow (Fig. 7.19a and e). The pulse repetition frequency (PRF) is used to define the frequency scale (in Hz) or velocities (in m/s or cm/s) of the flows studied. Because the flows of the ocular and orbital vessels are relatively slow, this scale of velocities is usually set from −5/6 cm/s to + 5/6 cm/s. If a vessel has a flow much faster than these speeds, there is risk of spectral ambiguity, or aliasing. In the orbit, with the velocity scale that is usually used, this artifact readily allows for differentiating the ophthalmic artery from its ciliary or muscular dividing branches.

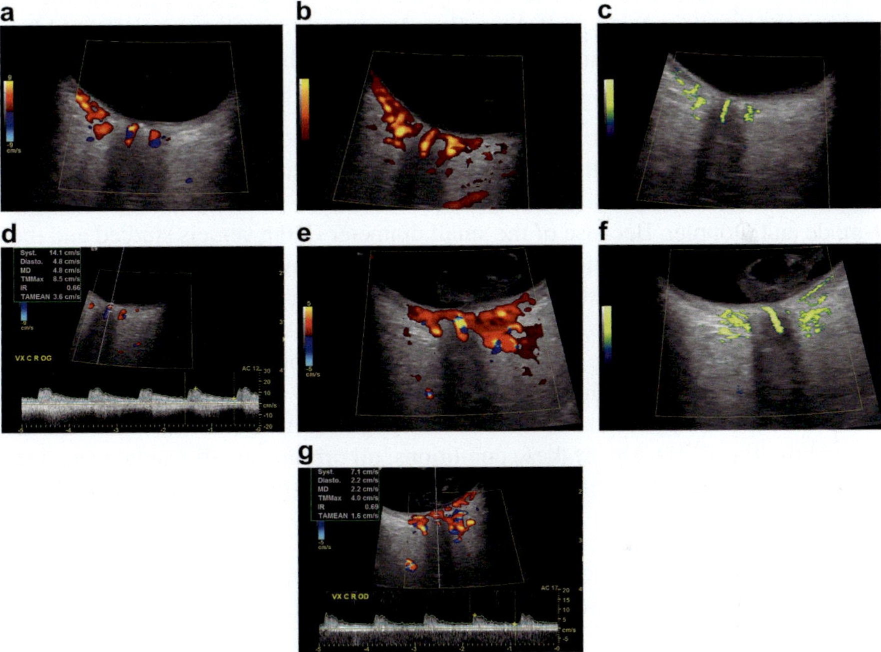

**Fig. 7.19** **Representation of the flows of the vessels of the optic nerve head**. **a**: OS, color mode—normal appearance; **b**: OS, power mode—normal appearance; **c**: OS, B-flow—normal appearance; **d**: OS, spectral mode—normal appearance; **e**: OD, color mode—pathological appearance after severe contusion of the eyeball—there is a large hemorrhage of the vitreous and diffuse retro equatorial ocular parietal thickening; **f**: OD, B-flow—pathological appearance after severe contusion of the eyeball; **g**: OD, spectral mode—pathological appearance after severe contusion of the eyeball. In color mode, the artery is coded in red and the vein in blue. In power mode and in B-flow, the two vessels are indistinguishable. In color mode and power mode, the vessels appear larger than in B-flow because of a blooming artifact (see Chap. 6), which does not affect B-flow. Spectral mode, which is quantitative, is ***essential*** for analysis of vascular flows, normal on the normal left side and exhibiting severe velocimetric disturbances on the contused right side: decrease in the peak systolic velocity (PSV) of the central retinal artery (CRA) (equal to half of the normal side) and discreet elevation of the resistive index; the flows represented in color mode and in B-flow appear to be entirely normal

- **Power mode**. The vessels appear according to gradients of a single color for which the intensity depends on the number of reflectors (red blood cells) circulating in the vessel and without information regarding the direction of the flow (Fig. 7.19b). Suitable for the study of very slow flows, the mode is rarely used in ophthalmology because it is very sensitive to movement artifacts.
- **B-flow** is a new mode of representation of blood flows without use of the Doppler effect (Fig. 7.19c and f). The presentation is similar to that obtained with the new micro-Doppler techniques.
- **Spectral mode** represents the characteristics of the blood flow from a particular vessel identified in color or power mode on a curve as a function of time. This is a quantitative mode ***necessary*** for all explorations (Fig. 7.19d and g). For arteries, the peak systolic velocity, end-diastolic velocity, and resistive index (IR) of blood flow within the vessel can be studied, and for veins, the maximum speed (Vmax), minimum speed (v min), and average speed (Vm) (Tables 7.1 and 7.2) [7].

The examination is performed with a suitable ultrasound device that must have a frequency probe greater than 7.5 MHz for B-mode and greater than 5 MHz for Doppler. On recent devices, the frequencies tend to be a little higher, both for the B-mode and Doppler. Because of the small diameter of the vessels studied and their low velocity flows, the device must have excellent temporal resolution as well as excellent spatial and contrast resolution. Variable focus, high-definition zooms, and the option of post-processing the image are desirable. At the technical level, to not modify the parameters of the vessels studied, a large amount of gel must be placed on the gently closed upper eyelid (Fig. 7.20) and the probe angled toward the posterior pole or the various vessels to be assessed, working in "immersion", without touching the eyelids (Fig. 7.21). Under these conditions, all orbital vessels can be visualized, but most often the vessels of the optic nerve head, central retinal vessels and short

**Table 7.1** Normal velocimetric constants of orbital arteries in color Doppler imaging

| | Oph A | CRA | Lateral sPCA | Medial sPCA |
|---|---|---|---|---|
| Peak systolic velocity (cm/s) | 45.3 ± 10.5 (31.4–39.6) | 17.3 ± 2.6 (8.8–12.6) | 13.3 ± 3.5 (9.8–11.4) | 12.4 ± 3.4 (8.6–14.2) |
| Resistive index | 0.74 ± 0.07 (0.77) | 0.63 ± 0.09 (0.70–0.76) | 0.52 ± 0.10 (0.63–0.68) | 0.53 ± 0.08 (0.63–0.68) |

Limit values found in the literature are indicated in brackets
Oph A = ophthalmic artery, CRA = central retinal artery, sPCA = short posterior ciliary artery
Data are mean ± SD

**Table 7.2** Normal velocimetric constants of orbital veins in color Doppler imaging

| | SOV | CRV |
|---|---|---|
| maxV (cm/s) | 8 ± 2 | 4 ± 2 |
| mV (cm/s) | 5.5 ± 2 | 3 ± 1 |

SOV = superior ophthalmic vein, CRV = central retinal vein
Data are mean ± SD

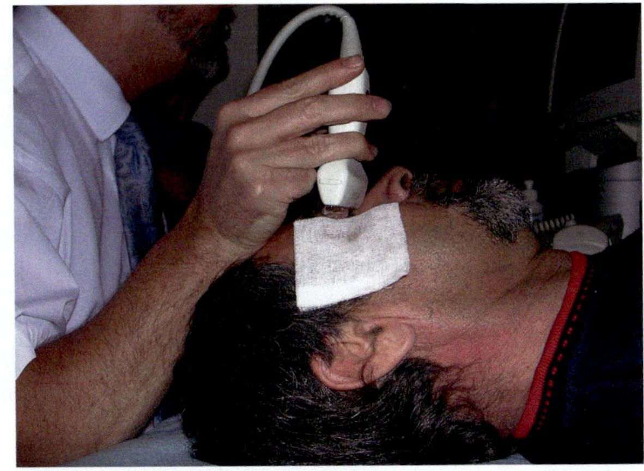

**Fig. 7.20  Color Doppler imaging of the vessels of the right optic nerve head: practical realization**. A large amount of gel is placed on the upper eyelid, and the patient is asked to look at a point on the ceiling nasally with the other eye, slightly on the left (as here it is the right side)

medial and lateral posterior ciliary arteries. Also, the ophthalmic artery at the level of the most posterior part of the third portion of its orbital segment, not far from the medial wall of the orbit, and the superior ophthalmic vein, are assessed. Some multipurpose ultrasound scanners have high-frequency probes, > 10 MHz, which are particularly suitable for assessment of tumors of the ciliary body.

CDI has shown its diagnostic utility in the following indications:

- **Eye masses and tumors**

    Positive and differential diagnoses of eye masses,
    Follow-up after conservative treatment

- **Vascular abnormalities of the optic nerve head**

    Chronic retinal ischemia and carotid stenosis
    Central retinal vein occlusion
    Central retinal artery occlusion
    Glaucoma
    Diabetes
    Retinal detachment
    Optic neuropathies

        vascular: arteritic anterior ischemic optic neuropathy, Horton's disease, complicated drüsen,
        inflammatory: multiple sclerosis or general diseases (sarcoidosis, etc.)
        Optic disc tumors

- **Orbital masses**

    Hypervascularized: capillary angioma,
    Vascularized: meningiomas, lymphomas, malignant tumors
    Hypovascularized: cavernous angioma, benign mixed tumor of the lacrimal gland,

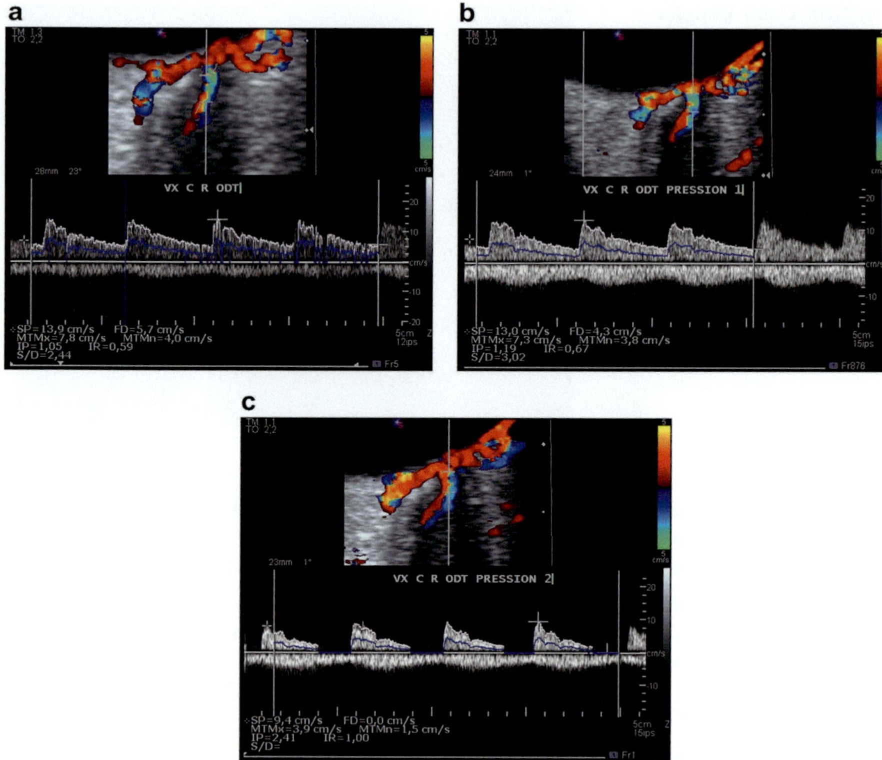

**Fig. 7.21** **Effect of pressure on the velocimetric constants of the central retinal vessels. a**: Proper recording technique, without any pressure; on the central retinal artery, the peak systolic velocity (PSV) recorded is 13.9 cm/s and the resistive index (RI) is calculated as 0.59, showing good diastolic flow. There is also a good flow in the central retinal vein. **b**: Recording while gently touching the upper eyelid: very discreet decrease in PSV, but a clear increase in RI, at the upper limit of normal. Still a good flow in the central retinal vein. **c**: Recording while exerting pressure, albeit moderate, on the upper eyelid: the PSV is further decreased, recorded to be 9.4 cm/s, but above all, there is no more diastolic flow, which results in an RI of 1.00. Note that the flow in the central retinal vein is decreased but still present

Cysts, non-vascularized

- **Cavernous carotid fistulas** (diagnostic and follow-up after endovascular treatment)

  High-flow, direct, post-traumatic fistula
  Low-flow, indirect, spontaneous fistula (dural fistula of the cavernous sinus)

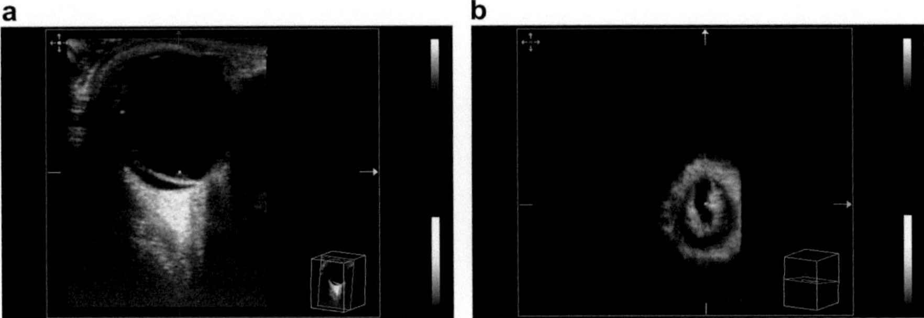

**Fig. 7.22   3D acquisition of a total retinal detachment of the right eye. a**: Para-axial 2D reconstruction mainly visualizing the 3 o'clock meridian. **b**: Frontal 3D reconstruction showing retinal detachment from the center of the eye in front of the posterior pole, revealing that the detachment is total, "macula-off", just sparing the 12 o'clock meridian

## 7.1.6   3D and Tissue Characterization

3D ultrasound is still underdeveloped, although many publications have demonstrated its usefulness:

- In oncological pathology (see Fig. 13.42), by allowing for more accurate and reliable assessment of tumor volume: increasing for small tumors that are monitored, decreasing after conservative treatment, which volume is known to be parallel to the percentage of local recurrence.
- In complicated vitreoretinal pathology, before surgery (Fig. 7.22).

An approach to tissue characterization can be obtained by analysis of quantitative ultrasound parameters such as the coefficient (or slope) of attenuation (see Chap. 1). Unfortunately, these quantitative parameters are not available on common imaging devices, only on research prototypes.

Therefore, ocular and orbital ultrasound involves a large number of different techniques, each of which answers specific questions and is tailored to the clinical presentation of the patient. Because systematic performance of all of these techniques each time is out of the question, one must have detailed clinical information before using any particular examination technique.

## 7.1.7   Indications

The frequency of indications varies according to the centers and changes from year to year. Most indications are represented by biometry before cataract surgery, with diagnostic indications representing no more than 25% of all indications. We provide, on an indicative basis, the respective frequency of the main entities encountered in our unit during the first 6 months of 2019 (Fig. 7.23).

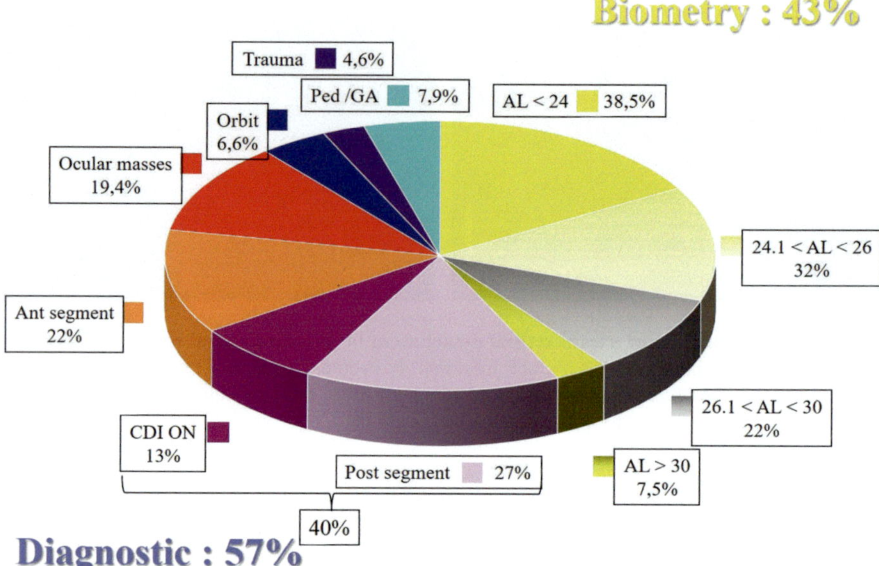


**Fig. 7.23 Respective indications of ophthalmic ultrasound**: 1248 examinations performed between January 1, 2019 and June 6, 2019

Biometry was performed in 43% of the cases and the other 57% had diagnostic indications.

Among the diagnostic indications were non-tumor pathologies of the posterior segment of the eye, mainly vitreoretinal pathologies but also exploration of the vascularization of the optic nerve head, representing 40% of these indications; anterior segment analysis, approximately 22%; eye masses and tumors, slightly less than 20%; orbital pathologies, nearly 7%; traumatic, ocular and orbital pathologies, approximately 5%; and pediatric pathologies requiring general anesthesia, 8%.

## References


1. Berges O, Puech M, Assouline M, Letenneur L, Gastellu-Etchegorry M. B-mode-guided vector-A-mode versus A-mode biometry to determine axial length and intraocular lens power. J Cataract Refract Surg. 1998;24(4):529–35.
2. Ossoinig KC. Evolution of standardized echography in: ultrasonography in ophthalmology 18. In: Bergès O, Perrenoud F Siahmed K, editors. Proceedings of the 18th SIDUO meeting. Paris: 2003 Sauramps medical Montpellier; 2000.
3. Frazier Byrne S, Green RL. Ultrasound of the eye and orbit, 2nd ed. Mosby St. Louis; 2002.
4. Till P. Solid tissue model for the standardization of the echo-ophthalmograph 7200 MA (Kretztechnik). Doc Ophthalmol. 1976;41(2):205–40.
5. Pavlin CJ, Harasiewicz K, Foster FS. Ultrasound biomicroscopy of anterior segment structures in normal and glaucomatous eyes. Am J Ophthalmol. 1992;113(4):381–9.

6. Erickson SJ, Hendrix LE, Massaro BM, Harris GJ, Lewandowski MF, Foley WD, Lawson TL. Color Doppler flow imaging of the normal and abnormal orbit. Radiology. 1989;173(2):511–6.
7. Tranquart F, Berges O, Koskas P, Arsene S, Rossazza C, Pisella PJ, Pourcelot L. Color Doppler imaging of orbital vessels: personal experience and literature review. J Clin Ultrasound. 2003;31(5):258–73.
8. Leung CK, Weinreb RN. Anterior chamber angle imaging with optical coherence tomography. Eye (Lond). 2011;25(3):261–7. https://doi.org/10.1038/eye.2010.201.

# Chapter 8
# Normal Echo-Anatomy

Olivier Bergès

**Abstract** This chapter shows the normal ultrasound appearance of the different structures of the eye and orbit (the optic nerve and the extraocular muscles and the different orbital vessels: central retinal artery, posterior ciliary artery, ophthalmic artery, central retinal vein, superior and inferior ophthalmic veins, connecting veins, with their normal variants); the eyeball, its anterior segment: the cornea (endothelium, stroma and endothelium), the iris, the ciliary body (pars plana and pars plicata), the zonular fibers, and the pupil, without forgetting the orbital fat, which is the largest constituent of the intra- and extraconal orbital cavity.

## 8.1 The Eyeball

It occupies the anterior part of the musculoaponeurotic cone and is approximately spherical. Arbitrarily, the eye is divided by a vertical-frontal equator that separates it into two hemispheres with an anterior pole (the center of the cornea), a posterior pole (centered by the macula), and meridians. An axial section at reduced gain allows the entire eyeball to be analyzed and to locate these various hallmarks (Fig. 8.1).

The ocular wall is formed by three layers, from the outside to the inside:

- the sclera, with the cornea extending forward
- the uvea, a vascular membrane comprising mainly the choroid at the rear and the ciliary body and the iris at the front
- the retina, which is a neurosensory membrane

At 10 MHz, differentiating between these three structures is difficult. However, they can be distinguished using a 20-MHz long focal probe (see Fig. 7.18).

The content is essentially comprised of transparent anechoic media in an axial section with reduced gain (the anterior chamber, between the posterior side of the

O. Bergès (✉)
Rothschild Foundation Hospital, Paris, France
e-mail: oberges@for.paris


O. Bergès (ed.), *Echography of the Eye and Orbit*,
https://doi.org/10.1007/978-3-031-41467-1_8

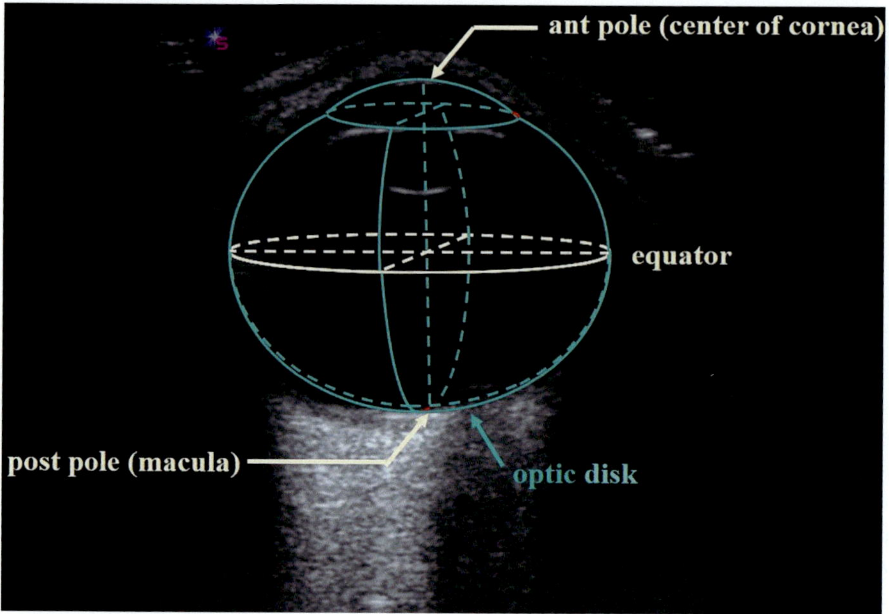


**Fig. 8.1 Axial section of the eyeball with a multipurpose ultrasound device**. The various hallmarks of this eyeball are readily visualized with its equator and its two poles. Note that with this type of device, the anterior side of the cornea can clearly be seen, even by a transpalpebral approach. In addition, the side walls of this globe, a full-fledged cyst, are not visualized

cornea and the irido-lenticular plane, the posterior chamber between the posterior pigment iris epithelium and the anterior crystalloid lenticular capsule, the cortex and the nucleus of the lens, and the vitreous):

- the anterior segment includes the cornea, the anterior and posterior chambers, the lens, the iris, and the ciliary body
- the posterior segment includes the wall of the globe and the vitreous body, which is a transparent mesenchymal gel, anechoic on an axial section with reduced gain

## 8.2 The Anterior Segment

It is best visualized with a (very) high-frequency probe at 25 or 50 MHz (see Chap. 4). The anterior surface (epithelium) and the posterior layer (endothelium) of the center of the cornea present as hyperechoic lines, whereas the stroma is less echogenic. At the periphery, the cornea can only be seen if the ultrasound beam is perpendicular to it. At 50 MHz, especially with high resolution, a small line is seen that is discreetly less echogenic between the epithelium and the Bowman membrane (see Fig. 7.15). However, such a presentation is not found between the endothelium and the Descemet membrane. The anterior chamber, filled with aqueous humor, is anechoic. With a high-frequency probe, the depth of the anterior chamber can be measured as well as the diameters from angle-to-angle and sulcus-to-sulcus (see Fig. 7.16). The anterior chamber angle is best assessed with a 50-MHz probe, with as the main reference the scleral spur, which is often represented by a small hyperechoic point at the intersection of curves emanating from the outer uvea and the corneal endothelium (see Figs. 7.17a and 11.3). The posterior chamber is also visualized, as is the zonule. However, due to its very structure, discerning the presence of a zonular rupture is almost impossible, except by 3D assessment. The lens, which is biconvex and anechoic, is limited by the anterior and posterior echogenic capsules (or crystalloids). The anterior capsule protrudes discreetly at the level of the pupil in relation to the plane of the iris. Although the architecture of the lens can be approximately evaluated with a 10-MHz probe, and slightly better with A-mode, it can only be studied in detail with a high-frequency probe, close to 20 MHz (Fig. 8.2 and see Fig. 10.1). The same applies to assessment of intraocular lens (IOL) (Fig. 8.3).

The posterior epithelium is straighter (Fig. 8.4). Its anterior convexity can be discerned. The ciliary body is moderately echogenic (see Fig. 7.17). Its location

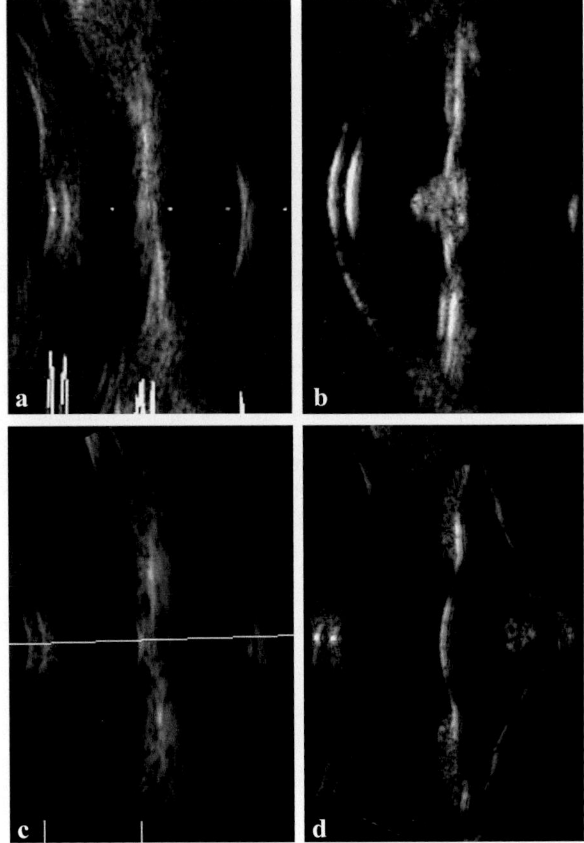

**Fig. 8.2 Congenital cataracts, special, unusual forms—superiority of 20 MHz. a, b:** Pyramidal cataract; **c, d:** posterior lenticonus; **a, c;** with a 10-MHz probe; **b, d:** with a 20-MHz probe. The pyramidal deformation of the anterior capsule, the posterior lenticonus, and the opacity of the nucleus are only discernable at 20 MHz

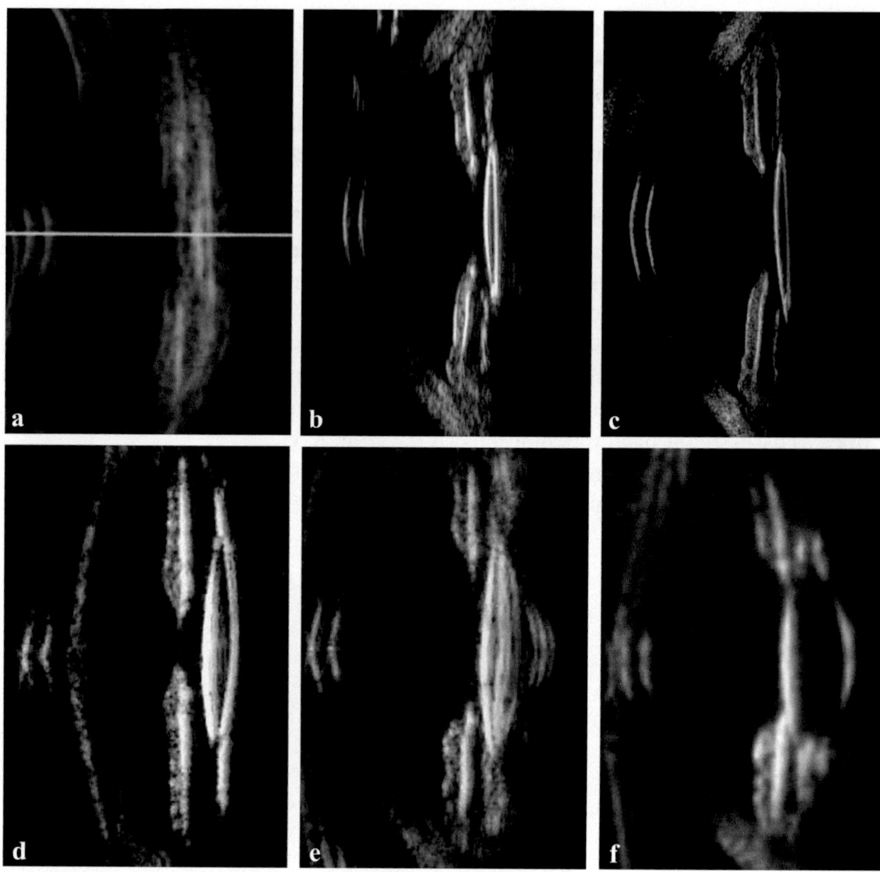

**Fig. 8.3** **Intraocular lens (IOL)—presentation at different frequencies. a, b, c, d:** acrylic IOL; **e:** PMMA IOL; **f:** silicone IOL; **a, e:** at 10 MHz; **b, d, f:** at 25 MHz; **c:** at 50 MHz. At 10 MHz, it can already be discerned that it is an intraocular lens, and even its nature, but individualizing the pupil from the iris plane is difficult, as is the measurement of the depth of the anterior chamber and the thickness of the IOL, and, therefore, the axial length could be inaccurate. High-frequency examination at 25 MHz helps to resolve both of these shortcomings. At 50 MHz, the posterior side of the optics of the IOL is sometimes not seen. For the acrylic intraocular lens, the posterior side is flat for **a, b** and **c** and slightly convex for **d**. The presentation of these IOLs differs greatly, as do their artifacts

(always in relation to the scleral spur), morphology, and structure should always be assessed.

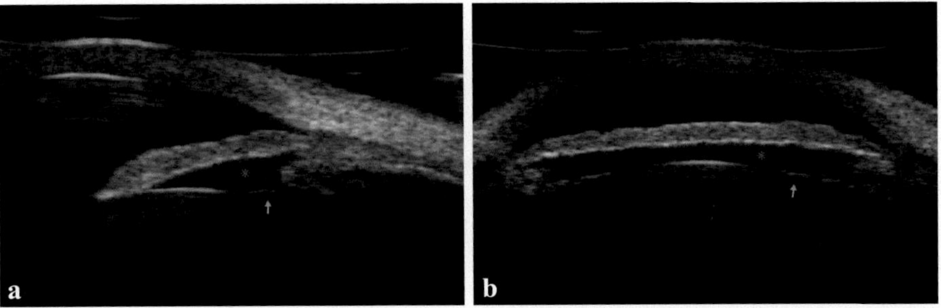

**Fig. 8.4  Iris at 50 MHz. a:** Section according to a meridian; **b:** orthogonal section. The probe is approximately perpendicular to the iris, which is visualized quite well. It is oblique to peripheral cornea, which is not well visualized. The stroma of the iris, moderately echogenic, like the ciliary body, is limited by two thin hyperechoic layers corresponding to the anterior epithelium and the posterior epithelium. Note the good visualization of the anterior zonular fibers (→ blue arrow) and of the posterior chamber (✳ red star)

## 8.3  Assessment of the Pupil

Multipurpose devices with small high-frequency probes can be used to visualize the iris and the pupil. They can be useful for assessing the pupillary reflex, if it cannot be clinically evaluated because of opacity of the cornea or anterior chamber, in the emergency or intensive care unit. Therefore, the pupil can be studied in myosis or mydriasis and its dimensions compared (Fig. 8.5).

## 8.4  The Optic Disc and the Optic Nerve

Their assessment must be systematic, bilateral and comparative, and part of the full clinical and paraclinical information: eye tension, visual field, and follow-up treatments. The optic disc is best assessed using a long focal  20-MHz probe in horizontal and vertical sections, with the probe placed on the conjunctiva at the temporal limbus. The optic disc presents as a small echogenic elevation, with a small depression at the center (corresponding to physiological cupping), which at 10 MHz, results in the appearance of an entity in the shape of an inverted omega (see Fig. 7.18a and b).

The optic nerve (visible in the form of a dark tunnel in an axial section) is best assessed by orthogonal (coronal) sections and must be measured on a section providing a strictly circular section of the nerve (see Fig. 7.6c). Optical fibers are hypo-reflective, with diameters of 2.9–3.5 mm. The diameter of the optical complex, including optical fibers, subarachnoid spaces, and meninges is 4.5–6 mm. The subarachnoid spaces and meninges become merged into a single, thick, hyperechoic layer. On such a coronal section, a small more echogenic point is sometimes seen in the center of the optical fibers, corresponding to the central retinal vessels, seen in cross-section.

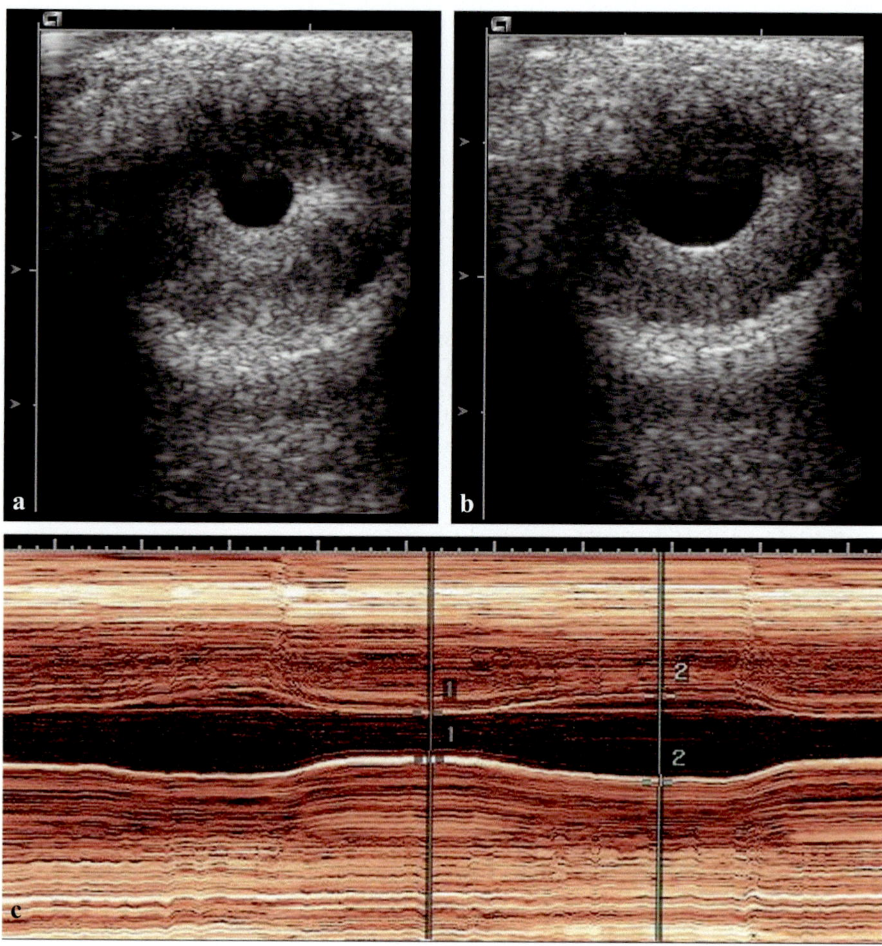

**Fig. 8.5** **Exploration of the pupil,** the patient being asked to look upward, and the probe placed on the lower eyelid and maximally tilted so that the ultrasound beam passes through the large axis of the iris. **a:** In myosis; **b:** in mydriasis; **c:** measurement of pupillary diameters in TM mode: the pupillary diameter in myosis is measured as 2.33 mm; the diameter in mydriasis is measured as 4.45 mm

## 8.5    The Muscles

These are assessed at a reduced gain. The rectus muscles are echogenic in their anterior part because of the many interfaces constituted by their microfibrils, and are surrounded by a thin hypoechoic border, corresponding to the fascia and the Tenon capsule. They appear hypoechoic at the orbital apex because of the angle of the ultrasound beam toward them. Their tendon, essentially fibrous, appears hypoechoic (Figs. 8.6 and 7.6). All of the muscles are visible; however, the medial rectus muscle

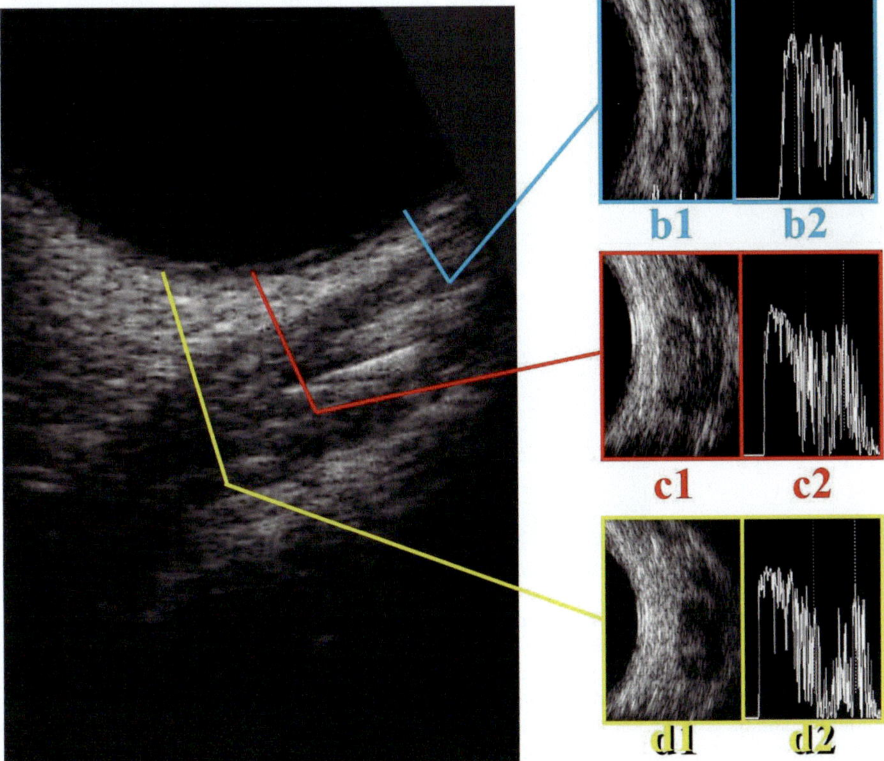


**Fig. 8.6 Left medial rectus muscle. a:** Longitudinal section of the medial rectus muscle; **b:** cross-section of the muscle tendon—1: B-mode, 2: A-mode; **c:** cross-section of the muscle belly—1: B-mode, 2: A-mode; **d:** cross-section of the posterior part of the muscle—1: B-mode, 2: A-mode

is the easiest to visualize along its entire length. In contrast, the inferior rectus muscle is rather difficult to follow, apart from its belly located behind the eyeball. The belly of the superior oblique muscle is visible against the orbital wall, above the medial rectus muscle. The tendons of the oblique muscles are clearly visible at the level of the lateral and medial walls of the eye. The reflected part of the superior oblique muscle and the inferior oblique muscle are more difficult to visualize.

## 8.6   Orbital Vessels

Color Doppler imaging, with color and spectral modes, is the only way to assess both the morphology and the function of orbital vessels. The vessels that are easiest to visualize are the vessels of the optic nerve head (see Figs. 7.19 and 8.7). Of note, no pressure should be exerted in order to properly examine orbital vessels (see Fig. 7.21).

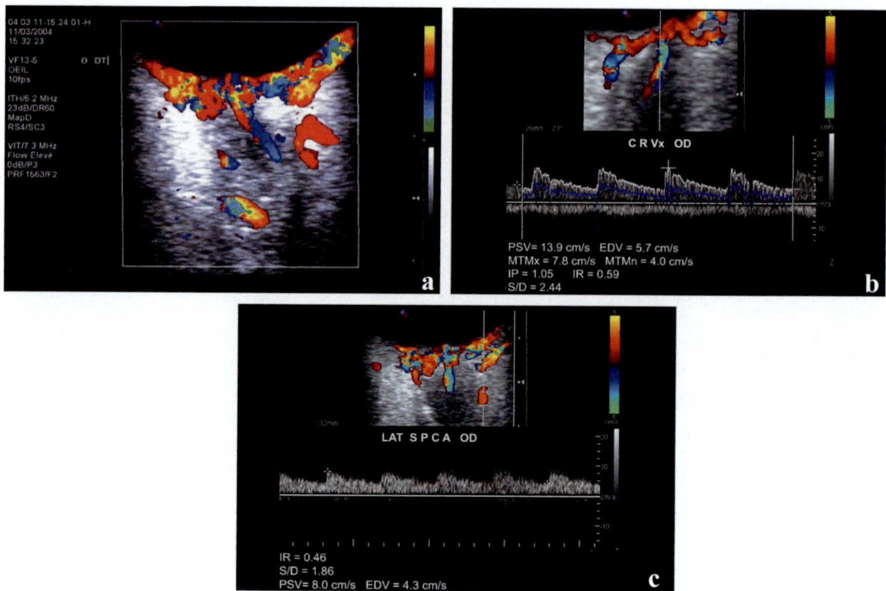

**Fig. 8.7** **Vessels of the optic nerve head—color and spectral Doppler a:** Color mode; **b:** central retinal vessels, spectral mode; **c:** lateral short posterior ciliary artery, spectral mode. The central retinal vessels (intertwined artery and vein) can be followed from their penetration into the optic nerve, 5–8 mm behind the optic disc. In spectral mode, the small Doppler gate should be placed just behind the lamina cribosa. On the central artery, the peak systolic velocity recorded is 13.9 cm/s and the resistive index is calculated as 0.59. In the vein, the maximum velocity recorded is 5.8 cm/s and the mean velocity is 2.2 cm/s. The resistive index of the short posterior ciliary arteries (sPCA), normally always lower than that of the CRA, is calculated as 0.46

The ophthalmic artery is normally encoded in red. Its direction is anterograde from the carotid siphon toward the globe (except for anatomical variants), and it can readily be detected at the level of its third portion near the medial wall of the orbit (Fig. 8.8). However, there are numerous anatomical variants (loops), so reproducing (and hence comparing the velocimetric constants of this artery) is difficult.

The superior ophthalmic vein should normally be coded blue and is directed toward the homolateral cavernous sinus. Its flow is linear or wave-like in spectral mode (Fig. 8.9). It can be visualized in 90% of cases by experienced operators. It can alternate, depending on respiration, the cardiac cycle, and the pressure gradient between the veins of the nasal cavity and the cavernous sinus (Fig. 8.10).

The inferior ophthalmic vein is only visualized in certain circumstances, such as with halogenated gas anesthesia (Fig. 8.11).

The connecting veins, connecting the superior and inferior ophthalmic venous systems, are usually not visible in color Doppler imaging because their path is perpendicular to the Doppler beam, but the medial connecting vein can often be discerned in B-mode, as well as the upper ophthalmic vein, seen in cross-section above the optic nerve (Fig. 8.12). More rarely, a lateral connecting vein can be seen.

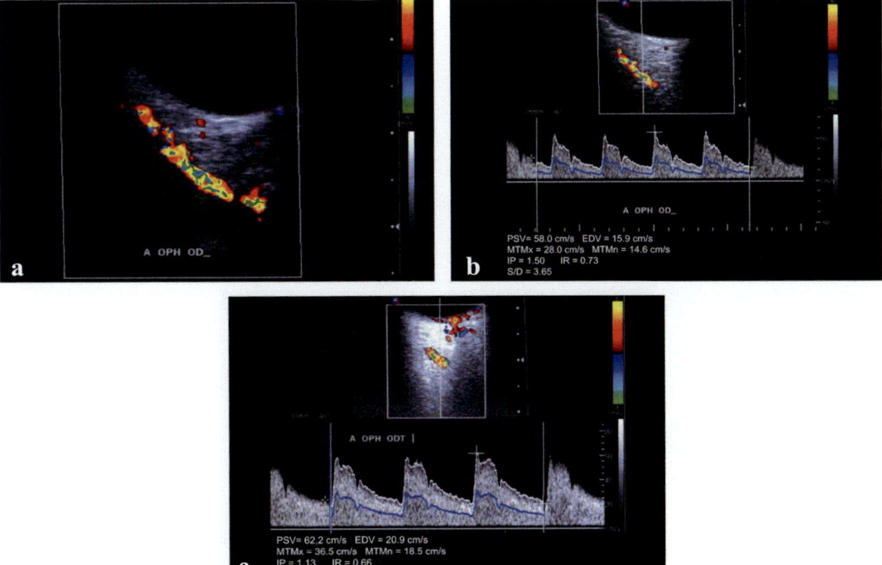

**Fig. 8.8** **Ophthalmic artery, color Doppler imaging. a:** Color mode; **b:** same patient, spectral mode; **c:** another patient, spectral mode. The artery is rarely visible over such a long distance as in **a** and **b**. In spectral mode, if the gate is located far posterior in the orbit, the peak systolic velocity is faster than in all of the other orbital arteries, most often close to 50 cm/s. Note the small protodiastolic incision, characteristic, less obvious at the level of the dividing branches. Its resistive index, higher than in the CRA, must be less than 0.85

The quantitative study of velocimetric constants is possible in spectral Doppler: the peak systolic velocity (PSV) and the resistive index (RI) for arteries, and the maximum velocity (Vmax) and mean velocity (Vm) for veins (see Tables 7.1 and 7.2) [1].

Two conditions must be met for a reliable and reproducible examination:

- a complete absence of pressure on the eyeball, requiring use of a *very* large amount of gel on the eyelids (the probe must not touch the eyelids) (see Figs. 7.20, and 7.21),
- angular correction of the Doppler pulse, except for posterior short ciliary arteries.

## 8.7  Orbital Fat

It is the largest constituent of the intra- and extraconal orbital cavity, serving as a natural contrast to other orbital structures because it is very hyperechoic due to its own structure and also because of the numerous vessels and nerves that cross it (see Fig. 6.5b).

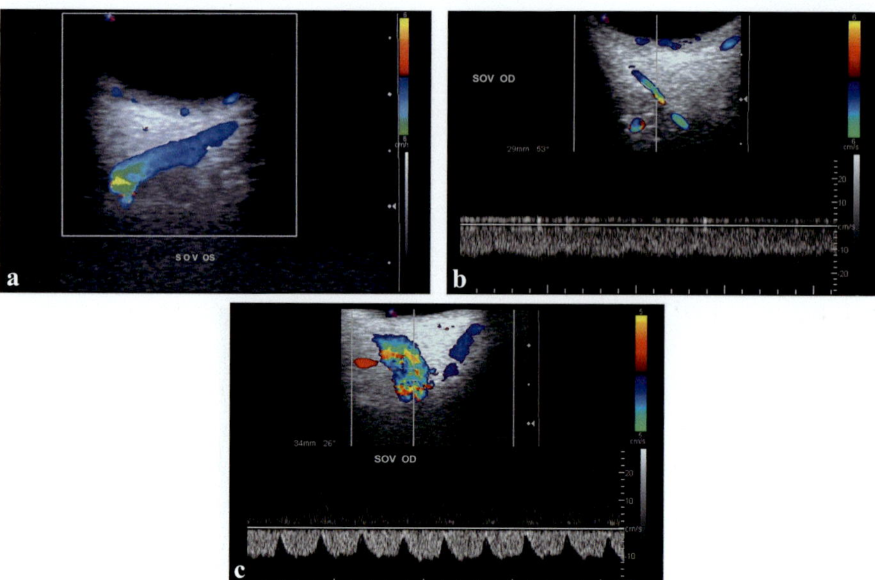

**Fig. 8.9 Superior ophthalmic vein, color Doppler imaging. a:** Color mode: the superior ophthalmic vein and its medial root have a slightly convex curvature forward and outward. At the typical settings, it is usually coded in blue, its flow going toward the cavernous sinus; **b:** another patient, spectral mode: almost a linear negative flow; **c:** a young child 3 years old examined under general anesthesia, color and spectral modes: the halogenated gases used lead to dilation of the superior ophthalmic vein and its medial root, where the flow, normal, is negative, wave-like, and well pulsed; however, also the lateral root can be seen, which is thinner and usually not visualized

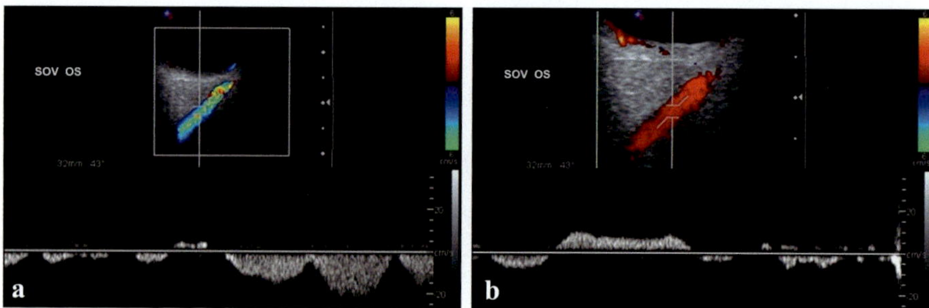

**Fig. 8.10 Alternating superior ophthalmic vein, color Doppler imaging a:** At a given moment, the vein appears blue in color mode, with a mainly negative flow in spectral mode. **b:** A few moments later, the vein is coded red in color mode, with a mainly positive flow in spectral mode. In both cases, the spectral analysis shows a typical venous flow, alternating positive and negative

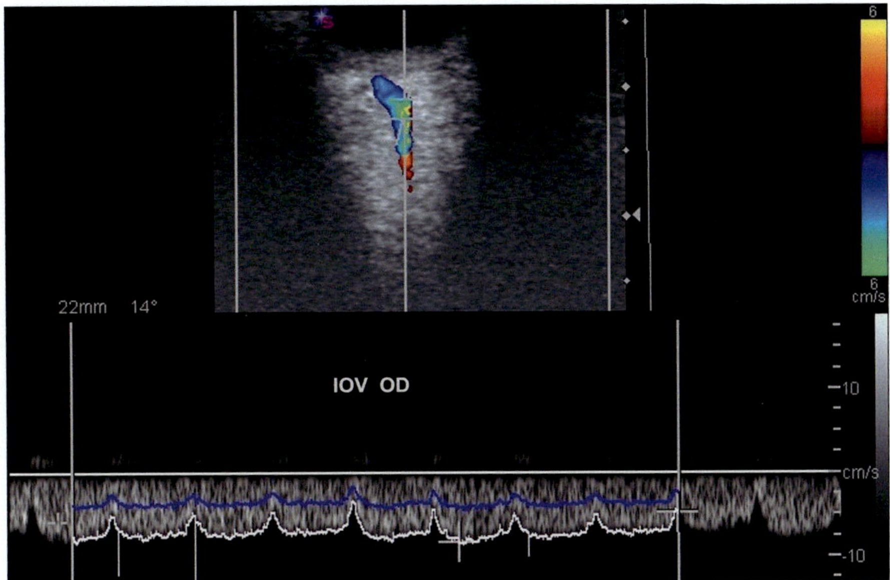


**Fig. 8.11  Inferior ophthalmic vein, spectral mode** in a young 4-month-old child examined under general anesthesia (halogenated gases) for persistent fetal vasculature of the other eye. It is thinner than the superior ophthalmic vein

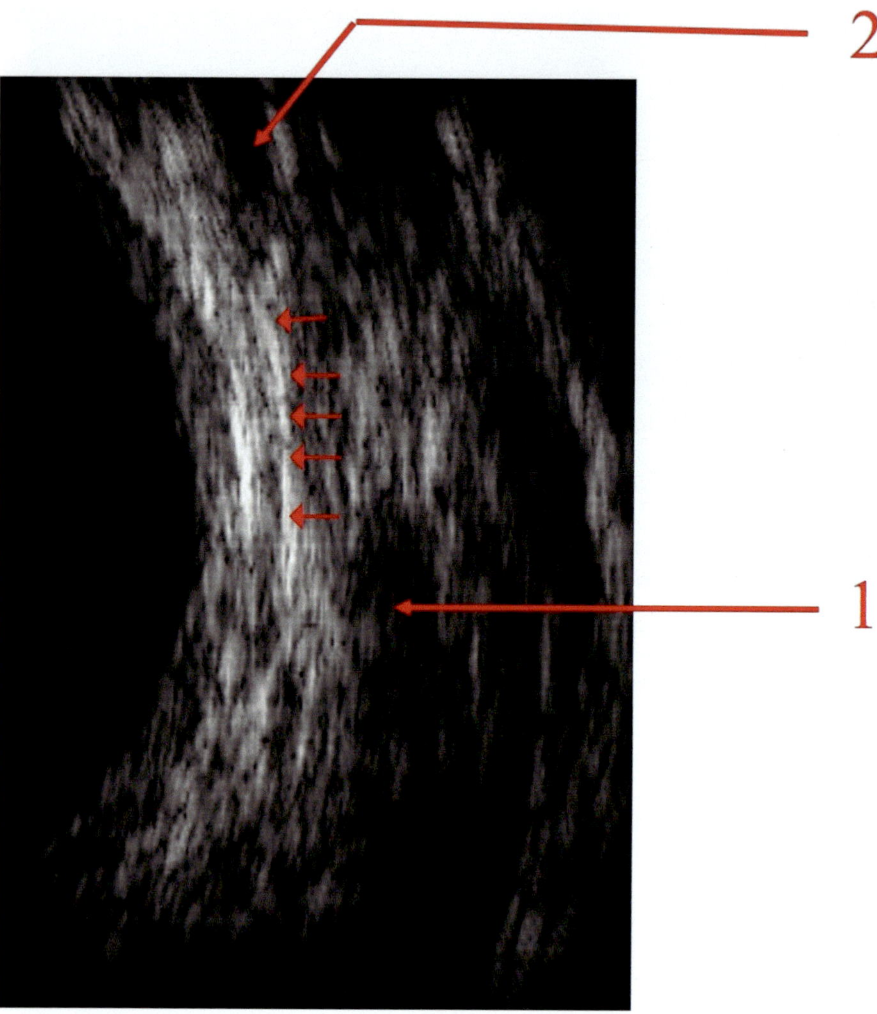

**Fig. 8.12 Medial connecting vein, B-mode.** Called the vertical vein by some authors, it is a tubular structure (⇇ red arrows) between the inner wall of the globe and the medial rectus muscle (←1) frequently encountered when the probe is placed without any pressure on the orbit. The superior ophthalmic vein seen in cross-section (←2) is visible at the upper part of this medial connecting vein. Their flow is necessarily perpendicular to the Doppler beam and, therefore, cannot be assessed using this technique

## Bibliography


1. Berges O, Puech M, Assouline M, Letenneur L, Gastellu-Etchegorry M. B-mode-guided vector-A-mode versus A-mode biometry to determine axial length and intraocular lens power. J Cataract Refract Surg. 1998 Apr;24(4):529–35.

2. Ossoinig KC. Evolution of standardized echography. In Bergès O, Perrenoud F, Siahmed K, editors. Ultrasonography in ophthalmology 18—proceedings of the 18th SIDUO meeting. Paris: Sauramps medical Montpellier; 2000.
3. Frazier Byrne S, Green RL. Ultrasound of the eye and orbit, 2nd ed. Mosby St. Louis; 2002.
4. Till P. Solid tissue model for the standardization of the echo-ophthalmograph 7200 MA (Kretztechnik). Doc Ophthalmol. 1976;41(2):205–240.
5. Pavlin CJ, Harasiewicz K, Foster FS. Ultrasound biomicroscopy of anterior segment structures in normal and glaucomatous eyes. Am J Ophthalmol. 1992;113(4):381–389.
6. Erickson SJ, Hendrix LE, Massaro BM, Harris GJ, Lewandowski MF, Foley WD, Lawson TL. Color Doppler flow imaging of the normal and abnormal orbit. Radiology. 1989;173(2):511–6.
7. Tranquart F, Berges O, Koskas P, Arsene S, Rossazza C, Pisella PJ, Pourcelot L. Color Doppler imaging of orbital vessels: personal experience and literature review. J Clin Ultrasound. 2003;31(5):258–73.
8. CK Leung RN Weinreb 2011 Anterior chamber angle imaging with optical coherence tomography. Eye (Lond). 2011;25(3):261–267.https://doi.org/10.1038/eye.2010.201

# Chapter 9
# Ultrasound Analysis Guide: Quantitative Ultrasound

Olivier Bergès

**Abstract** This small chapter presents considerations for performing a good ultrasound examination of the eye and orbit, morphologically (situation, shape, limits and contours) in B-mode and in color Doppler imaging but also to obtain functional information via spectral Doppler (presence of vessels [peak systolic velocity and resistive index]) and quantitative information via standardized echography (reflectivity, attenuation [angle kappa] internal echotexture and kinetic study (consistency, post-movements).

A well-performed ultrasound should be bilateral and comparative. In terms of the clinical symptomatology, it needs to be exhaustive. For this, one must successively analyze the overall shape of the eye, the anterior segment, the vitreous, the vitreo-retinal interface, the wall, retina, choroid and sclera, the optic disc, and the macular region, and, whenever possible, the vessels of the optic nerve head. In the orbit, the optic nerve, extraocular muscles, intra- and extraconal retrobulbar orbital fat should be visualized, and, if possible, also the flows of the orbital arteries and veins as well as the anterior paraocular space. When a lesion is discovered, and especially if it is a space-occupying entity, a semiological analysis must be performed following the steps of quantitative ultrasound [1]: first of all performing:

- a morphological study, the situation, the shape, the limits, and the contours of the lesion,
- a quantitative study, readily achievable in B-mode but better in standardized A-mode by assessing three parameters:

    - The reflectivity of the lesion, to be assessed on the first centimeter of the process if it is voluminous, at tissue sensitivity (T), in reference to the scleral peak, which can be zero, very weak, weak, medium, high, or very high
    - The attenuation of the ultrasound beam by the lesion, best expressed in dB/cm or as the kappa angle

O. Bergès (✉)
Rothschild Foundation Hospital, Paris, France
e-mail: oberges@for.paris



O. Bergès (ed.), *Echography of the Eye and Orbit*,
https://doi.org/10.1007/978-3-031-41467-1_9

- The internal echotexture of the lesion can be homogeneous or heterogeneous, regular or irregular
- A dynamic, or kinetic, study by assessment of:

  The consistency of an orbital lesion (hard, soft, or mixed) by assessing its deformability to the pressure from the probe, the Valsalva, the position in hyperdecubitus

  The mobile or solid nature of an intraocular lesion; assessment of post-movements

  The vascular nature of a lesion, best by color Doppler imaging because it provides precise quantification: Peak Systolic Velocity (PSV) and Resistive Index (RI) but also, more simply, by searching for rhythmic pulsations within the lesion in B-mode or in A-mode.

## Reference

1. Ossoinig KC. Evolution of standardized echography. In: Bergès O, Perrenoud F, Siahmed K, editors. Ultrasonography in ophthalmology 18—proceedings of the 18th SIDUO meeting. Paris: Sauramps medical Montpellier; 2003.

# Chapter 10
# Ocular Biometry and Calculation of IntraOcular Lens Power

Olivier Bergès, Jean-Brice Gauthier, François Perrenoud, Mickaël Sellam, and Maté Streho

**Abstract** This chapter first details the physical principle of ocular biometry, then presents results, with the distances, in millimeters, depending on the celerity in the different eye structures (cornea, anterior chamber and vitreous, lens) and finally the quality criteria of a "good" biometry: as high as possible peaks, on equal height, with repetition echoes and results consistent with refraction. Considering the technique, A-mode biometry (contact and immersion) is first presented, the manual acquisition mode being much more preferable. B-mode guided biometry is then presented and discussed; it has several advantages, particularly better intra- and inter-examiner reproducibility. Special cases are also discussed, according to age (neonates, infants and children), the refraction (myopia or hyperopia) or the pathology (aphakia, pseudophakia, phakic eye with a refractive phakik intraocular lens [pIOL], intravitreal silicone, melanoma and age-related macular degeneration, risk of closed angle glaucoma, hypotonic eye, and eye trauma). Then, pachymetry allowing the measurement of corneal thickness, and optical biometry using interferometry, are briefly presented. The second part of the chapter deals with the different formulas for IOL power calculation and how to use them. We successively present the historical method, also known as the 1.25 dpt correction; the first-generation theoretical formulas; and the regression formulas SRK and SRK II, to concentrate on the latest generation of theoretical formulas: SRK/T, Holladay, Hoffer-Q, Haigis, and Barrett's Universal II. The importance of the keratometry value on the result is then analyzed, and we discuss the biometry for toric IOLs, the special case of contact lens wearers, special cases when keratometry is not possible, IOL design for children and infants (congenital cataracts), and special cases of corneas modified by refractive surgery. We present tables for the advantages and disadvantages of ultrasound and optical axial length measurement techniques and the proposed choices of theoretical formulas to be used

O. Bergès (✉)
Rothschild Foundation Hospital, Paris, France
e-mail: oberges@for.paris

J.-B. Gauthier
Department chair of Ophthalmology, Laon Hospital, Laon, France

F. Perrenoud · M. Sellam · M. Streho
Explore Vision Diagnostic Center Paris, Paris, France

as a axial length function taking into account the optimal efficiency of each formula. These tables help readers master this subject of ocular biometry and IOL power calculation.

Ultrasound ocular biometry has become established in ophthalmology with the development of the implantation of intraocular lenses during phacoemulsification. First described by Gernet [1] in 1965, A-mode biometry has always accounted for a large proportion of eye ultrasound indications (see Fig. 7.23). Ultrasound has thus become the reference method for measuring the axial length and calculating intraocular lens (IOL) power to optimize results and avoid refractive errors.

However, ultrasound is not limited to this indication, as long as the ultrasound beam can be perpendicular to the interfaces delineating the structure/lesion to be measured. It is also useful for monitoring globes likely to progress toward atrophy, modeling of eyeballs before radiotherapy, and in high frequency, measuring transverse distances (anterior chamber angle to angle diameter and sulcus-to-sulcus diameter), and assessing the risk of angle-closure glaucoma. Measurements of the anteroposterior axes (depth, thickness, axial length, etc.) are more reproducible and more accurate than those of transverse axes (diameters) (Fig. 10.1).

## 10.1 Principle

Measurement of the axial length involves performing a linear echogram following the optical axis (which most often merges with the visual axis). Therefore, the corneal apex must be located and the macular region identified. Anatomically, the foveola (0.35 mm in diameter) is in the center of the fovea (1.5 mm or 1 papillary diameter), itself in the center of the macula, with a diameter of 5.5 mm centered at 4 mm temporally and 0.8 mm below the center of the optic disc. The foveolar depression should be searched for "outside" the vertical axis and slightly "below" the transverse axis to optimize, in most cases, the visual axis.

## 10.2 Results

The ultrasound beam will successively encounter the coupling medium (gel), the cornea, the anterior chamber, the lens, the vitreous cavity, the vitreoretinal interface, and then the ocular wall and the orbital contents, with a reflection echo for each interface, or:

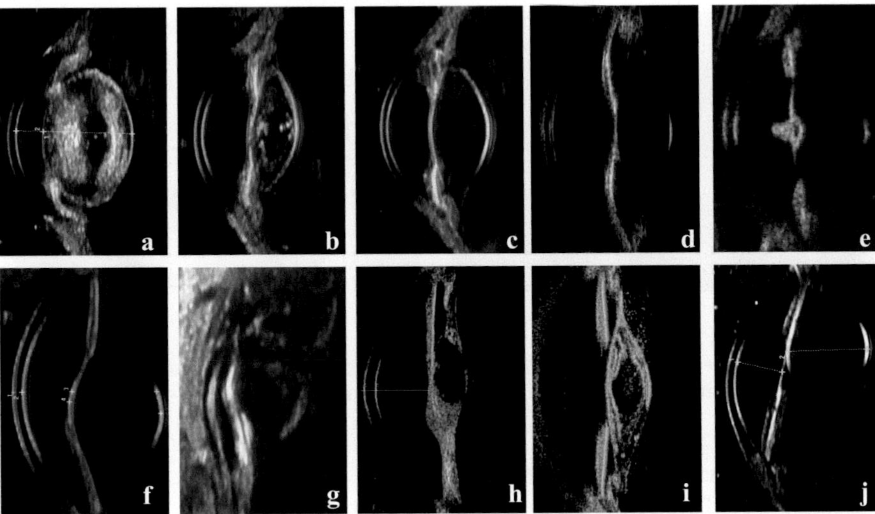

**Fig. 10.1 Lenses all exhibiting cataract, but with different morphologies, positions, and echo-textures.** For the presentation of the figures, the front is always located to the left of the image. **a** Hyperechoic intumescent lens (high-frequency ultrasound [HFU] with an 18-MHz probe). The entire lens is visible, 6.1 mm thick and 9.4 mm in diameter. The cornea has a normal thickness of 564 μm, and the anterior chamber is shallow, at 1.94 mm. The lens vault is greatly increased to 2.1 mm. HFU from 18 to 25 MHz is the best frequency to analyze these very large and very echogenic lenses. At 50 MHz, only the front half of the lens is visualized, and at 10 MHz the resolution is insufficient and only useful for ocular biometry. **b** A small echogenic lens (HFU with an 18-MHz probe). High frequency is used to analyze small echoes of the lens, which are not visible at 10 MHz but which can be discerned on reconstructed A-mode. The lens has a normal size, 4 mm thick. **c** Superior sectorial cataract related to melanoma of the iris treated by proton beam therapy (★). The lens capsules are slightly condensed around the equator of the lens (→). HFU with an 18-MHz probe, sagittal section. **d** Anechoic cataract in a 2-year-old child already operated on in the perinatal period for congenital glaucoma (HFU with a 25-MHz probe. The lens, which has a normal size and position, is anechoic, even with this frequency of 25 MHz. **e** Pyramidal cataract (HFU at 20 MHz with a short focal length). Invisible at 10 MHz, it does not cause a biometric error (see also Fig.8.2b). **f** Microspherophakia: axial section with a multipurpose ultrasound with a 5–15 MHz probe. This type of device is better for measuring the equatorial diameter of the lens, here at 5.1 mm for a thickness of 4.8 mm. **g** Post-traumatic fracture of the lens: parasagittal section of the lens with a multipurpose ultrasound device and an 18-MHz probe. In addition to echoes due to cataract, there are also small retrolenticular echoes in the anterior vitreous: lenticular masses or hemorrhage? **h** Congenital cataract and anterior persistent fetal vasculature (PFV)—very high frequency ultrasound [VHFU] at 50 MHz. The entire lens can be seen at 50 MHz because it is small in size. Its echotexture is very heterogeneous. Anterior PFV results in perilenticular echogenic thickening. **i** Inflammatory cataract in a child with juvenile polyarthritis: VHFU with a 50 MHz probe. The lens, with a small size and normal position, is echogenic and heterogeneous. On this superior para-axial section (the center of the cornea is not visualized), small punctiform echoes in the vitreous are seen, related to associated hyalitis. **j** Cataract with superior subluxation of the lens in a patient with Marfan syndrome (HFU with an 18-MHz probe, sagittal section)

                                                          

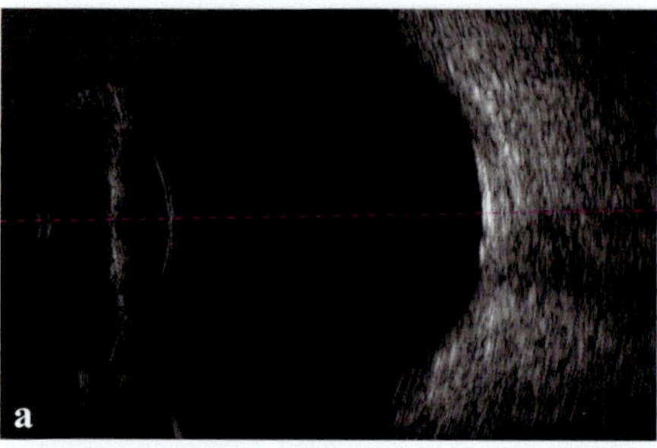
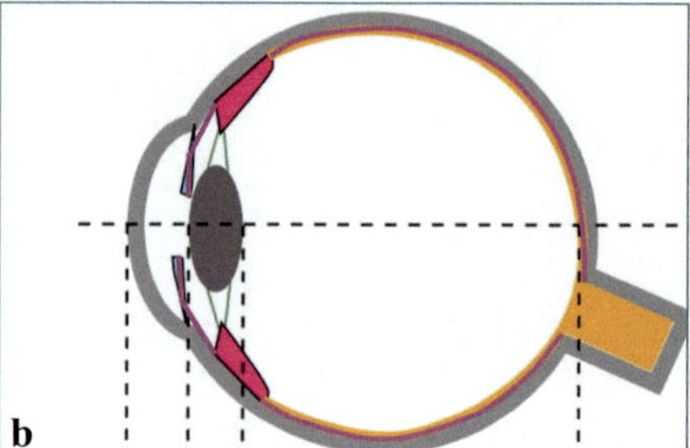


**Fig. 10.2 Right eye**, axial section. **a**: Ultrasound in B-mode; **b**: Schematic representation of an eye and the different segments that are traversed during an ultrasound

- medium/**anterior surface of the cornea**
- **posterior surface of the cornea**/aqueous humor
- aqueous humor/**anterior lens capsule**
- **posterior lens capsule** /vitreous cavity
- vitreous cavity/**vitreoretinal interface** (Fig. 10.2)

Very often, with only four markers, manufacturers have simplified the names, and the term **anterior chamber (AC)** then refers to the distance between the anterior surface of the cornea and the anterior surface of the lens; however, this measurement includes the thickness of the cornea and the depth of the AC. The current devices, with five markers, allow the two faces of the cornea to be individualized and thus determine the actual value of the depth of the AC, which is an essential parameter for some IOL calculation formulas. Otherwise, when the cornea is normal, the actual depth of the AC must be assessed by removing 0.5 mm from this AC value.

The positioning of the markers is important: for each interface, they should be positioned at the upper third of the ascending peak. Positioning in a non-rigorous manner leads to approximations on the order of ± 0.1 mm per marker. (Fig. 10.3), which can be even larger and lead to refractive errors of more than 1 dpt.

The chosen peak of the desired interface should be verified, especially for the posterior capsule of the lens, so it will not be confused with an intralenticular echo (Fig. 10.4), or the vitreoretinal interface.

In ultrasound, times ($\mu$s) are measured. Distances (mm) can be deduced if the speed of propagation of ultrasound (velocity) in the different media crossed is known. In practice, the default values used in biometers are usually as follows:

cornea: 1620 m/s
aqueous humor: 1532 m/s
lens: 1641 m/s
vitreous humor: 1532 m/s.

Ultrasound velocity in the lens is a little altered by the extent and type of cataract; however the mean value of 1641 m/s for the lens seem reasonable and give good

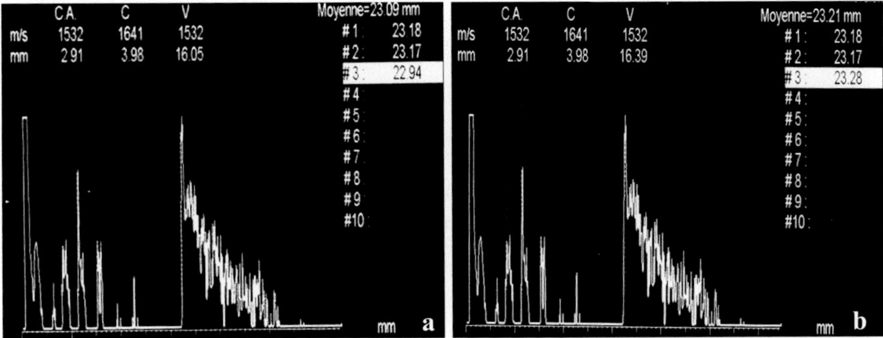

**Fig. 10.3 Variations in the measurement of axial length depending on the positioning of the caliper at the vitreoretinal interface**. **a**: The caliper is incorrectly placed below the peak; the axial length in this case would be 22.94 mm. **b**: The caliper is placed correctly at the upper part (and not at the top) of the peak. The actual axial length is measured at 23.28 mm. The difference of 0.34 mm corresponds to a refractive error of one diopter for this emmetropic eye!

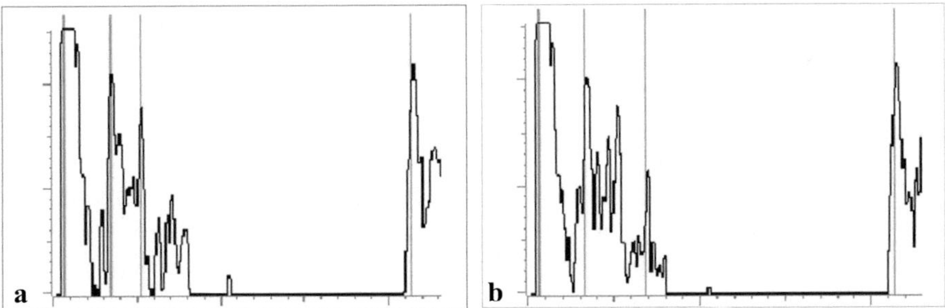

**Fig. 10.4 Measurements variations of the axial length depending on the positioning of the caliper of the posterior capsule of an echogenic lens**: A-mode biometry, contact method. **a**: The caliper dedicated to the posterior capsule of the lens was automatically placed on a very reflective intralenticular echo. Anterior chamber = 3.57 mm; lens = 2.78 mm; axial length = 22.86 mm. However, this acquisition is questionable because a lens that is this echogenic cannot, a priori, be this thin in an adult. This measurement should not be taken into account when averaging measurements. **b**: Another acquisition in which the caliper is placed correctly on the posterior capsule: Anterior chamber = 3.61 mm; lens = 4.96 mm; axial length = 23.22 mm. The difference of 0.36 mm corresponds to a final refractive error of one diopter

results. On the other hand, the use of an average value of 1550 m/s with only a corneal marker and a retinal marker is no longer possible because it is too approximate and a source of error.

Before each examination, the correct ultrasound velocities should be verified and checked that they have not been changed. Creating "profiles" for examinations involving pseudophakia or in the presence of silicone can be useful but increases the risk of using incorrect speeds.

## 10.3 Quality Criteria

It is customary to require at least 5 criteria before asserting that a biometry is correct:

- At least three different measurements yielding concordant values.

Biometers provide the standard deviation for different measurements. This must be less than 0.1 for the total axial length and for each distance.

- **The peaks vertices** of the corneal interfaces, the anterior and posterior faces of the lens, and the vitreoretinal interface are **as high as possible**.

Aside from cases of myopia, the ultrasound beam must approach the different interfaces orthogonally, thereby resulting in maximal reflection and, therefore, the highest possible peak height.

- The peaks are **all of the same height**, the absorption in the media crossed being almost zero, aside from very dense cataracts with no access to the retinal fundus and very echogenic lenses for which the posterior peaks can be attenuated.
- There are **repetition echoes** behind the lens.

Their presence, although not essential, indicates perpendicularity of the ultrasound beam to the capsules of the lens

- The measurements found are **consistent with refraction.**

Currently, under these conditions, ultrasound biometric measurements have an accuracy in the order of 0.1 mm, at the limit of the possible resolution at 10 MHz. Any biometric error will affect the calculation of the IOL power (and, therefore, the postoperative refraction).

This is easy to verify, using a "simple" formula such as SRK, where $P = A - 2.5L - 0.9\,K$: an error of 0.1 mm would result in a modification of $2.5 \times 0.1$ or 0.25 dpt, even for average values.

> Note that the tolerance is a little better in nearsighted people, possibly because of a smaller relative error and because the rule of 1 mm = 3D fully applies to only emmetropic eyes. However, hyperopia biometric errors, even when minor, can lead to significant refractive errors.

Biometry shall start with an **interrogation** phase to determine the patient's history: refractive surgery (technique and ametropia before surgery), use of contact lenses (type and duration of removal), and other prior eye issues.

The measurements mainly focus on keratometry and axial length. However, the formulas for the latter generations involve other parameters such as the thickness of the lens and the white-to-white diameter, the anterior chamber depth, etc.

## 10.4   Technique

**Axial length** is mainly measured by two techniques, an ultrasound technique and an optical technique, each of which has advantages and disadvantages (Table 10.1). For ultrasound biometry, two ultrasound techniques can be used: simple A-mode [2, 3], and B-mode guided A-mode [4].

### *10.4.1   The Conventional Method: A-Mode*

In A-mode, once again, two possibilities are available: a so-called contact method and an immersion method. The contact method can be performed with the patient sitting or lying down; the immersion method usually requires a reclined position.

#### 10.4.1.1   Contact A-Mode (Fig. 10.5)

The probe is placed on the cornea, after topical anesthesia by oxybuprocaine, while the presence of the tear film ensures the transmission of the ultrasound beam. Naturally, the cornea should not be depressed by pressing too hard or should not be in contact with excess tear film or eye drops (Fig. 10.6). In the past, to avoid these pitfalls, manufacturers designed probes with soft ends filled with water [3]. Currently, all biometric probes have a rigid end, slightly concave to match the convexity of the cornea.

**Table 10.1** Advantages and disadvantages of ultrasound and optical axial length measurement techniques

| Devices | Advantages | Disadvantages |
| --- | --- | --- |
| B-mode-guided ultrasound | • Independent of opacities<br>• Independent of fixation<br>• Analysis of the posterior segment (retinal detachment, staphyloma, optic disc, macula etc.) | • Operator-dependent<br>• Equipment<br>• Contact<br>• Silicone oil |
| Optical biometry | • No contact<br>• Comfort, fast<br>• Reproducibility<br>• "Delegable"<br>• Silicone oil | • No posterior segment analysis<br>• Cooperation required<br>• No gaze fixation<br>• Age ($< 6$ years)<br>• Limiting opacities<br>• Excessive axial length |

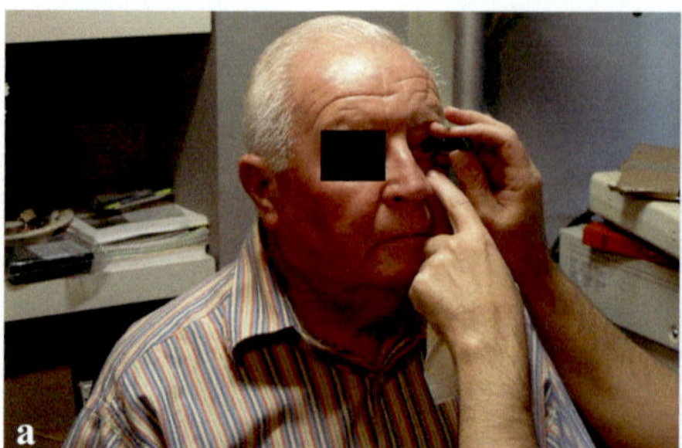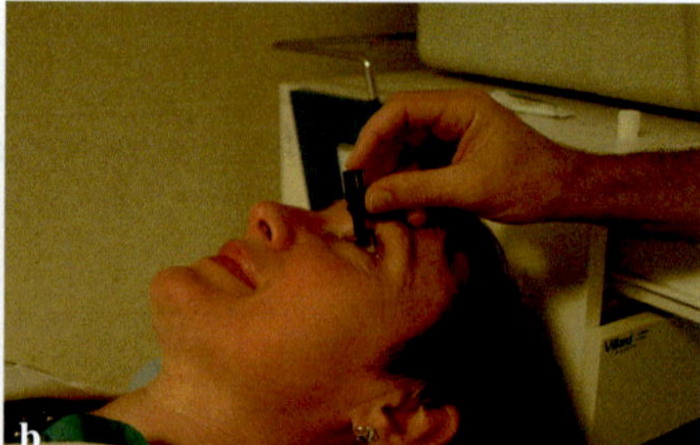

**Fig. 10.5 A-mode biometry, contact method. a**: In a seated patient; **b**: In a recumbent patient. It is obvious that when the patient is seated, the comfort of the examiner is "marginal", which tends to lead to less accurate measurements

### 10.4.1.2 Immersion A-Mode (Fig. 10.7)

An immersion cup, again placed after topical anesthesia, is filled with saline or liquid gel (Goniosol®), thereby ensuring the coupling [5]. Regardless of the method, the patient looks directly at a light inside the probe with their examined eye, or better yet, a point on the ceiling or on a wall with the contralateral eye. The measurements are taken by using manual mode, whereby the operator saves the image, analysis, and backup and then makes several other measurements, or in automatic mode, whereby the operator must analyze the results at the end of the X measurements.

How to recognize the optic nerve, which manifests on echograms by an acoustic vacuum behind the parietal echo, is useful. Once spotted, the operator can simply tilt the probe slightly toward the temporal region by approximately 15° in order to reach the macula.

### 10.4.1.3 Advantages and Disadvantages

Contact Method

The contact method is probably the most used, requiring little investment both in terms of equipment (A-mode biometer), premises (the measurements can be carried out in a consultation room), and time requirements (no need to place the patient in a recumbent position) (Fig. 10.5). Moreover, the method has appeal and seems reliable at first glance. Manufacturers have integrated aids into their machines: the modes for capture and recording of echograms can be automated, and the placement of markers and measurements is also automatic. A dozen measurements can be made in just 2–3 s, thus giving the impression of having fulfilled one of the quality criteria of a good biometry. However, most often, the method does not involve a dozen different measurements but rather repeats the same measurement 10 times in a row.

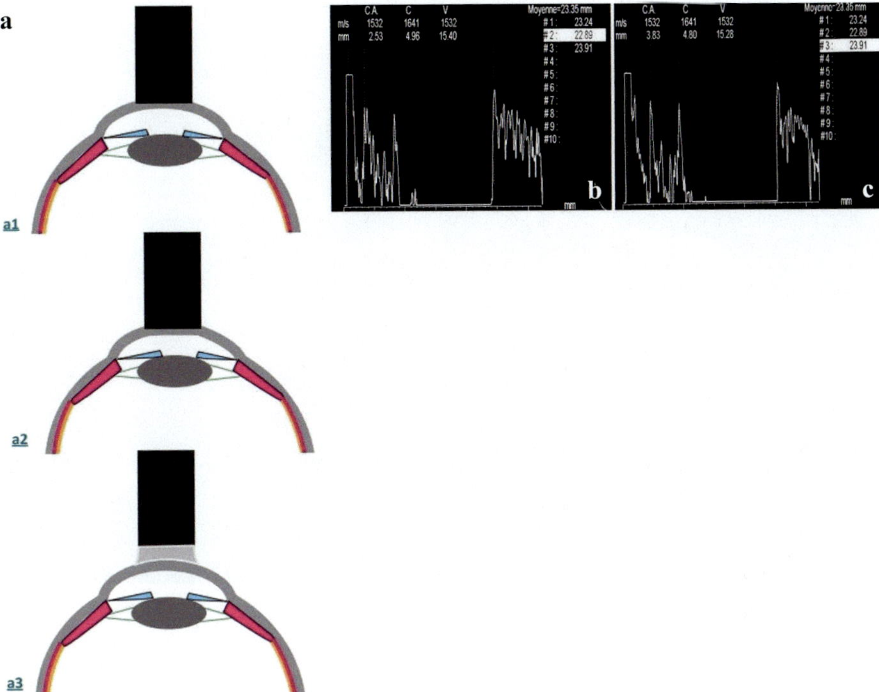

**Fig. 10.6  Contact problems. a**: Schematic showing (**a1**) the ideal contact between the probe and the cornea, (**a2**) too much contact, resulting in depression of the cornea, a decrease in the depth of the anterior chamber and the total axial length, (**a3**) insufficient contact related to a tear meniscus responsible for an increase in the depth of the anterior chamber and the total axial length. When the contact is ideal, anterior chamber = 3.02 mm/lens = 4.88 mm/vitreous = 15.34 mm/total axial length = 23.24 mm. **b**: A-mode biometry, with too much contact pressure: anterior chamber = 2.53 mm/lens = 4.96 mm/vitreous = 15 mm/total axial length = 22.89 mm. **c**: A-mode biometry in the same patient with insufficient contact: anterior chamber = 3.83 mm/lens = 4.80 mm/vitreous = 15.28 mm/total axial length = 23.91 mm. In both cases, the thickness of the lens, which is very echogenic, and the length of the vitreous are concordant, but the anterior chamber is very reduced in **b** and exaggerated in **c**. It is only the comparison of several measurements made successively by removal of the probe from the eye between each measurement that allows for eliminating the erroneous measurements. Note that for a trained eye, in absolute terms, the ultrasound **c** is reason to doubt the measurement because there are plenty of artifacts in the anterior chamber due to the poor contact between the probe and the cornea

Best practice is for the operator to lift the probe off the corneal contact between each measurement. **Therefore, the operator must remember this with the automatic acquisition mode, thus making the manual acquisition mode preferable.**

In addition to this shortcoming, which can readily be avoided with a bit of care, the problem with contact mode remains the pressure exerted by the operator:

Excessive pressure, in addition to the risk of abrasion, leads to depression of the cornea, a decrease in the anterior chamber depth and hence a shortening of the axial length. This would lead to an IOL being placed that is too powerful, resulting in myopia in the patient.

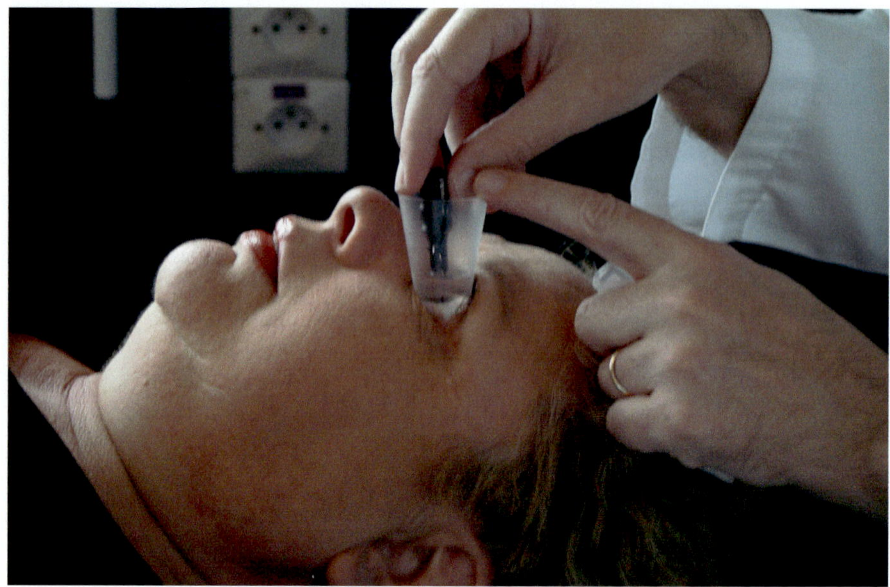

**Fig. 10.7 A-mode biometry**: immersion technique

However, if the contact is made by interposition of an excessive meniscus of tears or eye drops, the length of the eye will be artificially lengthened, and the IOL power will be less than the emmetropic power (Fig. 10.6), which would render the patient farsighted.

The study of the measurements obtained allows for visualizing this error: The variation in length in case of an error due to incorrect pressure will only affect the measurement C + CA, with the thicknesses of the lens and the lengths of the vitreous being perfectly reproducible. However, once the technique is mastered, the pressure exerted will remain identical, and analysis of the results will allow improvement of the postoperative refractive accuracy. This analysis of postoperative results is carried out on 50 consecutive files and must be done on a yearly basis. To overcome this issue, A-mode biometric probes are sometimes mounted on applanation tonometer supports or on a spring-loaded system to control the amount of pressure applied.

Immersion Method (Fig. 10.7)

Performing the immersion method requires placing the patient in a supine position [6]. These conditions are similar to those experienced when performing a B-mode guided biometry, unless a small handpiece, such as those sold by some manufacturers, is used [6, 7]. The main advantage of immersion is that it overcomes the problems related to corneal pressure. The disadvantages are the need to place the patient in a recumbent position and to learn to master a somewhat discreetly trickier technique.

With the probe at a distance from the corneal apex, achieving alignment with the visual axis is more difficult and requires being more thorough. Despite its strengths, its use remains limited.

## *10.4.2   B-Mode-Guided Biometry Method [4]*

### 10.4.2.1   Principle

Performing a cross-section in B-mode allows for visualizing the foveolar region. A control vector (CV) is generated on this section that follows a line that passes through the visual axis. Thus, the distances necessary for the calculation of the IOL power are perfectly individualized.

### 10.4.2.2   Implementation (Fig. 10.8, see Figs. 7.1 and 7.2)

In the space of the palpebral fissure, after optional placement of a drop of local anesthetic, and, a bead of tear gel (carbomer) is placed on the cornea, which is

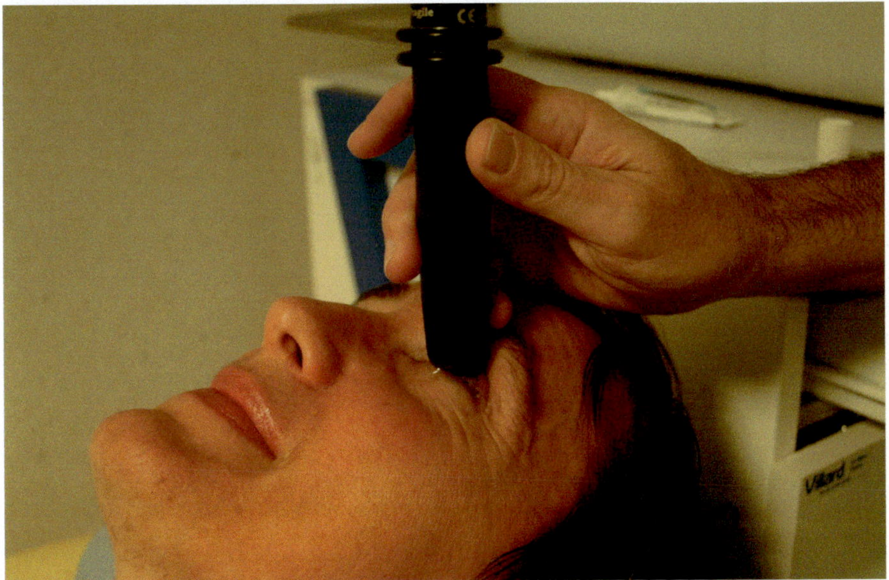

**Fig. 10.8  B-mode guided biometry with simplified immersion** [4], **without contact or cup**. In anxious or uncooperative patients, to keep the palpebral fissure open, the operator can hold the eyelids with the index and middle finger of the hand that does not hold the probe, or hold the upper eyelid and ask the patient to hold the lower eyelid

sufficient to ensure ultrasound coupling and to keep the probe off the cornea. To limit blinking, the eyelids should be held gently but firmly with the index and middle fingers of the hand that does not hold the probe The B-mode probe is placed transversely. Because of the position of the macular region, the operator must perform a discreet rotation of the outer part of the probe downward by 15° so that this cross-section passes through the optic disc and foveola. Acquisition of this section is performed in B + CV (cross vector) mode, which allows to position on the screen a line that will coincide with the visual axis: the image is frozen when this line is correctly positioned:

- at the front on the corneal apex (the presentation of the cornea can sometimes result in two small circular arcs with anterior paradoxical concavity),
- at the back on the foveola (Fig. 10.9).

Here again, these various acquisitions must be made in "manual" mode, and at least three sections must be obtained with concordant measurements (SD < 0.1). These acquisitions are facilitated by the ability of current devices to save sequences and to retain only a particular selected section.

One should not hesitate to replenish the bead of gel between each acquisition.

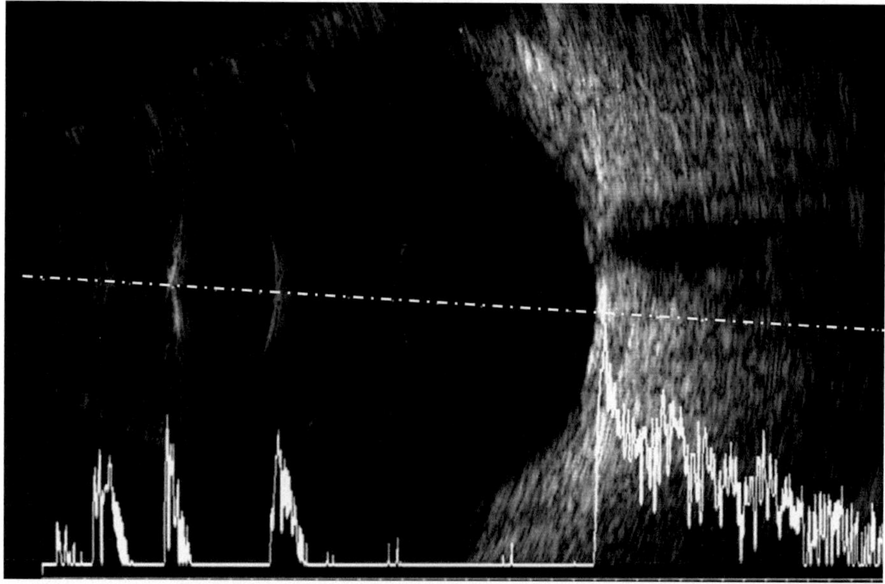

**Fig. 10.9 B-mode guided biometry of a left eye**: results. A B-mode axial section superimposed with A-mode passing through the optical axis (dotted line), passing through the center of the cornea and the foveola, temporal (so below for the left eye) to the optic disc. Note the existence of anechoic gel (immersion) in front of the cornea, which has an anterior "paradoxical" concavity with this 10-MHz probe related to the arciform scanning of the crystal of the mechanical probe

### 10.4.2.3   Result

From each section, A-mode can be reconstructed, which allows the different peaks and interfaces to be discerned and the biometric values to be obtained.

### 10.4.2.4   Advantages and Disadvantages

- The method simplifies the understanding of the principles of a good measurement by showing the various intraocular structures more readily than with A-mode alone.
- Intra- and inter-examiner reproducibility is significantly improved.
- Teaching the biometric technique is greatly facilitated, and the learning time is reduced.
- In the case of multiple intravitreal echoes (e.g., asteroid hyalosis), this is the only method that can readily provide reliable measurements.
- The risks of error are limited: the authors showed that the reproducibility of the measurements was much better, both for myopic, emmetropic and hyperopic eyes, and that the measurements were more accurate than with the A-mode method, the deviation from the desired postoperative refraction being smaller, again both for myopic, emmetropic and hyperopic eyes.
- However, the procedure takes longer, which also requires placing the patient in a recumbent position.

## 10.5   Special Cases

### 10.5.1   According to Age

- In neonates and infants, the eye measures approximately 17.2 mm at birth. It grows very rapidly during the first 3 months and still relatively fast during the first year, when it measures approximately 20 mm. However, a thorough biometric assessment should be performed in case of congenital cataracts, especially if implantation is considered, for the calculation of the IOL power and for the detection of associated abnormalities, which are more frequent in cases of microphthalmia.
- In children, a size of 22.5–23 mm is obtained at approximately 3 years of age, with the eye growing more slowly after the first year [8, 9] until 5 years of age, when it reaches a dimension closer to its final size.
- In adults, axial length is considered to be 23–24 mm for emmetropic eyes.

However, we must not forget that emmetropia is a function of the axial length as well as the keratometry value, which varies from 41 to 45 dpt (47 in children) and the power of the lens (from 18 to 22 dpt in adults, 38 dpt to 42 dpt in young children).

## 10.5.2 According to the Refraction

### 10.5.2.1 Myopia

Myopia is usually axial, resulting from an abnormal increase of the axial length. Myopia is often accompanied by deformation of the eyeball, whose shape shift from spherical to ± conical. There may or may not be associated localized parietal deformities (staphylomas), in connection with scleral thinning. These staphylomas can be peripheral, relatively anterior, or most often localized at the posterior pole, temporal, nasal, inferior to the optic disc, or may sometimes have a complex morphology [10].

In automated A-mode, the measurement is often performed at the more posterior part of this depression. If the staphyloma is located on the nasal side of the optic disc, or if the slope encompasses the macular region temporally, the echo of the macula will be weak, in relation to the angle of the macular plane with respect to the visual axis, and this echo may not be retained as significant by the machine.

B-mode guided biometry of such eyes solve this shortcoming because measurement errors in nearsighted people are mainly angulation errors. However, there are complex posterior staphylomas, for which even B-mode-guided biometry does not allow for determining the exact location of the fovea, which moreover is sometimes eccentric.

### 10.5.2.2 Hyperopia

Hyperopia is characterized by a shorter-than-average globe but with a mostly harmonious morphology, and biometric data are usually readily obtained.

However, a few issues should be highlighted:

- when the anterior chamber is very shallow, some machines have difficulty accepting the values, and in automatic acquisition mode, the operator must switch to manual or semi-manual mode, which, in any case, should always be preferred.
- errors in farsighted individuals are mainly errors in regard to the applied pressure and errors regarding the position of the markers, especially at the lens level.

## 10.5.3 Depending on the Pathology

### 10.5.3.1 Aphakia

Perpendicularity is not easy to assert in A-mode because of the absence of any lenticular peaks, so again it is best to use the B-mode guided technique. The velocity of ultrasound propagation in the aqueous and vitreous humor is 1532 m/s. The lens should not be taken into account: the measurement peaks that correspond to it are superimposed.

### 10.5.3.2 Pseudophakia

In the event of an IOL change, A-mode biometry is particularly difficult. The operator must first recognize the type of IOL that has been placed. It is useful to use B-mode at 10 MHz but also at 25 MHz for this (see Fig. 8.3) [11], because, unfortunately, the data for the placed IOL are not always available. Then, the ultrasound velocity in the IOL must be adapted (generally easy to set in modern biometers) and the positioning of the peaks of the lens verified to be in accordance with the average thickness of the same type of intraocular lens [6].

- **Polymethylmethacrylate (PMMA) IOLs**: the average thickness is close to 0.7 mm and the ultrasound velocity is 2718 m/s.
- **Silicone IOLs**: the average thickness is close to 1.3 mm and the ultrasound velocity is 1050 m/s.
- **Acrylic IOLs**: the average thickness is close to 0.8 mm and the ultrasound velocity is 1946 m/s.

With recent devices, IOL changes have been accounted for, and the operator can simply position the peaks corresponding to the lens on the anterior and posterior sides of the lens by selecting the material corresponding to it. Therefore, it is important to know how to recognize the material of the intraocular lenses.

PMMA IOLs induce major repetition artifacts that interfere with analysis of the posterior segment behind the IOL. Acrylic IOLs generate smaller, fewer, and less troublesome artifacts (see Fig. 6.1). Silicone IOLs appear thicker because the velocity of propagation is lower, and they cause a shadow that decreases the brightness of the echoes of the posterior pole (see Fig. 8.3).

### 10.5.3.3 Phakic Eye with a Refractive IOL (pIOL)

A personalized empirical method consists of positioning the anterior lenticular peak on the IOL, the posterior peak on the posterior capsule, and adding 0.1 mm to the axial length obtained. Indeed, this type of IOL, very thin in the center, has little influence on the axial length. However, the accuracy of this method is far from the greater accuracy of the IOLMaster®, even when corrective factors are not added.

Of note, the presence of these refractive pIOLs in an eye affects the axial length measurement in A-mode. They generate ultrasound reverberations that result in a succession of echoes projected between the posterior side of the IOL and the posterior wall of the globe, rendering analysis of ultrasound in A-mode very difficult, if not impossible. This phenomenon is pronounced with PMMA IOLs and is less with silicone and collamer (implantable collamer lens) IOLs. However, the latter cause absorption of the ultrasound signal that disrupts recognition of the vitreoretinal interface. Only B-mode–guided biometry can accurately locate the position of the posterior wall where the peak corresponding to this interface must be positioned.

#### 10.5.3.4 Intravitreal Silicone

The posterior segment is sometimes filled with silicone oil to treat complex retinal detachments. Some authors have proposed a technique involving A-mode [12]. Indeed, during the measurements performed with the patient in a dorsal recumbent position, the silicone bubble, which rarely completely occupies the posterior segment, floats, and there is most often a space filled with aqueous humor between its posterior surface and the posterior wall. (The opposite phenomenon is observed in the case of heavy silicone). The propagation velocity of ultrasound in silicone oil is 940 m/s. This relative decrease in velocity leads to an apparent lengthening of the globe. If the posterior interface of the silicone bubble can be clearly seen, the anterior segment should be measured the conventional way, and then the distance of the silicone bubble with a speed of 940 m/s and the space behind the bubble with a speed of 1532 m/s is added (see Fig. 6.15c) [13]. However, silicone oil also disrupts the propagation of ultrasound (dispersion), and recognizing this posterior interface is often impossible. In addition, in case of a high degree myopia, given the low velocity of ultrasound in silicone, the eyeball may not entirely fit on the ultrasound screen. Very often, the measurements cannot be reliable, so measurement by helical CT scanner (CT) can then represent a good option [14]. For this method, a biometry of the contralateral eye is first performed; then, one verify that the measurement of the contralateral eye are identical by ultrasound and by CT; then the affected eye is measured on the optimal CT scan section, taking the precaution of positioning the markers in the same way as for the contralateral eye (Fig. 10.10). As long as the lenticular opacity is not too dense, biometry by interferometry can also be considered. The use of corneal topography as the basis for the keratometry is preferable.

#### 10.5.3.5 Melanoma and Age-Related Macular Degeneration

Measurement of the axial length is used by radiotherapists to model the eyeball and thus define the therapeutic protocol. The technique is standard if the melanoma is at a distance from the macular region. If it is located at the posterior pole, this measurement can only be achieved by B-mode guided biometry: One must know how to recognize the double scleral peak and the estimated position of the normal retina to best estimate the axial length. This also applies in case of maculopathy, where placement of an IOL can be considered, for example in case of non-progressing exudative age-related macular degeneration to improve ambulatory peripheral vision.

#### 10.5.3.6 Risk of Angle-Closure Glaucoma (ACG)

Measurement of the depth of the anterior chamber is one of the predictive measures of the risk of acute primary angle closure. Although the best method for studying this risk remains very high-frequency ultrasound) (see Chap. 11), 10 MHz biometry allows this depth to be measured with a reasonable accuracy, keeping in mind the

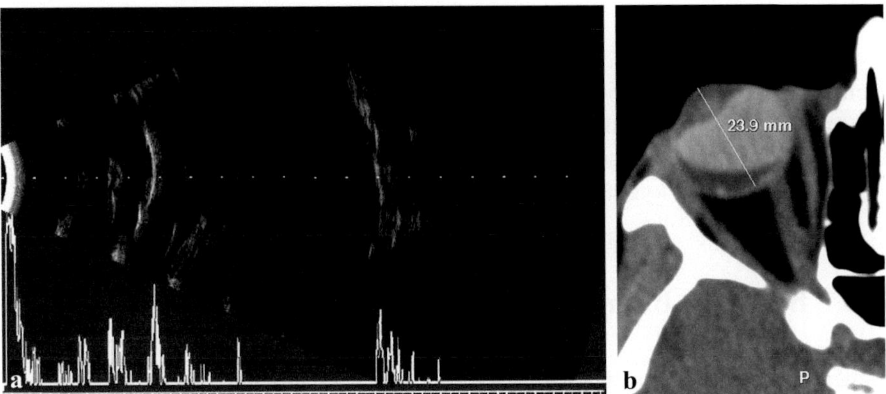

**Fig. 10.10   Biometry of a right eye with an intraocular silicone bubble. a**: B-mode guided biometry; **b**: CT Scanner, axial section. The disturbances of the ultrasound beam by the silicone bubble impede finding the posterior interface of the silicone bubble and recognition of the posterior pole (optic disc, optic nerve, and macula) by ultrasound, while they are seen perfectly well by a scan. However, the anterior segment is better visualized using ultrasound (lenticular echoes and densification of the posterior lens capsule)

precautions described above, and it would be a shame not to use it. For the record, the risk for a depth of 2.0–2.1 mm is 3% but increases to 12% for a depth of 1.8–1.9 mm, 36% for a depth of 1.6–1.7 mm, and 100% for a depth of 1.1–1.3 mm [15].

### 10.5.3.7   Hypotonic Eye

Using the contact method, the existence of hypotonia, if substantial, can lead to a reduction in the axial length, by corneal deformation. The usual pressure would indeed be too important relative to the counter-pressure exerted by the hypotonic globe. Immersion A-mode or B-mode guided biometry (which uses simplified immersion) counteracts this disadvantage.

### 10.5.3.8   Eye Trauma

In case of a penetrating trauma, the axial length can be measured. However, one should be aware of infectious risks and pressure, with the possibility of the Seidel phenomenon and hypotonia. Therefore, B-mode guided biometry is to be preferred.

## 10.6  Pachymetry

Pachymetry uses single-purpose devices to measure the corneal thickness. The measurement is performed in contact mode on a dozen central points. It is mainly used before refractive surgery. To increase the use of tonometers for measurements, its use in glaucoma is a consideration, for which the central measurement is sufficient.


## 10.7  Biometry by Interferometry

Rather than an ultrasound beam, this method uses a 780 nm light beam. Developed by Haigis [16] and marketed by Zeiss as the original model under the name IOLMaster®, it offers many advantages: easy to perform and measurements resembling those taken with a refractometer: the patient sitting in front of the device looks at a target inside an aiming system. The measurement does not require contact, and the measurements are automatic (keratometry value and axial length).

The results are excellent. Keratometry seems to compensate for the fact that the axial lengths are slightly increased by the reflection on the pigment epithelium and not on the vitreoretinal interface.

However, in approximately 10% of cases, this technique fails:

- Patient unable to achieve a steady gaze (cooperation), tremor, severe respiratory failure;
- Nystagmus, serious problems with tears or the cornea;
- Dense cataract, palpebral abnormalities;
- Vitreous hemorrhage, synchysis scintillans and asteroid hyalosis, intraocular membranes, maculopathies, and retinal detachment.

Since then, new devices have been developed and provide the accuracy of an optical measurement for biometry. Finally, the latest generation of optical biometers combine the advantages of optical biometers and the precision of a "swept-source" device.

> Of note, the A constants of the IOLs are refined by the manufacturers according to the technology used.

## 10.8  Formulas for Calculating the Power of an Intraocular Lens (IOL)

The power of the artificial lens depends on three factors:

- The power of the cornea
- The precise position of the IOL in the eye
- The axial length.

The power of the cornea and the axial length are determined by oculometry. The position of the IOL in the operated eye is determined by theoretical calculations and statistical data. The first IOL had to be explanted because of an error in the evaluation of its power [17].

**Optics reminder**: An artificial lens, if placed in a position more anterior than that of the natural lens, must have a lower power than that of the latter. This more anterior position, by lengthening the focal length image, generates a retinal image larger than that which would have formed in the same contralateral eye.

Several methods have been used to determine the power of a lens.

### 10.8.1  Historical Method, Known as the 1.25-dpt Correction [6]

Before the days of ultrasound biometry, calculation of the emmetropizing IOL was based on the only available data: anterior refraction. Starting with a lens power thought to be fixed and arbitrarily compensated by an IOL with standard power, the calculation adjusted this value by 1.25 times the anterior refraction:

$$\text{Emmetropizing P} = \text{Standard P} - 1.25 \text{ anterior refraction}$$

where standard P = 17 dpt for an anterior chamber IOL, 18 dpt for an iris-fixated IOL, and 19.5 dpt for a posterior chamber IOL.

Example: a myopic eye of − 2 dpt would have its preoperative ametropia restored by a posterior chamber IOL with a power of 19.5 dpt. Myopia would be corrected by placing an IOL of $19.5 - (2 \times 1.25) = 17$ dpt etc.

This coarse and very approximate method led to frequent errors because it ignored the refractive variations induced by cataracts and it did not take into account the extreme variability of the lens power. We nevertheless mention this empirical and imperfect rule here because it allows for rapid evaluation of a calculation that yields a surprising result.

Many formulas can be used to calculate the power of an intraocular lens: In the beginning, at the end of the 1960s, two approaches existed, a theoretical approach and a more pragmatic one.

## 10.8.2 The First-Generation Theoretical Formulas

Fyodorov [18] in 1967, then Colenbrander [19], Binkhorst [20], Thijssen [21], and Van der Heijde [22] developed these first theoretical formulas that used data from ocular biometry. The formulas are all based on optical principles applied to simplified eyes for thin lenses:

By knowing the convergence power of the cornea and the axial length, the power of the lens necessary to focus the image on the retina can be deduced.

They can all be summarized by the following algebraic formula:

$$P = (n\,/l - C) - [(n - K)/(n - KC)]$$

where n represents the refractive index of aqueous humor and vitreous; l, the axial length; K, the power of the curvature of the cornea in diopters; and C, the estimated depth of the anterior chamber postoperatively [3].

Although these formulas are of intellectual interest, their main shortcoming was the need for calculations that at the time were not straightforward because microprocessors were not ubiquitous. This is what led to the success of the so-called regression methods.

## 10.8.3 Regression Formulas

These formulas are based on the a posteriori statistical analysis of the results of the refraction of a large cohort of pseudophakic patients, to determine the constants necessary to relate the power of the emmetropizing IOL to readily measurable factors: keratometry value and axial length.

### 10.8.3.1 The SRK Formula

The pooling of several studies results gave rise in 1980 to the SRK formula [23], named after three ophthalmic surgeons Sanders, Retzlaff, and Kraff. In this formula, a linear relationship unites the power of the emmetropizing intraocular lens (IOL) to the main biometric parameters:

$$P = A - 2.5\,L - 0.9\,K$$

A is a constant that accounts for the geometry and position of the IOL, which is greater as the IOL has a more posterior position: approximately 115 for an anterior chamber IOL, and in the order of 119 for a posterior chamber IOL placed in the capsular bag.

L is the axial length measured in mm, and K is the value of the mean keratometry, expressed in diopters.

Results: The SRK formula and the theoretical formulas largely provide the same results when the eyes are 22.5–24 mm long. Other than these values, the results differ greatly. For hyperopic eyes, the SRK formula underestimates the power of the IOL, resulting in hyperopia in the patient. Conversely, for myopic eyes, the power of the IOL is too strong, resulting in myopia.

An adaptation by the authors resulted in the SRK II formula.

### 10.8.3.2   The SRK II Formula [24]

$$P = A - 2.5\,L - 0.9\,K + C$$

where:
  $C = +3$ if $L < 20$ mm,
  $C = +2$ if $L = 20 - 21$ mm,
  $C = +1$ if $L = 21 - 22$ mm,
  $C = -0.5$ if $L > 24$ mm, and
  $C = -1.5$ if $L > 26$ mm.

## 10.8.4   *The Latest Generation of Theoretical Formulas [25]*

The integration of computing modules of sufficient power into biometers and/or ultrasound devices has led to generalizing the use of theoretical formulas, allowing for the use of more sophisticated formulas, adapted to new materials and architectures and to the increased requirements of obtaining emmetropia, particularly with regard to multifocal IOLs. All sonographers agree that *one or more of these latest-generation formulas should be used today and that regression formulas should no longer be used.*

### 10.8.4.1   SRK/Theoretical (SRK/T) Formula [23]

The same authors have established their new formula SRK/T (Fig. 10.11). This formula combines the elements of the theoretical optical formula of Hoffer-Collenbrander and Binkhorst with estimation of the physiological iris plane and the use of A constants as determinants of IOLs. It also takes into account the depth

## SRK/T Formula

$$P_{ame} = \frac{1336 \text{ x } [(1.336 \text{ x } r) - (1/3 \text{ x LOPT}] - 0.001 \text{ x ame x } [V \text{ x } (1{,}336 \text{ x } r - 1/3 \text{ x LOPT}) + \text{LOPT x } r)]}{(\text{LOPT} - \text{ACD}) \text{ x } [(1.336 \text{ x } r) - 1/3 \text{ x ACD})] - 0.001 \text{ x ame x } [V \text{ x } (\{1.336 \text{ x } r\} - \{1/3 \text{ x ACD}\}) + \text{ACD x } r)]}$$

$r = 337.5 / K_m$
$n_a = 1.336, n_c ml = 0.333$
   if AL $\leq$ 24.4
      LOPT $= AL + $ Retthick
      Retthick $= 0.65696 - 0.02029 \text{ x AL}$
   if AL $\leq$ 24.4
      LOPT $= Al_{cor} + $ Retthick
      Retthick $= 0.65696 - 0.02029 \text{ x } Al_{cor}$
$Al_{cor} = 3{,}446 + 1.716 AL - 0.0237 \text{xALxAL}$
$V = 12$

**Fig. 10.11 SRK/T formula**

of the postoperative anterior chamber, the refractive index of the cornea, and the thickness of the retina.

### 10.8.4.2 Holladay Formula [26]

This formula is also widely used (Fig. 10.12). It integrates the position of the IOL in the eye. This is determined by adding the value of the anatomical anterior chamber depth (the space between the cornea and the iris plane in the aphakic eye) and the distance from the anterior iris plane to the optical plane of the IOL. This constitutes the surgeon factor "sf". Therefore, the surgeon can customize this formula by altering this factor according to the statistical analysis of their personal postoperative results.

### 10.8.4.3 Other Formulas

Other formulas are used, such as that of Shammas [27], which some use more readily for hyperopic eyes, as well as that of Hoffer [28] (Fig. 10.13).

More recently, Haigis [25] (Fig. 10.14) and Olsen [29] developed formulas based on the axial length and also the depth of the anterior chamber and the thickness of the lens (for Olsen's formula). These parameters were also introduced into Holladay's second-generation formula.

Finally, with a calculation algorithm accessible on the Asia Pacific Association of Cataract and Refractive Surgeons website (Fig. 10.15), Barrett's Universal II formula can be used, which appears to provide extremely accurate results, for all types of eyes [30–32], but has, unfortunately, not been published. This Australian surgeon from

---

$$\text{Holladay 1 Formula}$$

$$P_{ref} = \frac{1336\ (1.336R\text{-}1/3Lh - 0.001\ Ref\ [V(1.336R - 1/3Lh) + LhR]}{(Lh - ACD - SF)\ (1.336R - 1/3(ACD+SF) - 0/001Ref\ [V(1.336R - 1/3(ACD+SF) + (ACD + SF)R]}$$

R = 337.5 / K$_m$ (dpt)
Ref = desired refraction, for emmetropia Ref = 0
Lh = AL +0.2 (mm)
SF = (A x 0.5663) – 65.60
ACD = 0.56 + Rag – [SQRT (Rag$^2$ – AG$^2$/4)]
Rag = R outside if R < 7mm, then Rag = 7mm
AG = 0.5333AL outside if AG>13.5 then AG = 13.5
V = 12mm

---

**Fig. 10.12 Holladay 1 Formula**

---

$$\text{Hoffer Q Formula}$$

**If AL<23**

$$P_{Rx} = [1336\ /(AL - P_{acd} - 0.05] - [1.336\ /\ [(1.336\ /K+R) - (P_{acd} + 0.05)/1000]]$$

Pacd = ACD + 0.3(AL - 23.5) + (tanK)2 + 0.1 (23.5 - LA)2 tan [0.1 (28-AL)2] - 0.99166

But if AL < 18.5 →AL = 18.5
ACD = (SF + 3.595) /0.9704
SF = (A x 0.5663) – 65.60

Rx = Desired postoperative ametropia
If Rx = -1 → R = -0.988
If Rx = +1 → R = 1.012

---

**Fig. 10.13 Hoffer Q Formula**

the Perth region has also provided access to the Barrett Toric Calculator (Fig. 10.16) on the American Society of Cataract and Refractive Surgery (ASCRS) website.

For these formulas, when the parameter of the depth of the anterior chamber is needed, in case of an aphakic or pseudophakic eye, the measurements at the time the eye was phakic need to be found. If this is not possible, the depth of the anterior chamber of the contralateral eye can be used, or if need be, one can apply arbitrary values: 2.7 mm for small eyes, 3.1 mm for normal eyes, and 3.5 mm for long eyes.

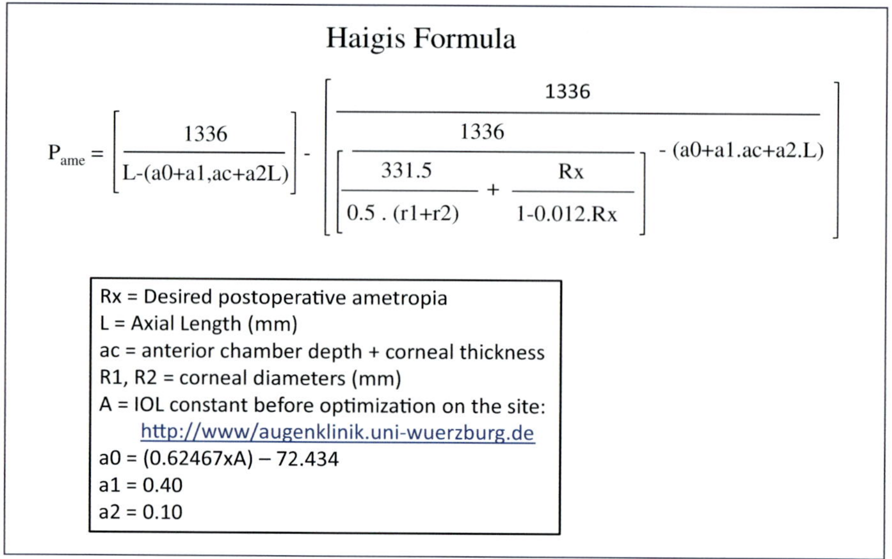



$$P_{ame} = \left[ \frac{1336}{L-(a0+a1,ac+a2L)} \right] - \left[ \frac{1336}{\dfrac{1336}{\dfrac{331.5}{0.5 \cdot (r1+r2)} + \dfrac{Rx}{1-0.012.Rx}}} - (a0+a1.ac+a2.L) \right]$$

**Fig. 10.14 Haigis Formula**



**Fig. 10.15 Barrett Universal II Calculator**. The parameters allowing the calculation are axial length, keratometry in diopters (note that a refractive index of 1.3375 or 1.332 can be selected), the measurement of the depth of the anterior optical chamber, and the refraction

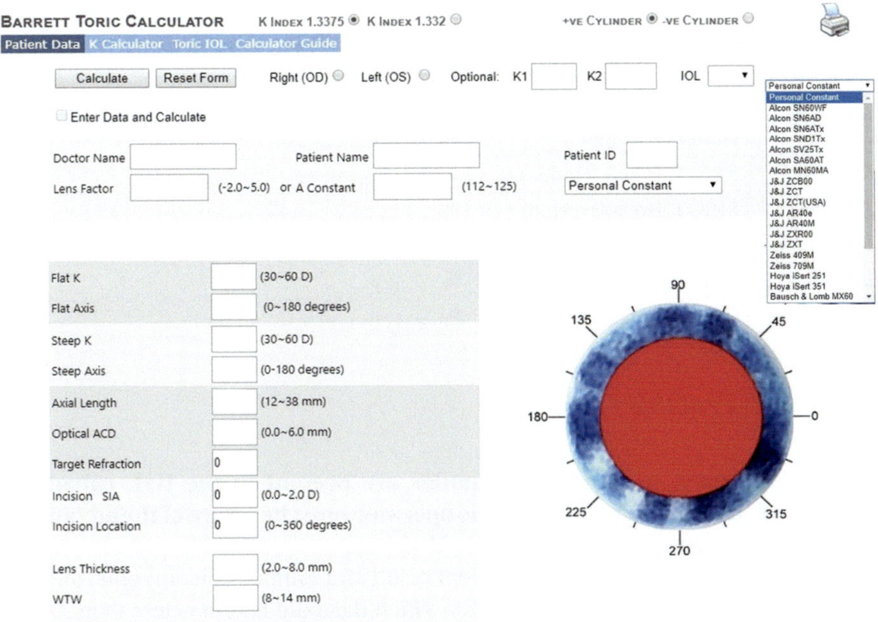

**Fig. 10.16  Barrett Toric Calculator**. Note that it can be entered as a crystalline factor, either a personal constant or a constant associated by the laboratory, with the main toric IOLs used. In addition, instead of average keratometry values, the powers in diopter of the flattest and steepest meridians of the cornea need to be entered

### 10.8.4.4  Calculation for Emmetropizing IOLs

Current biometers provide the IOL powers for emmetropia and also for a whole series of ametropias. Otherwise, the power of the measured keratometry value can be altered by adding the power of the desired ametropia (e.g., if the keratometry value is 42 dpt and the desired residual ametropia is − 1 dpt, one can enter 41 dpt in the calculation formulas). However, the results are approximate. Similarly, ametropia can be estimated according to the theoretical emmetropizing IOL and the one to be installed. It is equal to two-thirds of the difference between the two: 2/3 (Pe − Pp).

### 10.8.4.5  Calculation for Iseiconizing IOLs

The goal is to calculate the IOL power that will provide the same retinal size image as that of the other eye. The Mawas curves [33], which have the ametropia on the abscissa and the magnifications induced by the different types of lens correction or IOL on the ordinate, allow for predicting and adapting the IOL calculation to enhance the comfort with binocular vision.

**Table 10.2** Proposed choices of theoretical formulas to be used as a function of axial length to account for the optimal efficiency of each formula

| Axial length | Average of the formulas | Powers to be provided, the surgeon/patient couple chooses |
|---|---|---|
| < 22 | Hoffer Q, Haigis | $P_E$, $P_{-1}$, $P_{+1}$ |
| 22–22.8 | SRK-T, Haigis, Hoffer Q | $P_E$, $P_{-1}$, $P_{+1}$ |
| 22.8–24.5 | SRK-T, Holladay, Hoffer Q | $P_E$ |
| 24.5–26 | Haigis, Holladay | $P_E$, $P_{-1}$ |
| 26–30 | SRK-T, Haigis | $P_E$, $P_{-1}$, $P_{-3}$ |
| ≥ 30 | SRK-T, Haigis | $P_E$, $P_{-1}$, $P_{-3}$, $P_{-5}$ |

## *10.8.5   In Practice*

**Many of the most widely used formulas are present in the IOL calculation program of current biometers, and the operator must be aware of the advantages and disadvantages of each to optimize their use.**

The SRK/T formula provides excellent results for emmetropic, myopic, and very nearsighted eyes. For farsighted eyes, for which the axial length is less than 22 mm, the formulas of Haigis and Hoffer Q appear to be more accurate. Therefore, the following master plan can be proposed (Table 10.2), which takes into account the recommendations of the Royal Society of Ophthalmology and of Haigis.

## *10.8.6   Factors Influencing Calculation Power of the IOL*

### 10.8.6.1   Importance of the Keratometry Value on the Result

A keratometry measurement error of 0.1 mm results in a 0.5 dpt error in postoperative refraction. The surgical procedure does not influence the average keratometry value and, by extension, the postoperative spherical equivalent. The conversion factor between the radius of curvature of the cornea (in mm) and the power of the cornea (in diopters) is slightly variable, depending on the device used (keratometers and biometers). In addition, the refractive index of the cornea can also vary according to the formulas, most using a value of 1.3375. Therefore, the operator must strive to always work in the same manner and understand the influence of these parameters on postoperative results. Because keratometers measure radii of curvature, keeping measurements in millimeters makes sense and allows standardization and easier comparison of different formulas. Also, the operator must be wary of averages, which are generally not the same between automatic keratometers and biometers Here again, inserting the two measurements, up to the second decimal place, is preferable.

**Table 10.3** The "10 golden rules" for optimizing biometry

| 1 | Avoid A-mode contact technique |
|---|---|
| 2 | The optical biometer is the reference (but if impossible, B-mode guided) |
| 3 | Verify the consistency of the measurements (axial length, keratometry [K]) |
| 4 | Determine the patient's mean axial length (SD < 0.10) on at least three concordant measurements |
| 5 | Preferably use K values in millimeters |
| 6 | Keep in mind contact-lens wearers |
| 7 | Use optimized A constants |
| 8 | Avoid using the SRK II formula |
| 9 | Tailor the formula to the axial length (and K) |
| 10 | Be cognizant of the degree of accuracy of biometry |

**In conclusion,** 10 logical rules can be proposed to optimize the biometry (Table 10.3).

### 10.8.6.2  The Special Case of Toric IOLs

The placement of a toric IOL provides even better refractive results than with a monofocal IOL [34]. In addition, regular corneal astigmatism can frequently (25%) be compensated by toric implantation by positioning the markers of the IOL according to the most arched corneal axis [35].

The spherical power calculation complies with the usual rules of calculation; but at least two elements strongly determine the accuracy of toricity: these are the total corneal power, including the power of the anterior surface of the cornea and also the posterior surface and the effective lens position (ELP), a point in common with aspherical monofocal IOLs, fitting into all the formulas of the latest generation.

Regarding the total corneal power, we can now measure it (using optical coherence tomography [OCT] or Scheimpflug technologies) or estimate it (using nomograms: Baylor, Goggin, etc.) with several formulas using ray tracing as the mathematical tool to improve its accuracy, as in Olsen's formula for example.

The influence of the ELP here is two-fold since it can affect both the accuracy of the spherical power and the toric power because a toric lens compensates for the cylindrical power of the cornea. To minimize errors, Han Bor Fam proposed a meridional analysis, now integrated into all algorithms and universally accepted [36].

However, the operator must be thorough (because an error of 1 degree in the measurement leads to a decrease in the cylindrical correction of 3.3%, on average!). Once the measurements have been made, the values must be entered into an algorithm that is provided online by several laboratories (Fig. 10.16) [37]. In addition, the surgical technique, and in particular the size and location of the incision, are determinants to recognize and minimize astigmatism.

### 10.8.6.3 The Special Case of Contact Lens Wearers

In these cases, keratometry must be performed after a certain period of time of not wearing contact lenses because they can modify the corneal curvature. The time limit is 3 days for hydrophilic soft lenses and at least 1 week for rigid lenses.

### 10.8.6.4 Special Cases When Keratometry is not Possible

Sometimes the measurement is not possible, for example, in case of corneal scarring, edema, or keratoconus: by default, the keratometry value of the contralateral eye is taken, although an arbitrarily chosen value of 43.5 dpt can also be selected (this should be specified in the report).This arbitrary value can be 44.5 dpt in case of hyperopia and 42.5 dpt for severe myopic eyes.

### 10.8.6.5 IOL Design for Children and Infants (e.g. Congenital Cataracts)

Implantation is performed more frequently in a primary care manner at the time of the intervention. The choice of an IOL for a child depends on the age at the time of surgery and the age at which emmetropia is desired. The eye grows very rapidly during the first 3 months of life, still relatively rapidly during the first year, and more slowly thereafter (it approximately reaches its adult size at 5 years of age). Generally, achieving emmetropia at 5 years of age is desirable. Therefore, the power of the IOL must be undercorrected at the time of the intervention [38]:

before 3 months, by 40%
from 0 to 3 months by 40%
from 3 to 6 months, by 35%
from 6 to 12 months, by 30%
from 12 to 18 months, by 25%
from 18 to 24 months, by 20%
from 24 to 30 months, by 15%
from 30 to 36 months, by 10%
from 36 to 48 months, by 5%
and from 5 to 7 years of age, by 1 dpt.

At nearly 7 years of age, the power of the IOL is provided by the theoretical calculation.

Indeed, this approach is effective for children undergoing surgery after 1 year of age; for children undergoing surgery earlier, there is often a "myopic shift", which could be better balanced if the growth of small eyes, large eyes, and operated eyes (versus non-operated eyes) was better known.

### 10.8.6.6   Special Cases of Corneas Modified by Refractive Surgery

Refractive surgery induces changes in the cornea that make difficult the calculation of its power. And it is not possible to rely on simple keratometry.

Three main mechanisms, sources of errors, are possible, leading to an underestimation of the power of the emmetropizing IOL, and thus giving rise to hypermetropization: one error on the keratometry, one on the assimilation of the cornea as a plane dioptre, and the third on the error of measurement of the depth of the anterior chamber and therefore of the ELP (Effective Lens Position).

As early as 1986, Markovits [38] reported the first case of miscalculation of the power of an IOL after radial keratotomy. Radial keratotomy, by making radial corneal incisions, induced modification of the curvatures of the cornea and a flattening of the central zone. Although this technique is no longer used, there are still corneas that have been treated as such, and it is therefore important to know that when the measurement is made with a Javal-type keratometer, the site of the measurement is too far from the center and corresponds to the area of the inner end of the incisions, where the curvature of the cornea is accentuated. Overestimation of the power of the cornea results in a calculation that underestimates the power of the IOL required. The IOL power can be either calculated [39] by decreasing the keratometry value by 1 dpt and aiming for a result of $-\,0.75$ dpt using a last-generation theoretical formula or taking the central value of the corneal topography, and using the Haigis formula.

The two current techniques for refractive surgery (photorefractive keratectomy and LASIK) use an excimer laser and aim to correct myopia or hyperopia by modifying the convergence power of the cornea. Modification of the corneal curvature is obtained by removing a part of the corneal stroma. This stromal ablation causes flattening or bulging of the anterior curvature of the cornea and, therefore, a loss of the parallelism of the two faces of the cornea, prohibiting its assimilation in formulas to a dioptre with parallel sides. Keratometers and even corneal topographers measure only the radii of curvature of the anterior surface of the cornea using the projection of it on a Placido disc with analysis of the Purkinje image and are not able to calculate its effective power.

Methods for Determining the Value of K

*Refractive History Method (Holladay)*

This method requires to know the power of the cornea and the value of refraction before and after performing refractive surgery.

Example: An eye has myopia corrected by a lens of $-\,6$ dpt and a corneal power of 44 dpt before surgery; if the residual myopia, is $-\,3$ dpt, the difference in power induced by the operation is $-\,6 - (-\,3) = -\,3$ dpt. The power of the cornea taken for the calculation of the IOL will be $44 - 3$ dpt $= 41$ dpt, 3 dpt corresponding to the correction of myopia by surgery.

*Contact Lens Method (Sopper and Gauffman)*

A contact lens of known power was placed on the cornea of the eye to be operated on. If the value of the refraction was unchanged, the power of the cornea corresponded to that of the contact lens. This method was difficult to carry out and is now rarely used.

*Method Using Corneal Topography*

Corneal topography has the advantage of providing measurements at many points of the central cornea. It reflects the diversity of radii of curvature observed after radial keratotomy.

Comparing these different methods, Celikol [40] found that the best postoperative results are obtained with keratometry provided by the refractive history method, in which the power of the artificial lens varies from $-0.16$ to $+0.50$ dpt, and with corneal topography, in which the power of the IOL varies from $-0.13$ to $+0.54$ dpt, compared to the ideal value. The results obtained by the contact lens method are considered unreliable and those obtained by a Javal-type keratometer provide an underestimation of the power of the IOL of 2.32 dpt, on average.

The most commonly used corneal refractive index is 1.3375. This overall index remains valid when the two faces of the cornea remain parallel, as in radial keratotomy. However, only the values of the central keratometry, 1 mm from the center, should be retained. For post-radial keratotomy corneas, topographers can be used to determine the value of the corneal power; for post-excimer corneas they provide erroneous results. Brancato et al. [41] favor the use of a variable refractive index, tailored to the case, and which, when introduced into the calculation graphs of corneal topographers, allows for more reliable results.

*Method Using Keratometry by Optical Coherence Tomography (OCT)*

The latest-generation anterior segment OCTs, by permitting the measurement of the radii of curvature of the anterior and posterior surfaces of the cornea, should allow for obtaining its true power that can then be integrated into the calculation formulas.

Therefore, in practice, one must know the values of keratometry and refraction before and just after refractive surgery by radial keratotomy, photorefractive keratectomy, and LASIK to preserve them and to entrust them to the patient. The method using the history of the refraction is proving to be the most reliable to determine the power of the cornea necessary for the IOL power calculation. However, refraction can be modified by cataracts:

- If the patient's refractive assessment is available, that is to say, keratometry and refraction values before photorefractive keratectomy or LASIK, the method involving the clinical history, universally recognized as the "gold standard", recommends subtracting the difference in spherical equivalent to the corneal plane (CRc) from the initial corneal power (before any operation). CRc = postoperative refraction at the corneal plane – preoperative refraction at the corneal plane. Most authors recommend then calculating the IOL power with several third-generation formulas (Haigis, Hoffer Q, Holladay 2, SRK/T) and selecting the highest value [6, 42].

- If values are available in the biometer, it may be preferable to use a Double K formula [43]. More recently, Haigis [44] has proposed a formula (Haigis-L) that is useful after corneal refractive surgery, for both myopic and hyperopic LASIK. In this case, the central value given by the corneal topography must be retained as the keratometry value.
- If the patient's refractive assessment is not available, there are several possibilities: the method for hard contact lenses of known power can be used, or the formula proposed by Shammas [45]: K = 1.14 Kpost − 6.8.

Thus, there are many methods for IOL power calculation after refractive surgery and a choice needs to be made regarding these different options. A consensus is desirable [46], and there is merit in being able to average the different values proposed. Various calculators, including the one proposed on the American Society of Cataract and Refractive Surgery website, taking into account the work of Drs. Hill, Wang, and Koch, offer an easy approach to this consensus (Fig. 10.17).

However, even with all these precautions, the prediction of the obtained refractive result is not as accurate as for an eye that has not undergone any corneal surgery.

### 10.8.6.7 The IOL Position in the Eye

The position of the IOL has a large influence on the calculation of the IOL power. The difference between the actual final refraction expected in the spectacle lens and that obtained in reality is of the order of 1 dpt/mm of error in the position of the IOL [47]. However, this correspondence is only true in eyes close to emmetropia. The calculation error is greater with more powerful IOLs, potentially reaching 2.5 dpt/mm. The same applies in cases where the cornea is of low power (hyperopia of curvature). Similarly, the calculation error is greater when the anterior chamber is deeper: if the calculation error is approximately 1 dpt/mm for a distance at the apex of 2–3 mm, it can reach 1.25 dpt/mm for a distance of 3–4 mm.

Thus, the risk of error related to a poor prediction of the position of the IOL is greater with posterior than anterior chamber IOLs and with farsighted than myopic eyes.

### 10.8.6.8 Other Factors

**The material of the IOL** is also important: in the case of a flexible IOL, retraction of the capsular bag, by changing the position of the IOL, can explain some notable variations in refraction several months after surgery.

In case of very pronounced myopia, beyond 31–32 mm the IOLs have a negative power. However, **the geometry of positive IOLs** (of the thin type) differs from that of

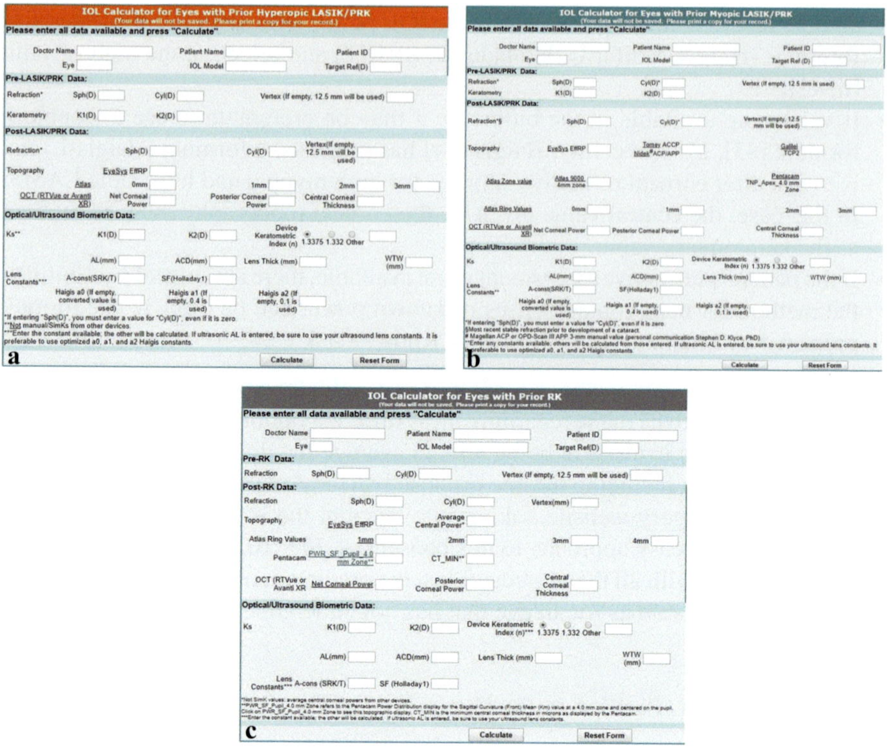

**Fig. 10.17 Calculator of the ASCRS for eyes after refractive surgery**. **a**: After LASIK/photorefractive keratectomy for hypermetropia; **b**: After LASIK/photorefractive keratectomy for myopia; **c**: After radial keratotomy. For each type of anterior refractive surgery performed, data should be entered

negative IOLs (of the thick type) and therefore, their constants are probably different [48].

**Acknowledgements** I would like to dedicate this chapter to Dr. Wolfgang Haigis from Würzburg, a colleague and friend, who passed away on October 21, 2019. He did not only pass on his formulas and the IOL Master, but since the SIDUO XIV in Iguazu in 1988, he succeeded in passing on to us during his regularly awaited lectures at every meeting, the rigor and enthusiasm necessary to master this part of ocular ultrasound. Moreover, his good mood, his dynamism and his availability made him easily approachable and pleasant to meet.

# References


1. Gernet H. Biometrie des Auges mit Ultraschall. Klin Monatsbl Augenheilkd. 1965;146:863–4.
2. François J, Goes F. Ocular biometry. In: Thijssen JM, Verbeek AM, editors. Ultrasonography in ophthalmology—proceedings of the 8th SIDUO congress—Nijmegen. Boston, London: Dr W Junk Publishers, The Hague; 1981, pp. 135–165.
3. Bergès O, Torrent M. Echographie de l'œil et de l'orbite. Paris: Vigot; 1986.
4. Bergès O, Puech M, Assouline M, Letenneur L, Gastellu-Etchegory M. B-mode-guided vector A-mode versus A-mode biometry to determine axial length and intraocular lens power. J Cataract refract Surg. 1998;24:529–35.
5. Shammas HJ. Axial length measurement and its relation to intraocular lens power calculations. J Am Intraocul Implant Soc. 1982;8(4):346–9.
6. Shammas HJ. Intraocular lens power calculations. Thorofare, NJ, USA: Slack Inc.; 2003.
7. Shroff NM, Ray S, Dutta, Kumar K. A practical device to aid in immersion A-scan biometry. J Cataract Refract Surg. 2004;30(6):1386–7.
8. Fledelius HC, Christensen AC. Reappraisal of the human ocular growth curve in fetal life, infancy, and early childhood. Br J Ophthalmol. 1996;80(10):918–21.
9. Luyckx J, Delmarcelle Y. Biométrie du globe oculaire en fonction de l'âge et de la réfraction. In: Poujol J, Massin J, editors. Ultrasonography in ophthalmology—proceedings of the 4th SIDUO congress—Paris. Paris: CHNO des XV–XX ; 1973, pp. 269–275.
10. Curtin BJ. The posterior staphyloma of pathologic myopia. Trans Am Ophthalmol Soc. 1977;75:67–86.
11. Bergès O, Nau E, Lafitte F, Koskas P. 20 MHz Echography of Intra Ocular Lenses. Usefulness for biometry. In: Nehmeth J, Csakany B, Barcsay G, editors. Ultrasonography in ophthalmology 20—proceedings of the 20th SIDUO meeting—Budapest. Nyctalus, Budapest; 2006, pp. 60–1.
12. Murray DC, Potamitis T, Good P, Kirkby GR, Benson MT. Biometry of the silicone oil-filled eye. Eye (Lond). 1999;13(Pt 3a):319–24.
13. Nepp J, Krepler K, Jandrasits K, Hauff W, Hanselmayer G, Velikay-Parel M, Ossoinig KC, Wedrich A. Biometry and refractive outcome of eyes filled with silicone oil by standardized echography and partial coherence interferometry. Graefes Arch Clin Exp Ophthalmol. 2005;243(10):967–72.
14. Takei K, Sekine Y, Okamoto F, Hommura S. Measurement of axial length of eyes with incomplete filling of silicone oil in the vitreous cavity using x ray computed tomography. Br J Ophthalmol. 2002;86(1):47–50.
15. Alsbirk PH. Anatomical risk factors in primary angle-closure glaucoma. A ten year follow up survey based on limbal and axial anterior chamber depths in a high risk population. Int Ophthalmol. 199216(4–5):265–72.
16. Haigis W, Lege B, Miller N, Schneider B. Comparison of immersion ultrasound biometry and partial coherence interferometry for intraocular lens calculation according to Haigis. Graefes Arch Clin Exp Ophthalmol. 2000;238(9):765–73.
17. Apple DJ. Sir Nicholas Harold Lloyd Ridley: 10 July 1906–25 May 2001. Biogr Mem Fellows R Soc. 2007;53:285–307.
18. Fyodorov SN, Kolonko AI. Estimation of optical power of the intraocular lens. Vestnik Oftalmologic (Moscow). 1967;4:27.
19. Colenbrander MC. Calculations of the power of an iris clip lens for distant vision. Br J Ophthalmol. 1973;57(10):735–40.
20. Binkhorst RD. The optical design of intraocular lens implants. Ophthalmic Surg. 1975;6(3):17–3.
21. Thijssen JM. The emmetropic and the iseikonic implant lens: computer calculation of the refractive power and its accuracy. Ophthalmologica. 1975;171(6):467–86.
22. van der Heijde GL. The optical correction of unilateral aphakia. Trans Sect Ophthalmol Am Acad Ophthalmol Otolaryngol. 1976;81(1):OP80–8.
23. Retzlaff J, Sanders DR, Kraff MC. Development of the SRK/T intraocular lens implant power calculation formula. J Cataract Refract Surg. 1990;16(3):333–40.

24. Sanders DR, Retzlaff J, Kraff MC. Comparison of the SRK II formula and other second-generation formulas. J Cataract Refract Surg. 1988;14(2):136–41.
25. Haigis W. The third-generation formulas: application to post-refractive surgery IOL work-up and to new available equipment. In: Bergès O, Perrenoud F, Siahmed K, editors. Ultra-sonography in ophthalmology 18—proceedings of the 18th SIDUO meeting—Paris. Sauramps Medical, Montpellier; 2003, pp 55–71.
26. Holladay JT, Musgrove KH, Prager TC, Lewis JW, Chandler TY, Ruiz RS. A three-part system for refining intraocular lens power calculations. J Cataract Refract Surg. 1988;14:17–24.
27. Shammas HJ. The fudged formula for intraocular lens power calculations. J Am Intraocul Implant Soc. 1982;8(4):350–2.
28. Hoffer KJ. The Hoffer Q formula: a comparison of theoretic and regression formulas. J Cataract Refract Surg. 1993;19:700–12.
29. Olsen T. Theoretical, computer-assisted prediction versus SRK prediction of postoperative refraction after intraocular lens implantation. J Cataract Refract Surg. 1987;13(2):146–50.
30. Chong EW, Mehta JS. High myopia and cataract surgery. Curr Opin Ophthalmol. 2016;27(1):45–50.
31. Cooke DL, Cooke TL. Comparison of 9 intraocular lens power calculation formulas. J Cataract Refract Surg. 2016;42(8):1157–64.
32. Gökce SE, Zeiter JH, Weikert MP, Koch DD, Hill W, Wang L. Intraocular lens power calculations in short eyes using 7 formulas. J Cataract Refract Surg. 2017;43(7):892–7.
33. Prevost G, Bonnac JP, Mawas E. L'aniséïconie: Importance de la mesurer pour le contactologue et le chirurgien de la cataracte. Bull Soc Ophtalmol Fr. 1980;80(4–5):349–53.
34. Visser N, Beckers HJ, Bauer NJ, Gast ST, Zijlmans BL, et al. Toric vs aspherical control intraocular lenses in patients with cataract and corneal astigmatism: a randomized clinical trial. JAMA Ophthalmol. 2014;132(12):1462–8.
35. Joshi RS, Jadhav SA. Frequency of corneal astigmatism in patients presenting for senile cataract surgery at a teaching hospital in Indian Rural Population. Asia Pac J Ophthalmol (Phila). 2020.
36. Fam HB, Lim KL. Meridional analysis for calculating the expected spherocylindrical refraction in eyes with toric intraocular lenses. J Cataract Refract Surg. 2007;33(12):2072–6.
37. Abulafia A, Koch DD, Wang L, Hill WE, Assia EI, Franchina M, Barrett GD. New regression formula for toric intraocular lens calculations. J Cataract Refract Surg. 2016;42(5):663–71.
38. De Laage de Meux P. Pathologie du cristallin. In: De Laage de Meux P, editor. Ophtalmologie pédiatrique. Masson, Paris; 2003, pp. 94–111.
39. Markovits AS. Extracapsular cataract extraction with posterior chamber intraocular lens implantation in a postradial keratotomy patient. Arch Ophthalmol. 1986;104(3):329, 331.
40. Lyle WA, Jin GJ. Intraocular lens power prediction in patients who undergo cataract surgery following previous radial keratotomy. Arch Ophthalmol. 1997;115(4):457–61.
41. Celikkol L, Pavlopoulos G, Weinstein B, Celikkol G, Feldman ST. Calculation of intraocular lens power after radial keratotomy with computerized videokeratography. Am J Ophthalmol. 1995;120(6):739–50.
42. Gobbi PG, Carones F, Brancato R. Keratometric index, videokeratography, and refractive surgery. J Cataract Refract Surg. 1998;24(2):202–11.
43. Seitz B, Langenbucher A, Haigis W. Intraocular lens power calculation in eyes after corneal refractive surgery. J Refract Surg. 2000;16(3):349–61.
44. Aramberri J. Intraocular lens power calculation after corneal refractive surgery: double-K method. J Cataract Refract Surg. 2003;29(11):2063–8.
45. Haigis W. Intraocular lens calculation after refractive surgery for myopia: Haigis-L formula. J Cataract Refract Surg. 2008;34(10):1658–63.

46. Shammas HJ, Shammas MC, Garabet A, Kim JH, Shammas A, LaBree L. Correcting the corneal power measurements for intraocular lens power calculations after myopic laser in situ keratomileusis. Am J Ophthalmol. 2003;136(3):426–32.
47. Qin B, Huang D. Intraocular lens power calculation after corneal refractive surgery. https://www.ncbi.nlm.nih.gov
48. Hill W, Wang L, Koch DD. M.D. IOL power calculator in post-myopic LASIK/PRK eyes. https://iolcalc.ascrs.org

# Chapter 11
# (Very) High-Frequency Ultrasound of the Anterior Segment

Michel Puech, Olivier Bergès, Jacques Laloum, Audrey Feldman, Pierre Pégourié, and Elisabeth Nau

**Abstract** After having shown the applications of (very) high frequency ultrasound (VHFU/HFU) to refractive surgery, in this chapter, we mainly consider the study of the anterior chamber angle/iridocorneal angle (ACA) in case of glaucoma, the corneal opacities and the traumas of the anterior segment. For the study of the ACA, we first define the scleral spur, a structure that must be recognized because in relation to this structure, we can evaluate and measure the opening of the ACA. The practical realization is then detailed: bilateral and symmetrical, the examination following ocular biometry and biometry of the anterior segment. A quantitative approach is preferred for the analysis of the angle and study of the risk of closure. This angle should be systematically measured in the light (photopic condition) and the dark (scotopic light level). The measurement in degrees is to be banished because of the too-variable morphology of the angle and root of the iris. The most frequently used measurement is the angle opening distance at 500 $\mu$m from the scleral spur (AOD500) or sometimes at 750 $\mu$m (AOD750) or even sometimes at the distance where the angle is the narrowest; however, we can also measure surfaces: angle recess area (ARA) and trabecular iris surface area (TISA), the most frequently used angular surfaces being ARA500 and TISA750. We can also measure the thickness of the iris (mainly at 750 $\mu$m from the scleral spur), as well as its morphology, central convexity or peripheral angulation. Finally, the situation of the ciliary body should be studied and the lens vault should be measured. We then describe the different mechanisms of chronic narrow angle glaucoma: pupillary block, plateau iris, basal insertion of the iris and creeping angle glaucoma, then pigmentary glaucoma. This VHFU is also useful after treatment: laser peripheral iridotomy, iridoplasty, filtering

M. Puech
Explore Vision Ophthalmic Diagnostic Centers, Paris, Rueil, France

O. Bergès (✉) · J. Laloum · E. Nau
Rothschild Foundation Hospital, Paris, France
e-mail: oberges@for.paris

A. Feldman
Centre Lyon Est Ophtalmo, Saint-Priest, France

P. Pégourié
University Hospital of Grenoble, Grenoble, France


O. Bergès (ed.), *Echography of the Eye and Orbit*,
https://doi.org/10.1007/978-3-031-41467-1_11

surgery or drainage implants. We then review the contribution of VHFU to the study of corneal opacities, mainly neonatal (Peters syndrome 1 and 2, glaucoma, sclerocornea, Rieger anomaly, Axenfeld, or Axenfeld-Rieger syndrome, and dermoids) but also in adults. VHFU is also useful for anterior segment trauma. Then we cover corneal edema, hyphema, angle recession, iridodialysis and iris tears; cyclodialysis and lens anomalies: intumescence; cataract; capsular rupture and (sub) luxation with or without vitreous herniation in the anterior chamber. Finally, the VHFU allows for localizing the foreign bodies with great precision.

## 11.1  Introduction

High-frequency ultrasound (HFU) of the anterior segment has only been possible since the pioneering work of Charles Pavlin, in the early 1990s [1], and the development of a new technique that he called ultrasound biomicroscopy, which became very popular in light of its many applications but also because of its easy-to-remember acronym: UBM. This UBM device became the benchmark for high-resolution imaging in ophthalmology, using a 50-MHz ultrasound transducer, with ocular ultrasound devices for posterior segment exploration using 10-MHz transducers.

The main benefit of high-frequency probes is that they improve the resolution of images and allow for greater magnification of the observed area. The resolution of the UBM device is approximately 50 $\mu$m.

Within a few years, other devices appeared that allowed for exploring the anterior segment with comparable resolution:

- The first was the Artemis device (UltraLink), developed by the team of Professor Jackson Coleman in the mid-1990s. With this device, the analysis resolution was even higher (approximately 20 $\mu$m), and the anterior segment could be visualized in its entirety (see Fig. 4.2). For example, one could identify the depth of a corneal flap by LASIK procedure. These researchers called this technique very high-frequency ultrasound (VHFU). The work of Dan Reinstein and Ron Silverman showed the value of this very high-resolution imaging in refractive surgery [2–10] (Fig. 11.1).

These applications can also be performed with modern optical coherence tomography (OCT) devices. Both techniques allow for determining the thickness of the residual stroma before a retreatment decision for myopic correction, for example.

Another application, intended for the anterior segment, is monitoring of phakic myopic intra ocular lens (pIOL). These intraocular lenses tend to cause secondary effects on the cornea or cause iris contact and the consequent risk of pupillary ovalization or sandwich effect. This results in greater vigilance for future candidates for implantation and regular monitoring of implanted patients.

The most widely used pIOLs have been angle supported or iris fixated anterior chamber IOLs.

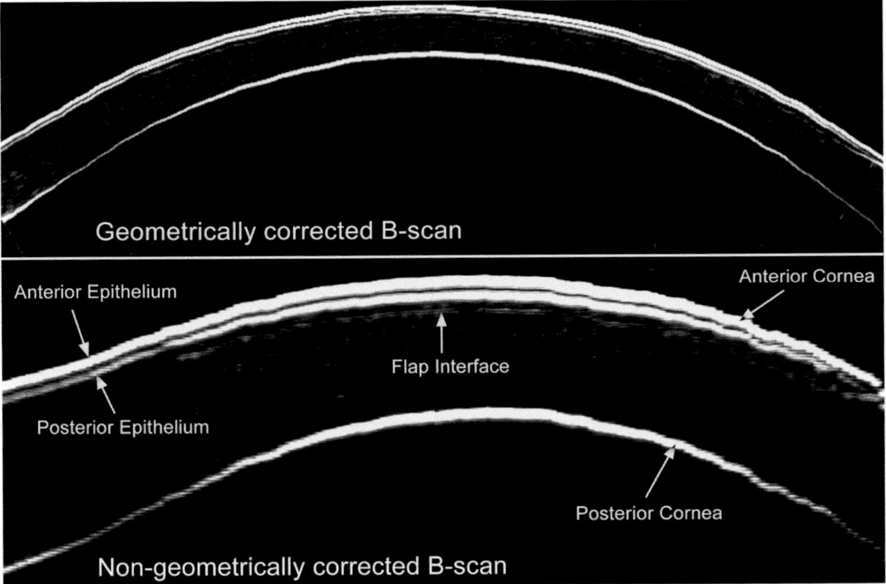


**Fig. 11.1  Visibility of the flap interface 9 years after LASIK with ultra high resolution using Artemis very high-frequency digital ultrasound B-scan (ArcScan, Inc).** Geometrically corrected (top) and non-geometrically corrected (bottom) VHF digital ultrasound B-scan of a cornea 9 years after LASIK with an Automated Corneal Shaper microkeratome (Bausch & Lomb). The flap interface can still be clearly identified along its entire length 9 years after surgery. The bottom scan has been zoomed to emphasize the interfaces, so that the image width represents 10 mm and the image height represents 1.2 mm. Reprinted with permission from Reinstein DZ, Archer TJ, Gobbe M, Silverman RH, Coleman DJ. Repeatability of layered corneal pachymetry with the Artemis very high-frequency digital ultrasound arc-scanner. J Refract Surg. 2010;26(9):646–659

VHFU allows for measuring the safe distances between the IOL and the cornea or the IOL and the lens for regular follow-up of patients who have already undergone implantation. Analysis of the position of haptics is also an important element of the follow-up of these patients (Fig. 11.2).

For patients who are candidates for this surgery, the progression of imaging techniques allows for considering superimposing the shape of the implant to be used on the cross-sectional image of a given patient, with its geometry directly dependent on the ametropia that is to be treated.

For this surgery, Georges Baïkoff described a parameter as a risk factor for the Sandwich effect in the case of an iris-fixated IOL: the lens vault, when greater than 600 µm, there is a risk of compression of the iris between the IOL material located in front and the anterior lens capsule behind the iris.

- A second category of instruments is represented by more multipurpose devices that allow for analyzing the posterior segment with conventional probes but also, by changing probes, the anterior segment with transducers of 20, 35, or 50 MHz.

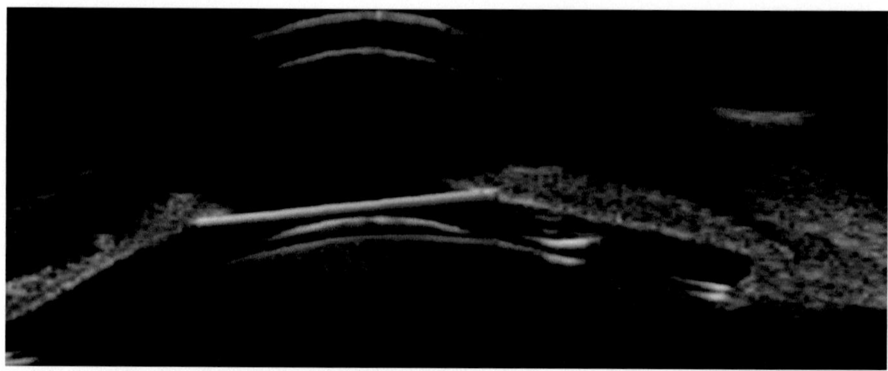

**Fig. 11.2  Very high frequency ultrasound of a phakic myopic intraocular lens of the posterior chamber** with visualization of the haptic of the IOL in the posterior chamber almost in contact with the ciliary body

Gradually, the term UBM, which corresponded to the name of the first device developed by Pavlin and the Zeiss-Humphrey Company, then Paradigm, became an umbrella term to encompass ocular analysis by HFU. **However, it seems more accurate to reserve the term UBM for examinations carried out with the ultrasound device designed by Pavlin and to reserve the term VHFU for examinations carried out with other devices if the frequency used is greater than or equal to 50 MHz and HFU if the frequency used is 20–50 MHz.**

VHFU is mainly indicated for:

- Assessing the anterior chamber/iridocorneal angle (ACA) in glaucoma
- Tumors of the iris and/or ciliary body
- Refractive surgery.

The applications in refractive surgery have mainly been described with the Artemis device. We will not describe all of them in this chapter, but we have provided two examples (see above). The application of VHFU to the study of tumors of the anterior segment, iris, and ciliary body will be discussed in Chap. 13. In this chapter, we mainly discuss the contributions of VHFU to the study of the ICA in glaucoma as well as the applications of VHFU to the study of corneal opacities and trauma of the anterior segment.

## 11.2 Analysis of the Iridocorneal/Anterior Chamber Angle (ACA)

From the beginning, Charles Pavlin [1] noted that measurements of the ACA in degrees were easy to make but difficult to define and not reproducible because of the large anatomical variation of the ACA. Therefore, he proposed measuring the angle opening distance (AOD) at 500 or 750 μm from the scleral spur.

Hence, the scleral spur is the anatomical pivot for this anterior chamber angle. It is a structure to be recognized with a significant degree of certainty, which is the case with good inter- and intra-rater reproducibility [11]. Sometimes manifesting as a very echogenic micro nodule, it is the point of convergence of two curved lines: that of the corneal endothelium and that of the inner side of the sclera (Fig. 11.3).

Of all the distances that Pavlin proposed for measurement characteristics of the ACA (Fig. 11.4) [12], only the AOD500 and, on request, the thickness of the iris remain routine. Several studies have shown the very good reproducibility of ultrasound measurements [13], as well as a good correlation between ultrasound measurements and measurements obtained by OCT of the anterior segment (AS-OCT) [14–16].

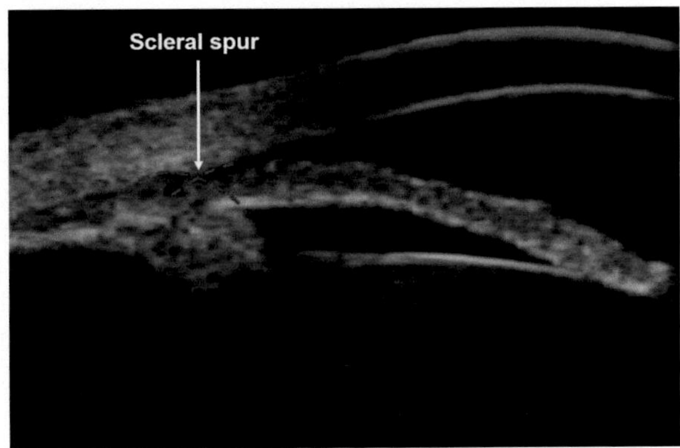


**Fig. 11.3 Location of the scleral spur,** very high frequency ultrasound at 50 MHz: at the point of convergence of the curved lines corresponding to the corneal endothelium and the interface between the sclera and the uvea

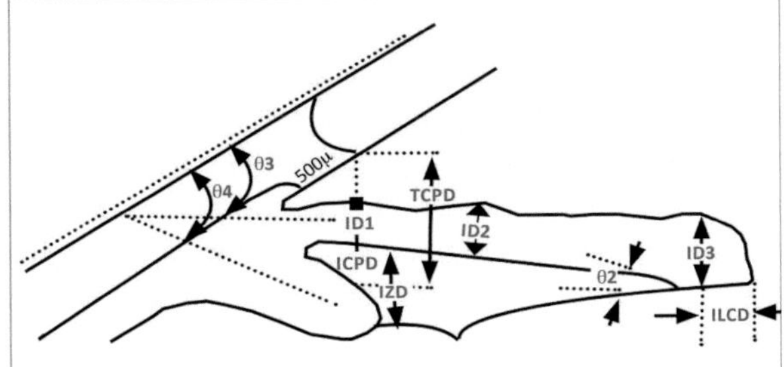


**Fig. 11.4 Various measurements possible at the level of the anterior chamber angle.** Reprinted with permission from Pavlin CJ, Harasiewicz K. Ultrasound biomicroscopy of anterior segment structures in normal and glaucomatous eyes. Am J Ophthalmol. 1992 Apr 15;113(4):381–9

AS-OCT, which became available in 2003, also allows for imaging the ACA, with very discreetly higher resolution (18 $\mu$m vs 25 $\mu$m for VHFU at 50 MHz), which is not a decisive factor, but especially with a less constraining character for the patient due to the non-contact technique and a seated position, which gives it an advantage, especially for the study of filtration blebs. However, the pigment epithelium of the iris is an obstacle for AS-OCT, and only VHFU allows for visualization and analysis of the structures located behind the pigment epithelium of the iris, so VHFU is the examination method of choice for diagnosing plateau iris syndrome or an angle closure in relation to iridociliary cysts. Therefore, these two technologies are complementary and not in competition with each other [17].

With AS-OCT, and its very high popularity, new values have emerged that seem even more suitable for evaluating the ACA. These are surface measurements of up to 500 or 750 $\mu$m from the scleral spur (ARA and TISA). We will also analyze these surfaces that modern ultrasound scanners now allow to calculate:

- The angle recess area (ARA)
- The trabecular-iris surface area (TISA).

## *11.2.1 Practical Implementation*

### The examination should always be bilateral and symmetrical

It is carried out in immersion, the probe always remaining far from the ocular structures, which is easy to check by visualization of an anechoic space in front of them. After careful topical anesthesia, a fairly large amount of carbomer gel can be placed on the cornea, possibly using a small lid speculum to keep the eyelids open, the probe only being closed off by a solidified gel plate, or with the ClearScan device fixed to the anterior part of the open probe, a small pouch with a very thin wall of acoustic impedance equivalent to that of the medium analyzed being filled with water (see Fig. 7.14).

### 11.2.1.1   Ocular Biometry

The examination always begins with the collection of biometric values for each eye with a 10/15 MHz probe: the depth of the anterior chamber, the thickness of the lens, and the total axial length from the center of the cornea to the fovea. This axial section, following the B-mode guided biometric technique [18] (see Fig. 10.9), allows for its immediate assessment whether the eye is emmetropic or hyperopic (more rarely myopic in these narrow-angle indications), to determine whether the depth of the anterior chamber is normal, borderline, or narrow and whether the lens is not large, especially for the size of the eye (Fig. 11.5a).

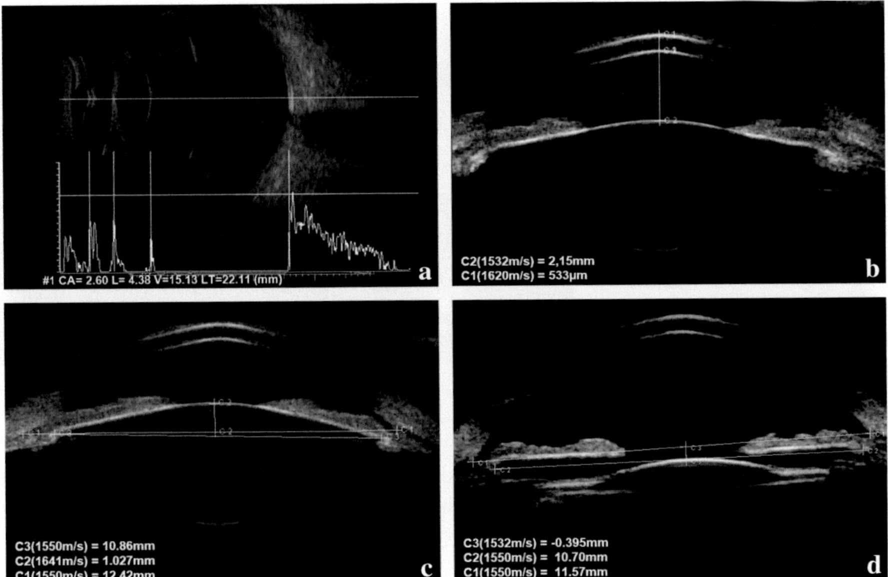


**Fig. 11.5  Biometry of the eye and the anterior segment before a very high frequency ultrasound for assessing a narrow angle. a: B-mode guided biometry with a 10 MHz probe.** The eye is hyperopic (axial length = 22.11 mm), with a borderline anterior chamber (2.1 mm) and a normal lens (4.4 mm). **b: Biometry of the anterior segment with a 50 MHz probe.** The thickness of the cornea and the depth of the anterior chamber are measured. Whether the two lines corresponding to the epithelium and the Bowman's membrane should be verified as well as whether a small arc corresponding to the posterior part of the posterior lens capsule can be clearly seen. Note that the depth of the anterior chamber corresponds to the value found at 10 MHz. **c: Biometry of the anterior segment according to the 3–9 o'clock axis, with a 50 MHz probe.** Angle-to-angle diameter and sulcus-to-sulcus diameter values are consistent with hyperopia and the lens vault is very important, superior to 1 mm, being in favor of a lens extraction versus peripheral iridotomy, a treatment for angle closure glaucoma would be considered

### 11.2.1.2   Anterior Segment Biometry

Then, on an axial section performed with a 50 MHz probe, one measures the thickness of the cornea in the center (from the epithelium to the endothelium/Descemet membrane interface) and the depth of the anterior chamber in the center, from the endothelium to the anterior lens capsule. The measurements provided by the ultrasound system are usually based on an ultrasound velocity of 1550 m/s. Therefore, the different values must be recalculated according to the velocity of ultrasound in these different structures: 1620 m/s for the cornea and 1532 m/s for the anterior chamber. This distance needs to be consistent with the depth of the anterior chamber measured with the 10/15 MHz probe, but it is more accurate at 50 MHz (Fig. 11.5b). If an IOL is present, the distance between the endothelium and the anterior surface of the optic and the distance between the endothelium and the pupillary plane should be measured. The diameter from angle-to-angle, the diameter from sulcus-to-sulcus,

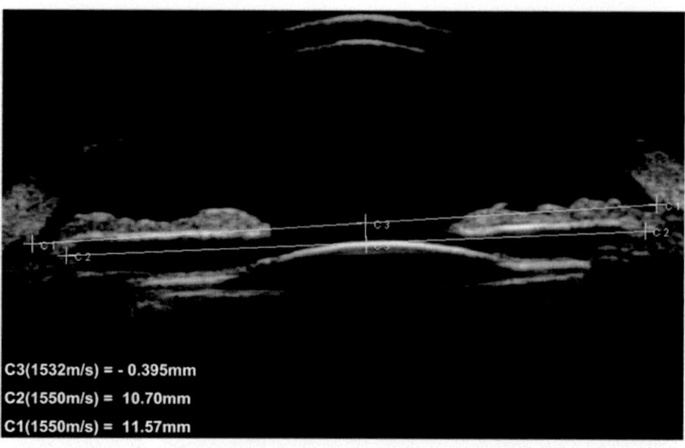


**Fig. 11.6 Measurement of the lens vault after phacoemulsification and posterior chamber intraocular lens (IOL) implantation**. Naturally negative here, measuring − 0.395 mm with a velocity of 1532 m/s

and the lens vault are also measured (Figs. 11.5c, and 11.6). Of note, the anterior segment is not strictly circular but, rather, discreetly oval, with a greater almost sagittal axis. Hence, one must specify in the report at which meridians the diameters are measured.

### 11.2.1.3 Analysis of the Anterior Chamber (Iridocorneal) Angle (ACA)

Assessment of this angle is very well achieved by gonioscopy, which provides an irreplaceable element: coloration of the angle and in dynamic gonioscopy, which allows one to consider reopening the angle, mainly by analysis of the angle over the entire circumference, with, owing to the dynamic indentation, the distinction between reversible closures by simple apposition and closures by synechiae.

The use of meridian cross-section angle imaging is useful because it provides a different perspective of the closing mechanism.

The four cardinal meridians of each eye must be studied in the light and the dark [14, 19]. Their practical realization is always possible, including for vertical meridians. However, it is advisable, to warn the patient at the beginning of the examination that it is a long procedure, and that the time required will be minimized if they carefully follow the instructions that they are given; that they fully execute all the gaze directions that they are told to follow, and especially that they do not move their eyes when the light is turned on or off.

To study a meridian, the probe has to be positioned according to it, in front of the limbus. The angulation should not be too great. Ideally, the ultrasound beam should be perpendicular to the surface of the iris root. To be sure that the section passes through the meridian and is not oblique, it is necessary, on the same section, to have the iris as short as possible and at the same time visualize the two hyperechoic lines corresponding to the epithelium and endothelium of the cornea. It is also necessary to visualize the zonule, which appears as weakly echogenic because the zonular fibers are thin and not sufficiently orthogonal to the ultrasound beam in this incidence to study the ACA.

As for AS-OCT, the study of horizontal meridians is easy, and the reproducibility of the measurements is good [20]. However, exploration of the vertical meridians is slightly easier with ultrasound because the eyelids are not an obstacle.

## 11.2.2 Measurements of the Angle

### 11.2.2.1 Qualitative Approach

Analysis of the risk of angle-closure glaucoma (ACG) is carried out preferentially by gonioscopy and dynamic visualization of the angle using dynamic gonioscopy lenses designed to exert pressure on the top of the cornea and determine the possibility of reopening of the angle. However, in case of clinical doubt, the use of angle imaging by meridian cross-sections can provide a different perspective regarding the closing mechanism. This examination can be carried out by OCT or by VHFU, which allows the examination to be carried out in the dark, comparable to the conditions of nocturnal attacks of ACG, whereas gonioscopy is carried out with lighting from the slit lamp.

In case of clinical doubt about the existence of a closure, OCT is the key examination. The risk of angle closure is judged on the number of quadrants that present a disappearance of hyporeflectivity of the aqueous humor between the cornea and the iris with a contact between the two structures. More than half of the quadrants exhibiting a closed appearance indicate a more or less proven risk of angle closure. However, the absence of penetration through the pigmented tissue of the iris prevents visualization of the position of the ciliary processes in relation to the scleral spur and thus determination of the mechanisms of primary closure other than that of a pure pupillary block.

VHFU (Fig. 11.7), which benefits from better penetration behind the iris, is the only method to allow analyzing the iridociliary component on the mechanism of angle closure. Therefore, its role is essential in case of persistence of closure after removal of the pupillary block.

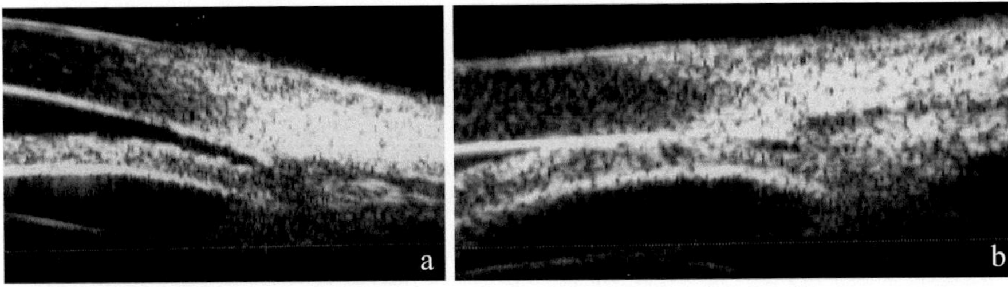


**Fig. 11.7 Dynamic test by ultrasound biomicroscopy (UBM)** of variation of the anterior chamber angle (ICA) as a function of the lighting in the room. **a: In ambient light, the angle is narrow; b: In the dark,** the angle closes, demonstrating the risk of acute glaucoma

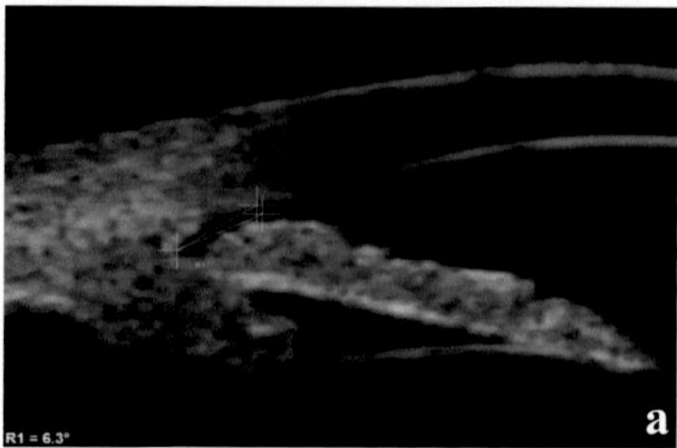
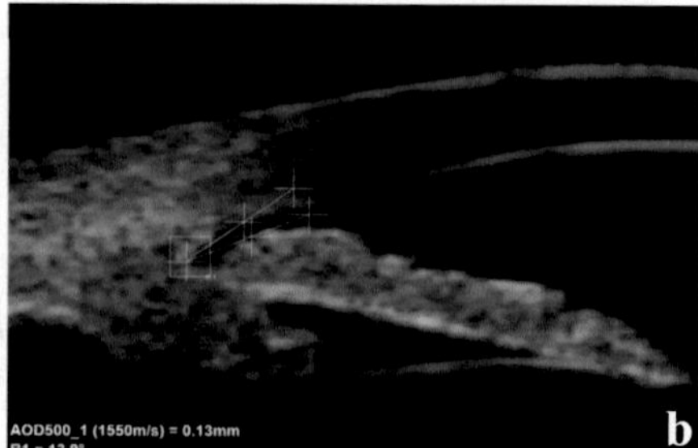


**Fig. 11.8** **Measurement of the angle in degrees. a: Measurement appearing correct but erroneous**, at 6.3°, compatible with a very narrow angle; **b: Correct measurement passing through the corneoscleral junction at 500 μm from the scleral spur and through the iris**. The angle now measures 13.9°, which corresponds to an angle opening distance of 0.13 mm (i.e., simply a narrow angle)

### 11.2.2.2 Quantitative Approach

**A quantitative approach to ACA measurements should be preferred over a purely qualitative approach** if comparisons are to be made in the same center and *a fortiori* in different centers, even if working on a console or computer may seem long and tedious. In addition, a quantitative approach allows for precise epidemiological studies, owing to advances in computing, and quantification that is usually automatable, which will lead to an increasingly extensive database. This is the reason to believe that increasingly relevant predictive parameters will be identified.

For measurements, the most important point is to be able to readily recognize the scleral spur (Fig. 11.3). This is easy when the angle is open but can sometimes be more complex when the angle is filiform or closed.

Angular Value in Degrees

Given the high variability of the morphology of the ACA, in particular the degree of convexity of the iris root and the undulations of its anterior surface, one must have benchmarks to measure this angle (Fig. 11.8), because otherwise the measurement obtained is too variable and not very useful, as expressed by Pavlin as early as 1992 [12].

The angle between the line crossing the corneal-scleral interface could a priori be measured at 500 μm (or 250 μm, or 750 μm) from the scleral spur and the line crossing the anterior surface of the iris at the point crossed by a line below and orthogonal to the previous corneoscleral point. However, this measurement is long and tedious to carry out and it is easier and more useful to measure the following.

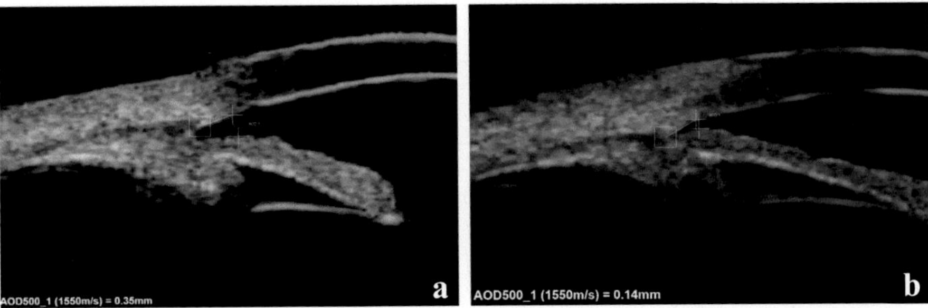


**Fig. 11.9 Angle measurement using angle opening distance 500 (AOD500). a: Normal angle:** AOD500 is quite open, equal to 350 μm, well above 250 μm; **b: Narrow angle:** AOD500 = 140 μm

**Fig. 11.10 Angle measurement using AOD750. Angle limit,** AOD750 measuring 160 μm

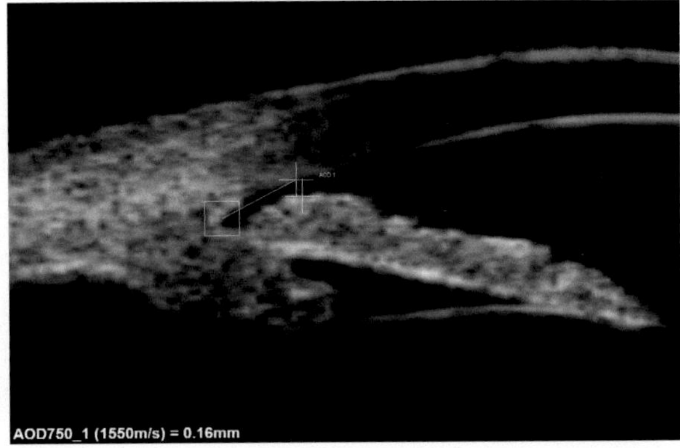


Angle Opening Distance (AOD)

Instead of measuring the angle in degrees, Charles Pavlin proposed to measure the distance of the lowered perpendicular between the corneoscleral point located 500 μm from the scleral spur and the anterior surface of the iris. Quite naturally, he called this distance the AOD500, for Angle Opening Distance at 500 μm from the scleral spur. This measurement very soon became the reference measure to characterize the aperture of the angle (Fig. 11.9). However, very quickly too, the various users realized that the AOD500 was insufficient because of the high variability of the morphology of the ACA. This gave rise to the fairly widely used AOD750 value for an AOD at 750 μm from the scleral spur (Fig. 11.10). As in practice, it is necessary to measure the narrowest distance at the place where the convexity of the iris root is maximal, it is sometimes necessary to measure angle "customized" opening distances at 600 μm, 650 μm, 800 μm, or even higher (Fig. 11.11).

When the ACA is closed, in addition to the closing distance (in mm or μm), one must specify whether this is a simple contact, with the creation of a small sinus of Mapstone, or a total extended closure (Fig. 11.12). Although VHFU has difficulty

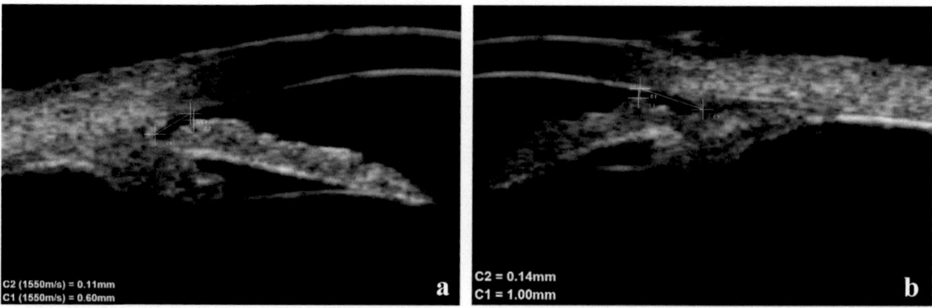



**Fig. 11.11 Measurement of the angle using customized AODs**: in both cases, the narrowest AOD was measured between the apex of the iris and the corneoscleral junction: **a: Narrow angle,** AOD600 equal to 110 μm. It would appear more open at 500 μm and 750 μm from the scleral spur. **b: Narrow-angle, AOD1000** equal to 140 μm. It would be larger, marginal, at 750 μm from the scleral spur

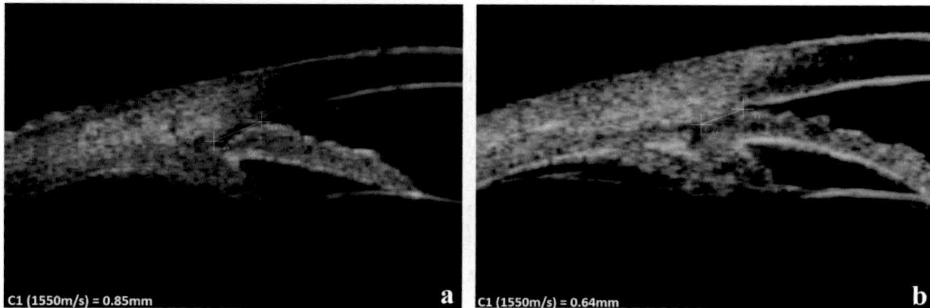



**Fig. 11.12 Closed angle. a: Persistence of a small fluid sinus of Mapstone** between the scleral spur and the apposition of the apex of the iris and the corneoscleral junction, 0.85 mm from the scleral spur. **b: Fully closed angle** over a distance of 0.64 mm

picking up synechiae, they must be carefully searched for [21], especially if the angle is always closed in the light.

## Angle Recess Area (ARA)

Measurement of a surface appears to provide more accuracy for ACA assessment than that of a simple line. The credit goes to Friedman and He [22] for having insisted on the advantage of studying the ARA which can, again, be measured up to 500 μm or 750 μm from the scleral spur. Naturally, measurement of this area is slightly more complex than that of the AOD and requires appropriate software. In addition, characterization of this area must be facilitated by the automatic proposal of an area, the operator simply having to modify certain points to achieve a perfect fit to the corneoscleral junction and the anterior surface of the iris root (Fig. 11.13). Even so, working on a console or computer can be time-consuming.

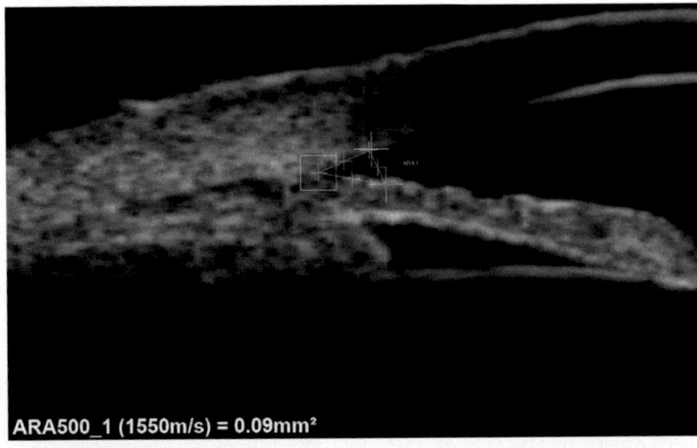

**Fig. 11.13  Angle recess area 500 (ARA500). Angle limit,** the ARA500 area is calculated automatically after repositioning the different calipers at 0.09 mm$^2$, corresponding to a borderline value because it is between 0.06 and 0.10 mm$^2$



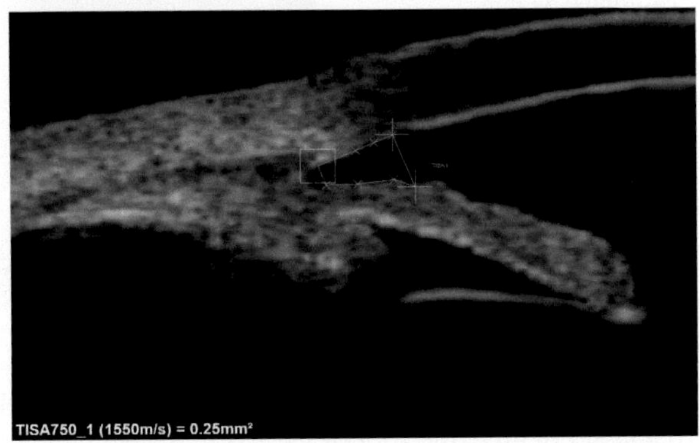

**Fig. 11.14  Trabecular iris surface area 750 (TISA750). Normal angle:** the TISA750 area is calculated automatically after repositioning the different calipers at 0.25 mm$^2$ (> 0.14 mm$^2$)



Trabecular-Iris Space Area (TISA)

This surface does not go to the apex of the angle but is a parallelepiped starting at the scleral spur and going up to to 500 μm or 750 μm from the latter (Fig. 11.14). According to their authors, it corresponds more, to the surface where the aqueous humor is in contact with the trabeculum [23].

The most frequently used angular surfaces are ARA500 and TISA750. Table 11.1 lists the various values that characterize an angle according to the different measurements available.

Other Values

*Iris Thickness (IT)*

As early as 1992, Pavlin noted the importance of measuring the iris. It is reasonable to measure it at its root, at its middle part, and near the pupillary edge, but of course, at the level of the root, a thickening will be able to lead to an engorgement and an

**Table 11.1** Quantitative evaluation of the angle according to the various measurements used

|  | AOD500 ($\mu$m) | ARA500 (mm$^2$) | TISA 750 (mm$^2$) |
|---|---|---|---|
| Filiform | x < 100 | x 0.00–0.03 | x 0.00–0.08 |
| Narrow | x 100–150 | x 0.03–0.06 | x 0.08–0.10 |
| Borderline | x 150–250 | x 0.06–0.10 | x 010–0.14 |
| Normal | > 250 | > 0.10 | > 0.14 |

*AOD* angle opening distance; *ARA* angle recess area; *TISA* trabecular iris surface area

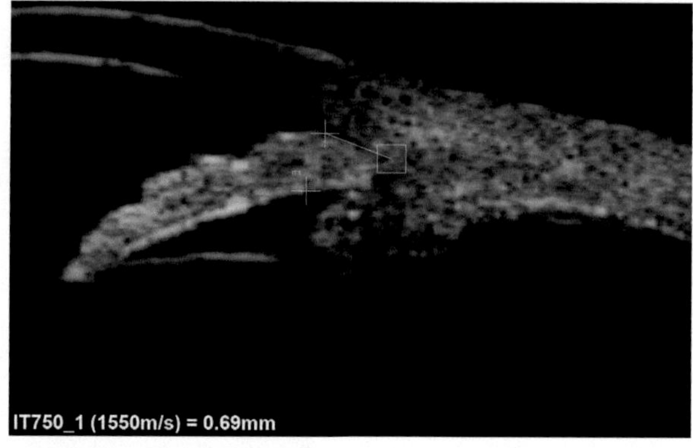


**Fig. 11.15 Iris thickness 750 (IT750). Moderate thickening of the iris** at 750 $\mu$m from the scleral spur, measuring 0.69 mm

impediment to the filtration of the aqueous humor as seen in creeping angle glaucoma. To a lesser degree, the root of the iris may also be thickened in plateau iris [24, 25]. Pavlin proposed measurement of this thickness at 500 $\mu$m from the scleral spur. With time and experience, the 750 $\mu$m measurement of the scleral spur has become the reference measurement (Fig. 11.15).

*Iris Morphology*

Although these are not measurements, the morphology of the iris needs to be systematically assessed. In pupillary block, the latter is convex forward (in AS-OCT, an iris vault is described, but this measurement is not yet available in VHFU), with a harmonious curvature, the maximum convexity being central. In plateau iris, it is angled with a maximum peripheral convexity, and a "stiff" medial part. Lastly, in pigmentary glaucoma, it appears concave with an increased contact distance with the anterior lens capsule, especially in accommodation. In the presence of a functional peripheral iridotomy, it is flat, which reflects the absence of a gradient between the anterior and posterior chambers. This sign is fundamental and takes precedence over measuring the diameters of the peripheral iridotomy that can be carried out by VHFU.

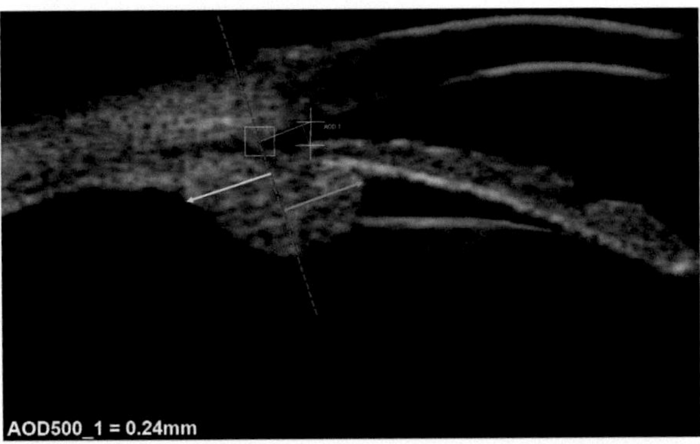


**Fig. 11.16  Anteriorization of the ciliary body** as part of a plateau iris configuration. Already evident without the measurements, the surface of the ciliary body in front of the red line perpendicular to the sclera and passing through the scleral spur is larger than the surface behind this line. Despite the anteriorization of the ciliary body, the angle is only marginal: AOD500 = 240 μm, because there is neither shifting nor indentation of the iris root by the ciliary body

## Position of the Ciliary Body

The surface of the ciliary body is compared in front of and behind a line perpendicular to the sclera passing through the scleral spur. Normally the pars plicata does not exceed this line by more than one third. Otherwise, the ciliary body is anteriorized, which is seen in plateau iris configuration. This anteriorization of the ciliary body is then accompanied by disappearance (or medialization) of the ciliary sulcus (Fig. 11.16).

## The Lens Vault

The lens vault has become a value that is systematically assessed during an examination for a narrow angle. It is defined as the distance between the apex of the anterior lens capsule and the angle-to-angle diameter. The value provided by the device (with an ultrasound velocity of 1550 m/s) should be corrected according to the velocity of ultrasound in the lens, which is 1641 m/s. One can now perform a semi-automatic fast calculation of this value, which automatically corrects the value found according to the velocity of ultrasound in the lens (Fig. 11.5c). More than 250 articles have been published on this value, its importance, and its usefulness. Epidemiologically [26, 27], it is greater in narrow angles than in open angles. However, there is no correlation with pupillary block or plateau iris. It increases with age and is greater in women than men. It is related, but not linearly, to the thickness of the lens found on the initial biometry performed with the 10/15 MHz probe. It is normal from 0 to 500 μm, moderately increased from 500 to 750 μm, greatly increased from 750 μm to 1 mm, and very strongly increased above 1 mm (Fig. 11.5c). With a posterior chamber IOL (Fig. 11.6), in the absence of a complication (malignant glaucoma), the lens vault is negative and the distance needs to similarly be recalculated with the velocity of ultrasound in the aqueous humor, which equals 1532 m/s. There is a close relation between the increase in the lens vault and the risk of angle closure [28]. Above 1 mm, in case of angle closure, and even if there are no lens opacities, the indication for peripheral iridotomy and phacoemulsification must be balanced [29, 30].

## 11.3 Mechanisms of Chronic Narrow-Angle Glaucoma

### *11.3.1 Pupillary Block*

To pass from the posterior chamber to the anterior chamber, the aqueous humor encounters resistance at the level of the pupillary edge next to the lens. Although the term is ambiguous, this resistance is called the pupillary block.

Pupillary block is present and permanent in all phakic patients. The pressure gradient it causes is responsible for the anterior convexity of the iris. Certain anatomical elements can make this convexity dangerous, by causing the apposition of the peripheral iris against the trabeculum [31].

When the root of the iris is pushed forward, it can stick to the periphery of the anterior surface of the cornea, causing a pretrabecular obstacle to the evacuation of the aqueous humor. This angle closure can occur in a brutal way, characterizing the acute angle-closure crisis, or more progressive, pernicious, leading to chronic ocular hypertonia whose clinical picture is close to chronic open angle glaucoma (Fig. 11.17).

In ultrasound, the iris has a centered convex anterior curvature, and the ciliary body has a normal position with a well-delineated, normal sulcus.

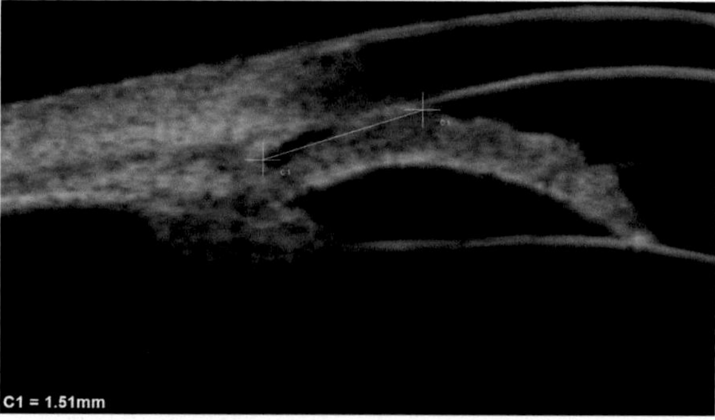


**Fig. 11.17 Closed-angle by pupillary block.** The angle is closed at 1.51 mm, with a small Mapstone sinus behind the irido-corneo-trabecular apposition. The entire iris is quite convex, with a peak centered on its middle part. Also note an average insertion of the iris on the ciliary body, the root of the iris of normal thickness, and also a perfectly normal sulcus

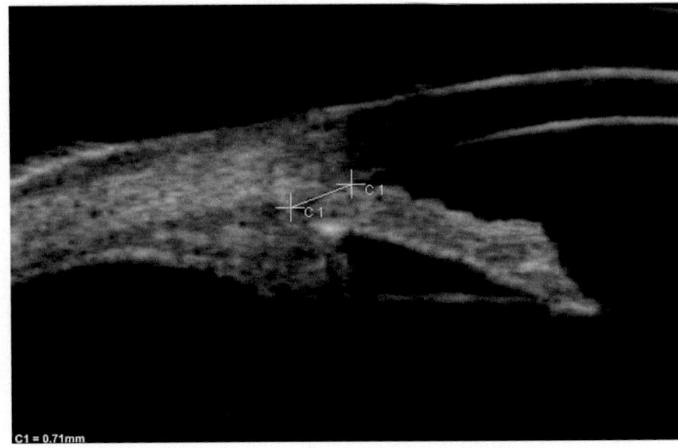


**Fig. 11.18 Plateau iris configuration**. The angle is closed at 0.71 mm. The ciliary body is anteriorized with disappearance (medialization) of the sulcus; the iris, stiff, is angled with a peripheral vertex

Peripheral laser iridotomy, a simple procedure, achievable on an outpatient basis, allows for removing this blockage. This shows the importance of early detection and treatment of primary angle-closure glaucoma.

After removal of the pupillary block by peripheral iridotomy, the persistence of significant closure requires additional treatment of the pretrabecular obstruction. This treatment depends on the etiology [32].

### 11.3.2 Plateau Iris

Plateau iris is a form of primary angle-closure glaucoma caused by a large or anteriorized ciliary body that indents the iris against the trabeculum, and leads to mechanical obstruction of the trabeculum, with disappearance of the peripheral sulcus as a cardinal sign on ultrasound [24, 25, 33]. This also leads to a peripheral angulation of the iris that is clearly visible by ultrasound (Fig. 11.18) as compared with the central harmonious curvature observed in pupillary block. One refers to plateau iris syndrome after peripheral laser iridotomy (Fig. 11.19); otherwise, if the same signs are observed without peripheral iridotomy, it is called plateau iris configuration.

### 11.3.3 Basal Insertion of the Iris

Another anatomical configuration that can lead to a narrow-angle and angle-closure glaucoma is basal insertion of the iris (Fig. 11.20), frequently associated with peripheral thickening of the iris, a narrower anterior chamber, and higher intraocular pressure before treatment than with middle or apical insertion [34].

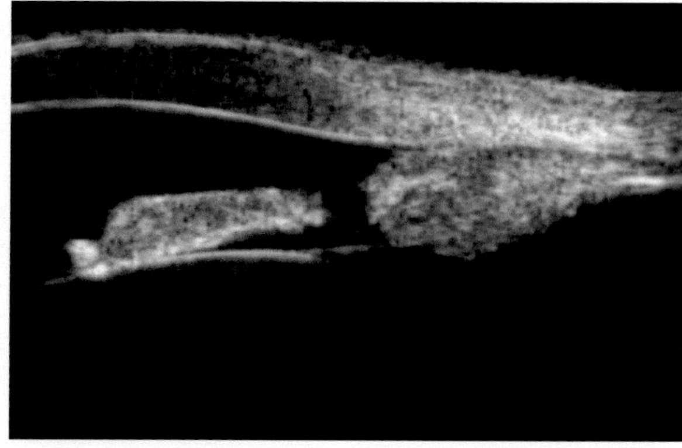

**Fig. 11.19 Plateau iris syndrome,** meridian of 11:30 o'clock, left eye, where the peripheral iridotomy is located, fortunately not too peripheral, but slightly anterior to the ciliary body which compresses the angulated iris root, with no reopening of the angle

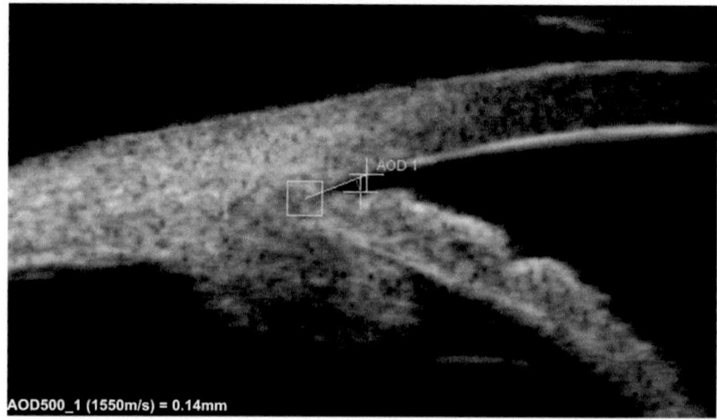



**Fig. 11.20 Anterior (peripheral), or basal insertion of the iris on the ciliary body,** causing a narrow-angle (AOD500 = 0.14 mm). There is slight anteriorization of the ciliary body, but the sulcus, which is narrow, is in a normal position

### 11.3.4 Creeping Angle Glaucoma

This form, common in the Asian-Mongoloid population, is related to the formation of peripheral synechiae moving the insertion of the iris forward (Fig. 11.21) to the trabeculum [35]. Several mechanisms are involved in producing this situation: pupillary block, anomaly of the thickness and position of the iris, and a plateau iris configuration.

## 11.4 Pigmentary Glaucoma

Pigment dispersion syndrome is characterized by the release of constituents of the iris pigment epithelium, which are then transported by the aqueous humor and deposited on various structures of the anterior segment, obstructing of the trabecular meshwork. This can lead to an increase in intraocular pressure, and then, in 15% to 25% of cases, to a particular form of open-angle glaucoma called pigmentary glaucoma. This mainly affects young, myopic, white adult males [36].

**Fig. 11.21  Creeping angle-closure glaucoma.** The angle is fully closed, with synechiae, beyond the trabeculum, associated with a thickening of the root of the iris to 0.67 mm

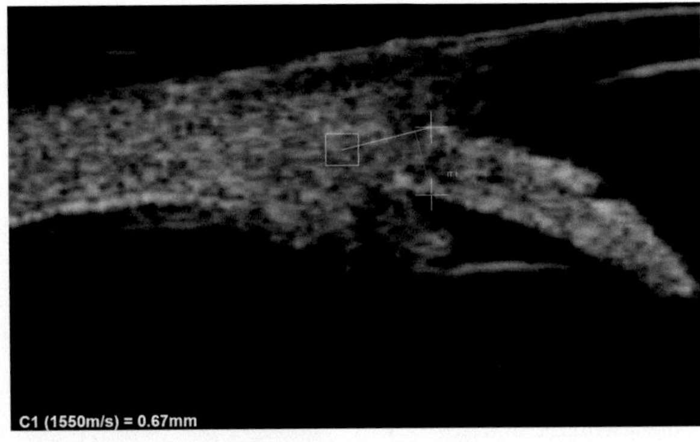


The release of pigment is thought to be related to a particular anatomical configuration of the iris: a concavity of the iris (Fig. 11.22) would lead to a close contact between the posterior surface of the iris and the anterior lens capsule and the anterior zonular fibers. During variations in pupil size, especially in mydriasis, the zonular fibers and the lens erode the iris pigment epithelium, thereby leading to the release of pigments [37]. The presentation being not characteristic in ultrasound, it may be useful to potentiate this concavity of the iris by performing a section in accommodation, quite tricky however to realize. Pigment dispersion is usually bilateral, and it is often discovered by chance.

At the stage of pigment dispersion without glaucoma, a peripheral iridotomy is recommended [38] when iris is concave. At the stage of pigmentary glaucoma, one should consider a trabeculoplasty ± of medical treatments, if it is moderate, or filtration surgery, if it has evolved [39].

## 11.5  Check-Ups After Surgery/laser Surgery

### 11.5.1  *After Laser Peripheral Iridotomy (PI)*

An orifice made at the periphery of the iris prevents or alleviates the permanent or definitive apposition of the iris against the trabeculum. The success is assessed by a flow of aqueous humor and pigments and deepening of the anterior chamber on the periphery [40]. The purpose of PI is to suppress the pressure gradient between the anterior and posterior chambers. Therefore, its functional nature is assessed not by visualization and quantification of the peripheral iridotomy itself but by a much more precise indirect sign: flattening of the iris.

Once the functional nature of the peripheral iridotomy has been established, the second step is to evaluate its effectiveness in reopening the angle. This effectiveness will depend on the absence or not of a mechanism added to that of closure by pure pupillary block.

**Fig. 11.22 Pigment dispersion syndrome in a discreetly myopic patient (axial length = 24.80 mm). a**: 9 o'clock meridian OS in the dark, **b**: 9 o'clock meridian OS in the light, **c**: 9 o'clock meridian OS in accommodation. Already in the light, the iris is concave but even more so in accommodation, the epithelium being in broad contact with the anterior capsule of the lens. The angle is marginal in the dark, open in the light, and wide open in accommodation

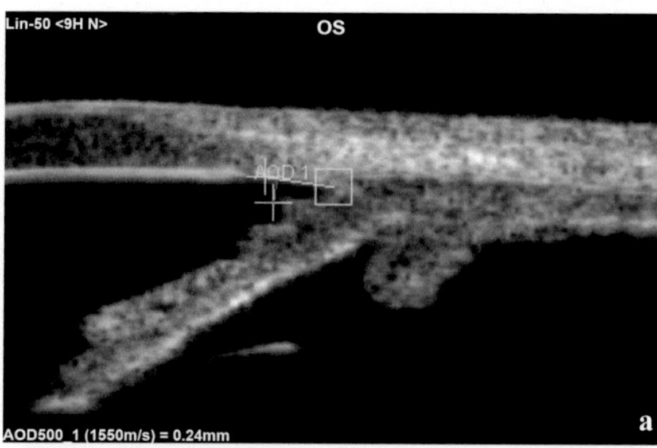


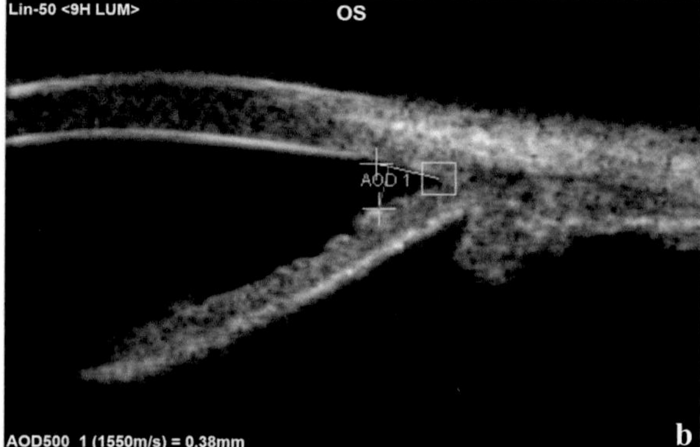


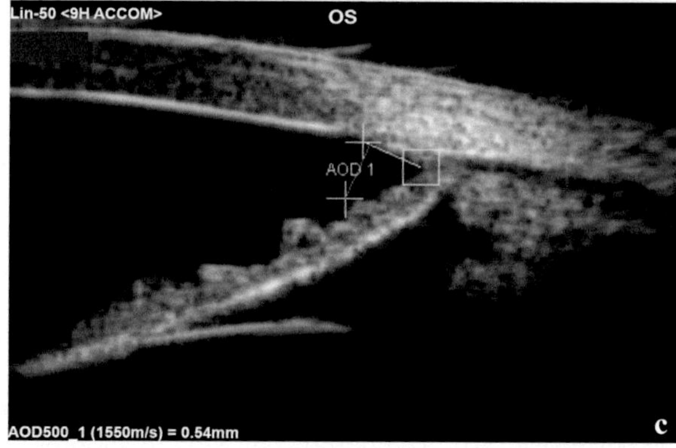


Imaging is mainly useful if there is no flattening of the iris or reopening of the angle, especially if plateau iris is suspected. Even if in these cases the main goal is the analysis of the relationship of the ciliary body and the iris, one must not forget to assess the peripheral iridotomy, in both planes, according to the meridian in question, but also according to the orthogonal quadrant.

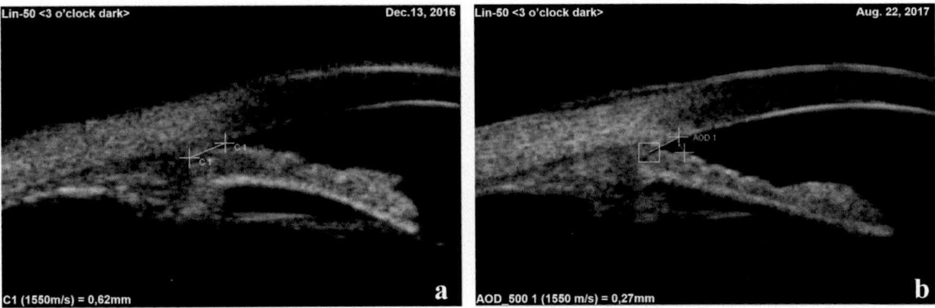


**Fig. 11.23 Opening of the angle after peripheral iridotomy (PI). a:** Before PI, the angle is fully closed, at 0.62 mm, and the iris is convex. **b:** After PI, the angle has opened, AOD500 has a normal value of 270 μm, and the iris has "flattened", reflecting the decrease in pressure in the posterior chamber

The width of the solution of continuity should be assessed, which can be quite small, even less than 400 μm, but also the disappearance of the anterior convexity of the iris, which reflects the functionality of a peripheral iridotomy and the angle opening, which reflects its effectiveness (Fig. 11.23). However, in all cases, scanning the area in both perpendicular directions is useful as is taking several images to analyze the morphology of the peripheral iridotomy and possibly measure it.

Even if the YAG laser is preceded by Argon laser, the laser readily causes dispersion of stromal cells that tend to organize themselves into thin membranes, which can sometimes produce real synechiae (Fig. 11.24). Regular edges of the iris and a larger size are characteristic of a surgical iridectomy (Fig. 11.25).

### 11.5.1.1 Non-transfixing/Non-permeable Character of Peripheral Iridotomy

Sometimes, even if the operator has noticed a flow of aqueous humor at the time of the procedure, the iris does not flatten and there is the concern that the PI is not fully transfixing (Fig. 11.26).

### 11.5.1.2 Polycystic Iridociliary Dysplasia

Another reason for an ineffective peripheral iridotomy can be that it was performed at a cyst of the posterior pigmented iris epithelium, in the context of iridociliary polycystic dysplasia. Whether it is discovered during an examination performed for assessing a narrow angle or during exploration of bulging of the iris, if peripheral iridotomy is indicated, one must specify which meridian(s) contain no cysts; indeed, when they are small, they are usually not clinically suspected (Fig. 11.27).

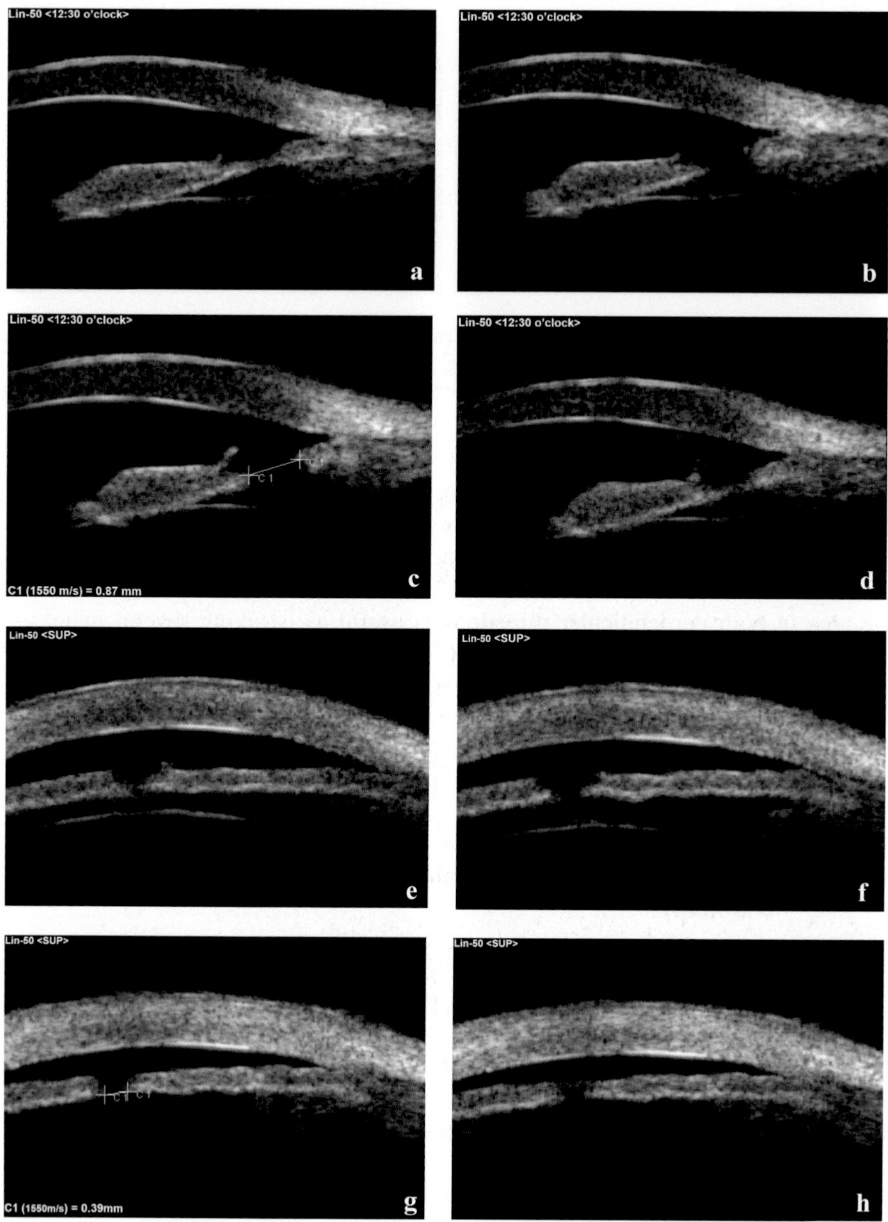

**Fig. 11.24 Ultrasound scanning around the PI** along the meridian considered (12:30 o'clock): **a**, **b**, **c**, and **d**, and in orthogonal quadrant section (superior): **e**, **f**, **g**, and **h**. The central sections (**b** and **c**, **f**, and **g**) pass at the center of the PI and the lateral sections (**a** and **d**, **e** and **h**) pass at the edge of the solution of continuity, which is perfectly transfixing at the ultrasound level and effective (absence of residual bulging of the iris). Note that the PI is higher than wide (0.87 vs 0.39 mm). Also note that although the PI is quite permeable, the ciliary body still compresses the root of the iris, which is characteristic of plateau iris syndrome. The laser burst on the stroma is responsible for the formation of iridocorneal membranes (**d**)

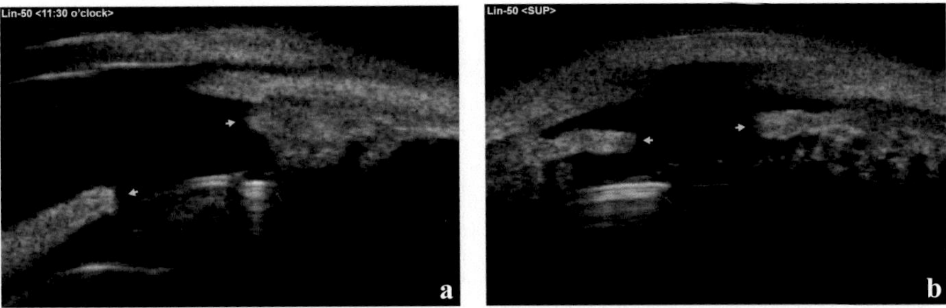

**Fig. 11.25 Surgical iridectomy as part of combined surgery,** cataract and trabeculectomy 15 years ago. **a**: Along the 11:30 o'clock meridian. **b**: Along the orthogonal superior quadrant. The solution of continuity is wider and the edges (➡ light blue arrows) are more regular than with the laser. The loop of the implant (→ thin purple arrow) is well positioned in the bag

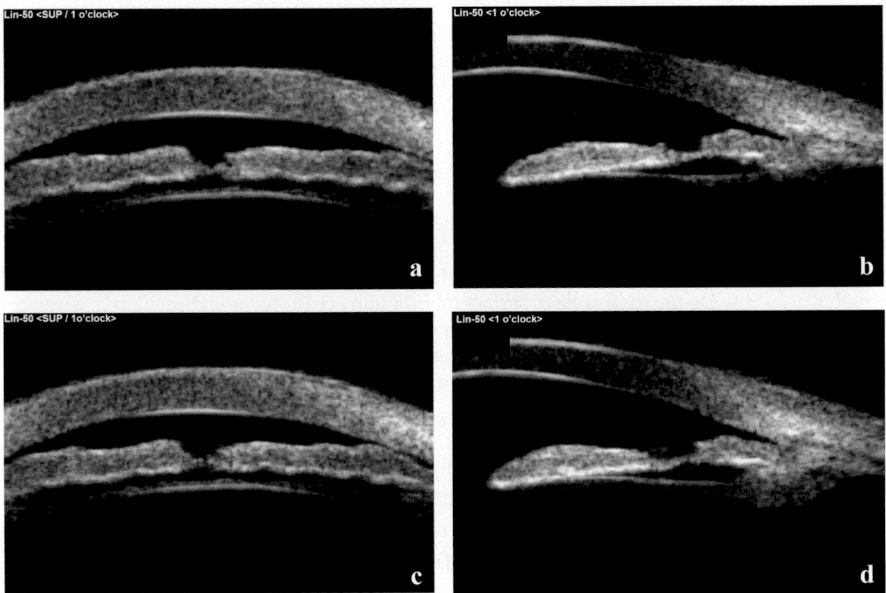

**Fig. 11.26 Non-transfixing peripheral iridotomy.** Either on quadrant (**a** and **c**) or meridian (**b** and **d**) sections, all the different sections pass through the center of the crater created by the laser, and all show the absence of solution of continuity at the posterior epithelium of the iris

## 11.5.2 After Iridoplasty

Iridoplasty is a technique performed with an argon laser on the periphery of the iris, which aims to retract the root of the iris to obtain reopening of a narrow angle after an iridotomy, to avoid filtration surgery for patients with plateau iris syndrome,

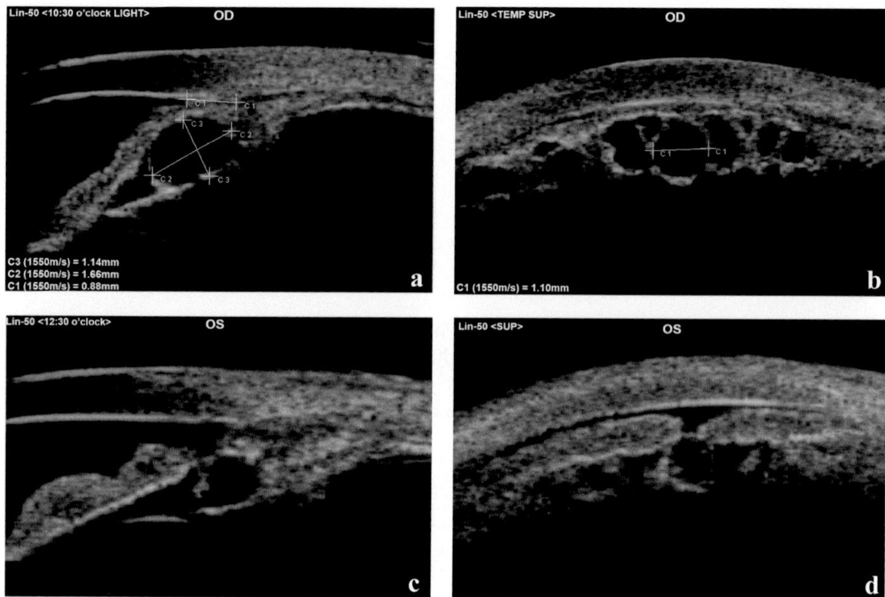



**Fig. 11.27** **Iridociliary polycystic dysplasia. a**: 10:30 o'clock meridian OD; **b**: superior temporal quadrant OD; **c**: 12:30 o'clock meridian OS; **d**: upper quadrant OS. On the right, the cysts are medium in size and cause discreet bulging of the periphery of the iris. On the left, the cyst is smaller, measuring 0.8 mm × 0.6 mm in diameter and 0.7 mm thick, and was clinically undetectable. The angle is closed on the right and on the left. On both sides, a cyst is responsible for the appearance of pseudoplateau iris. On the right, a laser peripheral iridotomy (LPI) being indicated, it is necessary to inform the correspondent of the exact location of the cysts; in particular, the superior temporal quadrant should be avoided. On the left, the already performed LPI is ineffective because it abuts the mini cyst, precluding communication between the posterior and anterior chambers

even though its long-term effectiveness remains to be demonstrated [41]. At a checkup performed 6 months after the procedure, VHFU can clearly show the stiff and retracted appearance of the iris root due to the action of the laser and the discreet reopening of the angle (Fig. 11.28), an effect that would tend to be worn out with time.

## 11.5.3 After Filtration Surgery

Monitoring of filtration surgery can benefit from VHFU exploration, with very good visualization of the filtration bleb, and the presence or absence of the decompression chamber. Trabeculectomy and deep sclerectomy can be identified in imaging of the angle as well as determining the mechanism of poor filtration.

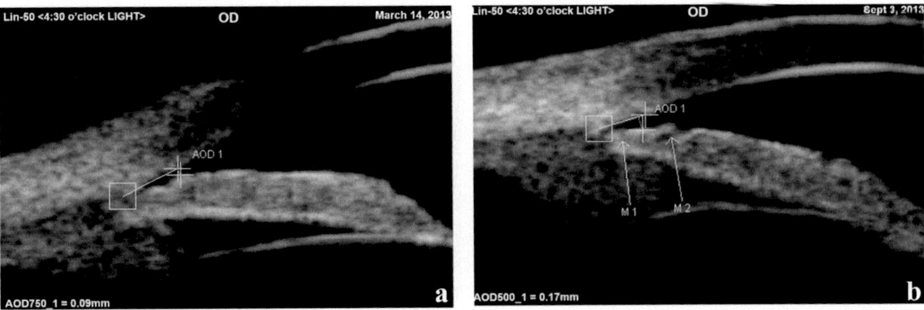


**Fig. 11.28  Iridoplasty performed for plateau iris syndrome: presentation before (a) and after (b) the procedure**. After laser peripheral iridotomy (LPI) (**a**), and despite it, the angle remained very narrow, even in the light, throughout the lower hemifield. After iridoplasty (**b**), the angle reopened very slightly: it became borderline and the stiff appearance of the root of the iris can be noted (M1 and M2)

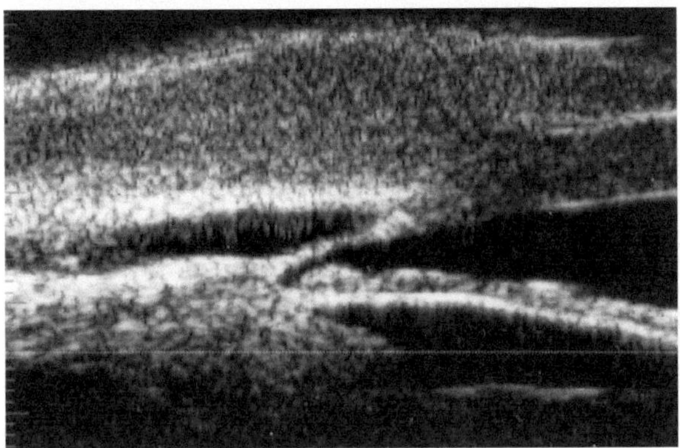

**Fig. 11.29  Non-perforating deep sclerectomy. UBM**: visualization of the trabecular leaflet left in place

In the case of a deep sclerectomy, the trabecular leaflet left in place can sometimes be highlighted (Fig. 11.29). A functional conjunctival bleb results in thickening of the conjunctiva, which acts as a sponge for the aqueous humor [42] (Fig. 11.30). A protruding conjunctival bleb but with fibrosis of the conjunctiva is a sign of less good evacuation of the aqueous humor (Fig. 11.31).

## *11.5.4  After Drainage Implants*

Used to treat refractory glaucoma, there are many models, such as the Molteno Tube, Ahmed valve, Baerveldt implant, etc. They are alternatives to cyclodestruction by

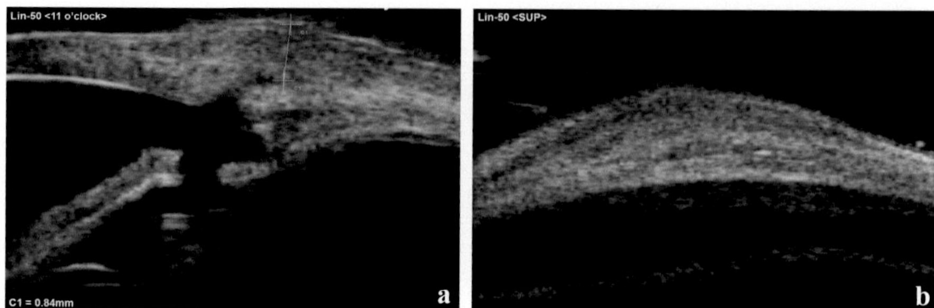

**Fig. 11.30** **Satisfactory filtration bleb**. **a**: Along the 11 o'clock meridian; **b**: orthogonal transverse view of the superior quadrant. The regular subconjunctival thickening is quite echogenic and mostly homogeneous

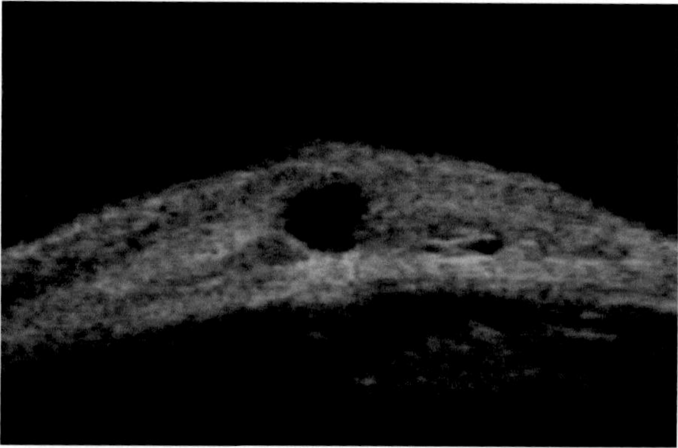

**Fig. 11.31** **Encysted filtration bleb**. The cyst within the filtration bleb is associated with a reduced filtration and a rise in intraocular pression despite multi-daily massages of the patient

micropulsed laser. Because of their superficial location, drainage implants are clearly visible by VHFU (Fig. 11.32), which sometimes helps to explain a complication.

## 11.6 Corneal Opacities

VHFU has been found useful particularly for neonatal corneal opacities (NCOs). This examination should be performed under general anesthesia after a careful clinical examination, very often limited however to the measurement of corneal diameters (sometimes imprecise) and determination of the IOP (sometimes insignificant). Irido-corneal synechiae can sometimes be discerned behind a corneal opacity, but most often access to the ocular fundus is not possible.

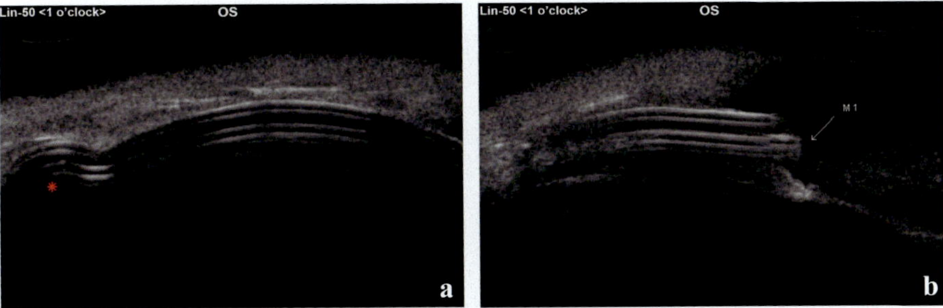


**Fig. 11.32 Ahmed valve with diffuse hyphema**. This diffuse hyphema is represented as a hypoechoic presentation of the entire anterior chamber, without a tendency to declivity. **a**: Posterior part, with the reservoir (∗) of the valve, **b**: Anterior part of the tube in the anterior chamber, without contact, neither with the endothelium nor the iris

VHFU is good for analysis of the abnormalities of the anterior segment and allows for analysis of the various morphological abnormalities of the cornea, iris, and lens.

Several authors have written reference texts on this subject. One of the first, Waring [43], focused the classification and recognition of the different entities on the location of the various afflictions, mostly central (Peters) or more peripheral (Rieger). In contrast, Nischal [44] based his classification on the pathogenesis, the surgical options, and the prognosis, contrasting primary NCOs, including corneal dystrophies and choristomas present from birth, and secondary NCOs, including kerato-irido-lenticular dysgenesis (KILD) and infectious, iatrogenic, and developmental causes.

### *11.6.1  Peters Anomaly Type 1*

It is the single most frequent entity, yet far from being a catch-all summing all the neonatal opacities of the cornea [43]. It is in fact a kerato-irido-lenticular dysgenesis (KILD) [44] (Fig. 11.33).

#### 11.6.1.1  Opaque Cornea

The opaque cornea is hyperechoic in its entirety, or more rarely partially. However, there is still a good correlation between clinical opacity and ultrasound hypere-chogenicity (Fig. 11.34).

When this opacity is sectorial, localized to a quadrant, a corneal rotation can be considered, with ultimately a better prognosis than with a transplant. In addition, there is often a degree of central or paracentral thinning and a thickening at a distance from the center. Finally, a rather characteristic defect of the posterior side of the cornea is often noted, the extent of which is extremely variable, from a simple irregularity to a *bona fide* deep posterior defect (Fig. 11.35).

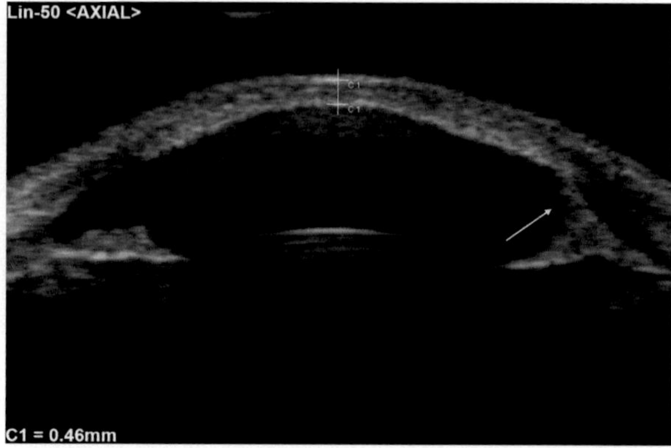

**Fig. 11.33 Kerato-irido-lenticular dysgenesis (KILD): Peters anomaly type 1.** Irregular thickness of the cornea with central thinning and pericentral thickening. More or less central irido-lenticular adhesion ($\rightarrow$ yellow arrow)

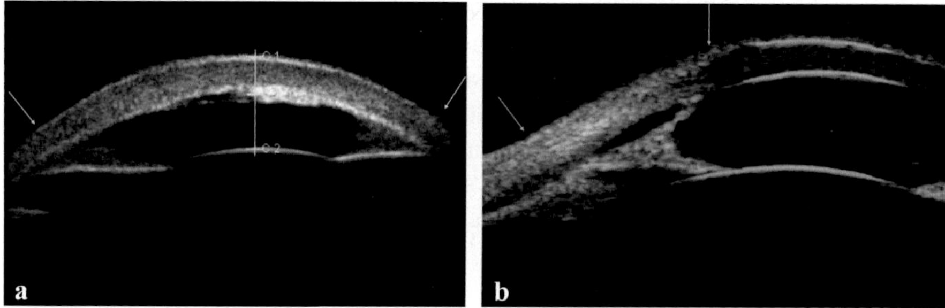

**Fig. 11.34 Peters anomaly type 1: variability in corneal hyperechogenicity. a:** Diffuse; **b:** sectorial. This hyperechogenicity (between the arrows) is parallel to the optical opacity

## 11.6.1.2 The Iris

Characteristically, iridocorneal adhesions (Fig. 11.36) are dense, thick, rigid, between the middle part of the iris and the periphery of the posterior defect of the cornea; but they can be thinner; and sometimes, rarely, they produce a real felting of the whole peripheral part of the anterior chamber; and finally, they may appear peripheral.

## 11.6.1.3 The Lens

The lens has to be studied with a lower frequency probe, close to 20 MHz. Most often it does not present an anomaly, but it is sometimes echogenic in connection with a cataract.

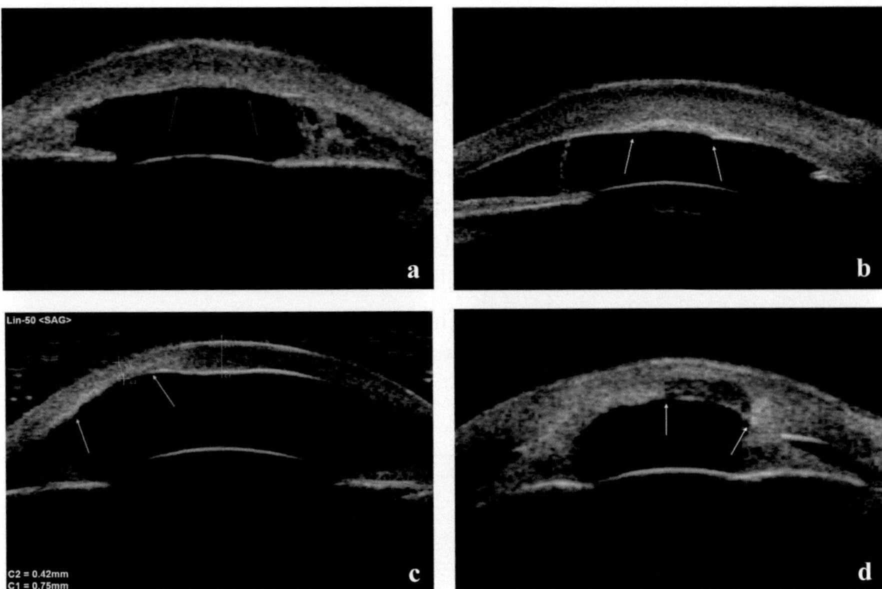

**Fig. 11.35 Peters anomaly type 1: variable extent of posterior corneal defect. a:** Minimal; **b:** moderate; **c:** moderate, extensive and eccentric; **d:** very substantial

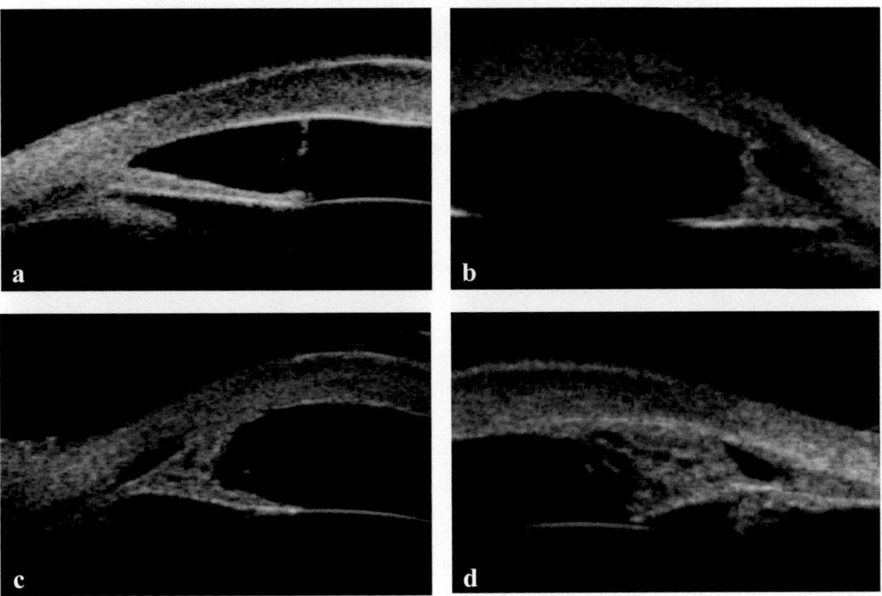

**Fig. 11.36 Peters anomaly type 1: variability of iridocorneal adhesions. a:** Very thin; **b:** wide at the iris and thin at the cornea; **c:** wide at the iris and thick; **d:** very thick and appearing as a real felting. In all cases, the iris is pulled forward by this synechia, mostly central, attaching to the cornea on the periphery of the posterior corneal defect

## 11.6.2   Peters Anomaly Type 2

It is characterized by non-separation of the lens and the cornea (Fig. 11.37).
To differentiate from:

- a separation between the cornea and the lens but without development of the latter,
- a separation between the cornea and the lens and the normal formation of the latter but a secondary late adhesion between the two [45] (Fig. 11.38),
- a defect in the formation of the lens (Fig. 11.39).

These anomalies of the lens are sometimes visible by VHFU at 50 MHz but are best assessed with a high-frequency probe, close to 20 MHz, allowing penetration, and acceptable resolution.

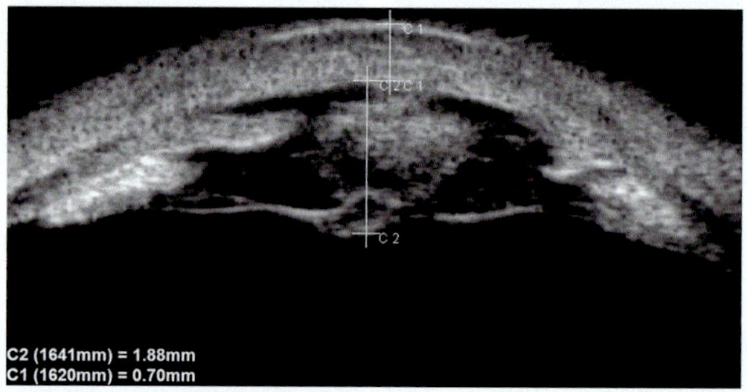


**Fig. 11.37   Peters anomaly type 2.** Incomplete separation of the lens from the cornea, the lens otherwise being echogenic, cataractous, and the cornea thick and very echogenic. This anterior segment dysgenesis is associated with microphthalmos, the axial length measuring 13.7 mm, and glaucoma

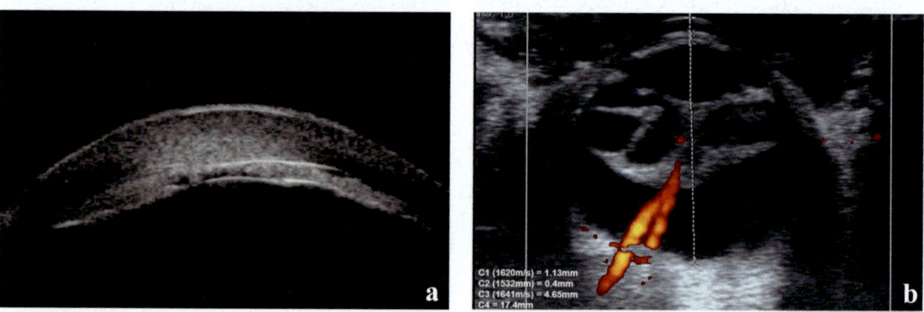


**Fig. 11.38   Corneal opacity secondary to contact with a large lens for the size of this microphthalmic eye, with vitreoretinal dysplasia. a:** Axial section at 50 MHz; **b:** axial section in color Doppler imaging, power mode at 12 MHz. In **a**, the cornea is thickened and very echogenic, and the compressed iris can clearly be seen between the endothelium and the anterior lens capsule. In **b**, the large lens can be seen, subluxated forward, as well as the total vascularized retinal detachment

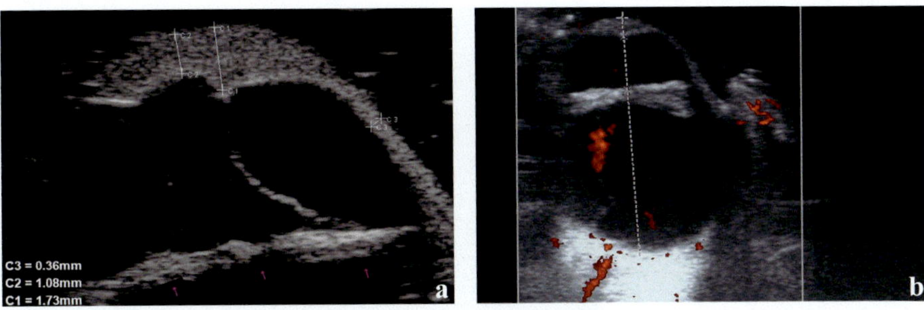

**Fig. 11.39 Complex dysgenesis of the anterior segment with glaucoma. a**: Axial section at 25 MHz; **b**: axial section in color Doppler energy mode at 12 MHz. In **a**, the cornea is thick and very irregular as well as quite echogenic, with disappearance of the posterior hyperechoic line corresponding to the endothelium and the Descemet membrane. Thin membranes can clearly be seen between the iris and the cornea, crossing the anterior chamber, which is very deep (4.8 mm). In **b**, the malformation of the lens can be appreciated

## 11.6.3 Glaucoma

Whether congenital glaucoma or glaucoma associated with iris abnormalities, Nischal [46] includes them in the same way as Peters' syndrome in "secondary" congenital opacities, because it is also a dysgenesis, iridotrabecular in this case. The opacity, most often moderate, can sometimes be dense. Other signs of buphthalmia should always be searched: an increase in the depth and diameters of the anterior chamber (Fig. 11.40). Sections centered on the angle often show an impasto appearance of the angle.

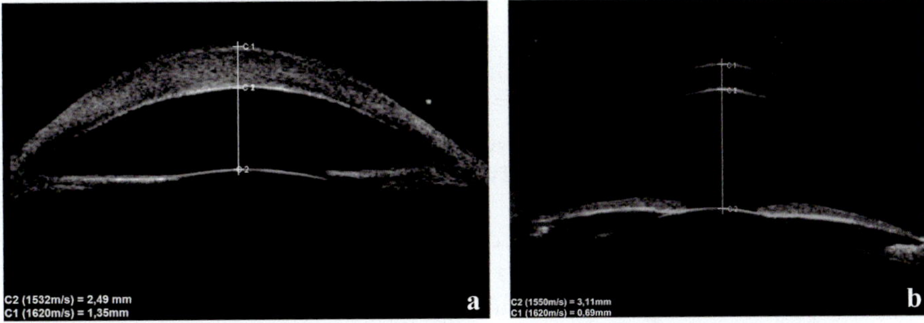

**Fig. 11.40 Infantile glaucoma with buphthalmia. a**: Glaucoma with a very thin iris and very thick and very echogenic cornea. **b**: Congenital glaucoma with a cornea of moderately increased thickness. In both cases there is a clear increase in the angle-to-angle diameter, 12.78 mm in **a** and 12.34 mm in **b**, sometimes difficult to image on a single section, the exploration cell having a diameter of 15 mm

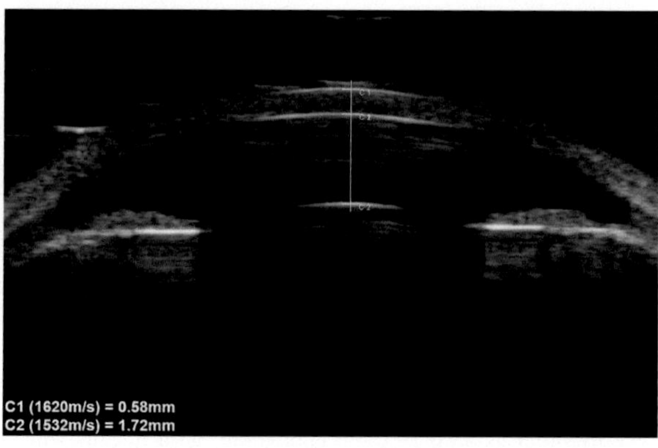



**Fig. 11.41 Sclerocornea associated with cornea plana**. The not very convex appearance of the cornea is obvious, as is its slightly increased thickness and significant peripheral echogenicity, and a shallow anterior chamber, with no detectable iridocorneal adhesion

## 11.6.4 Sclerocornea

Always according to the Nischal classification [46], as opposed to dysgenesis, the primary opacities include dystrophies, dermoids, conditions related to the CYP1B1 gene, and sclerocornea, always peripheral and associated with a cornea plana (Fig. 11.41), with its total secondary opacification, often associated to severe microphthalmia.

The opaque cornea is less echogenic than in Peters anomaly type 1, more peripheral, and there is usually no iridocorneal adhesion.

## 11.6.5 Rieger Anomaly, Axenfeld Syndrome, Axenfeld-Rieger Syndrome

### 11.6.5.1 Rieger Anomaly

It is an irido-trabeculo-dysgenesis characterized by bilateral iris abnormalities, asymmetrical or not, which can be associated with glaucoma: thinning of the iris, polycoria, and corectopia (Fig. 11.42).

### 11.6.5.2 Axenfeld-Rieger Syndrome

Rare, its prevalence being 1/200,000, it associates ocular and extraocular abnormalities. The ocular abnormalities are identical to those observed in Rieger anomaly but are associated with a posterior embryotoxon: a prominence with anterior displacement of the Schwalbe line and peripheral synechiae or iris attachments from the angle to the trabecular meshwork (Fig. 11.43). This dysgenesis can cause glaucoma,

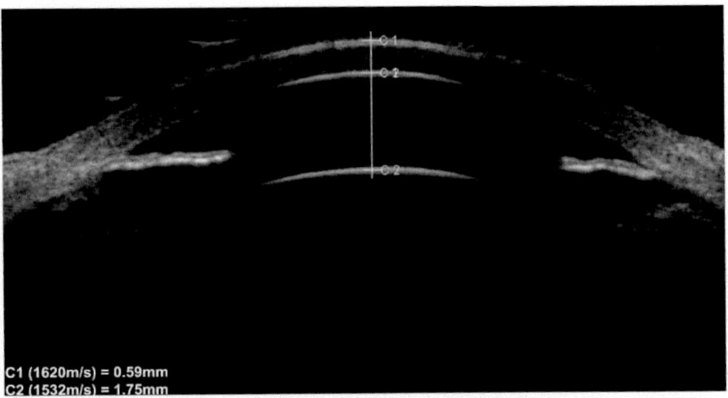


**Fig. 11.42 Rieger anomaly**. On this axial section of the anterior segment, there is a slight thickening of the cornea, normally convex, and a shallow anterior chamber, but mainly a very thin and very short iris

occurring at a young age or in older children. The most typical extraocular abnormalities are craniofacial dysmorphism and dental abnormalities, but many others can be encountered [47]: genitourinary, pituitary, etc.

## 11.6.6 Dermoids

The clinical and ultrasound diagnosis is straightforward at the limbus, or rarely central (Fig. 11.44). Dermoids can sometimes be associated with / extend into a *bona fide* extraconal dermoid cyst (see Chaps. 23 and 26). By ultrasound, the appearance is hyperechoic, often poorly delineated, and attenuating, so the examination to assess the cornea behind it is often difficult (Fig. 11.45). Using CDI, intrinsic vascularization may sometimes be disclosed, which is surprising for such a choristoma (Fig. 11.46).

## 11.6.7 Other Causes

Lastly, there are also acquired secondary opacities, including viral (herpes) and bacterial (*Neisseria gonorrhea*) infections, trauma (Fig. 11.47), and metabolic disorders (mucolipidosis IV).

**Finally**, it should be emphasized that in all these cases of NCO, the anterior segment should be examined at 50 and 25 MHz but also the whole eye explored at 10/15 MHz and with color Doppler imaging, because these eyes frequently exhibit microphthalmos, in approximately one quarter of cases, hence the need to measure their axial length. Also, they frequently present, in almost half of cases, associated abnormalities, hemorrhage, persistent fetal vasculature, retinal detachment, coloboma etc. and very often glaucoma, hence the usefulness of looking for disturbances in the flows of the vessels of the optic nerve head.

**In adults**, VHFU is of course not essential in preoperative assessment before a corneal transplant, but an ultrasound of the posterior segment as well as a CDI of the optic nerve head vessels is very useful. It can be useful for diagnostic purposes

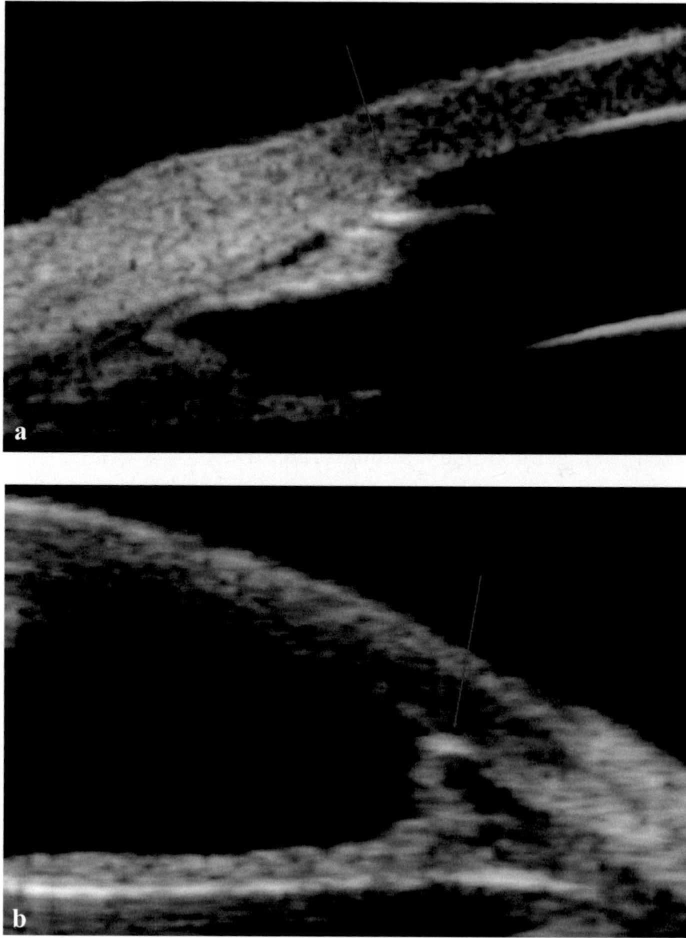

**Fig. 11.43** **Axenfeld-Rieger syndrome**. Two types of peripheral iridocorneal adhesions. **a**: Associated with morphological abnormality of the iris; **b**: with a morphologically normal iris. In both cases, there is a small hyperechoic nodule corresponding to the embryotoxon (→ purple arrows)

or to assess, with OCT, the extension to the different layers of the cornea, as in Salzmann's nodular degeneration (Fig. 11.48). However, in some cases, the changes are so unusual that interpretation becomes difficult (Fig. 11.49).

Some conjunctival lesions are frequent, often asymptomatic, observed fortuitously at the level of the limbus on examinations carried out for exploring a narrow angle, such as pingueculae (Fig. 11.50). **Pinguecula** is a conjunctival degeneration, often related to ultraviolet rays and wind, manifested by a small yellowish-white limbic thickening. In ultrasound, this slight bump is most often not very echogenic and well delineated, but it can be moderately echogenic, heterogeneous, even protruding, remaining quite superficial, however.

**Fig. 11.44  Central corneal dermoid**. Hyperechoic appearance of the lesion as a helmet, without peripheral extension. Note the slightly echogenic appearance of the underlying corneal stroma, which is quite thin

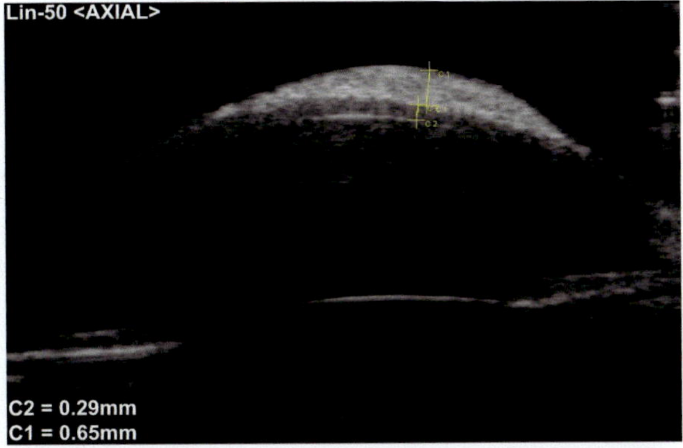



**Fig. 11.45  Limbal dermoid**. The lesion partially encroaches on the corneal stroma, but on the periphery, it reaches the scleral spur

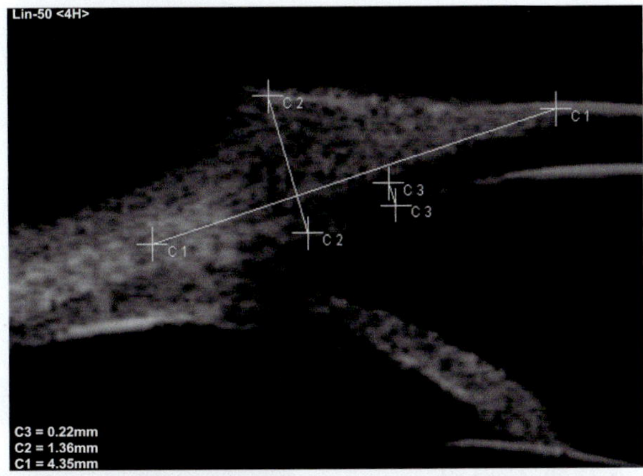



**Fig. 11.46  Limbal dermoid**. Color doppler imaging. Evidence of very low flows: peak systolic velocity < 5 cm/s and resistance index = 0.43, inside this small choristoma

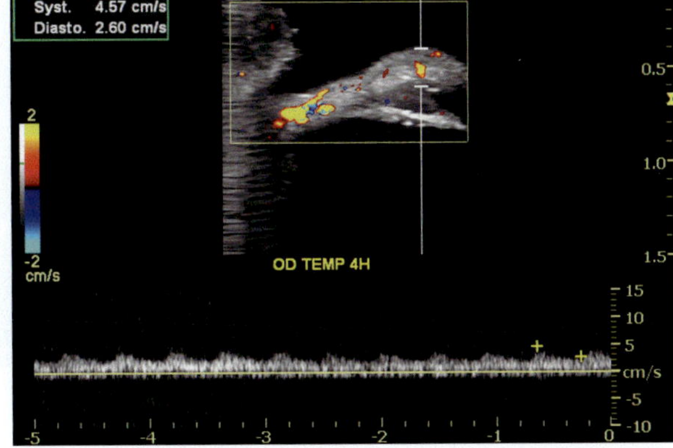

**Fig. 11.47 Post-traumatic opacity**. Disappearance of the visibility of the endothelium and anterior chamber fully filled with a fibrinous mass preventing assessment of the lens due to the attenuation

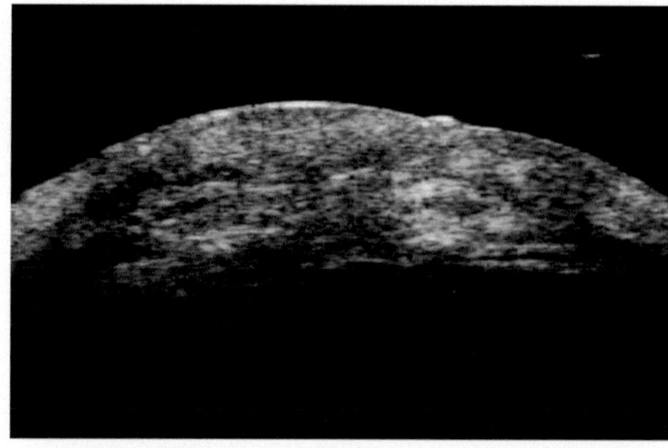

**Fig. 11.48 Salzmann subepithelial nodule**. This degeneration occurred 1 year after phacoemulsification intervention with IOL implantation. The very superficial position of the very echogenic and attenuating lesion can clearly be seen, thicker than the underlying stroma

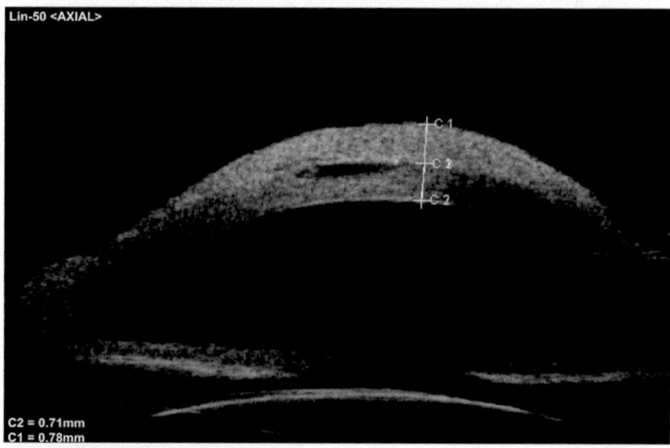


**Fig. 11.49 Corneal rearrangement after a wasp sting**. Assessment before corneal transplantation: total disorganization of the different layers of the cornea

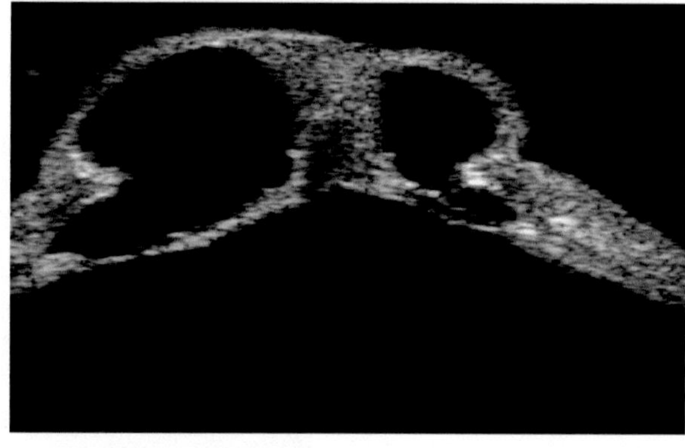

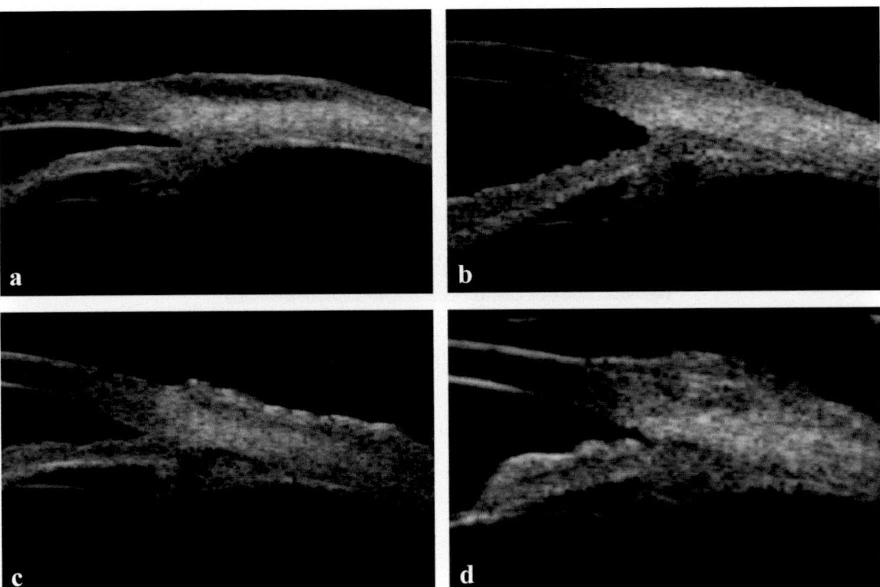

**Fig. 11.50 Pinguecula, different ultrasound presentations**. **a**: Small, hypoechoic, and well-delineated, by far the most common presentation; **b**: Small size, moderately echogenic, and heterogeneous, with a very echogenic and irregular surface; **c**: Thin, moderately echogenic, and heterogeneous, with a very echogenic, irregular, scalloped surface; **d**: Thick, protruding, moderately echogenic but well delineated; Note that in all cases the thickness of the sclera is strictly normal

In contrast, **pterygium** extends to the cornea, which can exert traction and extend toward the visual axis (Fig. 11.51) and can be treated by surgical excision.

The difference is most often clear, both clinically and with ultrasound, with a **keratoconjunctival tumor** (Fig. 11.52).

Equally unnoticed at the clinical level, one must highlight crossing of the sclera by vessels (Fig. 11.53), most often observed in the inferior quadrant.

## 11.7 Anterior Segment Trauma

Eye injuries and contusions are often accompanied by lesions of the anterior segment that are sometimes difficult to assess exhaustively because of associated disturbances: cloudy cornea, hemorrhage, or inflammation of the anterior chamber. Ultrasound is useful in these cases [48], best by immersion at 50 MHz, but depending on the pain, also through the eyelids with a high-frequency probe close to 20 MHz. In any case, it is certainly only feasible after suturing the wound. The following are some examples.

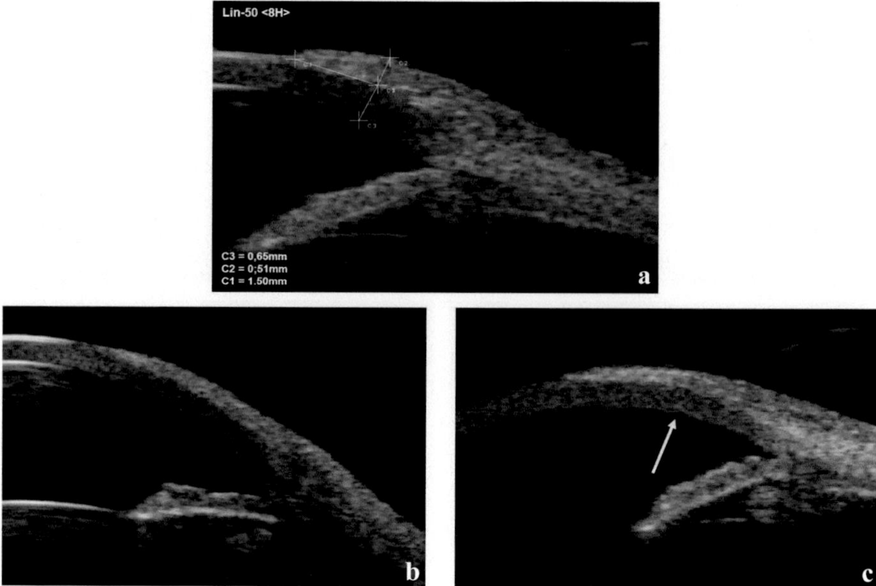

**Fig. 11.51 Pterygium. a**: Echogenic and thick (0.51 mm), quite homogeneous, extending not far from the visual axis but without repercussion on the thickness of the corneal stroma with a thickness of 0.65 mm. The fibrovascular tissue of the pterygium causes traction on the cornea, resulting in an arching of the cornea, already appreciable in the primary gaze (**b**) but above all in an increase in the opening of the angle (arrow) in the 45° lateral gaze (**c**)

**Fig. 11.52 Invasive squamous cell carcinoma.** The angle of connection with the cornea, the impact on the underlying cornea, and the very heterogeneous echotexture of this carcinoma are very different from pterygium

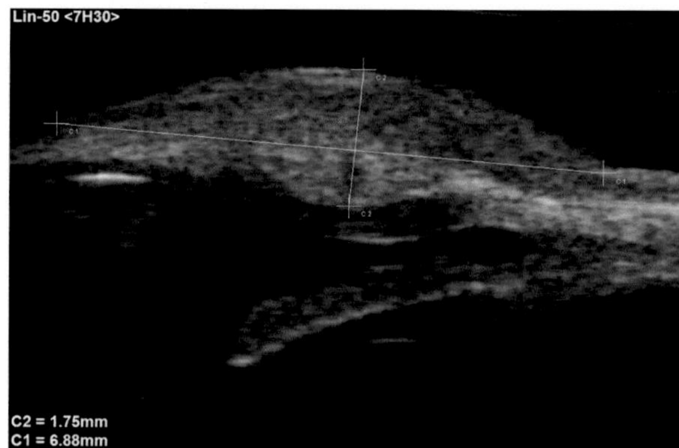

## 11.7.1 The Cornea and the Anterior Chamber

Corneal edema and hyphema are common (Fig. 11.54). Corneal edema does not always result in hyperechogenicity of the cornea, especially as it is at a distance from the focal area, and the thickening can be moderate, only becoming apparent when

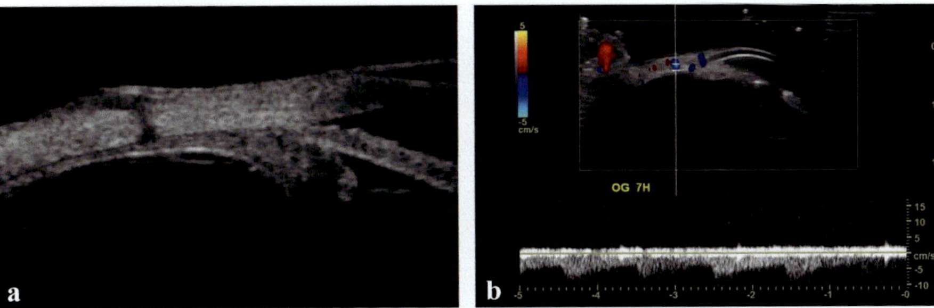


**Fig. 11.53 Peripheral transscleral vessel. a**: VHFU section according to 7 o'clock; **b**: High frequency CDI, color and spectral modes according to 7 o'clock. The linear path of the vessel is associated with a subconjunctival microprotrusion. CDI clearly shows that it is a small arterial capillary

its thickness is measured. When hyphema is diffuse, many small poorly echogenic spots can be seen in the anterior chamber, mainly in the vicinity of the focal zone, identical to those seen in a retrohyaloid hemorrhage (see Chap. 12). However, not much may be seen in the event of sedimentation.

## 11.7.2   The Iris

### 11.7.2.1   Angle Recession

This is caused by pressure from contusion causing a tear on the ciliary body. It can cause glaucoma if the lesion has also affected the trabeculum. The ultrasound presentation is quite characteristic (Fig. 11.55).

### 11.7.2.2   Iridodialysis

This is the consequence of a tear of the iris at its root, where it is thinnest (Fig. 11.56). Unlike a peripheral iridectomy, the tear is in contact with the scleral spur and not at a distance.

### 11.7.2.3   Other Traumas

Iris tears can be seen at full thickness, at the middle part of the iris (Fig. 11.57), associated or not with adjacent hematomas (Fig. 11.58).

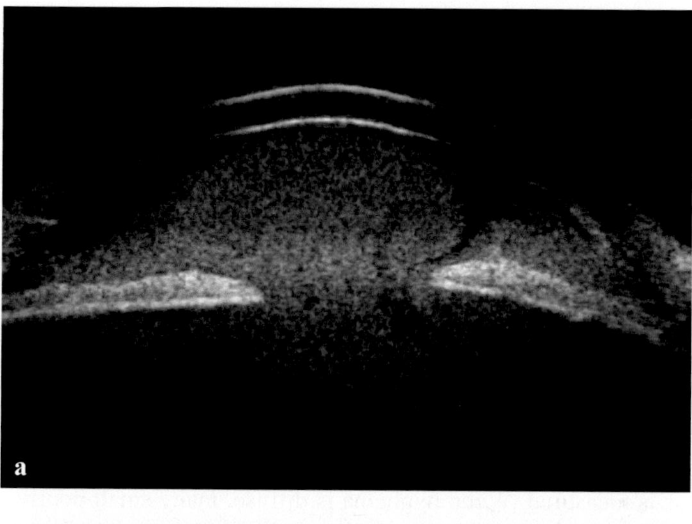

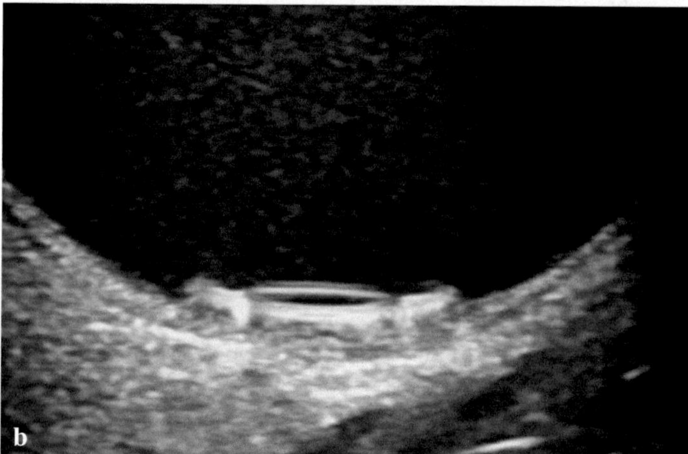

**Fig. 11.54 Post-traumatic corneal edema and hyphema** following a fall from a bicycle after hitting a lamp post. **a**: 50-MHz section of the anterior segment; **b**: sagittal section at 10 MHz of the posterior part of the eyeball. The many small, minimally echogenic dots filling almost the entire anterior chamber are especially visible at the level of the focal area. Edema causes thickening of the cornea in the center, without abnormality of its echotexture. Note that the small echogenic dots are finer at 50 MHz than at 10 MHz

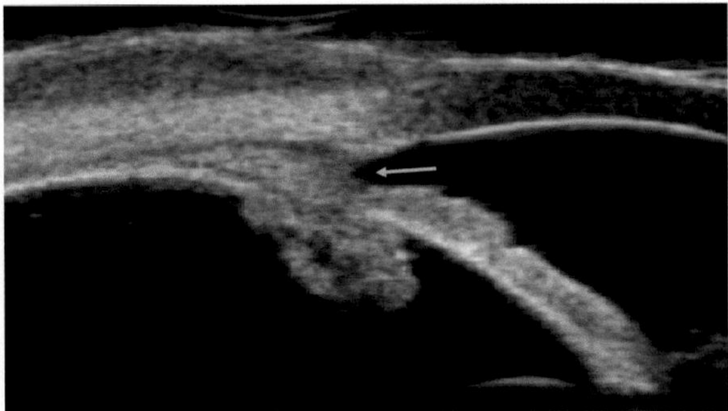

**Fig. 11.55 Angle recession**. VHFU section clearly showing a tear in the ciliary body (→), remaining attached to the scleral spur

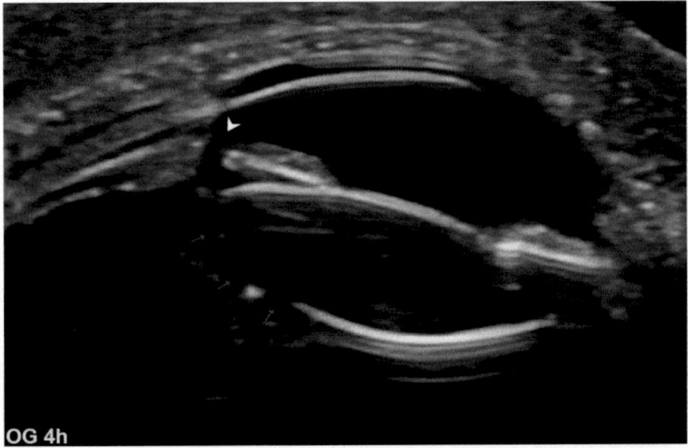


**Fig. 11.56 Post-traumatic peripheral iridodialysis, by an angle grinder**. Section along the 4 o'clock meridian with an 18 MHz probe. The tear is at the level of its root, where the iris is the thinnest (➤white arrowhead). Note that due to the obliquity of the structure to the ultrasound beam, the posterior capsule at 4 o'clock, appears irregular (→ red thin arrows), although it was perfectly normal and not broken. However, small intralenticular echoes related to the early stage of a cataract can be seen

**Fig. 11.57 Tear of the iris** in its middle part at 5 o'clock. Phacoemulsification and iris suture (two stiches) performed 3 months later with favorable progression

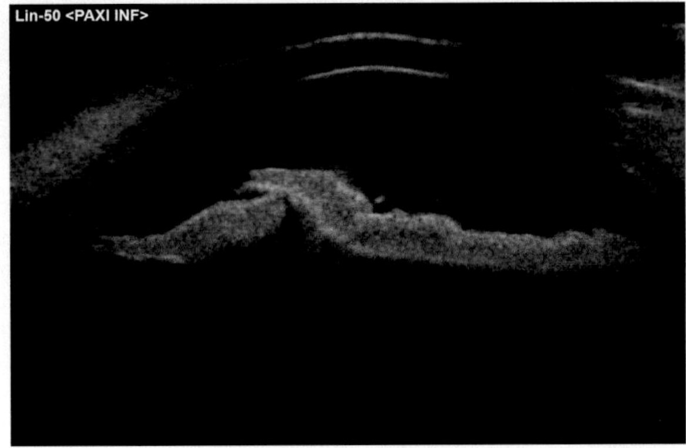

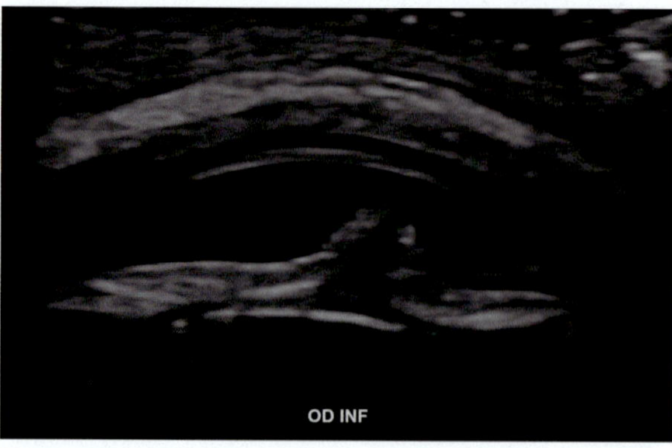

**Fig. 11.58 Tear of the iris** in its middle part at 7:30 o'clock. Transpalpebral section with an 18 MHz probe: hyphema and hematoma on contact, after a fall against a washbasin. Favorable progression at 8 weeks: still waiting for phacoemulsification and pupilloplasty, especially because of substantial irido-phacodonesis

### 11.7.3 The Ciliary Body

#### 11.7.3.1 Cyclodialysis

This involves separation of the ciliary body from the scleral spur. It usually leads to hypotonia. The ultrasound presentation is characteristic (Fig. 11.59). The pupil is readily moved to the site of cyclodialysis, with in this case a posterior displacement of the anterior ciliary body and the root of the iris. As in the case shown, there may be a space between the ciliary body and the sclera. The choroidal effusion is often more extensive, being visible on 360°. When cyclodialysis is of traumatic origin and is accompanied by hypotonia, the anterior chamber may be narrowed, and the angle closed.

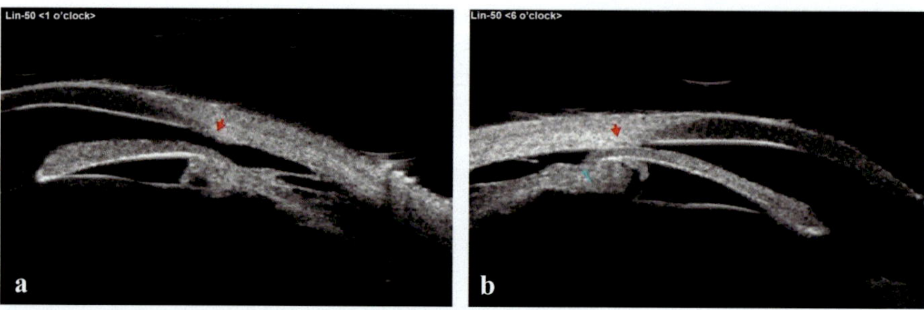

**Fig. 11.59 Post-traumatic superior cyclodialysis** after a severe road accident with very severe facial and eye trauma. **a**: Section according to the 1 o'clock meridian; **b**: section according to the 6 o'clock meridian. In **a**, there is disintegration of the ciliary body with posterior displacement of the root of the iris behind the scleral spur (→ red arrow), associated with a large space between the ciliary body and the sclera. In **b**, the presence of a supraciliary detachment can be discerned, which was visible on 360°. The root of the iris (→ blue arrow) has moved behind the scleral spur (→ red arrow), with the peripheral iris coming into contact with the scleral spur, and a narrow anterior chamber. Therefore, very-high-frequency ultrasound shows that the cyclodialysis is more extensive than what was suspected clinically

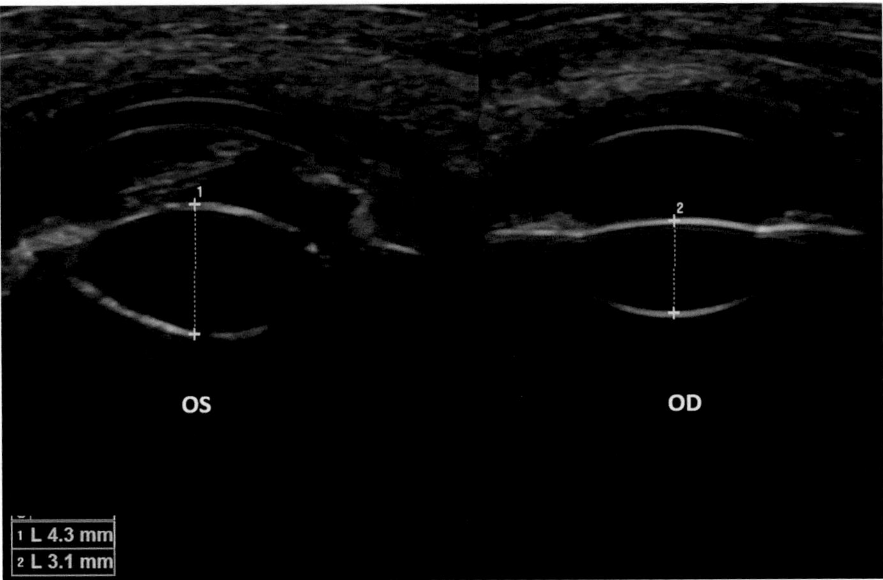


**Fig. 11.60 Intumescent lens**. Right eye contusion by a jump rope. The bilateral and comparative examination carried out on D3 shows several lesions of the anterior segment: corneal edema, trauma of the iris with fracture and vast disinsertion, the iris floating in the anterior chamber, and a clearly enlarged lens with an incipient cataract, the capsules being visible closer to the equator OD > OS, without signs of capsular rupture

## 11.7.4 The Lens

### 11.7.4.1 Intumescence/Cataract

This is a frequent sign, requiring comparative assessment of both lenses. Intraocular lens echoes occur only a few days (sometimes a few weeks) after trauma (Fig. 11.56), but the increase in size can occur very rapidly (Fig. 11.60).

### 11.7.4.2 Capsular Rupture

Most often, they are detectable at the posterior capsule because the iris can mask them at the anterior level. Of note, the integrity of a capsule can only be evaluated if the ultrasound beam is perpendicular to it (Fig. 11.56). Leakage of lens protein can cause phacolytic glaucoma by obstructing the trabeculum (Fig. 11.61).

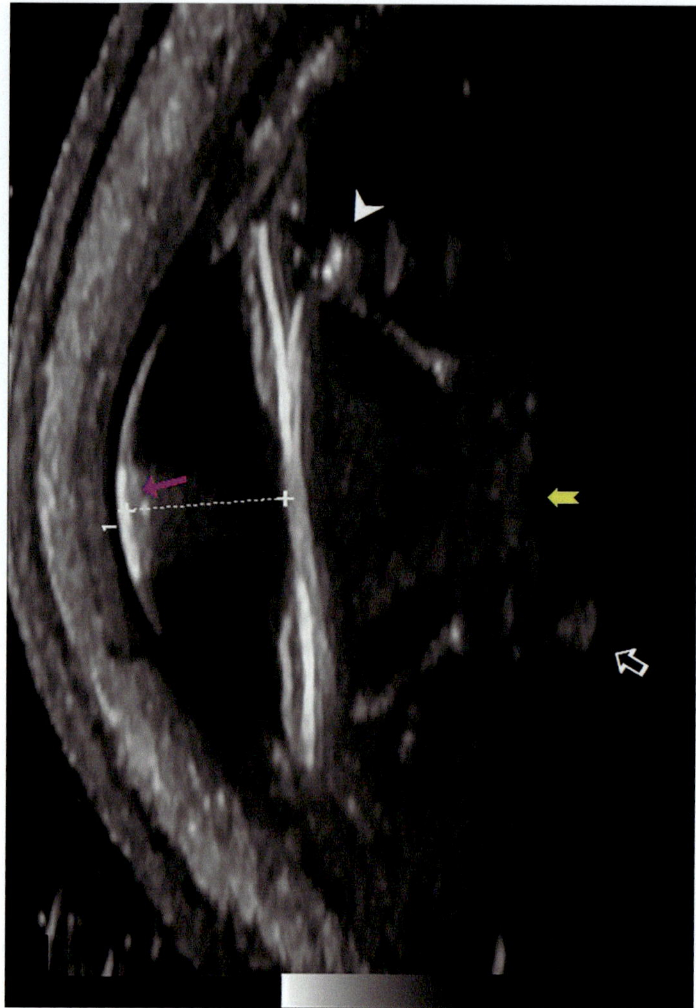

**Fig. 11.61** **Post-traumatic posterior capsular rupture** after mild contusion: fall from his height, in a patient who had surgery for retinal detachment with tamponade by silicone oil that was removed secondarily: sagittal section of the anterior segment at 18 MHz. A solution of continuity of the posterior capsule (➡ yellow arrow) reflects the capsular rupture; however, the anterior capsule appears to be intact. The lens is weakly echogenic, cataractous, but without calcification. In the background, a very echogenic micro-nodule (➤ white arrowhead) can be seen with a comet-tail artifact related to a silicone minibubble as well as some small hemorrhagic echoes (⇨ white arrowhead). A thin silicone blade (→ purple arrow) behind the apex of the cornea, non-mobile, with a posterior fog artifact can also be seen. The leakage of lens protein was the cause of phacolytic glaucoma with an intra-ocular pressure of 60 that led to the consultation. Favorable progression after phacoemulsification on day 5, although visual acuity was limited to 100/200 because of the previous surgery for retinal detachment

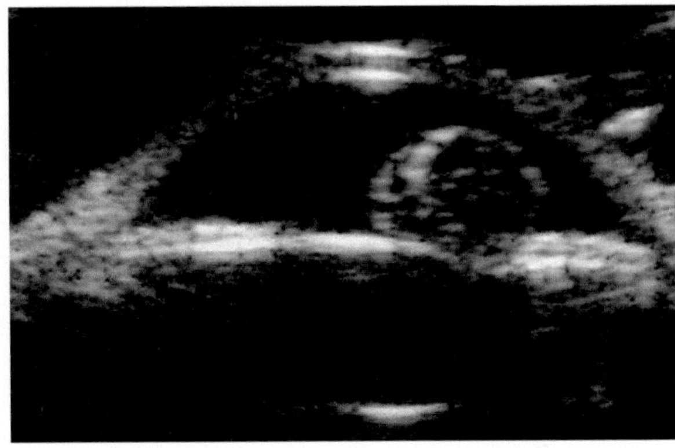

**Fig. 11.62  Vitreous hernia in the anterior chamber.** After a contusion with minimal subluxation: axial section with a short focal length 20 MHz probe

### 11.7.4.3   Dislocation

In addition to size and echotexture anomalies, position anomalies should also be noted. Sometimes it is only a minimal subluxation, but associated with a zonular hiatus, which can be the cause of a vitreous hernia in the anterior chamber (Fig. 11.62).

## *11.7.5   Intraocular Foreign Bodies (IOFBs)*

VHFU is of course not useful for an already visible FB, such as very common corneal foreign objects. The increase in spatial resolution by the (very) high frequency allows even more precise localization than for FBs of the posterior segment (see Chap. 12), followed by a posterior shadowing (Fig. 11.63) or by a posterior enhancement such as behind a tantalum clip, FBs that are very frequent after proton beam therapy (Fig. 11.64) (see Figs. 6.3 and 13.45).

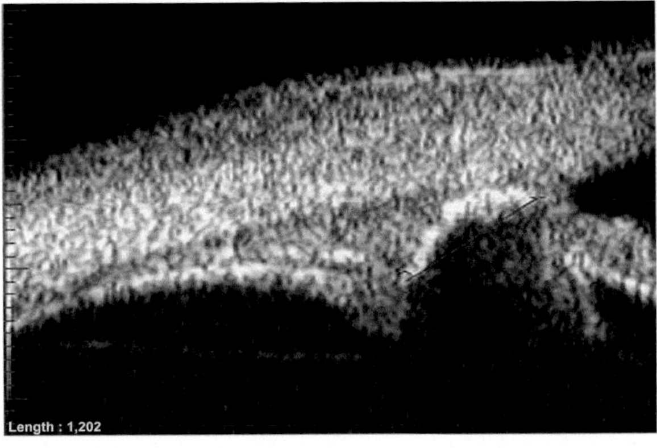


**Fig. 11.63  UBM of a foreign body (FB) located in the ciliary body.** Metallic, arciform, hyperechoic FB resulting in a posterior shadowing

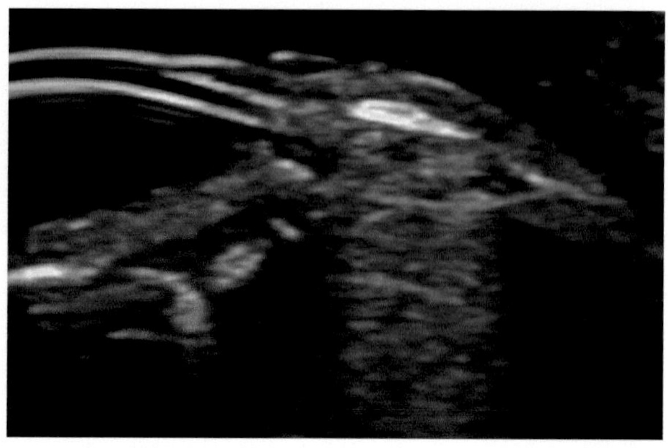

**Fig. 11.64 Externalized tantalum clip**, 2 months after proton beam therapy, with its very long procession of posterior comet tail artifacts. Para-axial section with a 18 MHz probe

Here, we have provided some indications for HFU and VHFU of the anterior segment. Other applications will be discussed in Chap. 13 for assessing eye masses of the iris and the ciliary body.

The other axis of development of HFU is represented by analysis of the posterior segment with very high-resolution probes with a long focal length allowing for visualizing the macula. This technical progression stems from the work of Michel Puech in 1998 (Patent FR98/02788).

**Acknowledgements** I would like to dedicate this chapter to Dr. Charles Joseph Pavlin, from Toronto, who passed away on November 14, 2014. He has taught us so much. His dynamism and his enduring research will forever be a role model for all of us. His legendary expertise, kindness, and availability allowed for navigating within these microscopic structures with a degree of ease, which before him, we did not know how to image. Fortunately, his numerous research articles [88] and his book will always remain accessible to everyone.

# References


1. Pavlin CJ, Harasiewicz K, Sherar MD, Foster FS. Clinical use of ultrasound biomicroscopy. Ophthalmology. 1991;98(3):287–95.
2. Kim DY, Reinstein DZ, Silverman RH, Nadajafi DJ, Belmont SC, Hatsis AP, Rozakis GW, Coleman DJ. Very high frequency ultrasound analysis of a new phakic posterior chamber intraocular lens in situ. Am J Ophthalmol. 1998;125(5):725–9.
3. Reinstein DZ, Sutton HF, Srivannaboon S, Silverman RH, Archer TJ, Coleman DJ. Evaluating microkeratome efficacy by 3D corneal lamellar flap thickness accuracy and reproducibility using Artemis VHF digital ultrasound arc-scanning. J Refract Surg. 2006;22(5):431–40.
4. Allemann N, Chamon W, Silverman RH, Azar DT, Reinstein DZ, Stark WJ. High-frequency ultrasound quantitative analyses of corneal scarring following excimer laser keratectomy. Arch Ophthalmol. 1993;111(7):968–73.

5. Reinstein DZ, Silverman RH, Trokel SL, Allemann N, Coleman DJ. High-frequency ultrasound digital signal processing for biometry of the cornea in planning phototherapeutic keratectomy. Arch Ophthalmol. 1993;111(4):430–1.

6. Reinstein DZ, Silverman RH, Sutton HF, Coleman DJ. Very high-frequency ultrasound corneal analysis identifies anatomic correlates of optical complications of lamellar refractive surgery: anatomic diagnosis in lamellar surgery. Ophthalmology. 1999;106(3):474–82.

7. Reinstein DZ, Silverman RH, Raevsky T, Simoni GJ, Lloyd HO, Najafi DJ, Rondeau MJ, Coleman DJ. Arc-scanning very high-frequency digital ultrasound for 3D pachymetric mapping of the corneal epithelium and stroma in laser in situ keratomileusis. J Refract Surg. 2000;16(4):414–30. Erratum in: J Refract Surg 2001;7(1):4.

8. Reinstein DZ, Srivannaboon S, Holland SP. Epithelial and stromal changes induced by intacs examined by three-dimensional very high-frequency digital ultrasound. J Refract Surg. 2001;17(3):310–8.

9. Rondeau MJ, Barcsay G, Silverman RH, Reinstein DZ, Krishnamurthy R, Chabi A, Du T, Coleman DJ. Very high frequency ultrasound biometry of the anterior and posterior chamber diameter. J Refract Surg. 2004;20(5):454–64.

10. Reinstein DZ, Ameline B, Puech M, Montefiore G, Laroche L. VHF digital ultrasound three-dimensional scanning in the diagnosis of myopic regression after corneal refractive surgery. J Refract Surg. 2005;21(5):480–4.

11. Cumba RJ, Radhakrishnan S, Bell NP, Nagi KS, Chuang AZ, & al Reproducibility of scleral spur identification and angle measurements using fourier domain anterior segment optical coherence tomography. J Ophthalmol. 2012;2012:487309.

12. Pavlin CJ, Harasiewicz K. Ultrasound biomicroscopy of anterior segment structures in normal and glaucomatous eyes. Am J Ophthalmol. 1992;113(4):381–9.

13. Ishikawa H, Liebmann JM, Ritch R. Quantitative assessment of the anterior segment using ultrasound biomicroscopy. Curr Opin Ophthalmol. 2000;11:133–9.

14. Dada T, Sihota R, Gadia R, Aggarwal A, Mandal S, Gupta V. Comparison of anterior segment optical coherence tomography and ultrasound biomicroscopy for assessment of the anterior segment. J Cataract Refract Surg. 2007;33(5):837–40.

15. Wang D, Pekmezci M, Basham RP, He M, Seider MI, Lin SC. Comparison of different modes in optical coherence tomography and ultrasound biomicroscopy in anterior chamber angle assessment. J Glaucoma. 2009;18(6):472–8.

16. Mansouri K, Sommerhalder J, Shaarawy T. Prospective comparison of ultrasound biomicroscopy and anterior segment optical coherence tomography for evaluation of anterior chamber dimensions in European eyes with primary angle closure. Eye (Lond). 2010;24(2):233–9.

17. Ishikawa H. Anterior segment imaging for glaucoma: OCT or UBM? Br J Ophthalmol. 2007;91(11):1420–1.

18. Bergès O, Puech M, Assouline M, Letenneur L, Gastellu-Etchegorry M. B-mode-guided vector-A-mode versus A-mode biometry to determine axial length and intraocular lens power. J Cataract Refract Surg. 1998;24(4):529–35.

19. Pavlin CJ, Harasiewicz K, Foster FS. An ultrasound biomicroscopic dark-room provocative test. Ophthalmic Surg. 1995;26(3):253–5.

20. Maram J, Pan X, Sadda S, Francis B, Marion K, Chopra V. Reproducibility of angle metrics using the time-domain anterior segment optical coherence tomography: intra-observer and inter-observer variability. Curr Eye Res. 2015;40(5):496–500.

21. Yoo C, Oh JH, Kim YY, Jung HR. Peripheral anterior synechiae and ultrasound biomicroscopic parameters in angle-closure glaucoma suspects. Korean J Ophthalmol. 2007;21(2):106–10.

22. Friedman DS, He M Anterior chamber angle assessment techniques. Surv Ophthalmol. 2008;53(3):250–73.

23. Radhakrishnan S, See J, Smith SD, Nolan WP, Ce Z, Friedman DS, et al. Reproducibility of anterior chamber angle measurements obtained with anterior segment optical coherence tomography. Invest Ophthalmol Vis Sci. 2007;48(8):3683–8.

24. Pavlin CJ, Ritch R, Foster FS. Ultrasound biomicroscopy in plateau iris syndrome. Am J Ophthalmol. 1992;113(4):390–5.

25. Stefan C, Iliescu DA, Batras M, Timaru CM, De Simone A. Plateau iris—diagnosis and treatment. Rom J Ophthalmol. 2015;59(1):14–8.
26. Sun JH, Sung KR, Yun SC, Cheon MH, Tchah HW, Kim MJ, Kim JY. Factors associated with anterior chamber narrowing with age: an optical coherence tomography study. Invest Ophthalmol Vis Sci. 2012;53(6):2607–10.
27. Lee RY, Chon BH, Lin SC, He M, Lin SC. Association of ocular conditions with narrow angles in different ethnicities. Am J Ophthalmol. 2015;160(3):506-515.e1.
28. Kim YK, Yoo BW, Kim HC, Aung T, Park KH. Relative lens vault in subjects with angle closure. BMC Ophthalmol. 2014;21(14):93.
29. Masis Solano M, Lin SC. Cataract, phacoemulsification and intraocular pressure: Is the anterior segment anatomy the missing piece of the puzzle? Prog Retin Eye Res. 2018;64:77–83.
30. Yan C, Han Y, Yu Y, Wang W, Lyu D, et al. Effects of lens extraction versus laser peripheral iridotomy on anterior segment morphology in primary angle closure suspect. Graefes Arch Clin Exp Ophthalmol. 2019;257(7):1473–80.
31. Lachkar Y. Glaucomes primitifs par fermeture de l'angle. EMC Ophtalmologie [21-280-A-10] 2000.
32. Laloum J. Situations cliniques particulières, formes mixtes (ch20) *in* Rapport SFO 2014: Glaucome Primitif à Angle Ouvert. In: Renard J-P, Sellem E, editors. Elsevier-Masson, Paris; 1994. p. 671–6.
33. Liebmann JM, Ritch R. Laser surgery for angle closure glaucoma. Semin Ophthalmol. 2002;17(2):84–91.
34. Hong JW, Yun SC, Sung KR, Lee JE. Clinical and anterior segment anatomical features in primary angle closure subgroups based on configurations of iris root insertion. Korean J Ophthalmol. 2016;30(3):206–13.
35. Cassoux N, Lemaitre C, Hamard P, Tuil A, Lehoang P, Baudouin C. Uvéite antérieure aiguë à hypopion bilatérale révélant un «creeping angle-closure glaucoma». J Fr Ophtalmol. 2003;26(6):622–5.
36. Lehto I, Vesti E. Diagnosis and management of pigmentary glaucoma. Curr Opin Ophthalmol. 1998;9(2):61–4.
37. Campbell DG, Schertzer RM. Pathophysiology of pigment dispersion syndrome and pigmentary glaucoma. Curr Opin Ophthalmol. 1995;6(2):96–101.
38. Küchle M, Nguyen NX, Mardin CY, Naumann GO. Effect of neodymium: YAG laser iridotomy on number of aqueous melanin granules in primary pigment dispersion syndrome. Graefes Arch Clin Exp Ophthalmol. 2001;239(6):411–5.
39. May F. Diagnostic différentiel I-Glaucome pigmentaire (ch14) *in* Rapport SFO 2014: Glaucome Primitif à Angle Ouvert. I: Renard J-P, Sellem E, editors. Elsevier-Masson, Paris; 1994. p. 461–8.
40. Stamper RL, Lieberman MF, Drake MV, Berlin M. In Becker-Shaffer's diagnosis and therapy of the glaucomas. 8th ed. St Louis: Mosby; 2009.
41. Bourdon H, Aragno V, Baudouin C, Labbé A. Iridoplasty for plateau iris syndrome: a systematic review. BMJ Open Ophthalmol. 2019;4(1).
42. El Salhy AA, Elseht RM, Al Maria AF, Shalaby SMAE, Hossein TR. Functional evaluation of the filtering bleb by ultrasound biomicroscopy after trabeculectomy with mitomycin C. Int J Ophthalmol. 2018;11(2):245–50.
43. Waring GO, Rodrigues MM, Laibson PR. Anterior chamber cleavage syndrome. A stepladder classification. Surv Ophthalmol. 1975;20(1):3–27.
44. Nischal KK. Congenital corneal opacities—a surgical approach to nomenclature and classification. Eye (Lond). 2007;21(10):1326–37.
45. Martinet V, Dureau P, Bergès O, Caputo G. Vitreoretinal dysplasia masquerading as Peters' anomaly. Eur J Ophthalmol. 2010;20(1):228–30.
46. Nischal KK. A new approach to the classification of neonatal corneal opacities. Curr Opin Ophthalmol. 2012;23(5):344–54.
47. Bengarai W, Chokrani H, Berraho A. Axenfeld-Rieger syndrome. J Fr Ophtalmol. 2018;41(5):470–1.
48. Pavlin CJ, Foster FS. Ultrasound biomicroscopy of the eye. New York: Springer; 1994.

# Chapter 12
# Ultrasound of the Posterior Segment


**Kamal Siahmed, Olivier Bergès, Mario de La Torre, Elisabeth Nau, and Dominique Satger**



**Abstract** Assessment of the posterior segment is one of the most frequent indications for diagnostic ultrasound. The review must be systematic and comprehensive. One must successively analyze the vitreous, which plays a major role in many retinal conditions. Its role is diagnostic and also pathogenic and prognostic. Subsequent assessment of the vitreoretinal interface, the retina, the choroid, the sclera, the optic disc, and the macula allows for detailed analysis of each structure in terms of morphological, quantitative, and kinetic criteria using current 10/15 MHz and 20 MHz B-mode probes that offer the advantage of image post-processing, kinetics, and excellent spatial and density resolution, and also standardized A-mode echography and color Doppler imaging.


## 12.1 Normal and Pathological Vitreous

- *Importance of examination of the vitreous*

The vitreous plays a major role in many retinal conditions. The role of posterior vitreous detachment (PVD) in the occurrence of rhegmatogenous retinal detachment has been known for a long time. Significant therapeutic advances have been made since the recent, and still imperfect, identification of the pathological role of the vitreous in a number of maculopathies [1–3].


K. Siahmed
Ophthalmic Center Vernon, Vernon, France

M. de La Torre
Instituto Nacional de Oftalmologia, Lima, Perú

O. Bergès (✉) · E. Nau
Rothschild Foundation Hospital, Paris, France
e-mail: oberges@for.paris

D. Satger
University Hospital of Grenoble, Grenoble, France



© The Author(s), under exclusive license to Springer Nature Switzerland AG 2024     219
O. Bergès (ed.), *Echography of the Eye and Orbit*,
https://doi.org/10.1007/978-3-031-41467-1_12

Partial detachment of the vitreous, readily demonstrated by ultrasonography during vasculopathies such as diabetic retinopathy or venous obliteration greatly influences the progression, the prognosis, and the therapeutic decisions to be made.

Therefore, its examination is indispensable. Assessment of the condition of the vitreous can help with diagnosis and treatment.

The review protocol should be rigorous and methodical [4–6]:

- *Settings*

In B-mode, all structures should be assessed at high and reduced sensitivity settings. Maximum gain mainly allows assessment of the vitreous. Maximum gain is the setting at which no intraocular artifacts are produced although very small low reflective floaters can still be detected. Reduced gain is a gain at which the different layers of the wall of the globe can be discerned (see Fig. 7.9).

- *Position of the probe*

After administration of a few anesthetic eye drops, it is sometimes useful to place the probe directly on the conjunctiva. This allows for gaining a few decibels that would otherwise be absorbed by the eyelids and to not disorganize the homogeneity of the ultrasound beam.

- *Immersion*

Assessment of the anterior vitreous is generally facilitated by an immersion technique for this anterior area to be at the focal point. Given the septic risk, these two methods, transconjunctival and immersion, are only possible on relatively unperturbed eyes; they are contraindicated in case of perforating trauma, a recent surgical procedure, or an eye infection.

- *Incidences*

Two types of sections are used: meridian and quadrant sections. With the probe placed behind the limbus, the meridian section distinguishes the ocular wall and the vitreous from the ciliary region to the posterior pole, according to the angulation of the probe. With its rotation around the limbus by 360°, all the meridians are exposed continuously (see Fig. 7.4).

The quadrant incidence creates sections parallel to the limbus and provides a detailed image of pathological areas. Hence, 3D mental reconstruction is possible. It allows for an accurate description of the condition of the vitreous and the vitreoretinal relationships in all sectors (see Fig. 7.5).

- *Dynamic*

To obtain the maximum amount of information, the examination of the vitreous should be dynamic and integrate a 3D approach. During movements of the globe, the mobility of the gel and the vitreous membranes provides information regarding the degree of liquefaction or organization of the vitreous; it can specify whether an adhesion or posterior vitreous detachment (PVD) is taut or loose.

At the end of the examination, one must reconstruct the various ultrasound sections produced to obtain the best possible representation of the vitreous in space, both in terms of its general configuration (the existence or not of a PVD) and, if possible, in terms of the details (e.g., evaluation of localized vitreous traction). A schematic representation is desirable, as for examination of the retina. It is best achieved with coronal and meridian sections spanning 360°.

## 12.1.1   Ultrasound Appearance of Normal Vitreous

The vitreous is a mesenchymal gel that is transparent and consists of 99% water. At maximum gain, the normal vitreous presents as an anechoic area. However, its reflectivity is slightly higher than that of a "cyst-like" structure filled with pure water. Like all "cyst-like" structures, the side walls of the eyeball are not visualized.

### 12.1.1.1   Vitreous Senescence

Age is the main cause of changes in the appearance of the vitreous. Senescence of the vitreous gel results in the appearance of more punctiform and mobile echoes because of liquefaction. It exhibits more mobility and also a certain degree of fibrillary structure. The condensation of collagen fibrils results in small, moderately echogenic, mobile dots. These floaters are sometimes organized into fine intravitreal membranes (Fig. 12.1), limiting anechoic lacunæ corresponding to liquefaction of the vitreous body.

This is called age-related fibrillary and lacunar degeneration of the vitreous. The posterior hyaloid membrane presents as a thin low reflective membrane, flexible,

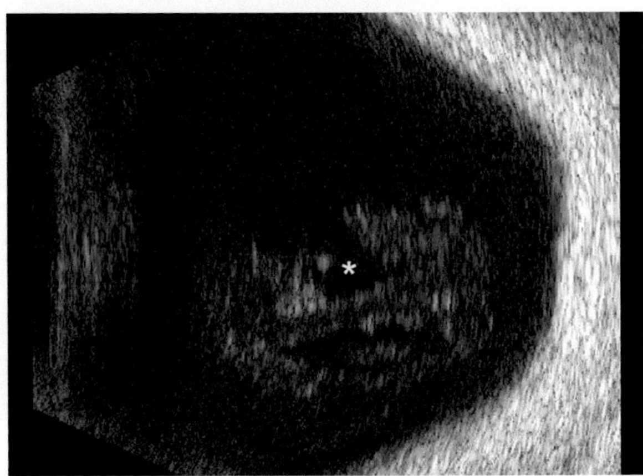

**Fig. 12.1  Intravitreal membranes.** Section at 10 MHz. Condensation of the vitreous with intravitreal membranes and a lacuna (*) within a myopic eye with staphyloma

and regular; its connection to the base of the vitreous should be identified [7, 8] (Fig. 12.2).

In high myopia, the vitreous echoes tend to be coarser, fuzzier, and more echogenic, making the diagnosis of PVD more challenging. The vitreous echoes exhibit movements of great amplitude, especially when the vitreous gel has detached. The hyaloid membrane may appear discontinuous and uneven. Myopia is a state that predisposes to accelerated liquefaction of the vitreous, with the formation of fibrillary condensation surrounded by large optically empty lacunæ (Fig. 12.3). Thus, it is difficult to diagnose with confidence a PVD in case of myopia.

The correlation between biomicroscopic examination and ultrasound is excellent [9, 10] Ultrasound is even more efficient than biomicroscopic examination when the media are not fully transparent as well as for the analysis of vitreoretinal relationships of the equatorial region [8].

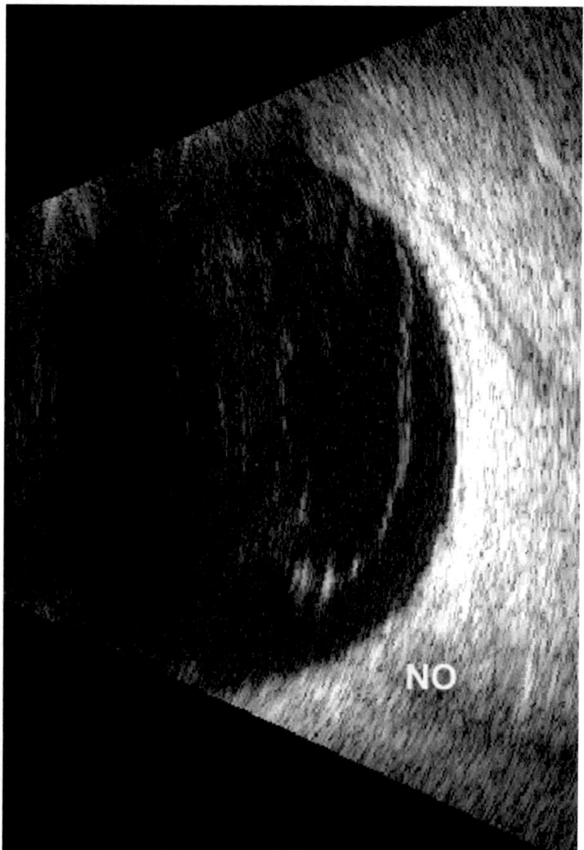


**Fig. 12.2 Insertion of the posterior hyaloid on the vitreous base: just behind the tendon of an extraocular muscle**. Section exploring a meridian at 20 MHz. In addition, the Weiss ring is visualized here by two hyperechoic spots in front of the optic disc. NO = optic nerve

**Fig. 12.3  PVD in a highly myopic patient, with an axial length of 32.3 mm**. In the highly myopic patient, the posterior hyaloid membrane appears thin and irregular, with the irruption of posterior lacunae (*) toward the retrohyaloid space. Sometimes distinguishing between an extended posterior vitreous detachment and a giant posterior lacuna is difficult

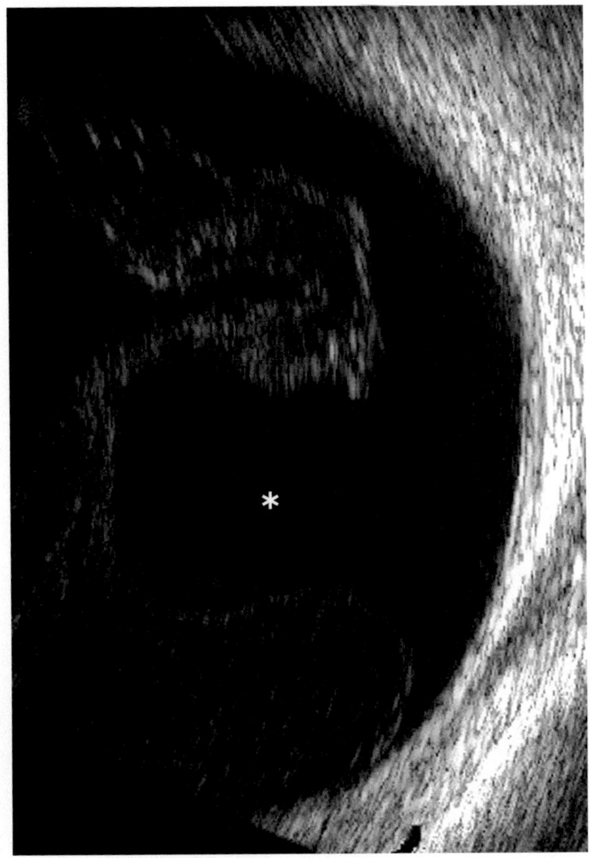

## 12.1.1.2  Ultrasound Criteria of PVD

- **Total PVD**: This is characterized by direct visualization of the posterior hyaloid membrane as a thin line, not very dense, of uneven thickness and echogenicity, passing over the optic disc without connecting to it. The retrohyaloid space is anechoic. The prepapillary ring (Weiss ring) commonly forms one or two hyperechoic spots facing, or slightly offset, often inferior, relative to the optic disc (Fig. 12.4); a single more echogenic spot along the posterior hyaloid; or, more rarely, an actual ring. Only meridian sections can reveal PVD, by showing the characteristic connection of the posterior hyaloid to the base of the vitreous and thus allowing elimination of an intravitreal cortical lacuna [11].
- **Partial PVD**: in this case, the posterior hyaloid membrane is only partially detached in one or more quadrants.
- **Subtotal PVD**: when persistent posterior hyaloid detachment is seen in all quadrants, with a papillary attachment (Figs. 12.5 and 12.7), or vitreoretinal adhesions to the posterior pole.

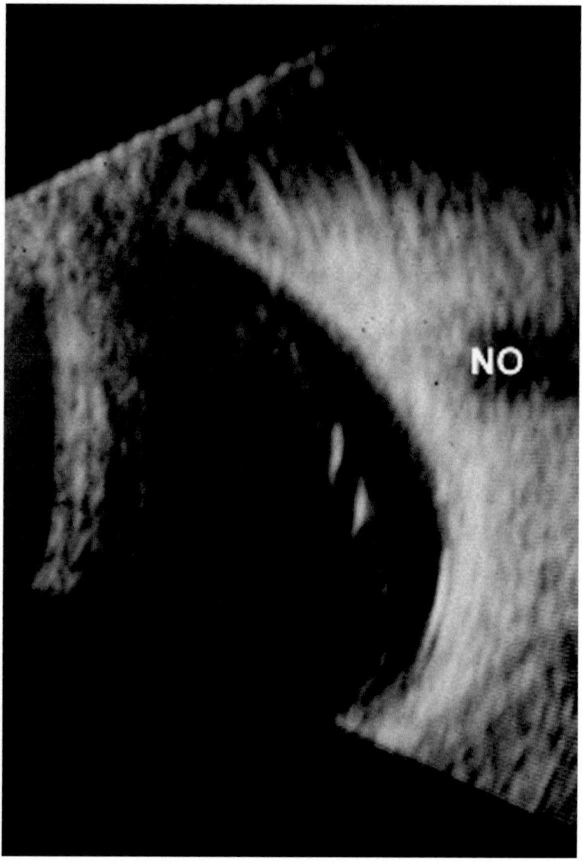


**Fig. 12.4** Posterior vitreous detachment (**PVD**) **and a Weiss ring next to the optic disc.** Section at 10 MHz. Facing the optic disc, there are two condensations on the posterior hyaloid membrane, which is totally detached. NO = optic nerve

- **Absence of PVD**: this is when the posterior hyaloid membrane is not visualized in any meridians.
- **Evaluation of the anterior vitreous**: It should not be neglected because it can provide abundant information regarding the overall degenerative status of the vitreous. One can discern the degree of echogenicity and the existence of lacunæ and fibrils. Its degree of mobility is a good indicator of its degree of liquefaction.

**Fig. 12.5 Subtotal PVD with intravitreal hemorrhage** in a diabetic patient. The attachment is thin to the parapapillary region; the membrane is insufficiently echogenic to be a retinal detachment

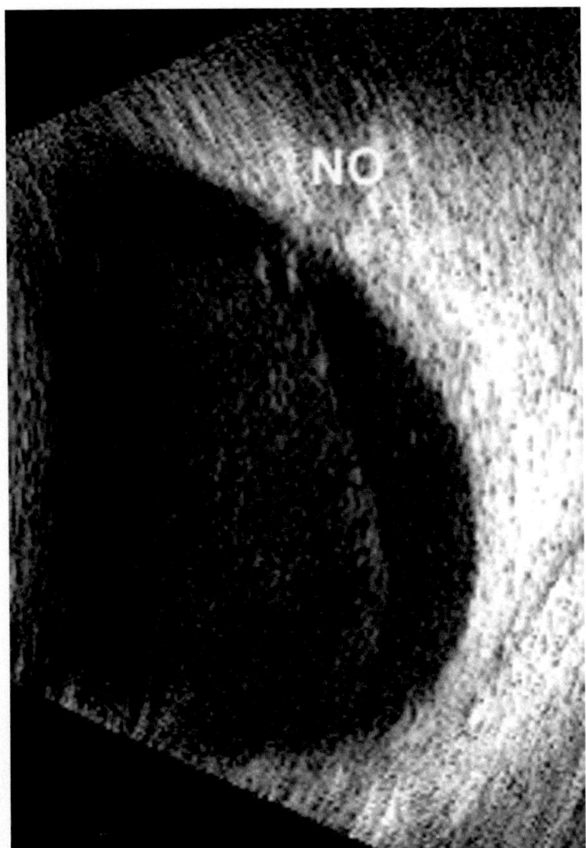


## *12.1.2 Pathology of the Vitreous*

### 12.1.2.1 Intraocular Hemorrhage

Intraocular hemorrhage can occur as part of a medical disorder or in a traumatic context. Because it results in poor visibility of the fundus, it is in itself an indication for ultrasound examination. The latter must not only search for retinal detachment but also try to determine the origin of the hemorrhage [12, 13] (PVD, retinal adhesion or tear, pre-retinal neovascular proliferation, macular degeneration, tumor). Comparison with the contralateral eye is sometimes useful. Similarly, the ultrasound should specify the degree of liquefaction or organization of the vitreous gel, the status of posterior vitreous detachment (partial (Fig. 12.6), or complete, with or without collapse), and the vitreoretinal connections (vitreoretinal adhesion, papillary attachment, etc.).

The initial examination and subsequent ultrasound monitoring provide valuable information regarding progression of the hemorrhage: organized and abundant, it

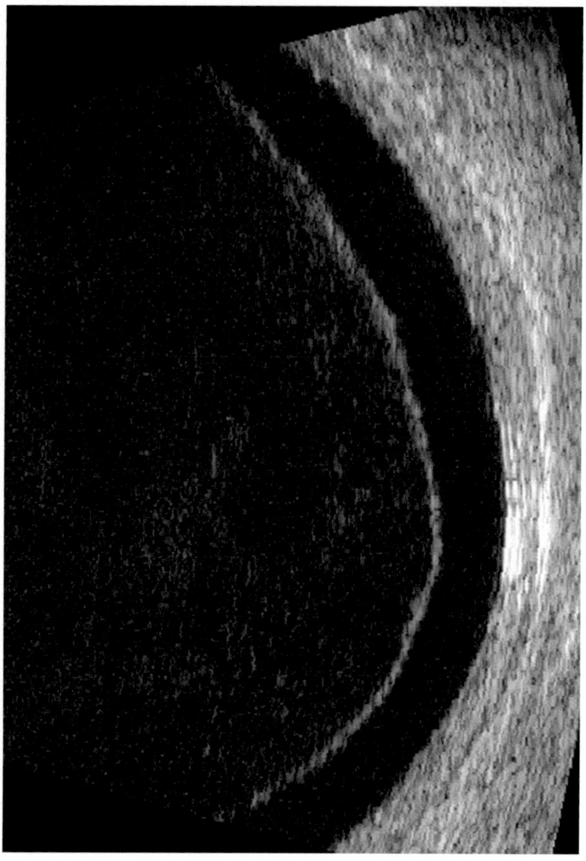

**Fig. 12.6 Hemorrhagic vitreous and partial PVD localized to one quadrant.** Exploration at 20 MHz. The vitreous gel has a frosted glass appearance and the posterior hyaloid is thickened in connection with intravitreal hemorrhage

warrants a vitrectomy if it persists. Therefore, ultrasound helps determine the timing of a surgical indication under the best conditions. Intravitreal hemorrhage (IVH) results in an increase in the reflectivity of the vitreous. Its appearance is variable, sometimes not much different from that encountered during hyalitis.

An IVH of low abundance is exceptionally anechoic; it is most often peripheral and localized inferiorly due to declivity. Formally eliminating it by ultrasound is difficult, even after careful assessment of the far periphery. In the beginning, the increase in the echogenicity of the vitreous is only moderately correlated with the amount of hemorrhage: at this stage, in the absence of organization, the echogenicity remains relatively low. Indeed, the blood cells have a diameter inferior to the wavelength of ultrasound within the vitreous (0.15 mm, or 150 $\mu$m): a diffuse and homogeneous hemorrhage initially only produces a few intravitreal echoes. Only the aggregation of red blood cells leads to the appearance of distinct echoes.

In some cases, when there is PVD, an early-stage IVH may only be visualized by the posterior hyaloid, which becomes thicker and more echogenic by precipitation of elements that form at this level (Fig. 12.6).

**Fig. 12.7  Low-abundance intravitreal hemorrhage and acute PVD**: small, moderately echogenic punctiform echoes within the vitreous. In this case, the vitreous is not fully detached, with persistence of a wide papillary attachment

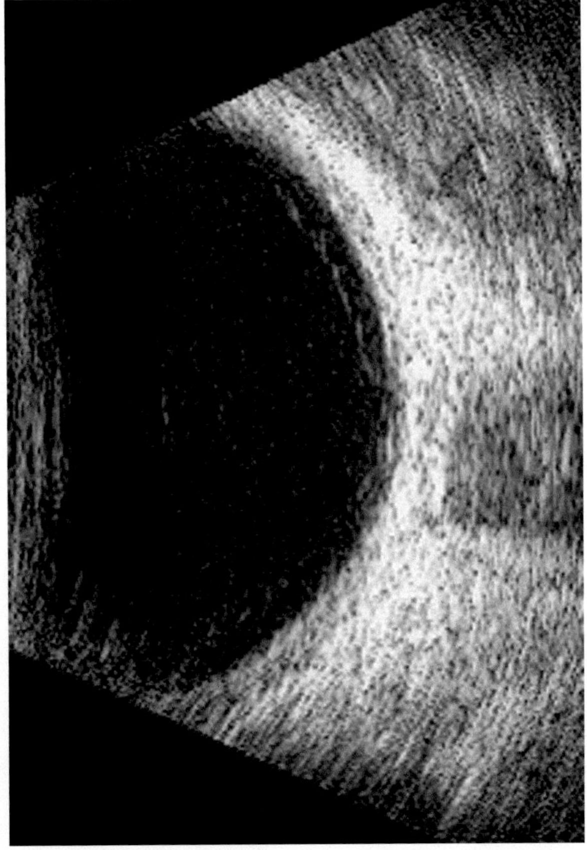

- **Subsequently**:

  - of low abundance, the IVH can be in the form of small punctiform diffuse echoes (Fig. 12.7).
  - of medium abundance, with the beginning of fibrino-hematic organization, areas of variable and inhomogeneous echogenicity appear. The vitreous dynamics is little modified: especially when there is a PVD. The vitreous, even hemorrhagic at its beginning, remains quite mobile and its harmonious undulations persist a few seconds after the globe has stopped moving.

- **The vitreous organization** that follows results in the appearance of highly echogenic membranes. The vitreous mobility then decreases significantly.
- **PVD secondary to hemorrhage**: if the vitreous is not initially detached, an IVH, by organizing the vitreous, promotes the occurrence of acute PVD.

### 12.1.2.2 Retrohyaloid Hemorrhage

This consists of fine echoes tightly packed together, of low to medium reflectivity, with possibly small and more echogenic sparse agglomerates. During eye movements, each particle is mobile and independent, thus confirming the appearance of an aqueous suspension. The blood condenses little on the hyaloid membrane but packs against it, thus highlighting the retro- and intravitreal spaces (Fig. 12.8). In places, the hyaloid can become thicker and more echogenic.

- The **phenomenon of posterior hyphema**: Sometimes, when a hemorrhage occurs in a retrohyaloid space that is a liquid space and not a gel like the vitreous, the blood cells can sediment and create a liquid/liquid level with a small echogenic lower part and the larger upper part little, or anechoic. By analogy with an anterior segment hemorrhage, this is called a posterior hyphema. The liquid//liquid level can act as a trap when one of its edges comes into contact with the optic disc, and this can look like a retinal detachment. Then horizontal sections of the posterior

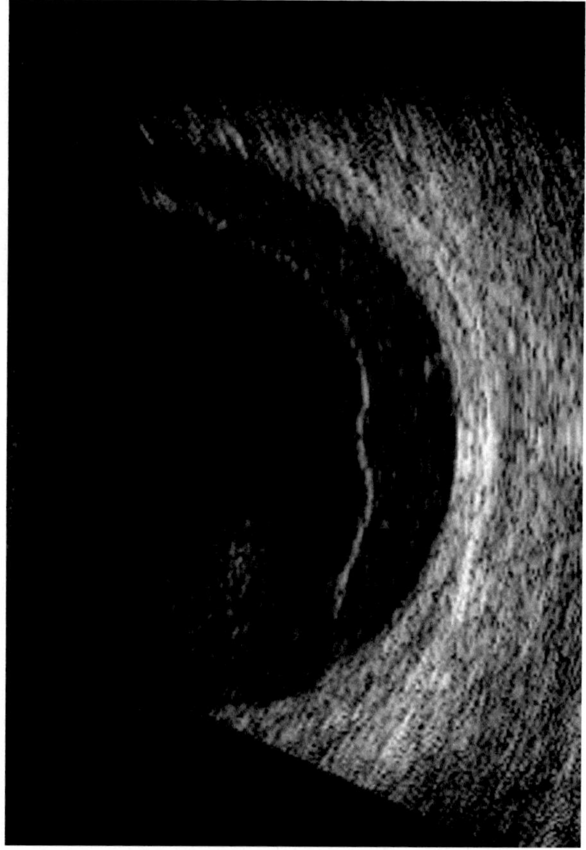

**Fig. 12.8 Intravitreal and retrohyaloid hemorrhage.** 10-MHz section of the nasal quadrant: small moderately echogenic punctiform echoes behind the posterior hyaloid. On this section, the vitreous is detached, the hyaloid is discreetly thickened, and the blood cells are pressed up against it, thus highlighting the retro- and intravitreal spaces. Most often, it is associated with intravitreal echoes, slightly more echogenic, coarser, and less mobile than the fine small retrohyaloid echoes

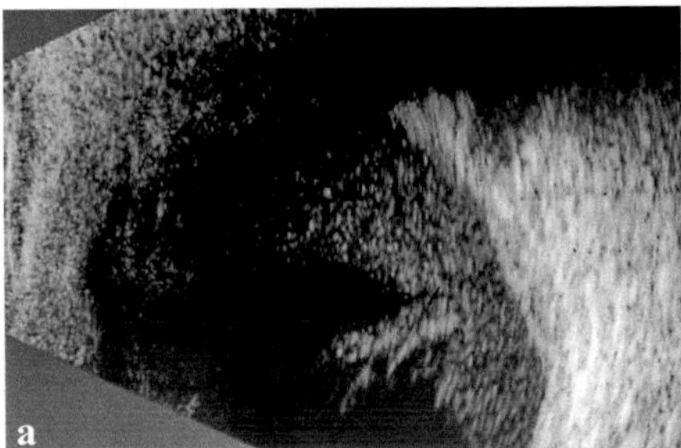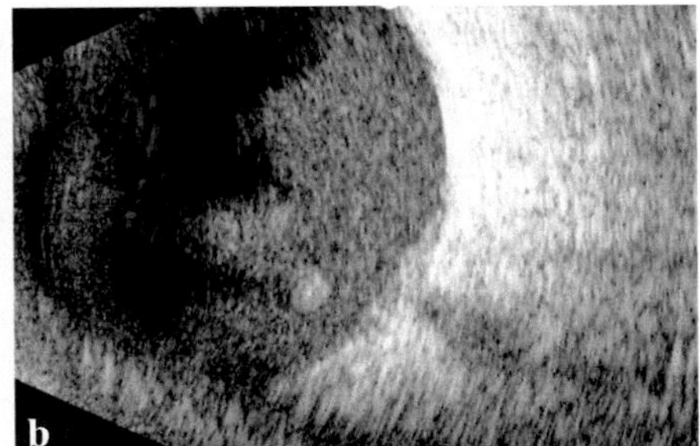

**Fig. 12.9** **Posterior hyphema secondary to an intraocular hemorrhage OS predominant at the level of the retrohyaloid space**. **a**: Section according to the 2 o'clock meridian, with intermediate gain: the hyphema appears to start at the optic disc and can resemble a retinal detachment; **b**: Section of the posterior pole in right lateral decubitus with high gain: the hyphema has moved, passing in front of the optic disc

pole can be acquired in right and left lateral decubitus to verify that it is not an authentic membrane, the level then passing in front of the optic disc and sliding above it (Fig. 12.9). This phenomenon can also be found in the subretinal space in case of total hemorrhagic retinal detachment.

### 12.1.2.3    Ocular Hematoma

Ocular hematoma is a major form of intraocular hemorrhage that occurs after severe trauma. It is difficult to examine with ultrasound due to the sensitivity of the eye and the presence of a large palpebral bruise that attenuates ultrasound.

The cavity is filled with a heterogeneous conglomerate formed by tightly packed and immobile echoes.

Any membranes are no longer discernible. Diagnosing retinal detachment becomes difficult or impossible. In any case, these major and complex intraocular rearrangements reflect lesions that most often cannot be managed with any of the currently available therapeutic resources. Ultrasound monitoring must then be performed regularly, to search for an associated complication (retinal detachment, vitreoretinal incarceration, athalamia, etc.).

Gradually, with parietal resorption, sedimentation, or organization, the ultrasound examination will become more precise. The condition frequently progresses to atrophy of the globe, with a decrease in axial length, retinal detachment, and cyclitic membrane as well as thickening and parietal ossification. Therefore, as a reference, one must measure the axial length and the parietal thickness during the initial examination.

### 12.1.2.4  Etiologies of Intraocular Hemorrhages

#### (a)  PVD

When it has formed, solid vitreoretinal adhesions at the periphery, can lead to vascular tearing or a retinal tear, which can cause intraocular hemorrhage. Therefore, such lesions should primarily be searched for at the periphery:

- **A vascular tear** is not visible by ultrasound;
- **A vitreoretinal adhesion may be detectable**, being very thin, not very echogenic or by contrast, manifesting itself as a pre-parietal hyperechogenicity toward which the hyaloid converges (Fig. 12.10).
- **A tear** appears as a short hyperechoic membrane, attached to the wall by its anterior part (Fig. 12.11). The hyaloid membrane adheres to its anterior end. The retina may be raised around this tear, and the extent of this should be determined.

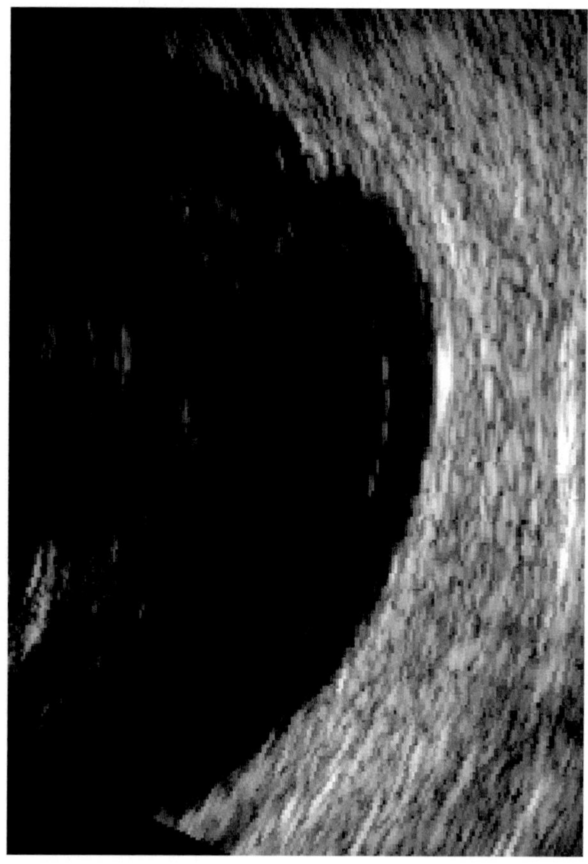

**Fig. 12.10  Vitreous traction**, resulting in pre-parietal hyperechogenicity with hyaloid adhesion

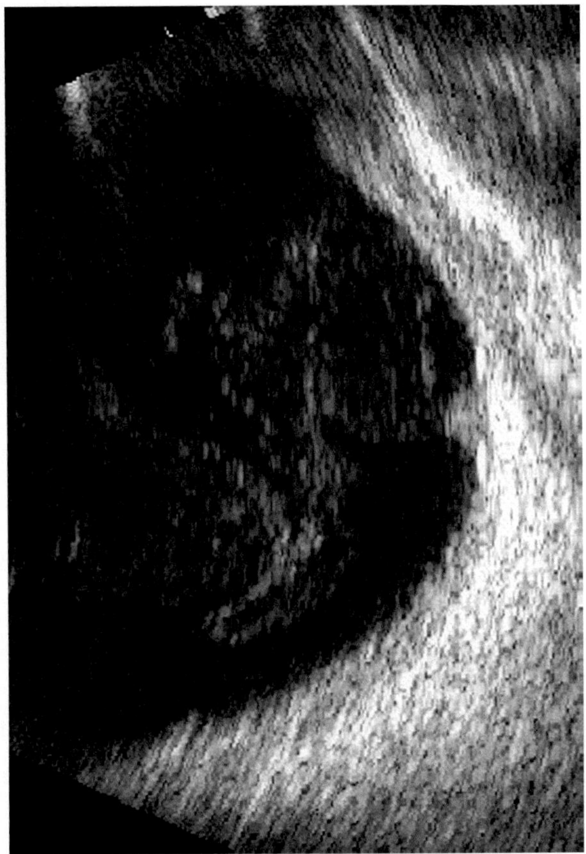

**Fig. 12.11  Retinal tear.** Section of OS according to 9 o'clock: short hyperechoic membrane, attached to the wall by its anterior part. The hyaloid adheres to its anterior end

## (b)  **Proliferative diabetic retinopathy**

The vitreous gel is altered in diabetics. PVD occurs earlier and frequently begins at the posterior pole, stretching between the temporal vascular arcades.

The existence of a pre-retinal neovascularization (predominant at the posterior pole near the vascular arcades and in the peripapillary region) strengthens the vitreoretinal attachments, which are already strong at this level: the PVD cannot become complete; it remains partial. Its retraction promoted by hemorrhage can induce localized traction retinal detachments starting at the posterior pole (Fig. 12.12). Its step-by-step progression is slow. Vitrectomy is then necessary because it alone can relieve the vitreoretinal traction [14]. Therefore, ultrasound is particularly useful [7, 15] to assess the status of the vitreous and vitreoretinal relationships. It provides the surgeon with the best information and helps determine how the operation will be performed.

The neovascular clusters are frequently visible by ultrasound in case of hemorrhage (Fig. 12.13). The posterior hyaloid membrane, which serves as a support for pre-retinal neovascularization, is partially detached. It is thicker and hyper-reflective,

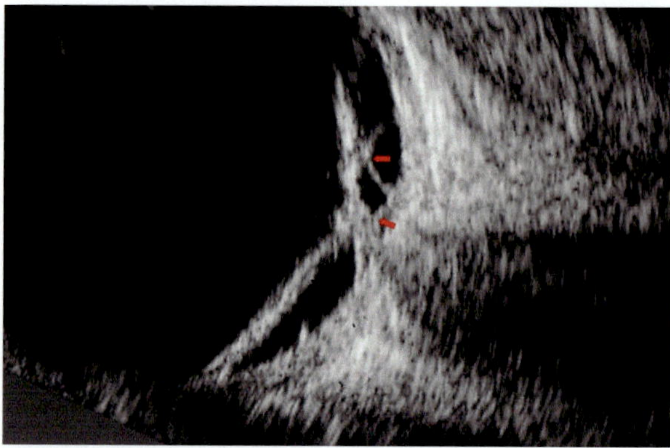

**Fig. 12.12 Proliferative diabetic retinopathy**. Section at 10 MHz showing detachment of the posterior hyaloid membrane, which is thickened with vitreoretinal tractions and highly elevated localized traction retinal detachments (➡ red arrows)

with many parietal attachments. The vitreous gel is most often heterogeneous, with the presence of many intravitreal membranes.

Concluding a retinal detachment under these conditions becomes difficult. Reflectivity criteria do not allow to conclude with certainty, and the interpretation is then more a matter of anatomical deduction.

### (c) Occlusion of the central retinal vein, ischemic type

As in proliferative diabetic retinopathy, this can lead to intraocular hemorrhage (retrohyaloid and/or intravitreal).

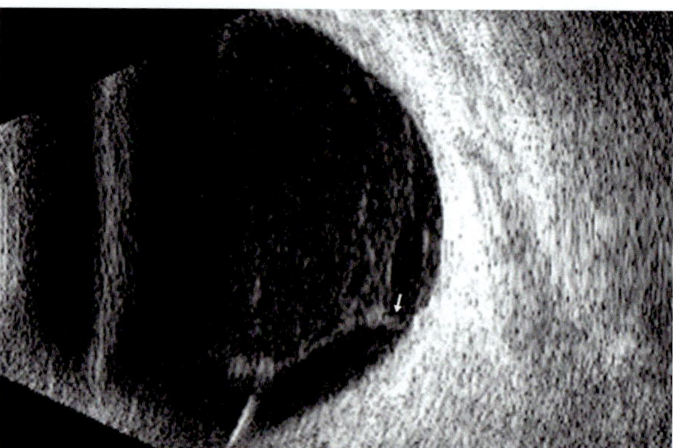

**Fig. 12.13 Advanced proliferative diabetic retinopathy, vitreous hemorrhage, PVD, and neovessels**. Para-axial section at 10 MHz: thickening of the posterior hyaloid membrane in relation to a semi-recent intravitreal hemorrhage that has resolved. This thickening makes the hyaloid membrane less mobile and rigid which in turn causes small areas of traction and possible localized traction retinal detachments. The image also shows a cluster of small pre-papillary neovessels (➡ white arrow)

The differential diagnosis with diabetic retinopathy is primarily clinical: non-diabetic patient, unilateral setting, and absence of signs of diabetic retinopathy on the contralateral eye [16].

(d) **Age-related macular degeneration**

This can be accompanied by IVH and/or retrohyaloid hemorrhage. In these older patients, the PVD is most often complete [17] and parietal hemorrhage can be extensive (Fig. 12.14).

(e) **Ocular tumors**

They are rarely revealed by an ultrasound examination performed for IVH. Nonetheless, one must look for an ocular tumor, in particular, to thoroughly assess the

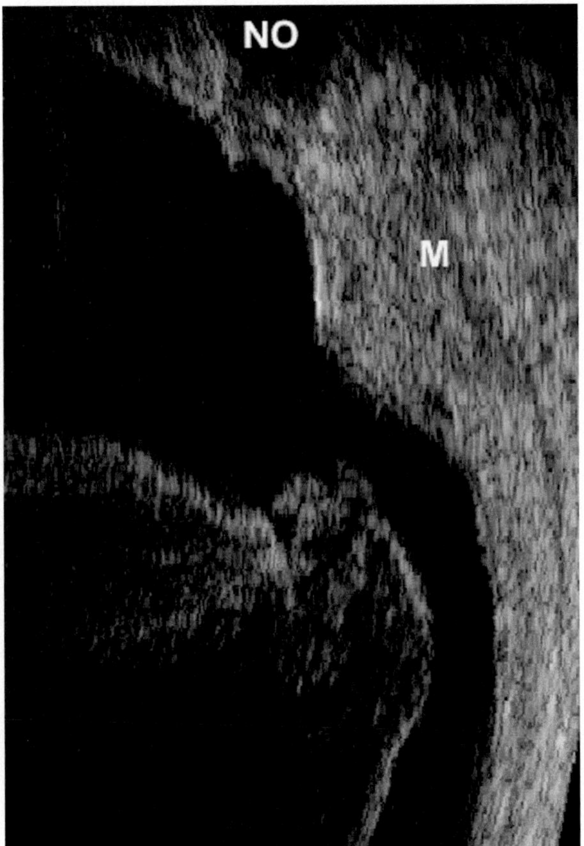


**Fig. 12.14 Junius-Kuhnt's senile disciform macular degeneration.** Section at 20 MHz revealing an intravitreal hemorrhage and an echogenic and heterogeneous lesion without signs of choroidal excavation. NO = optic nerve; M = macula

periphery if no other cause has been discovered (see Chaps. 13 and 14). The echo-texture characteristics of a parietal mass can be altered by hemorrhage if it is diffuse and highly reflective (Fig. 12.15). One should know how to differentiate a choroidal hematoma from a melanoma, using all the resources of B-mode, but also standardized A-mode and especially color Doppler imaging (see Chaps. 13 and 14) and, if there is any doubt, repeat the examination [18].

## (f)  Terson syndrome

This is IVH, uni- or bilateral, occurring as a result of a subarachnoid hemorrhage in younger patients whose vitreous is most often not detached. Unlike otherwise healthy individuals, in whom a hemorrhage tends to sediment inferiorly, the prolonged supine position in these patients explains a higher density of echoes in front of the posterior pole. In most cases, there is no hematic clotting. Ultrasound monitoring is necessary to look for a possible and rare organization of hemorrhage as well as for PVD (Fig. 12.16) [19] and RD (see Chap. 25).

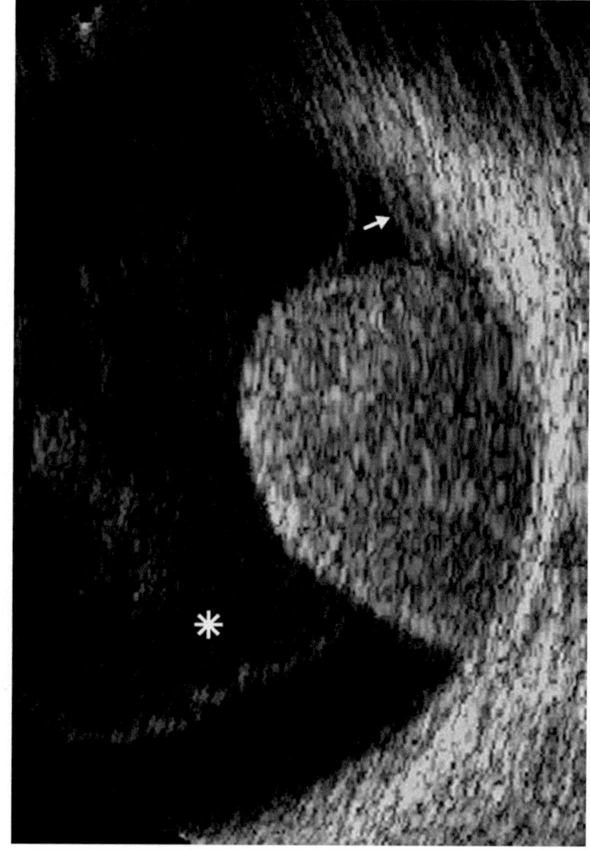

**Fig. 12.15  Choroidal melanoma**. Section at 10 MHz with fairly high gain: revealing a voluminous dome tumor, hypoechoic and homogeneous of the inferior quadrant, behind an intravitreal hemorrhage ( ✱white star) with extensive PVD. The choroidal attenuation and excavation were more readily visualized at a lower gain, as was a small inferomedial satellite retinal detachment ( →white arrow)

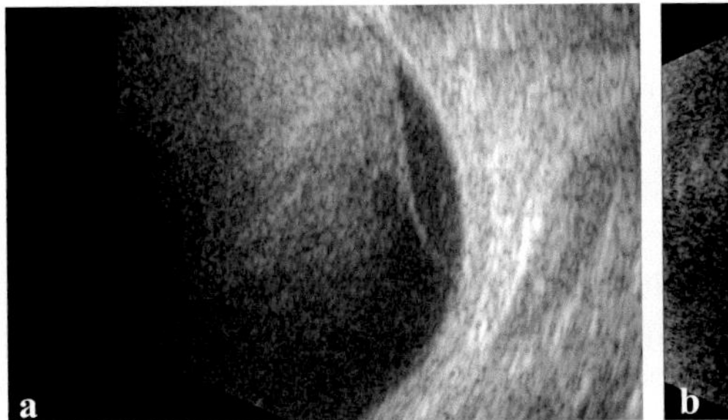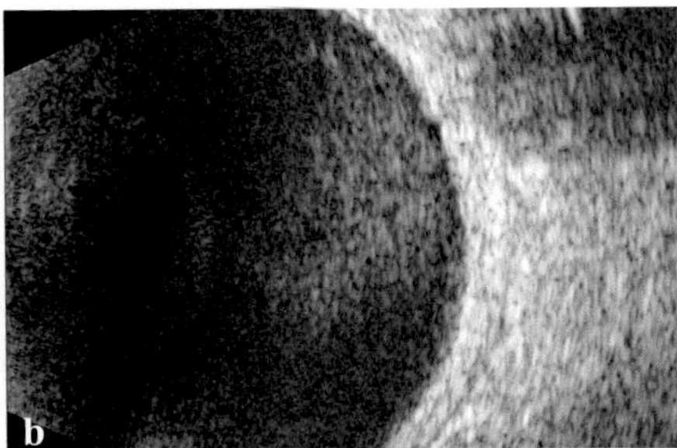

**Fig. 12.16 Terson syndrome. Bilateral intraocular hemorrhage in a patient hospitalized for a subarachnoid hemorrhage a month ago after a ruptured aneurysm. a**: Section of the right eye according to 3 o'clock, with maximal gain (110 dB); **b**: para-axial section of the left eye, with maximal gain (110 dB). In addition to the clinical circumstances and bilaterality, the denser nature of the hemorrhage in front of the posterior pole (due to sedimentation?) is very suggestive of the diagnosis. On the right (**a**), there is an extensive PVD, without collapse of the detached hemorrhagic vitreous gel, and an intravitreal and retrohyaloid hemorrhage

Other etiologies can be complicated by pre-retinal neovascularization, which can be a source of intraocular hemorrhage. However, they are rarer (Sickle cell disease, Eales' disease, etc.).

### 12.1.2.5 Differential Diagnosis of PVD – Membranes – Retinal Detachment (RD)

An uncomplicated PVD should not be confused with RD: the posterior hyaloid is much less thick and much less echogenic than a detached retina. In addition, if the PVD is total, it clearly does not connect to the optic disc.

In cases where the posterior hyaloid membrane is thick and echogenic, subtotal PVD, with persistence of a papillary attachment, may very well simulate a RD.

Thus, in certain circumstances, especially in case of complex vitreoretinal rearrangements with the presence of epiretinal membranes, the differential diagnosis between PVD-epiretinal membranes and RD may be difficult if not impossible, especially when localized.

In B-mode

Some general signs, technical rules, and misleading images need to be known. None of these are definitive.

### – General signs

*In favor of RD*: a continuous line, of consistent thickness and echogenicity, inserting itself into the ora serrata.

*In favor of PVD*: a continuous line, of lesser echogenicity, condensation of the peripapillary ring.

## – Technical rules

- *Gradual reduction of the gain*

It may be useful to gradually reduce the overall gain, allowing only the most echogenic structures to persist: in principle, a posterior hemorrhagic hyaloid (or an intravitreal) membrane remains less echogenic than a detached retina, itself a little less echogenic than the sclera. However, this is not definitive: an epiretinal membrane can be more echogenic than a detached retina.

- *Dynamic study*

In general, movements of the vitreous body are more extensive, slower, smoother and longer than those of a detached retina. However these criteria may no longer be valid in case of vitreous organization.

## Contribution of standardized A-Mode

Vitreous membranes and retina have different textures: the retina has a smooth surface and membranes have an uneven surface. Therefore, their reflectivity is different in ultrasound (and mainly in standardized A-mode). When the surface is smooth, all ultrasound is reflected. When the surface is uneven, only part of it is reflected; the others are diffracted [20–22].

The differential diagnosis between RD and intravitreal membrane can be particularly difficult when the media are opaque (dense hemorrhage, severe eye trauma, advanced proliferative diabetic retinopathy, endophthalmitis). Also, the diagnosis is best carried out by combining B-mode (four criteria) and A-mode (four criteria). In all cases, the ultrasound beam should be perpendicular to the interface studied.

B-mode is already of great help to assess the morphology and kinetics of membranes, but quantitative ultrasound in standardized A-mode provides the most valuable information to differentiate RD from a vitreous membrane.

- First of all (A1, surface echo), at tissue sensitivity (T), the reflectivity of the membrane is assessed, taking care to be perpendicular to it. The retinal peak has 100% reflectivity, whereas most membranes have a reflectivity of less than 100% (Fig. 12.17).
- In addition, a detached retina most often has few nodules (< 3) on the ascending edge of the membrane, whereas a dense membrane has more ($\geq$ 3) (Fig. 12.18).

The recent refinements of standardized echography have resulted in greater reproducibility and speed: displaying ultrasound of large amplitude in A-mode could be tedious and required attention and certain skills to maintain the perpendicularity (maximum signal) long enough on the screen to be able to evaluate its characteristics. The A1 software, during an examination, allows the equipment to "remember"

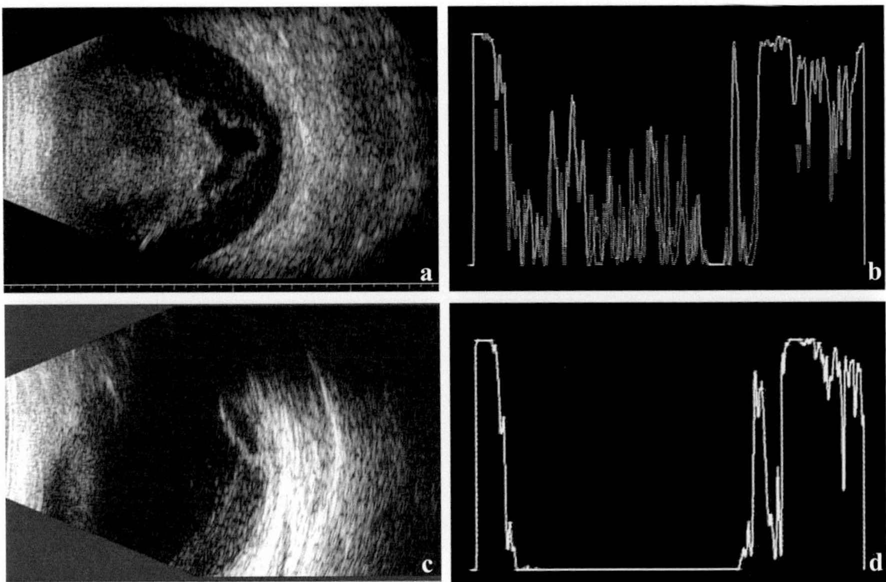

**Fig. 12.17   Retinal detachment (a, b) and vitreous membrane (c, d)**. Respective contributions of B-mode and standardized A-mode at tissue sensitivity (A1). **a, c**: B-mode; **b, d**: standardized A-mode (A1) at tissue sensitivity. In B-mode, the diagnosis is not obvious based on the morphology and the echogenicity, but it does not pose a problem in standardized A-mode: the detached retina has a very high reflectivity, greater than 95%, and the membrane has a reflectivity less than 90%

the maximum signal obtained from the examined surface. Then it selects the peak with the highest amplitude and calculates the signal height as well as the number of high-frequency nodules on the ascending edge.

- A2 corresponds to the reflectivity of the membrane, which must be greater than 95% when the probe is directed toward the ora serrata.
- A3 corresponds to assessment of post-movements: fast and fading rapidly (candlestick sign), more sensitive than in B-mode. However, they can evolve with the appearance of fibrosis/gliosis.
- Then A4 (Quantitative II), the difference in reflectivity between the membrane and the sclera can be compared, noting the reflectivity when the suspect membrane, then the sclera, produces a line positioned by the software at 50% of the height of the scleral peak at tissue sensitivity. If the difference in reflectivity is < 15 dB, it is a detached retina (Fig. 12.19); if the difference is > 20 dB, it is a vitreous membrane; between the two values, the diagnosis is uncertain.

However, even with recent technological advances, the interpretation of these curves is quite difficult and remains reserved for experienced operators: if the probe is not placed strictly perpendicular to the detached surface, the signal strength decreases significantly, which can result in diagnostic errors.

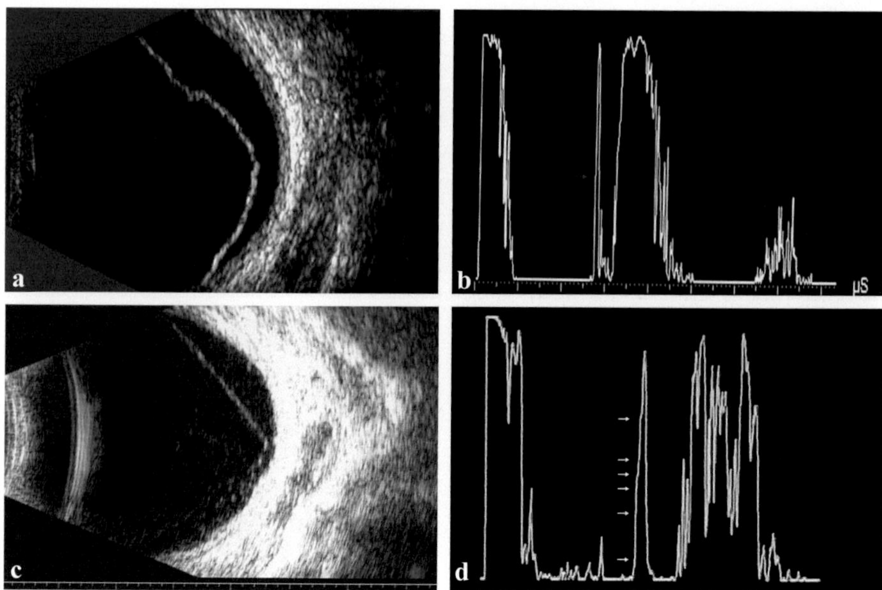

**Fig. 12.18  Retinal (a, b) and vitreous membrane (c, d)**. Respective contributions of B-mode and standardized A-mode. **a, c**: B-mode; **b, d**: standardized A-mode (A1) at tissue sensitivity. In B-mode, the diagnosis is already suggested by both the morphology and the echogenicity, but in standardized A-mode it is obvious: the detached retina has a very high reflectivity, greater than 95%, and has only one high-frequency nodule on its ascending peak, whereas the membrane has a reflectivity slightly less than 90% and, above all, has five high-frequency nodules on its ascending peak

### 12.1.2.6   Hyalitis and Endophthalmitis

**Hyalitis** corresponds to the development of an inflammatory process within the vitreous, regardless of its etiology (uveitis, endophthalmitis).

**Endophthalmitis** corresponds to infection of intraocular media. It is one of the most feared complications in ocular surgery and in case of perforating lesions of the globe with or without a foreign body.

The ultrasound presentations of hyalitis and endophthalmitis are similar.

When the opacity of the media prevents access to the fundus, ultrasound [23] completes the clinical examination by specifying the situation of the retina and the possible existence of papilledema or macular edema. It also helps with the etiological assessment by sometimes revealing a granuloma or a protruding parietal focus. However, once again, regardless of the transparency of the media, its role is also to evaluate the status of the vitreous and its degree of organization.

(a)  **Hyalitis**

- **Ultrasound presentation of clinical Tyndall effect**: homogeneous, it results in the appearance of fine diffuse spots with minimal echogenicity (Fig. 12.20).

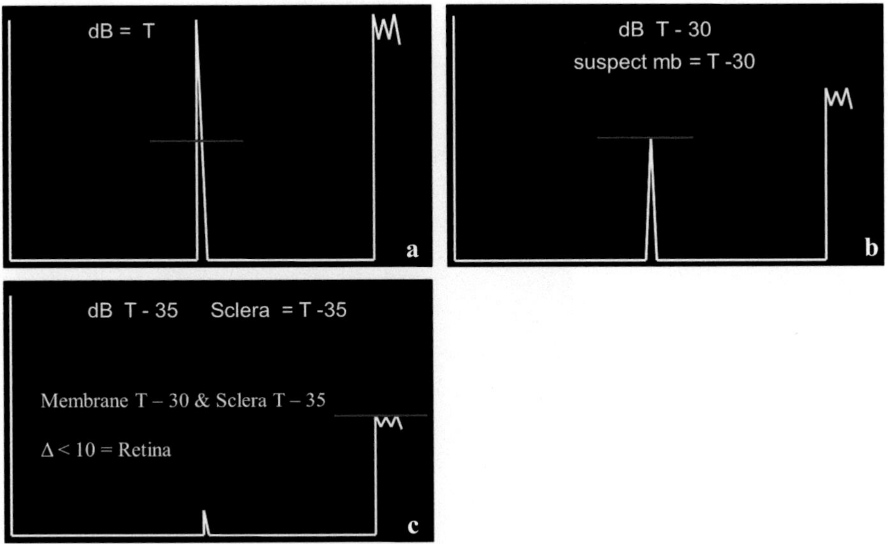


**Fig. 12.19  Retinal detachment (A4—Quantitative II),** comparing the difference in reflectivity between the membrane and the sclera. The operator must be perpendicular to the membrane and sclera to retain their greatest reflectivity. **a,** At tissue sensitivity (T), the membrane appears very reflective; the software positions a red threshold at 50% of the height of the scleral peak; **b,** by lowering the gain gradually, the peak of the membrane to be characterized is exposed by this red threshold. Note the gain: T-30; **c,** the reflectivity of the sclera is calculated in the same manner. Again, note the gain: T-35. The difference (T-35)–(T-30) is less than 10 dB, corresponding to a detached retina

Gradually, membranes with little or medium echogenicity appear and are arranged into networks.

- **If the inflammation is controlled,** the ultrasound Tyndall effect disappears, but the membranes often remain apparent. Vitreous syneresis accelerates, and PVD occurs earlier and more frequently. The existence of vitreoretinal adhesions in relation to former parietal foci then increases the risk of tractional RD or retinal tear. Therefore, they warrant regular clinical and ultrasound monitoring.

- **When the inflammation is more substantial or the infection is not controlled,** the vitreous organization increases, with the occurrence of more echogenic membranes that provide the vitreous with a more heterogeneous appearance. Its mobility decreases. In case of PVD, the thicker and more echogenic hyaloid membrane becomes immobile in places. The vitreous retracts. As long as the PVD is not total, the risk of tractional RD remains maximal. If the latter appears, only vitrectomy allows for retinal reapplication.

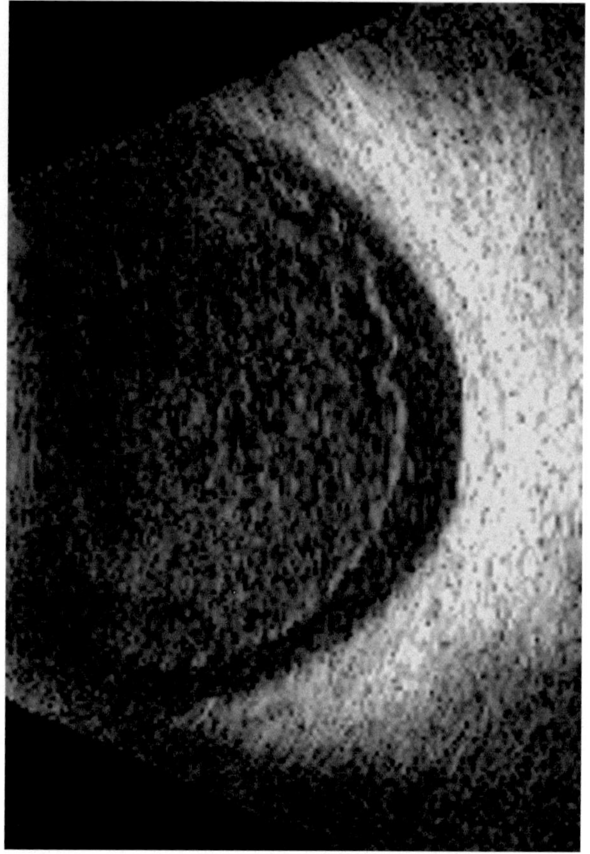

**Fig. 12.20 Hyalitis.** Section at 10 MHz, with maximum gain. The intravitreal echoes are weakly echogenic. The posterior hyaloid membrane is much less echogenic than a retina. It is thickened due to the inflammation of the vitreous

### (b) Endophthalmitis

In addition to the hyalitis that accompanies it, endophthalmitis is frequently marked by a diffuse choroidal thickening (Fig. 12.21). Searching for a foreign body is essential: it constitutes a microbial site that is refractory to antibiotic treatment. Therefore, its extraction is urgently required.

### 12.1.2.7 Degenerative Pathology

Asteroid Hyalosis

Is a rare, unilateral, degenerative condition of the vitreous, occurring mainly in the elderly. It can readily be identified by biomicroscopic examination.

With ultrasound, it manifests as scattered punctiform echoes that are very echogenic because of their high content of calcium stearate or palmitate. They can

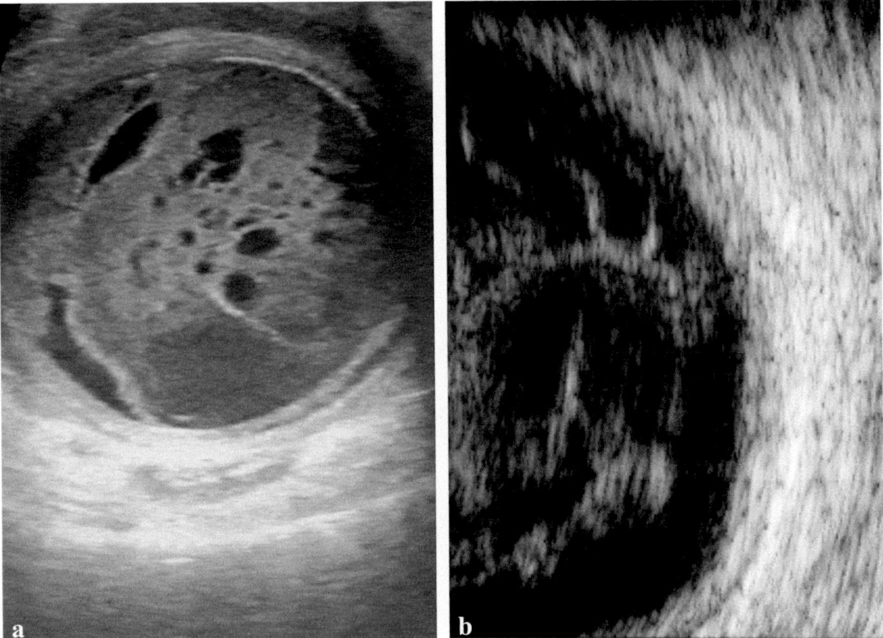

**Fig. 12.21 Endophthalmitis. a**: High gain section of the temporal quadrant with an 8–18 MHz probe; **b**: moderate gain section of the temporal quadrant at 10 MHz. The vitreous gel, which is not fully detached, is echogenic, heterogeneous, with membranes, and not very mobile. The risk of retinal detachment is high and there should be frequent ultrasound check-ups. Note the parietal thickening measured at 1.9 mm in **b**

have a focal distribution or occupy the entire vitreous. Although abundant, they are always separated from the wall of the globe by an anechoic area behind which a posterior vitreous detachment can sometimes be seen (Fig. 12.22).

However, PVD is less common in asteroid hyalosis, and Wasano [20] has noted that even without PVD, asteroid bodies do not usually extend to the retina and there may be confusion regarding the presence of PVD.

Although abundant and dense on ultrasound, the impact of asteroid hyalosis on visual acuity remains low. Therefore, in these conditions, one rarely performs vitrectomy.

Synchysis Scintillans

It results in punctiform echoes, more or less coarse and very reflective related to cholesterol crystals. It usually occurs on highly modified globes with little functionality (Fig. 12.23).

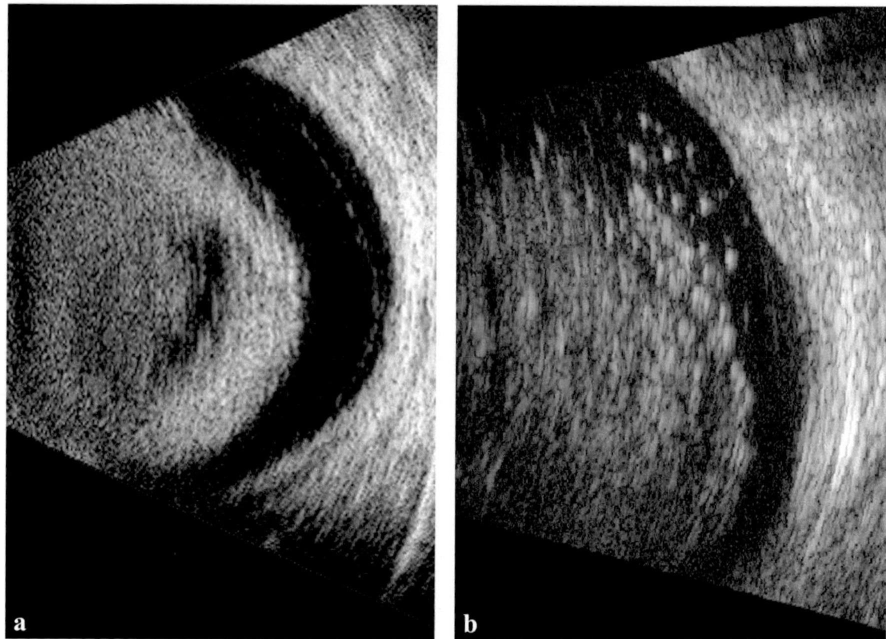

**Fig. 12.22 Asteroid hyalosis. a**: Section at 10 MHz showing a multitude of hyperreflective elements within the vitreous gel, surrounded by a hypoechoic peripheral crown. In this case, it is associated with a PVD, clearly seen within this peripheral hypoechoic crown. **b**: Section at 20 MHz. The hyperreflective calcium spots are much better defined than at 10 MHz, and those located near the wall of the globe in the vicinity of the focal zone are sharper than those located in the anterior vitreous. Moreover, in this case, PVD is absent

**Fig. 12.23 Synchysis scintillans.** Small hyperechoic dots with posterior microresonance readily visible in the superior field secondary to an inferior foreign body (➤ white arrowhead), complicated by retinal detachment (➜ black arrows)

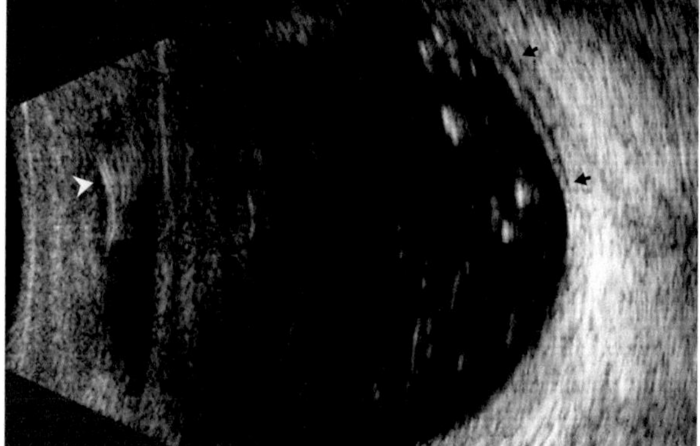

### 12.1.2.8 Traumatic Injury Pathology

A distinction is made between:

- Closed globe trauma or globe contusions.
- Open globe trauma or globe wounds requiring surgical treatment in emergency.
- Foreign bodies, which may be superficial, intraocular, or orbital, jeopardizing the visual prognosis.

Because the lesions often overlap, we have deliberately separated them, and in this chapter, we will only cover anomalies of the posterior segment. Lesions of the anterior segment are discussed in Chap. 11.

Contusions [25, 26]

Ocular damage is more likely to be more pronounced when the blunt agent is small and projected at high speed: a champagne cork, a golf or tennis ball, etc.

**At the level of the posterior segment**, one can see:

- posterior pole edema or Berlin's edema, which can lead to a transient or permanent decrease in visual acuity and sometimes progress toward a macular hole (Fig. 12.24);
- hemorrhage of the vitreous, by retinal vascular rupture, sometimes associated with luxation of the lens or implant (see Fig. 11.54; Fig. 12.25);
- retinal tears, which can lead to retinal detachment;
- hematomas or choroidal hemorrhagic detachments.

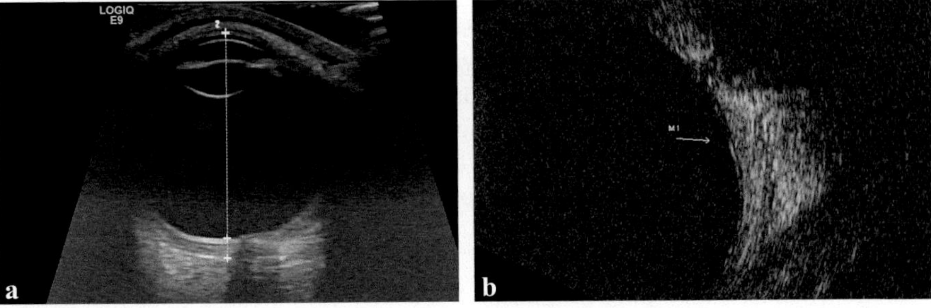


**Fig. 12.24 Ocular contusion with posterior pole edema (Berlin's edema). a:** Axial section, with a lot of gel on the eyelids with a multipurpose ultrasound unit; **b:** Section of the macular region with a long focal length 20-MHz probe. The posterior pole is thickened, to 2.2 mm, and very discreetly protruding (→m1)

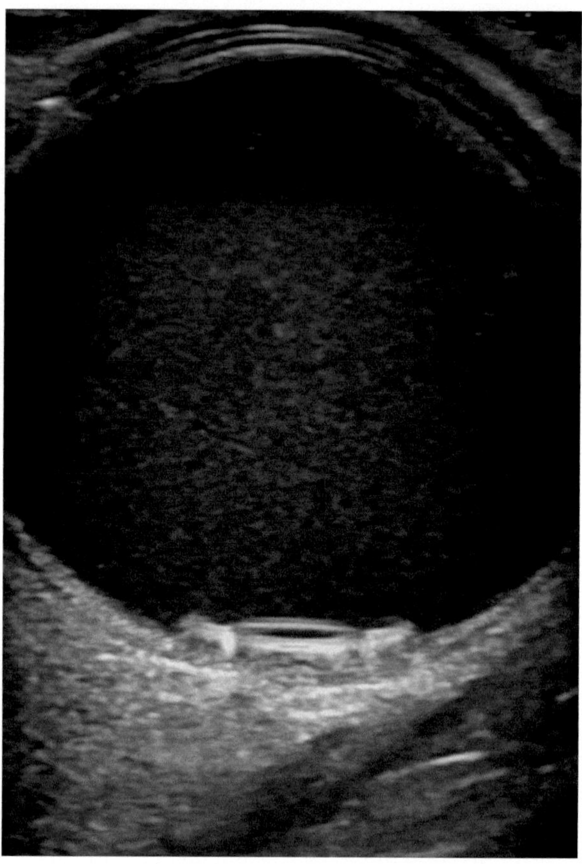

**Fig. 12.25 Intraocular hemorrhage with a luxated intra-ocular lens in front of the posterior pole** in a patient who already underwent vitrectomy for retinal detachment. The hemorrhage takes on the appearance of small, moderately echogenic dots like a retrohyaloid hemorrhage. The optics of the implant is readily visible on the posterior pole. Haptics were visible on other sections, causing many artifacts

## Perforating Wounds [27]

- These are observed in adults, during domestic accidents, DIY projects, workplace accidents, or in a context of physical aggression. They are also common in children (BB guns, bows and arrows, plant trauma, etc.).
- Ultrasound is performed after suturing the wound, without applying pressure, placing a large amount of gel between the probe and the eyelid.
- It can be a corneal injury, in association with lesions of the iris or the lens (see Chap. 11).
- Small scleral wounds.
- Large wounds, with a poor prognosis, frequently complicated by retinal detachment or even phthisis bulbi (Fig. 12.26).

**Fig. 12.26 Large corneoscleral wound in a 10-year-old child after direct trauma with a broomstick**. Para-axial section with a multipurpose ultrasound unit and plenty of gel on the eyelids. Rapid progression in less than 10 days toward a total retinal detachment (➡) and choroidal detachment (➤), then toward phthisis (a thick wall at 2.7 mm at the posterior pole and axial length of 14.2 mm/and 16.9 mm to the sclera). There was no other option but to schedule evisceration/ enucleation

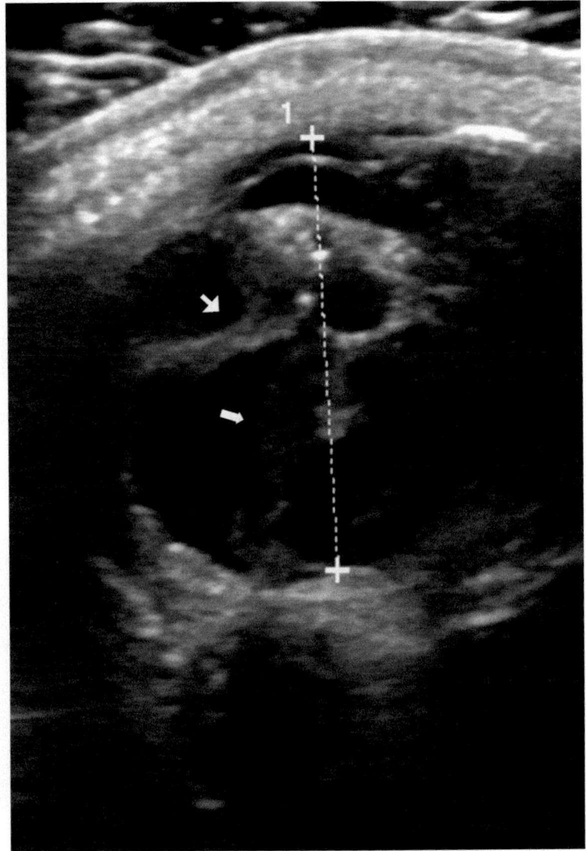

## Foreign Body (FB) Trauma

- In case of injury of the globe, a FB should not be ignored, and at the slightest doubt a CT scan without injection should be performed first: a spiral CT scan remains the technique for optimal imaging to assess oculo-orbital trauma [28]. FBs can be single or multiple, sometimes bilateral, of varying size and nature.
- Ultrasound is useful to complete the assessment, refine the precise location of intraocular FBs, and to assess intraocular lesions which affect prognosis [29, 30]. It is very efficient, more so than a CT scan, for detecting small FBs close to the wall. However, a CT scan is superior for orbital FBs.
- At the semiological level, FBs result in a hyperechoic nodule followed by artifacts, typically posterior resonance in the vitreous and a posterior shadowing on the orbit (see Figs. 6.6), (Fig. 12.27). Their localization, as with a CT scan, must be very accurate: with the distance to the optic disc and the scleral spur along the meridian where it is located (Fig. 12.28).

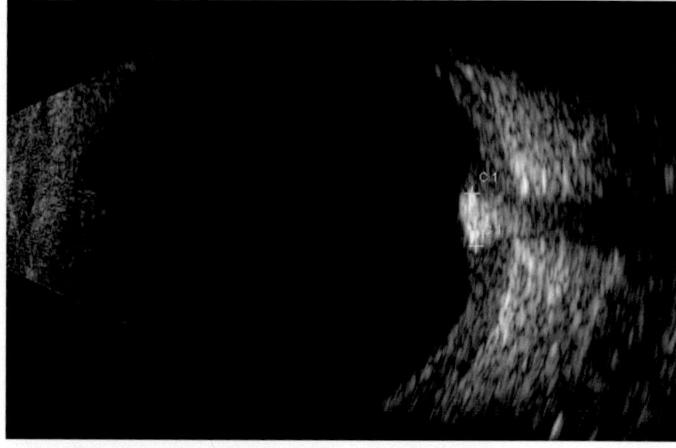

**Fig. 12.27 Metallic foreign body** (work accident with a hammer) of 3 mm in diameter, stuck in the wall, 7.3 mm from the optic disc, nasally, with reduced gain (83 dB). At this gain, the associated intravitreal hemorrhage cannot be visualized, but the posterior shadowing on the orbit is obvious

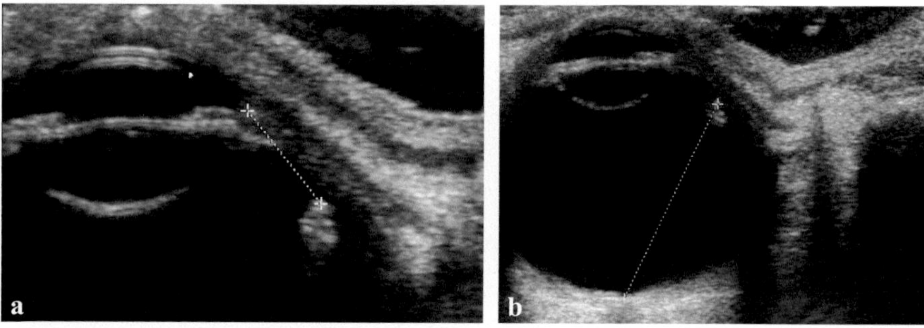

**Fig. 12.28** Foreign body (FB) located next to the ora serrata on the 7 o'clock meridian of the right eye. Sections with a multipurpose ultrasound unit: **a**: With an 18-MHz probe: distance between the FB and the scleral spur measured as 5.4 mm; **b**: With a 12-MHz probe: distance between the FB and the optic disc measured as 18.9 mm

- For parietal FBs, one needs to specify whether they are pre-parietal (and hence mobile), embedded in the retina, choroid, or sclera, or immediately behind the wall after having crossed it.
- When the resonance artifacts are very long and extend onto the orbit, a spherical FB should be considered, such as a pellet in ballistic trauma [31] (Fig. 12.29), for which the visual prognosis is unfavorable [32, 33].
- An intraocular air bubble, after the passage through the eye of a FB located in the orbit, can result in a presentation very similar to a FB. However, the artifacts are much shorter, restricted to the eye, and do not extend to the orbit [34]. In addition, they fade in a few hours or days, and of course, no FB is seen by CT scan.
- MRI is contraindicated in case of a suspected ferromagnetic metallic FB because it is potentially dangerous [35, 36], even if they are microscopic [37–39], but can

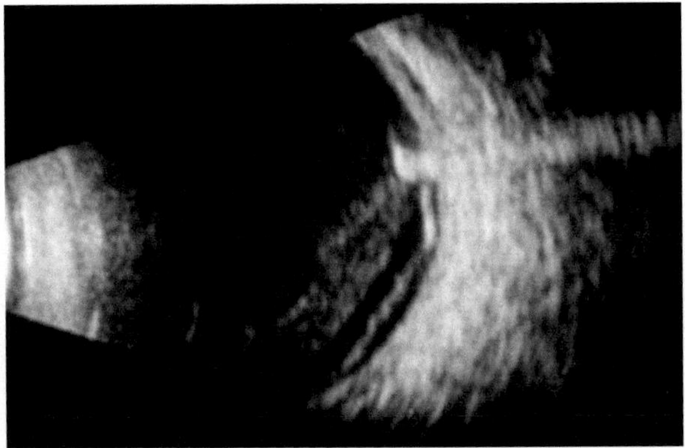

**Fig. 12.29  Spherical foreign body** (pistol bullet) in the inferior nasal quadrant on the periphery, with hemorrhage and retinal detachment. The spherical shape of the FB is responsible for the repeated back and forth movements, causing this very long posterior resonance artifact in the orbit

be done if the entity is made of lead, and is mainly relevant in the diagnosis of plant FBs [40], which are most often orbital.

- Intraocular FBs can cause early complications: endophthalmitis (Fig. 12.30), RD (Fig. 12.29), traumatic cataracts, etc. but also late complications if the FB is unknown: siderosis, chalcosis, remote infectious complications.
- Multiple foreign microbodies can be the consequence of mine explosions; they are characterized by small artifacts of short posterior resonance. The appearance is quite similar to what can be seen in synchysis scintillans (Fig. 12.23).

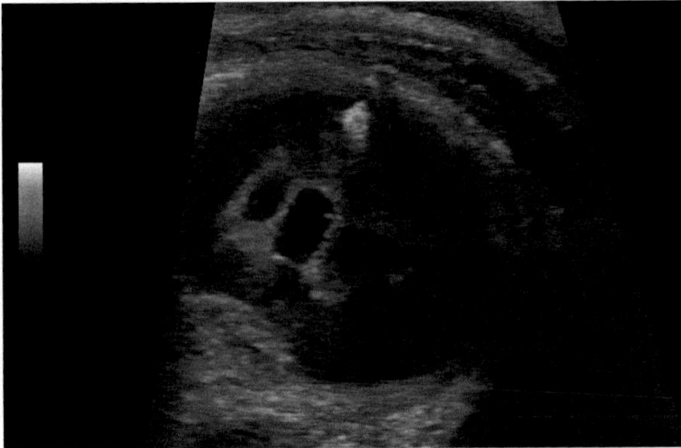

**Fig. 12.30  FB (from gardening) stuck in the wall at 5 o'clock, complicated very quickly by endophthalmitis**, with vitreous echoes, pseudomembranes, and thickening of the wall. Two months after removal of the FB, extraction of the lens (cataract), vitrectomy, endolaser on a tear, and gas: good morphological progression (a flat retina everywhere) and relatively satisfactory functional evolution (visual acuity = 20/120)

### 12.1.2.9   Tumor Spread in the Vitreous

This is mainly due to retinoblastoma in children (Fig. 12.31) and lymphomas in adults (see Chaps. 13 and 14). However, these cases are rare.

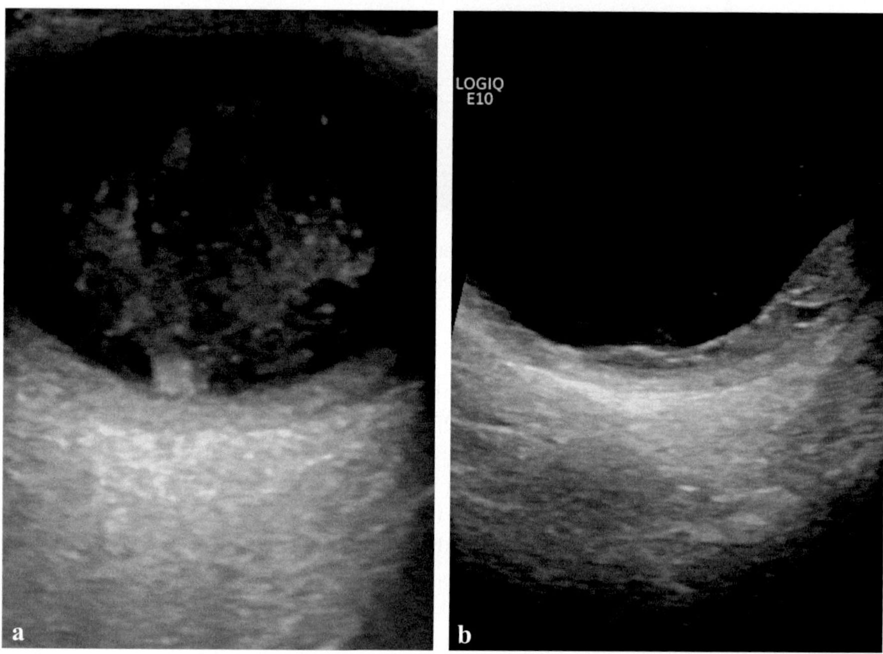


**Fig. 12.31   Tumor spreading in the vitreous of a retinoblastoma (stage D and Vb). a**: View of the inferior quadrant; **b**: View of the superior temporal quadrant. Tumor spreading in the vitreous, predominates in the inferior quadrant. These are coarser echoes than hematic clots, and one is calcified. The parietal mass is located in the superior temporal area and contains some barely visible microcalcifications

## 12.2   Retina

### *12.2.1   Retinal Detachment (RD)*

Different pathological circumstances can lead to separation of the neuroepithelium from the retinal pigment epithelium, which is typically referred to as RD.

The following are distinguished:

- **Rhegmatogenous RD**
- **Traction RD**
- **Exudative RD**
- **Tumoral RD**.

Ultrasound, in case of opaque media, provides fundamental help in this regard. Hence, one can:

- diagnose RD;
- accurately determine its extent and its borders;
- detect possible dehiscence;
- evaluate the degree of proliferative vitreoretinopathy;
- follow the postoperative changes.

Thus, when the media are hazy, ultrasound is used to establish the surgical plan.

### 12.2.1.1  Rhegmatogenous RD

The occurrence of rhegmatogenous RD results from the combination of several factors. The vitreous, as a result of its modifications leading to PVD, plays a major role. A peripheral vitreoretinal anomaly, not always visible, involving identifiable vitreoretinal traction, will promote the formation of a tear of the retina and allow the retrohyaloid fluid to flow into the subretinal space.

Ultrasound Diagnosis

- Morphology

The non-elevated retina is indistinguishable from the choroid. Once formed, at first, RD presents as a continuous, relatively thick, and highly echogenic membrane. It attaches to the optic disc and extends peripherally to the ora serrata. Then, when it is total, RD assumes a mobile V shape for all sections passing through the optic disc: biconcave when it is flat, biconvex when it is bullous.

The presence of multiple small punctiform echoes of low intensity behind a very echogenic flat RD is common. These then simulate a hemorrhage behind the retina but are compatible with simply serous subretinal fluid.

- Reflectivity

A detached retina is more echogenic than a posterior hyaloid membrane or an unaltered intravitreal membrane and less echogenic than the sclera (Fig. 12.32), provided that the ultrasound beam is perpendicular to it.

In standardized A-mode, at tissue sensitivity, the retinal peak has a reflectivity of 90% to 95% of the scleral peak. In B-mode, more difficult to quantify than in

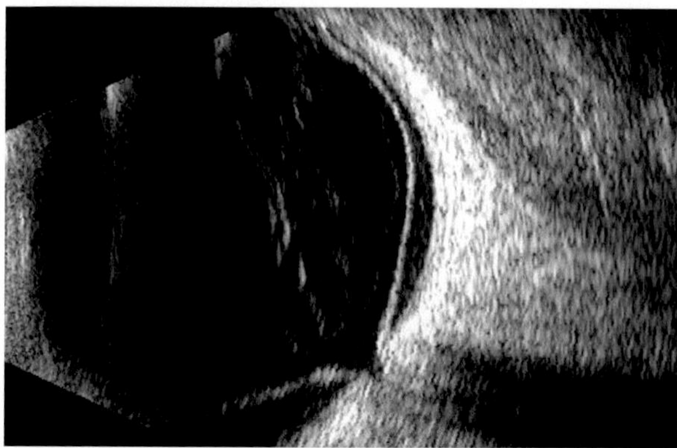

**Fig. 12.32  Total retinal detachment**. Para-axial section with a long focal-length 20-MHz probe. The membrane starts at the optic disc. It is hyperechoic along the temporal meridian because it is perpendicular to the ultrasound beam. However, it is slightly to moderately echogenic along the nasal meridian depending on the obliquity of the ultrasound beam. It is rather thin and more echogenic than the posterior hyaloid membrane, which is visible right in front of the detached retina

standardized A-mode, the differential quantification with respect to the scleral peak is less than 15 dB (see above, Sect. 12.1.2.5 and Fig. 12.19).

- Thickness

A detached retina is thicker than a normal posterior hyaloid membrane and thinner than a detached choroid.

- Mobility

As compared with an unaltered posterior hyaloid membrane, a raised retina displays less extensive movements, with faster, shorter, more jerky oscillations that do not persist much once the movements of the globe stop. They are not dampened. A detached retina is all the more mobile when the RD is recent and extensive. But all these criteria can be modified in case of proliferative vitreoretinopathy (PVR).

Extent and Limits

Is the RD localized or total? As always, the combination of radial and circular sections (taking care to bring the flat retina–raised retina transition area to the center of the screen) allows for determining its extent and borders with great precision.

It is also useful to inform about the status of macula: whether it is detached (macula-off) or not (macula-on), in particular when there is an IVH preventing access to the fundus. This information is sometimes difficult to provide and requires all possible technical tricks: horizontal and vertical sections of the posterior pole by lateral and medial approach, or even oblique sections, with reduced and medium gain.

## Ultrasound Detection of Retinal Tears

This is based on recognition of their direct signs (the tear itself) and indirect signs (retinal operculum–vitreoretinal adhesions). It is best achieved by circular sections allowing a fast and very wide sectorial scan by simple variation of the inclination of the probe. Meridian sections confirm the diagnosis and pinpoint their location acurately.

- **in a non elevated retina**

Different types of tears are found:

(a)  **Tear with a flap**

This is a horseshoe tear opening posteriorly (toward the posterior pole), whereby the flap remains attached to the peripheral (anterior) retina.

Detectable by ultrasound, the tear presents as a short hyperechoic membrane attached to the eye wall (Fig. 12.33).

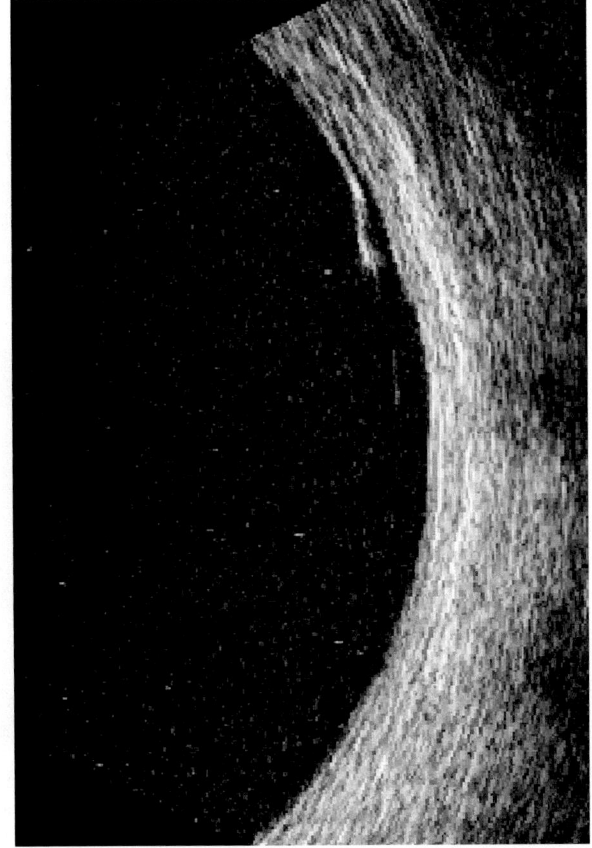

**Fig. 12.33  Flap retinal tear, and acute PVD.** Temporal field section at 20 MHz. Presence of a detachment of the posterior hyaloid membrane, which is thin. This membrane is attached to a short, highly echogenic, pre-parietal membrane corresponding to the tear

The vitreoretinal adhesion is sometimes visible owing to the hyaloid membrane that converges and remains adherent to its floating anterior end. The loss of visualized retinal substance is found inconsistently. It becomes visible especially when the edges of the tear become raised or a localized retinal detachment appears.

### (b)  Round holes with pulled-out operculum

The flap under traction from the vitreoretinal adhesion has completely detached from the retina. It remains adherent to the hyaloid membrane and constitutes the operculum.

The hole is impossible to discern by ultrasound when the retina is undetached. When the retinal edges are elevated, the loss of substance may be apparent if it is not too small. However, analysis of these breaks remains difficult because of their very peripheral location. The operculum, which is easier to detect, is manifested by a very localized hyperechogenicity on the detached hyaloid membrane. Therefore, it is an excellent indirect sign of retinal tear, thus allowing its presence to be suspected. Regardless, it cannot be differentiated from a small hyaloid clot if it is associated with a vitreous hemorrhage.

- **in a detached retina**

They manifest as a solution in the continuity of the retina, sometimes surmounted by a flap (Fig. 12.34). Wide and giant breaks (with a surface area greater than or equal to that of a quadrant) are readily detectable.

Anterior or posterior small breaks (holes, microflaps) are generally invisible. For these, many false positives are possible because of the frequent presence within the detached retina of uneven thickness (localized thinning).

Thus, only the most evocative aspects are retained: broad solution of continuity (Fig. 12.35) or a flap image found both in meridian and circular sections.

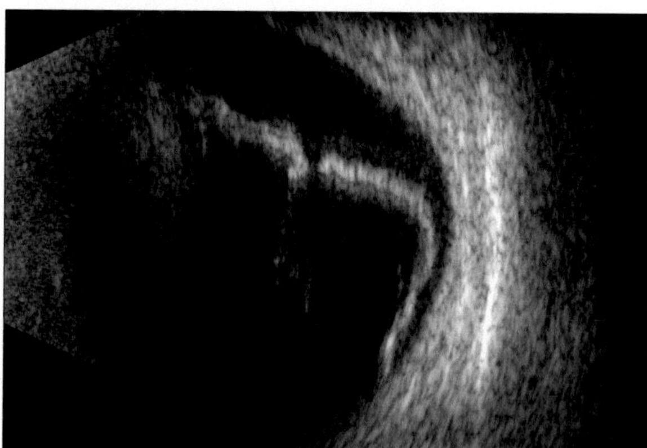

**Fig. 12.34  Flap retinal tear on a constituted superior retinal detachment**. Section at 10 MHz. Note the beginning of rolling-up of the tear (reflecting proliferative vitreoretinopathy [PVR]) and attachment of the posterior hyaloid membrane to the peripheral edge, anterior, of the tear

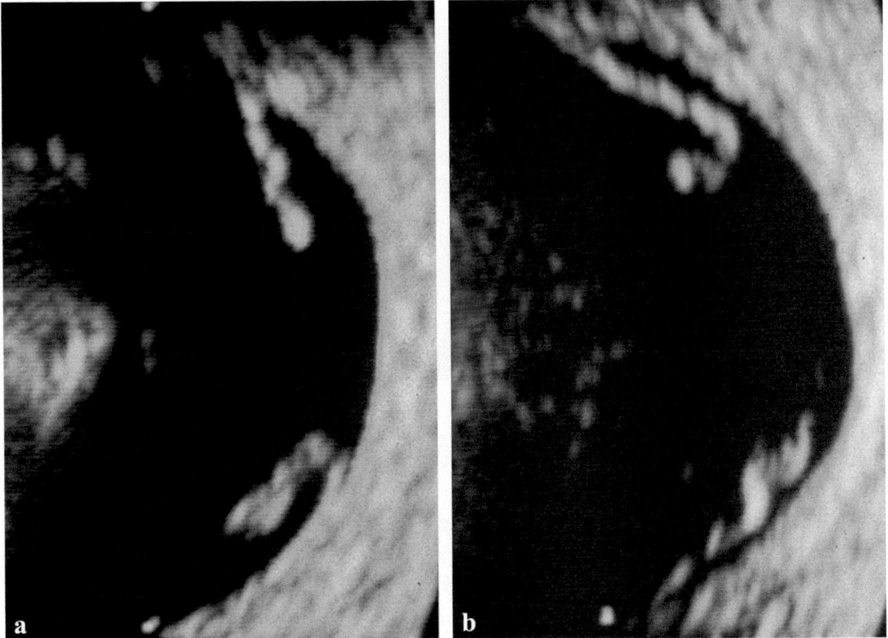

**Fig. 12.35   Giant tear. Section at 10 MHz. a**: Extensive retinal break, with broad solution of the continuity; **b**: Giant tear with curled-up edges

Hence the importance of indirect signs: essentially vitreoretinal adhesions exerting traction and converging toward the top of the dehiscence.

## Ultrasound Evaluation of Proliferative Vitreoretinopathy (PVR)

**The reference is the classification of proliferative vitreoretinopathy (from Machemer 1991)** [41].

Ultrasound evaluation of vitreoretinal proliferation can only be approximate as compared with ophthalmoscopy [42]: it is invisible by ultrasound in stage A. In stage B, the tear may have rolled edges, but these are rarely visible (large tears especially) (Figs. 12.34 and 12.35). In practice, only advanced PVRs (stage C, type 1 to type 5) are diagnosable.

This ultrasound evaluation is based on several criteria:

- **the presentation of the vitreous**

It becomes more echogenic with the appearance of echogenic preretinal membranes and a thickened posterior hyaloid. In case of PVR, its mobility decreases. This aspect is sometimes difficult to differentiate from a hemorrhagic organization of the vitreous.

- **the presentation of the retina**

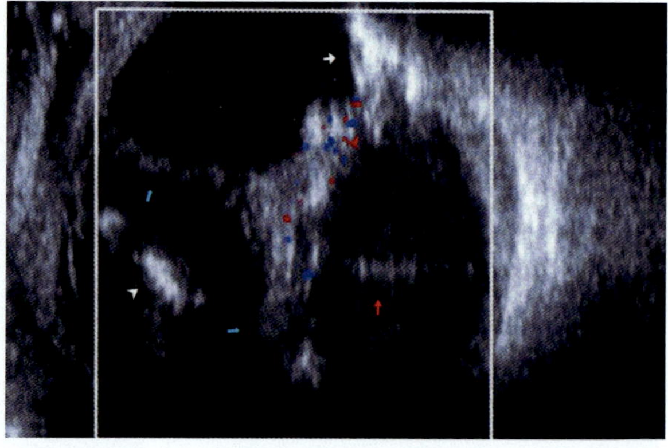

**Fig. 12.36 Subretinal strands (→ red arrow) and cyclitic membrane (→ blue arrows) visible on this highly advanced retinal detachment (RD) with massive PVR**. section exploring the 3 o'clock meridian of the right eye. There is also a calcified lens (▶ white arrowhead) and parietal calcifications around the optic disc (➜ white arrow)

Initially mobile, it gradually becomes fixed. Its less pronounced movements become short, like high-frequency tremors.

Readily visible fixed folds appear in case of significant PVR (type 1 and type 2). They lead to a gradual reduction of the retinal surface. In their absence, the retina can become thicker, sometimes discontinuous. Similarly, the visualization of stretched subretinal strands (Fig. 12.36) of varying echogenicity is possible (PVR type 3). Retinal reapplication can only be considered if they are cut.

A thick and echogenic frontal membrane then appears, referred to as a "cyclitic membrane". Associated with retinal detachment, it results in a triangle presentation, with an anterior base and papillary apex. It corresponds to the vitreous retracted toward the retrolental ciliary region and is a sign of anterior PVR (type 4 and type 5) (Fig. 12.36).

Using ultrasound, it is best visualized by an immersion technique. It is responsible for the gradual closure of the V: the retina then becomes almost completely immobile. The V turns into a Y and then into a T (a funnel blocking the optic disc). These aspects of RD can in most cases not be addressed with any of the currently available therapeutic resources and indicate an old and advanced-stage process.

Once type 5 is reached, if there is still traction, the detachment can extend to the ciliary retina and then to the ciliary body itself, a source of prolonged hypotonia causing phthisis.

Old RDs can assume a variety of ultrasound presentations: thin, not very echogenic, or, on the contrary, thick. Pseudocysts can appear (Figs. 12.37 and 12.38): they correspond to a closed retinal funnel sealed inside an epiretinal membrane.

**In summary**, the presence of a total V-shaped RD that is not very mobile with movements of the globe, to which fixed folds or intravitreal membranes are associated, has a poor prognosis and warrants vitrectomy.

A total V-shaped, or T-shaped, RD with cyclitic membrane and/or pseudocysts has very poor prognosis. In most cases, it cannot be addressed with any of the currently available therapeutic resources.

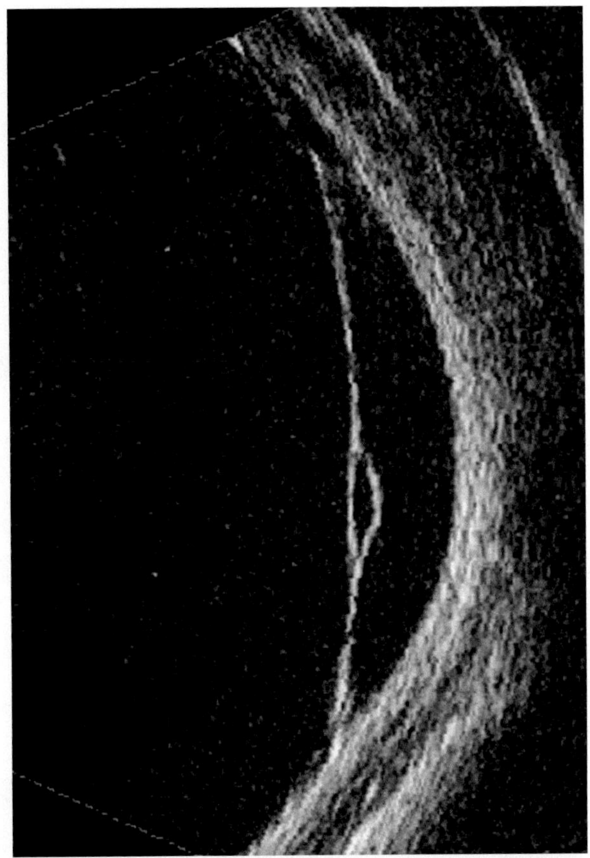

**Fig. 12.37  Retinal pseudocyst, small in size**, section at 20 MHz, complicating an old total retinal detachment

## Contribution of Color Doppler Imaging (CDI)

Although the difference between RD and vitreous membranes (VMs) was published as early as 1991 [43], over time and through technological improvements, CDI has acquired a sensitivity of 92.3%, specificity of 100%, and diagnostic accuracy of 96.3% by finding flows on the retinal leaflets when the RD is extensive or total while not finding any on VM [44]. Although it involves a slightly more cumbersome procedure, CDI with ultrasound contrast medium injection further increases this diagnostic accuracy [45] (Fig. 12.39).

The study of velocimetric constants of intraocular membrane flows also allows for differentiating RDs from a hyaloid artery in the case of uncomplicated posterior or mixed persisting fetal vasculature [46] (Fig. 12.40), with the difference in the walls of the two vessels and the difference in the area vascularized (neural for the retinal vessel and vitreous for the hyaloid artery) explaining this difference.

The postoperative visual acuity of a rhegmatogenous RD is related to the existence of PVR, macular involvement, and the duration of the detachment. It seems also

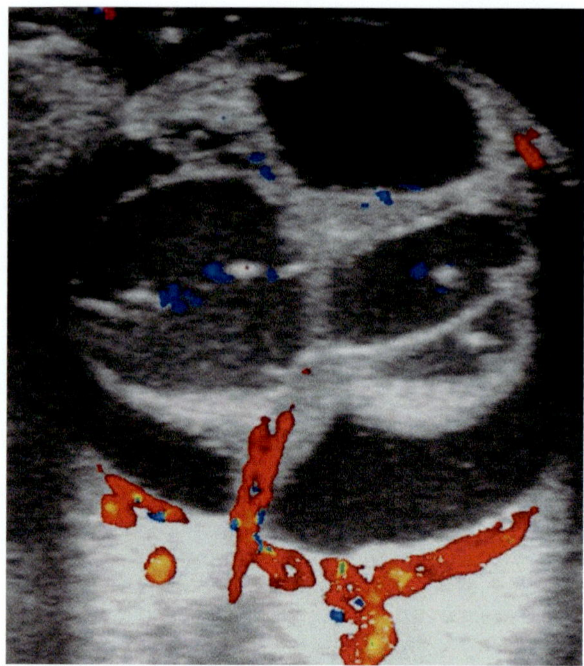

**Fig. 12.38  Retinal pseudocysts, echogenic, hematic, occurring in old vascularized retinal detachment**. Color Doppler imaging, axial section

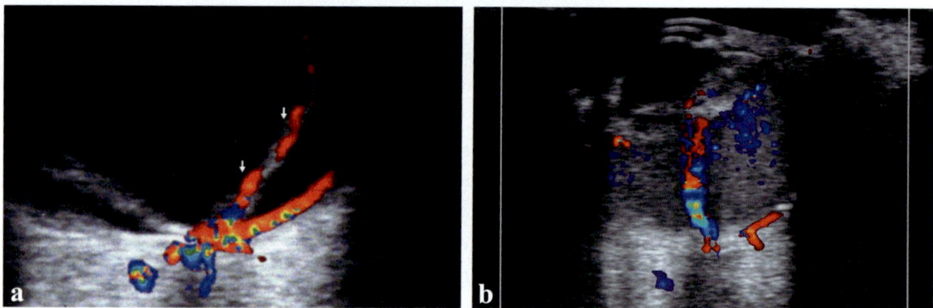

**Fig. 12.39  Retinal detachment**. CDI, color mode. **a**: V-shaped total retinal detachment, wide open at the front: the colored flows are visible on the side where the Doppler beam is slightly oblique to the detached retinal leaflet (→ white arrows), but not on the other side where it is almost perpendicular to it; **b**: Total T-shaped hemorrhagic RD following Coats' disease. The base of the RD, parallel to the Doppler beam, is highly vascularized, but the retrolental cyclitic membrane that is perpendicular to it, is not. Finally, note the small blue-colored dots at the level of the subretinal space in connection with the movement of the red blood cells "falling" toward the declive part of the eye

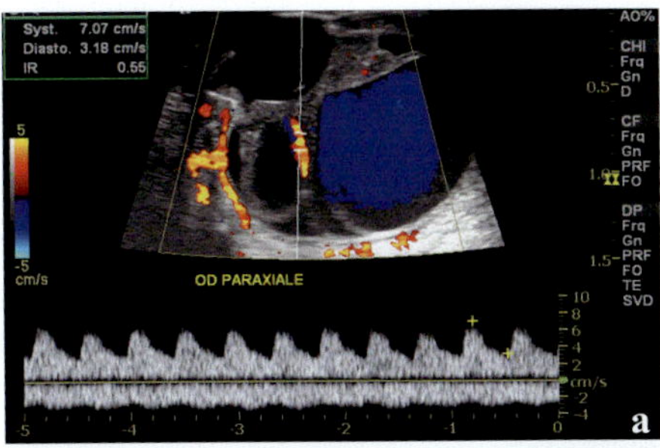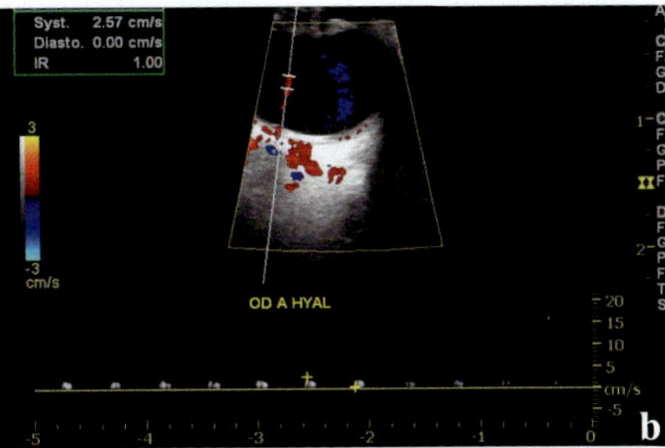

**Fig. 12.40  Contribution of spectral Doppler. a:** Color and spectral Doppler in a case of a mixed persisting fetal vasculature complicated by total retinal detachment with hemorrhagic retinal pseudocysts (the large blue pool corresponding to the movement of red blood cells "falling" toward the declive part of the voluminous hemorrhagic temporal pseudocyst. Within the retinal vessels of the base of the RD, the peak systolic velocity (PSV) is 7.07 cm/s and the resistive index (RI) 0.55, very close to that of the central retinal artery (CRA); **b:** Color and spectral Doppler in a case of mixed persisting fetal vasculature with a persistently permeable hyaloid artery. The PSV is 2.57 cm/s (much lower) and the RI is 1.00 by abolished diastolic flow.

related to low eye pressure and the existence of velocimetric disturbances in the central retinal artery and the ophthalmic artery.

A preliminary study [47] in the medical imaging department of the Rothschild Foundation Hospital has already shown a correlation between the Peak Systolic Velocity in the central retinal artery and postoperative visual acuity.

In RD, complications of PVR are associated with endothelin 1 (a very potent vasoconstrictor), intra-ocular pressure, and disruptions in the flow in the central retinal artery (CRA) [48]. When the RD is total, there is a slight decrease in peak systolic velocity (PSV) in the CRA on the side with the RD as compared with the contralateral eye (Fig. 12.41a and b). If the difference is very large, and the PSV on the side of the RD is less than half of the PSV of the contralateral eye, visual acuity after anatomically successful surgery is functionally ineffective (Fig. 12.41c and d). This poor functional prognosis, associated with these low flows within the CRA, seems parallel to the extent of the PVR [49].

Postoperative Follow-Up

Getting the thin leaflets to reconnect is performed by external indentation or internal tamponade. The two methods are sometimes combined in one or two steps.

### (a)  External buckling

This is indicated in simple forms. External compression is achieved by ligation of a synthetic material on the sclera that pushes the wall against the neuroepithelium. It is a strip of foam made of Silastic™ or solid silicone, with a round or oval section. This indentation is placed toward the pre-equatorial region in relation to the break.

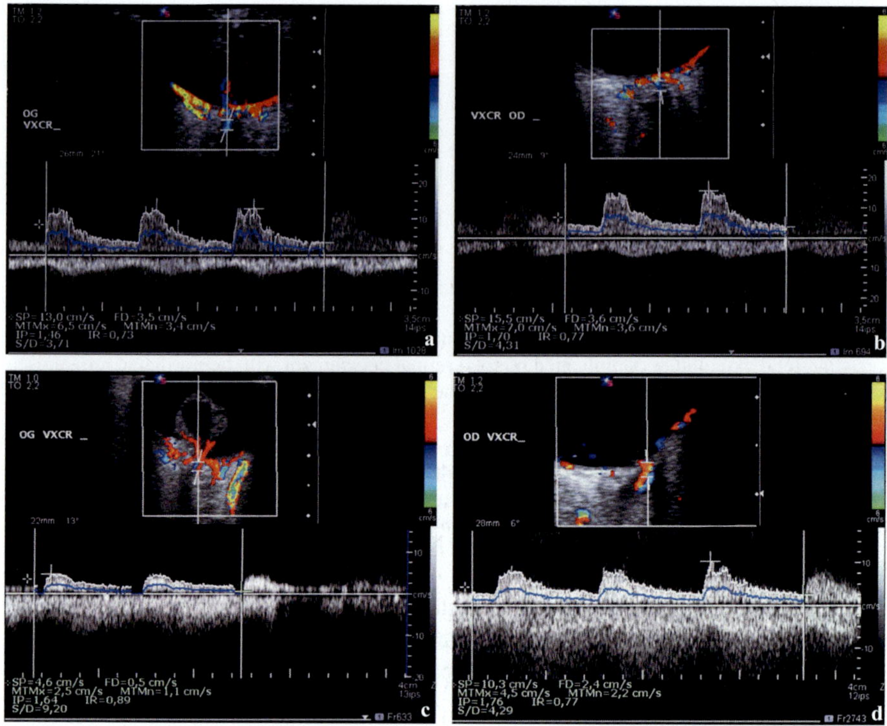

**Fig. 12.41 Contribution of spectral Doppler for assessment of the functional prognosis of RD after surgery. a and b**: Total RD with a good postoperative functional prognosis; **c and d**: total RD closed at its anterior part with a poor postoperative prognosis; **a and c**: recording of the central retinal vessels on the side of the RD; **b and d**: recording of the central retinal vessels of the contralateral eye; **In a and b**: with a good prognosis, there is only a small decrease in the PSV; **In a**: PSV = 13.0 cm/s and **in b** = 15.5 cm/s; **In c and d**: with a poor prognosis, the decrease is very substantial; the PSV on the side of the RD being less than half the value of that of the contralateral eye; **In c**: PSV = 4.6 cm/s and **in d** = 10.3 cm/s

In ultrasound, a sponge made of Silastic™ foam (Fig. 12.42) appears as highly echogenic. It results in a posterior acoustic shadowing and a discreet artifactual haze. By contrast, a solid silicone cylinder is anechoic (Fig. 12.43). Only its anterior interface is hyperechoic. It also causes a slight posterior acoustic shadowing.

### (b) Tamponade

This is performed by injection of silicone oil or gas into the eye cavity, thereby pushing the retina against the wall.

### • Silicone oil

This is used in complex or recurrent forms treated with buckles. Its injection is preceded by vitrectomy or even dissection of the epiretinal membranes.

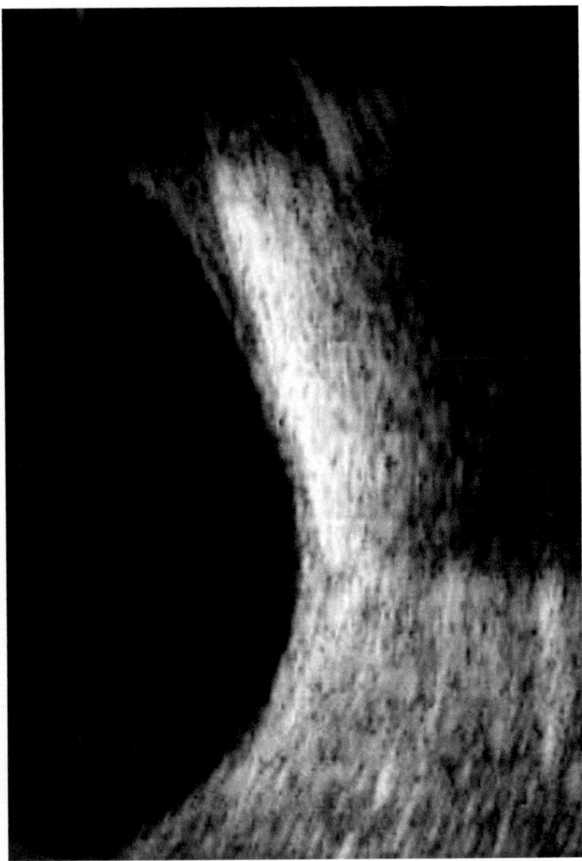

**Fig. 12.42  Silastic™ sponge**. View of the superior quadrant, revealing an upper temporal radial sponge. Hyperechoic, it gives rise to a total acoustic shadow behind it

Lighter than water, it should preferably occupy most of the posterior cavity. Silicone oil is anechoic. The slow propagation of ultrasound within it (900 m/s) explains an apparent increase in the size of the globe (the correction coefficient is 0.66). But silicone oil also disrupts the propagation of ultrasound (dispersion), and even at maximum gain, assessment of the posterior pole is difficult, and that of the ocular periphery impossible (see Figs. 6.15c and 10.10).

In these cases, it seems preferable to use MRI, which allows for evaluation of the filling of the posterior cavity by the silicone bubble and notes the absence or existence of recurrence of the detachment. Occasionally, it can demonstrate passage of silicone into the subretinal space.

The long-term toxicity of silicone on ocular structures (cataracts, corneal dystrophy, glaucoma) requires its removal after a few months. Ultrasound then detects small hyperechoic echoes floating in the eye cavity (Fig. 12.44). These correspond to silicone micro-bubbles in emulsion that are invisible on biomicroscopy. Sometimes

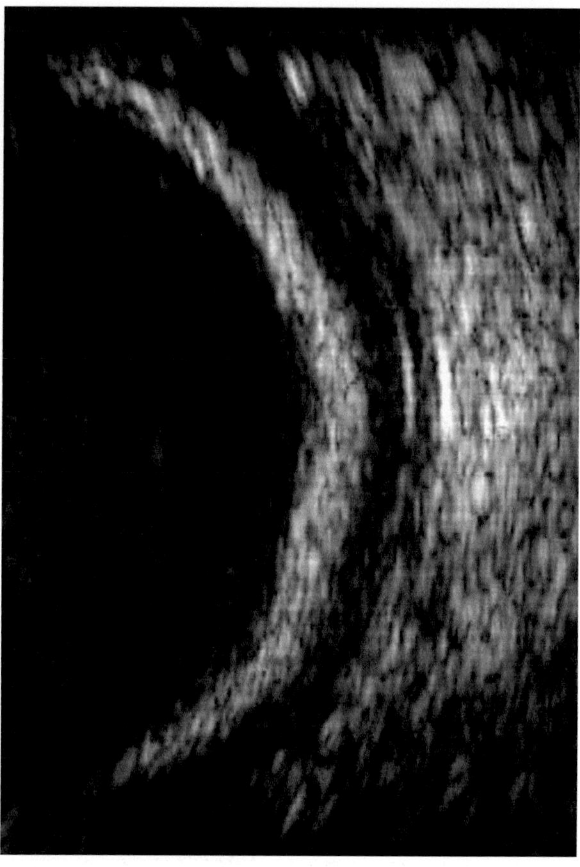

**Fig. 12.43 Circular silicone band**. View of the superior quadrant. The silicone band is hypoechoic, with a thin echogenic line in the center. The posterior attenuation is considerably less than with Silastic™

they are a little bit larger, and mini silicone bubbles can persist, located toward the region of the ciliary processes or in the anterior chamber. They give rise to posterior resonance artifacts (Fig. 12.45 and see Fig. 6.2).

- **Gases**

These are expansive, and they are injected with or without prior vitrectomy. Their expansion is maximal in 24 or 48 h; their resorption is spontaneous and gradual over the course of a few weeks.

They completely prevent the progression of ultrasound (see Fig. 6.15a, b). Thus, examination becomes impossible when the bubble occupies the entire posterior cavity (a rare possibility as a source of hypertonic complications). It can be conducted in part for bubbles of lesser volume, taking into account the physical properties of the gas that always occupies the highest part of the cavity:

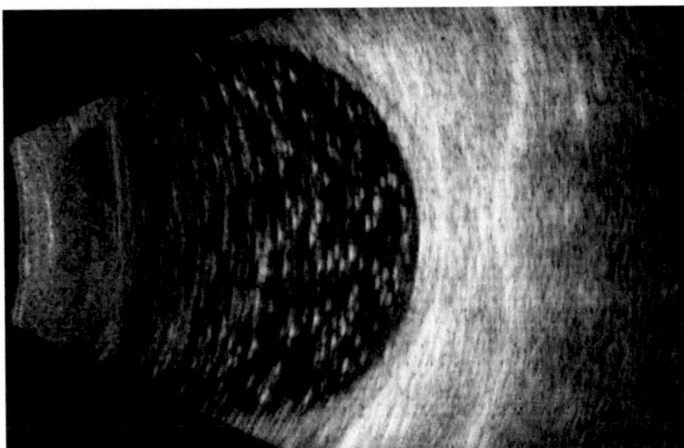

**Fig. 12.44 Silicone microbubbles in a vitrectomized eye**. As with asteroid hyalosis, the resolution of these echogenic and mobile microbubbles is greater near the focal zone, located near the ocular wall

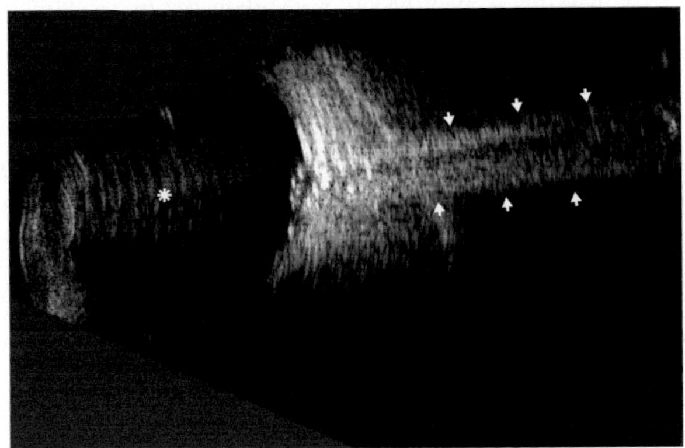

**Fig. 12.45 Silicone minibubble(s) located in the vicinity of the ciliary processes and perfluoro-carbon minibubbles near the posterior pole after vitrectomy**. Section of the right eye according to 9 o'clock. Silicone minibubbles are lighter than the aqueous humor that fills the posterior segment after vitrectomy and are located at the upper part of the eye. Therefore, they are not actually seen, but they are detected by the posterior resonance artifacts that are not very echogenic and visible throughout the posterior segment (✳). One can get a sense of the size of the bubble by the distance separating two interfaces of this artifact, which is gradually depleted throughout the vitreous. On the other hand, PFCL minibubbles, are heavy and are often located near the posterior pole and are characterized by rather echogenic comet-tail reverberation artifacts that can be seen very far in the orbit, provided the image is not zoomed too much (➤)

When it is partial and of modest size, mobilization of the gas bubble is readily achieved by a change in gaze direction and better yet, by moving the patient's head (lateral decubitus, sitting position) allowing for relatively satisfactory exploration of the area to be assessed. However, this is only possible at least 10 days after SF6 injection and 3 weeks after C3F8 injection. Thus, the image obtained is often mixed:

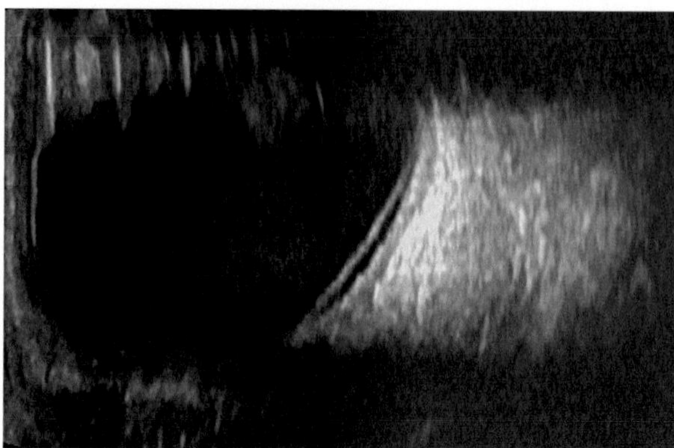

**Fig. 12.46 Recurrent retinal detachment under gas 3 weeks after C3F8**, a hemorrhage preventing access to the fundus is readily visible on this ultrasound section. Vertical parasagittal section; the patient is in a sitting position. The residual gas bubble is located at the top of the image. With its posterior artifacts, it precludes assessment of the superior quadrant in this position but nevertheless allows for detecting a small localized recurrent RD in the inferior quadrant, in the middle periphery

half consisting of vitreous acoustic silence corresponding to the part of the posterior segment being explored and the other half of a very echogenic image marking the location of the gas bubble (Fig. 12.46). In all cases, one can examine a patient within 24 to 48 h after the intervention (i.e., before maximum expansion of the gas). Again, MRI can be useful to assess the retinal situation behind the bubble.

- **Perfluorocarbon liquid (PFCL)**

Use of these heavy liquid gases is increasingly common in vitreoretinal surgery. They help to unfold the detached retinal leaflets and reapply them against the eye wall.

Because they are toxic, they must be completely removed at the end of the intervention. A few minibubbles of the product can sometimes persist, located at the most declived part of the globe or near the posterior pole: they are visible by ultrasound in the form of small hyperechoic nodules, followed by comet-tail reverberation artifacts that are very long and often mobile when located in front of the retina and, by contrast, almost immobile when stuck behind a retina that has almost completely been reapplied (Fig. 12.45 and see Fig. 6.2) if the gas bubble has passed under the retina by a wide dehiscence during the procedure.

Note that these highly reflective properties have been used for some ultrasound contrast media in Doppler.

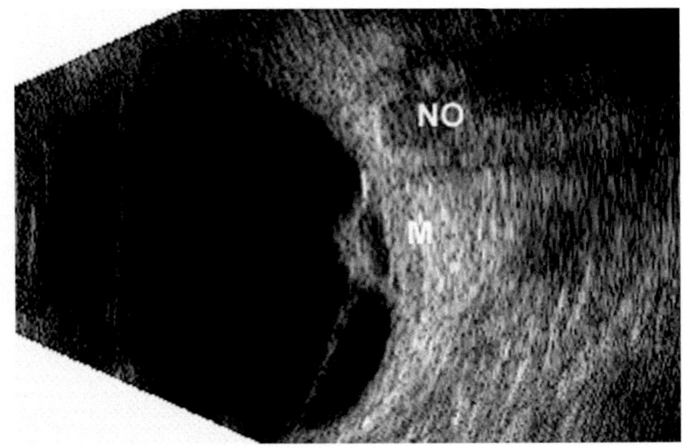


**Fig. 12.47  Traction RD**: Proliferative diabetic retinopathy. Section at 10 MHz showing detachment of the posterior hyaloid, which is thickened with vitreoretinal traction and localized tent-shaped retinal detachment, of the posterior pole. NO = optic nerve; M = macula

### 12.2.1.2  Tractional Retinal Detachment

It presents in ultrasound as an elevated and localized "tent-shaped" membrane, and is progressing slowly. The often reshaped posterior hyaloid (or echogenic membranes) converge(s) toward the top of the RD.

Proliferative Diabetic Retinopathy

Ultrasound is a major part of the examination of diabetic retinopathy, mainly in cases of vitreous hemorrhage. It allows for evaluating abnormalities and their progression, thereby assisting with determining the appropriate time for vitrectomy, guiding surgical procedures, and ultimately contributing to the prognosis (Fig. 12.47).

Inflammatory or Traumatic Vitreous Organizations

Inflammatory and especially traumatic vitreous organization can be rapid and require ultrasound monitoring once or twice a week. The retinal traction areas are much less systematized than in diabetic retinopathy.

When a parietal inflammatory focus exists, vitreous membranes can adhere to it and give rise to a retinal detachment.

With an ocular perforation, traction often takes place on the opposite side of the wound, but any area where the hyaloid remains adherent can be a site of a tractional retinal detachment (Fig. 12.48).

## 12.2.2  Exudative Retinal Detachment

The origin of the exudation can be as follows:

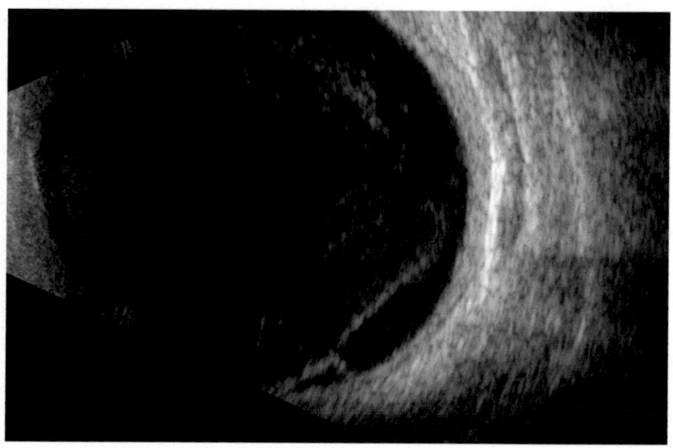

**Fig. 12.48 Localized peripheral tractional RD** at 4:30, discovered on an iterative ultrasound check-up 18 days after a scleral wound in the superior temporal quadrant of the right eye.

- Inflammatory (Vogt-Koyanagi-Harada [VKH] uveomeningitis) [51], which is frequently associated with choroidal thickening or detachment (Fig. 12.49);
- Hypertensive (eclampsia, renovascular hypertension, pheochromocytoma): the retina often appears thickened, the detachment is multifocal, bullous, and of variable size;
- Telangiectasia (Coats' retinopathy);
- Neovascular (choroidal neovascularization in the context of age-related macular degeneration). Retinal elevation is frequently serohemorrhagic.

## 12.2.3 Tumoral Retinal Detachment

A mass, most often choroidal (melanoma, metastasis, angioma), less frequently retinal (exophytic retinoblastoma), raises the neuroepithelium by its extension in the subretinal space. Retinal detachment can be localized, satellite (Fig. 12.50), more extensive, or even total.

The search for a tumor in the subretinal space must be systematic in case of any retinal detachment, especially when no tear has been found in the fundus.

## 12.2.4 Retinal Detachment in Children

It is rare (2% to 12% of RDs). The same mechanisms are encountered, but with different frequencies:

- **Rhegmatogenous RD (especially after 5 years)**

  - Traumatic
  - Degenerative (myopia; Wagner–Stickler, Marfan syndromes)
  - Postsurgical (congenital cataract)

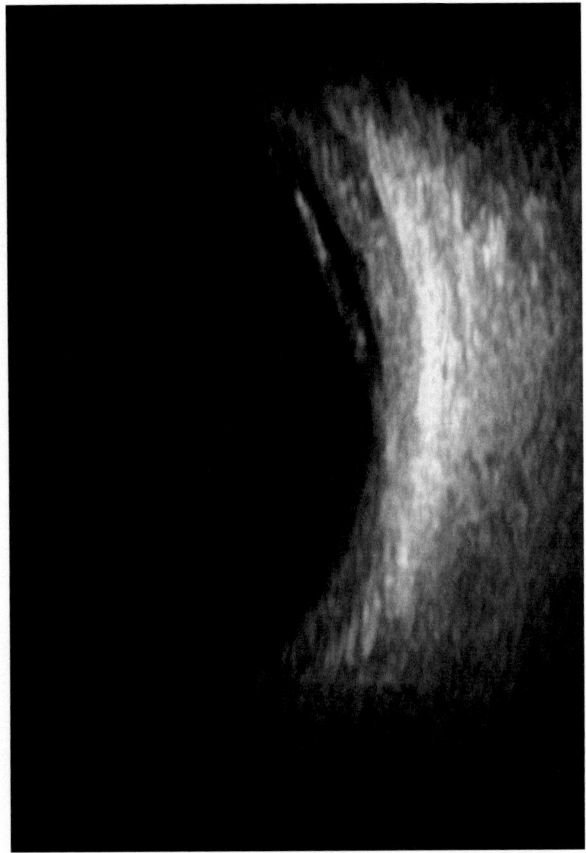

**Fig. 12.49 Exudative RD** and choroidal thickening; VKH. Section of the inferior temporal quadrant of the right eye

- Juvenile retinoschisis
- Coloboma

- **Tractional and/or exudative RD**

  - Before 5 years

    - Retinoblastoma
    - Coats' retinopathy
    - Retinopathy of prematurity (Fig. 12.51)
    - Persistent fetal vasculature

  - Regardless of age

    - Familial exudative vitreoretinopathy
    - Choroidal hemangioma
    - Optic disc pit

**Fig. 12.50  Tumoral RD.**
Choroidal melanoma with
inferior satellite retinal
detachment

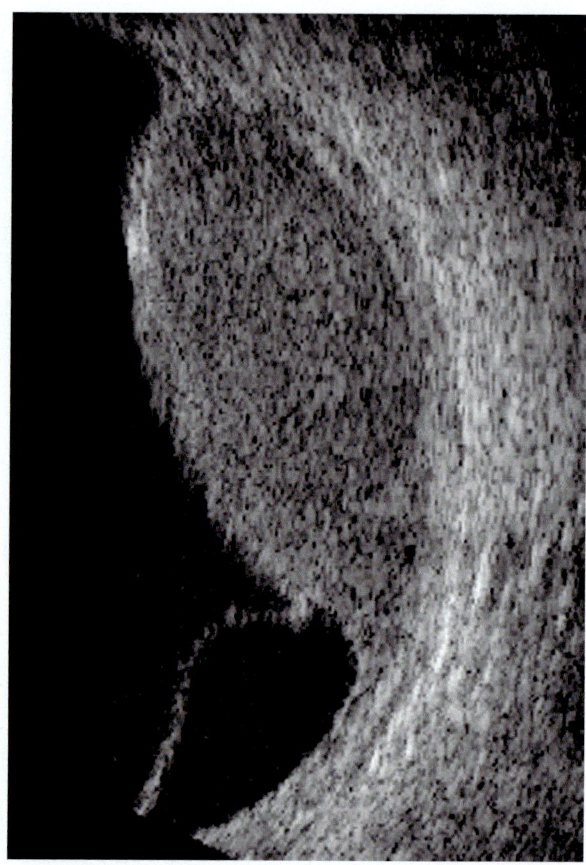

**Fig. 12.51  ROP Stage 5
with total traction RD,
"retrolental fibroplasia" in
an 18-day old baby
(27 weeks of gestation,
birth weight = 1.1 kg).**
CDI, color mode, para-axial
section. Slight
microphthalmos (AL =
16.3 mm). Vascularization of
RD is obvious, and the
subretinal blue dots are due
to hemorrhage

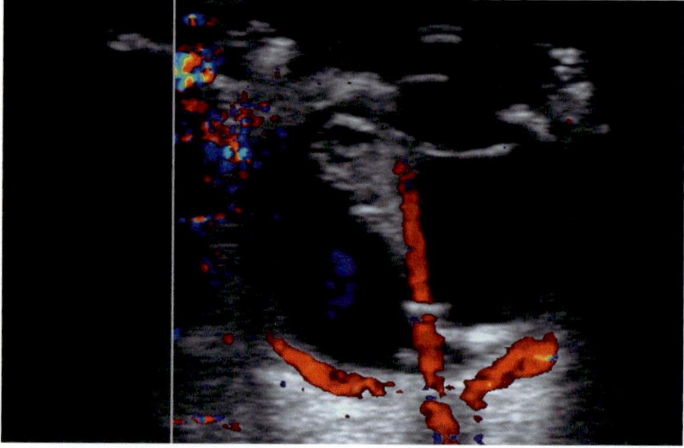

## *12.2.5   Degenerative Retinoschisis*

Retinoschisis corresponds to a cleavage of the neuroepithelium and not its detachment. Located in superior or inferior temporal region, with clear boundaries, it is frequently bilateral and occurs especially in older adults. It can be plane, peripheral or bullous, in which case, more posterior.

In ultrasound, its wall is hyperechoic, like the retina (Figs. 12.52 and 12.53). It can generally readily be differentiated from a retinal detachment or choroidal detachment, such as by its characteristic position and bilaterality. Its connections are more convex. Its wall is thinner than a peripheral localized RD and significantly less thick than a small choroidal detachment, which often has a double peak appearance in A-mode. Moreover, there is no "step sign".

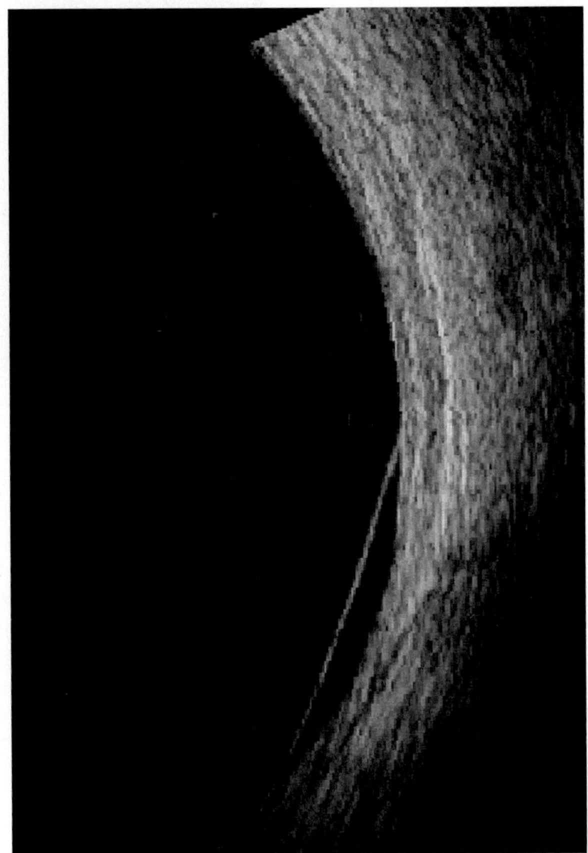

**Fig. 12.52   Relatively flat retinoschisis**. Section at 20 MHz. In addition to the very indicative inferior temporal position, the membrane, thinner than a peripheral localized retinal detachment and much less thick than a small choroidal detachment, adds to a favorable diagnosis. Absence of any step sign

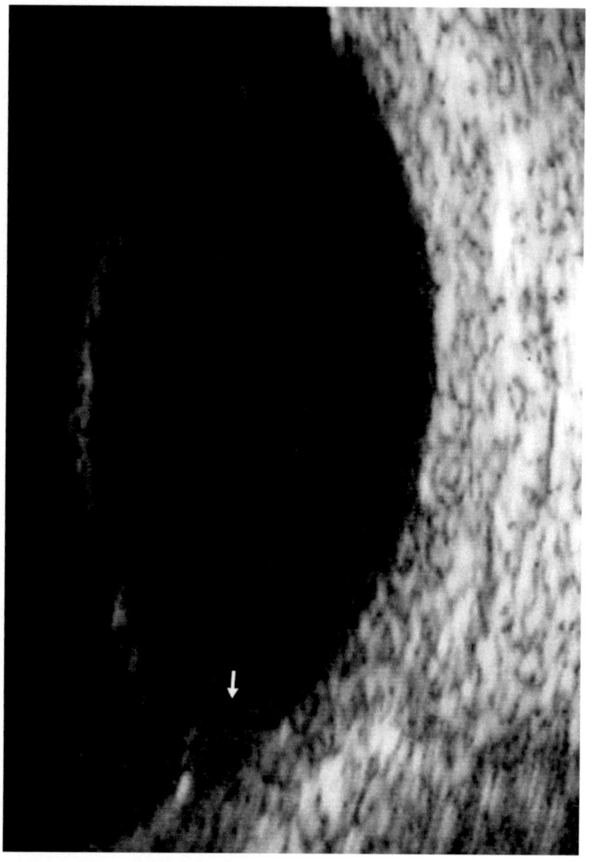

**Fig. 12.53 Extensive bullous retinoschisis**, with cleavage in the thickness of the neuroepithelium, clearly visible inferiorly with splitting of the membrane corresponding to the inner (→ arrow) and outer wall

## *12.2.6 Serous Detachment of the Retinal Pigment Epithelium*

This presents as a small protruding membrane at the posterior pole, for which the connections with the wall are acute. Differential diagnosis from choroidal melanoma can be difficult, especially because it can be hemorrhagic (secondary to age-related macular degeneration), with a low reflective appearance (Fig. 12.54). There is no intrinsic flow in CDI. In case of doubt, successive ultrasound controls show the collapse of the lesion.

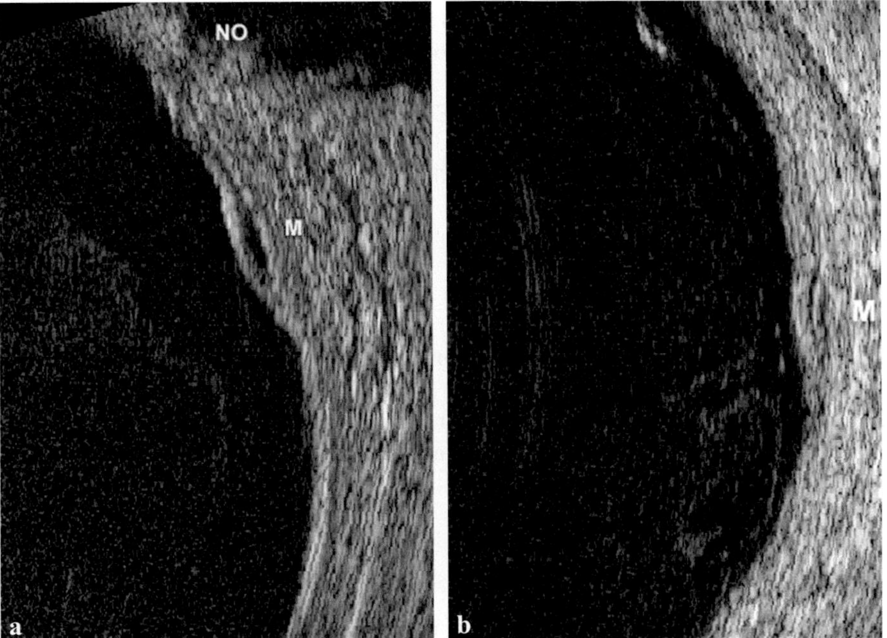


**Fig. 12.54 Serous detachment of the retinal pigment epithelium**. Exploration at 20 MHz. **a**: para-axial section; **b**: parasagittal section showing the small hypoechoic parietal protrusion at the level of the macular region, with an absence of choroidal excavation. NO = optic nerve; M = macula

## 12.3 Choroid

### *12.3.1 Choroidal Thickening*

In ultrasound, the total parietal thickness (sclera, choroid, and retina) varies from 1 mm in nearsighted individuals to 2.5 mm in individuals with hypermetropia. It is approximately equal to 1.5 mm in emmetropia. The choroidal thickness varies from approximately 0.5 mm to 1 mm at the posterior pole.

In general, these choroidal thickenings must be differentiated from minimally protruding choroidal tumors, such as melanoma, metastasis, lymphoma, or even diffuse choroidal hemangioma in the context of Sturge–Weber syndrome.

Choroidal thickening can be encountered in many pathologies:

### 12.3.1.1  Ocular Hypotony (Especially After Any Globe Filtration Surgery such as Trabeculectomy)

### 12.3.1.2  Inflammatory or Infectious Edema

- uveitis, sympathetic ophthalmia, Vôgt-Koyanagi-Harada syndrome;
- lymphoid hyperplasia;
- scleritis, inflammatory pseudotumor of the orbit;
- endophthalmitis.

### 12.3.1.3  Venous Stasis (Orbital Tumor, Carotid-Cavernous Fistula)

### 12.3.1.4  Post-traumatic: In Case of Trauma, Choroidal Thickening May Be Diffuse (Fig. 12.55) or Localized

Diffuse

This is a very mundane sign because, for some authors, it is almost constant.

(a) Moderate: less than 2.0 mm immediately present after the accident; it may be responsible for a transient and discreet decrease in visual acuity. When isolated, it generally disappears without leaving sequelae in 7 to 10 days. However, when associated, its prognosis is variable and depends on the other abnormalities.
(b) Substantial: greater than 2.0 mm.

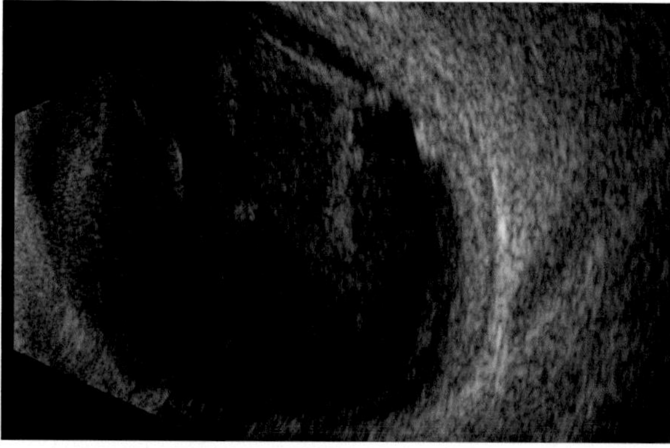

**Fig. 12.55 Diffuse choroidal thickening, after severe contusion** by a tensioner in a young man without PVD. Section at 10 MHz, with high gain of the inferior temporal quadrant: Massive intravitreal hemorrhage, already undergoing organization (membranes) only 24 h after the trauma, and diffuse choroid thickening, with the chorioretinal layer measuring 1.87 mm. There is also a discrete enlargement of the sub-Tenon episcleral space

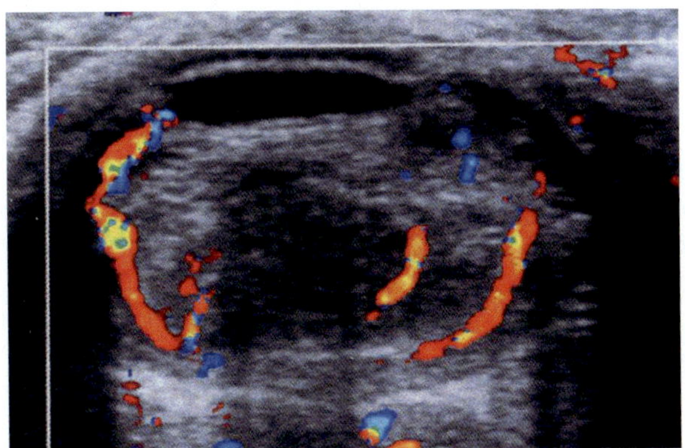

**Fig. 12.56  Globe atrophy (phthisis bulbi).** CDI, axial section. The globe has lost its spherical shape; its axial length is very diminished, measuring 18.2 mm up to the pigment epithelium and 20.7 mm up to the sclera (vs 24.2 mm on the contralateral eye). In addition, there is global hematic organization, with total retinal detachment and extended choroidal vascularization, and an absence of flow in the central retinal vessels

This can be the first ultrasound sign of progression toward atrophy of the globe. It can result from violent trauma with retinal detachment and also from inflammation and eye infections or even failures of retinal detachment surgery.

At the end-stage (phthisis bulbi), the long axis is greatly diminished (up to 16 mm). The very thickened wall can reach 3 mm (Fig. 12.56). More or less diffuse parietal calcifications associated with a total, V-shaped, retinal detachment with a cyclitic membrane are frequently seen. It is best appreciated by an immersion technique because of the small size of these atrophic eyes. The lens, if it has not been removed during a surgical procedure, is often voluminous and also calcified, thus resulting in a posterior shadowing. Under these conditions, eliminating an intraocular tumor is often difficult.

Localized

This is an induced sign reflecting a parietal pathology. It is often the consequence of the following:

- a significant vitreous traction exerted by a vitreoretinal adhesion;
- a small localized choroidal or suprachoroidal hematoma;
- an intraocular FB embedded in the wall;
- Berlin's edema (post-contusive macular edema).

## 12.3.2   Thinning of the Choroid

**Etiologies**

- certain congenital anomalies;
- myopic choroiditis and staphyloma (thinning, often uneven and with a varying degree of extensiveness) (see Fig. 13.39).

## 12.3.3   Choroidal Detachments (CDs)

These can be seen:

- after any open globe surgery, especially an antiglaucoma procedure (trabeculectomy), the consequences of which are frequently marked by prolonged hypotonia;
- during an ocular or orbital inflammatory syndrome;
- after trauma with or without effraction of the globe;
- and can also occur spontaneously.

**Ultrasound Diagnosis**

CD typically manifests as a thick, convex, and consistent internal bulging of the eye wall [52]. Its posterior connection angle, instead of being gently sloping as in a retinal detachment, is abrupt in relation to the thickness of the choroid. It generally inserts somewhat behind the emergence of vorticose veins and extends forward to the scleral spur at the level of the tendon of the ciliary body (Fig. 12.57). In addition, the wall underlying the CD becomes thinner. This variation in parietal thickness is particularly pronounced at the level of the connection, where it thins noticeably (**step sign**) (Fig. 12.58).

Its content is strictly anechoic or may present a few small echoes. Thus, a CD is different in almost all respects from an RD that starts from the optic disc and goes toward the ora serrata. Differential diagnosis is easy. Its morphology is also very different: there may be only one bullous dome-shaped lesion (Fig. 12.33), but most often, it is annular, circumferential with classic scalloped shape (Fig. 12.59). These may be very voluminous: bulging towards the vitreous, and then abut each other (kissing CDs). In A-mode, they present as a double peak: behind the choroidal detachment, only a thin membrane remains: the sclera, limiting the eyeball.

## 12.3.4   Hemorrhagic CDs

These can be secondary to "open globe" surgery [53]. They are voluminous, and their main form constitutes one of the most feared acute peri- or postoperative complications in eye surgery: expulsive hemorrhage. They can also be secondary to contusive

**Fig. 12.57 Ciliochoroidal detachment**. Para-axial section with an abundant layer of gel over the eyelids, using a multipurpose ultrasound unit and an 18-MHz probe. The IOL is pushed forward in connection with the hemorrhagic choroidal detachment lesions. The extension to the supraciliary space, here obvious, is sometimes difficult to demonstrate transocularly. However, it can readily be seen with high or very high frequency ultrasound, readily differentiating a fluid space from a cellular space (lymphoma for example)

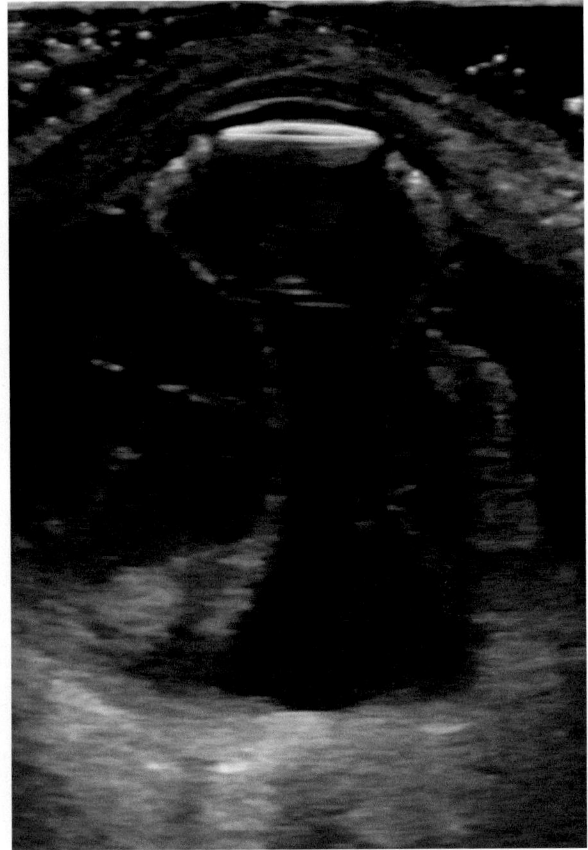

or penetrating violent trauma with or without a foreign body. As a general rule, the more voluminous, extensive, posterior, and echogenic in terms of content (blood), the worse its prognosis.

**Ultrasound Diagnosis**

They have a shape and topography similar to typical CDs described above, but their serohemorrhagic content has the same ultrasound characteristics as a retrohyaloid hemorrhage: moderately echogenic, sometimes with coarser more echogenic clots (Fig. 12.60).

Ultrasound should be able to specify whether or not it is associated with RD. Sometimes very large, the two main pouches can collid with each other, filling most of the posterior cavity. They can reach the posterior pole, making the functional prognosis very poor.

On average, 15 days after the acute episode, liquefaction of the hematoma can be considered, based on the appearance of a less echogenic and mobile aspect of

**Fig. 12.58  Choroidal detachment, "step sign".** The membrane, always very echogenic, is thicker than a detached retina, and the "step sign" at the level of the temporal pocket is very clear, in relation to the thickness of the choroid, which is lacking at the wall at this level (→ arrow)

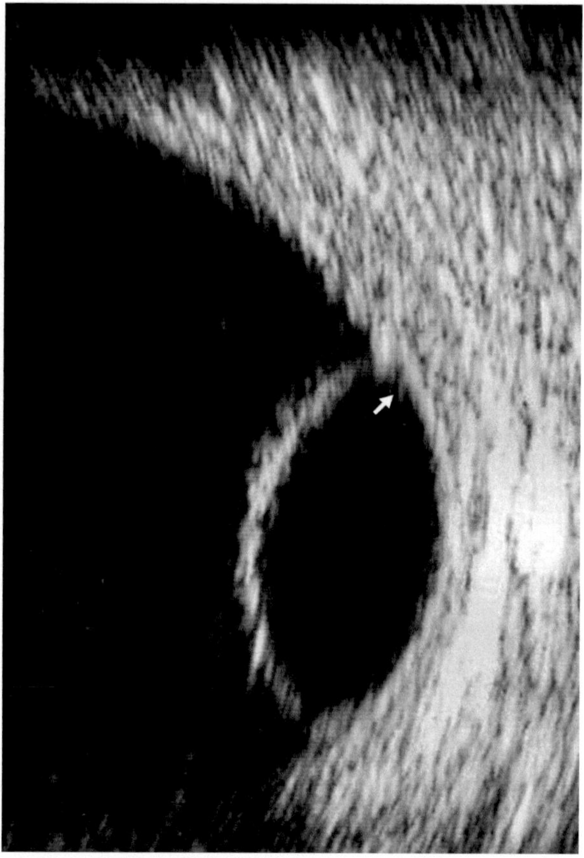

**Fig. 12.59  Choroidal detachment, frontal peripheral section** showing several very large scalloped shaped pouches, almost faced, with a thick wall

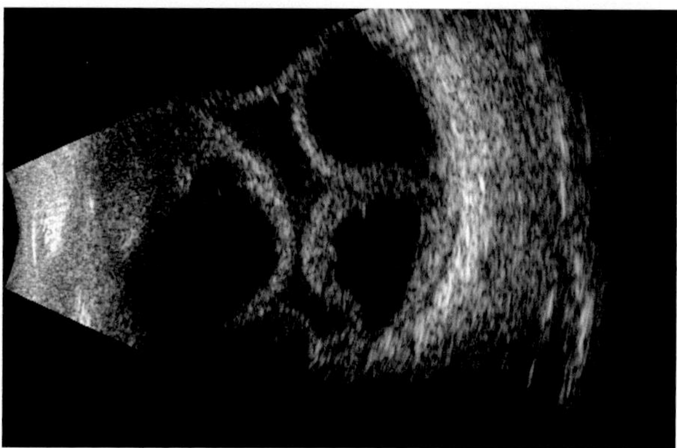

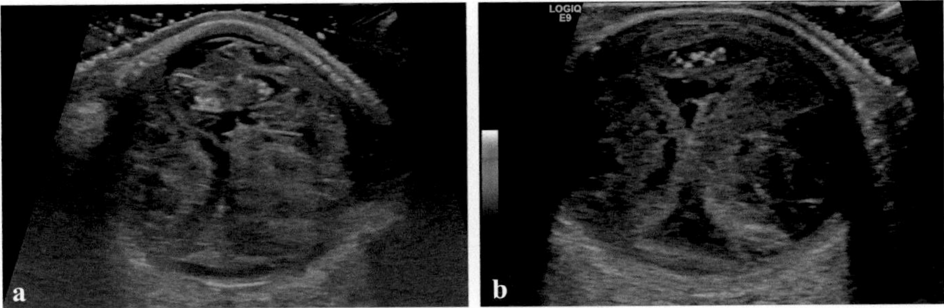

**Fig. 12.60** **Hemorrhagic choroidal detachment of the right eye following an expulsive hemorrhage that occurred at the very beginning of a cataract surgery and that interrupted it. a:** axial section performed on Day 1 after the event; **b**: axial control performed 14 days later. On the first examination, the persistence of echoes can be noted within the lens as well as an anterior hyphema. Behind these, there are voluminous pouches of choroidal detachment that are very echogenic and heterogeneous, facing each other. No sign of additional retinal detachment at the posterior pole. The largest, temporal pouch has a thickness measuring 12.5 mm, the nasal pouch is 8.5 mm. On the check-up carried out 14 days later, the appearance is quite similar, but the echotexture of the choroidal detachments, while still heterogeneous, is much less echogenic, which reflects liquefaction of the suprachoroidal hematoma, allowing its drainage

the echoes, which allows for considering surgical drainage (Fig. 12.60b). Video loop comparison is useful for the diagnosis.

### 12.3.5 Small Suprachoroidal Hematoma

Because it is small, a suprachoroidal hematoma takes on a significantly different appearance: its wall is still as thick and immobile, but it is flat, not convex, very peripheral, often ante-oral, and more or less annular. Its prognosis is then excellent.

## 12.4 Sclera

### 12.4.1 Scleritis

Ultrasound is an excellent examination to establish the diagnosis of posterior scleritis. It manifests as hyperechoic scleral thickening. Most often, it is associated with edema or inflammatory infiltration of the Tenon space as well as thickening of the choroid. This associated posterior tenonitis is readily visualized by ultrasound on either side of the optic nerve due to its acute connection angles with the wall. It thus assumes a characteristic "T-shaped appearance" [54, 55] (Fig. 12.61). The presentation is totally different from that of lymphoma (see Fig. 13.48).

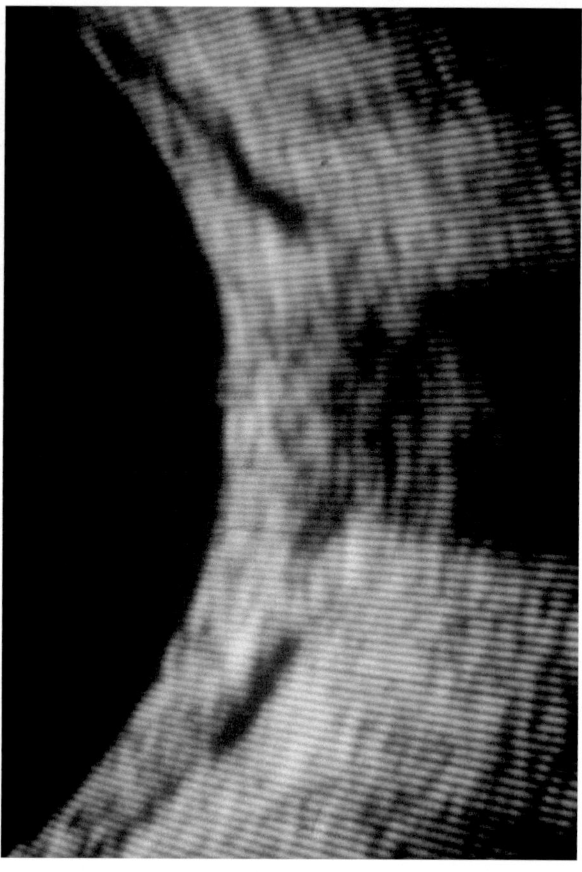

**Fig. 12.61  Posterior scleritis: T sign**. Para-axial section in B-mode: parietal thickening and enlargement of the sub-Tenon episcleral space, associated with an enlargement of the optic nerve, achieving a characteristic T-shaped appearance

Scleritis can be localized or diffuse. The localized, nodular form [56] (Fig. 12.62) can sometimes pose a difficult differential diagnosis problem with an intraocular tumor.

## 12.4.2  Sclerochoroidal Calcifications

Although they can pose a problem of differential diagnosis with ocular tumors at the fundus [57], their ultrasound presentation is characteristic: a small hyperechoic nodule, calcified, with a posterior shadowing, sometimes multiple, sometimes bilateral, preferentially localized in the superior temporal of the macular region [58]. They can sometimes be quite prominent (Fig. 12.63).

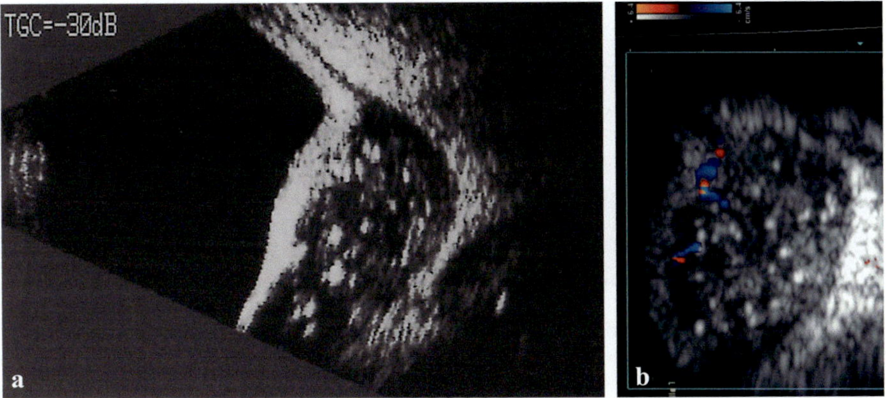

**Fig. 12.62  Posterior nodular scleritis secondary to a gorse thorn.** a: B-mode; b: CDI. It is clear that the voluminous mass, in the inferior temporal quadrant and very heterogeneous, is extraocular. The vascularization is inflammatory in nature. Thickening of the wall and the presence of sub-Tenon episcleral fluid adjacent to the mass can also be seen. Brightener coloration allowed affirmation of the origin of this inflammatory mass. Two years after the surgical excision, the patient was asymptomatic and had only a discrete sequellar parietal thickening

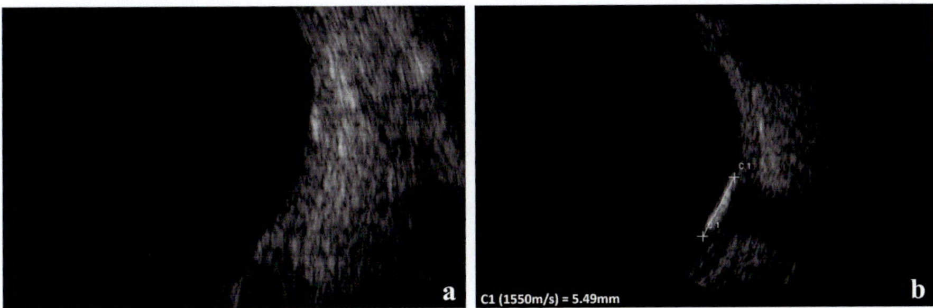

**Fig. 12.63  Idiopathic sclerochoroidal calcification.** a: 10-MHz section of the right eye along 10:30, with reduced gain; b: section at 10 MHz of the left eye along 1:30 at a reduced gain in another patient. In both cases, a small parietal calcification in superior temporal and at a distance from the macula is seen. It is more protrusive, and the posterior shadowing is more pronounced in b

They are most often idiopathic but can be associated, albeit rarely, with disorders of phospho-calcium metabolism, thus requiring a complete systemic assessment [59]. In rare cases, they can resolve over time [60] or become complicated, with neovascular membranes or even RD [61]. Less studied and presenting fewer differential diagnostic problems are peripheral scleral calcifications (Fig. 12.64), accidentally discovered on VHFU performed most often for a narrow angle evaluation. They are most often unilateral, but they can also be multiple and bilateral. We have not personally found an association between these peripheral scleral calcifications and para-equatorial choroidoscleral calcifications.

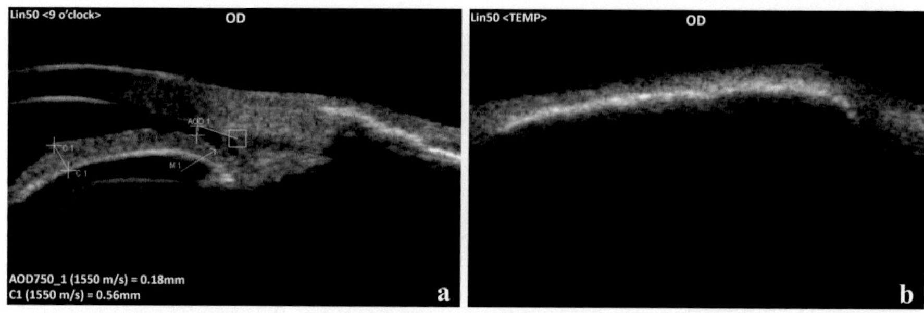



**Fig. 12.64  Peripheral scleral calcification. a**: 50-MHz section according to 3 o'clock (nasal meridian), OD; **b**: 50-MHz section according to the temporal quadrant, OD. In both cases, this small calcified scleral plate is responsible of the total posterior shadowing. Note the narrow angle which prompted the examination being undertaken

By analogy, albeit not as a general rule, a complete systemic assessment is recommended.

### *12.4.3  Scleral Thinning*

Ultrasound can also reveal ectatic scleral thinning protruding through the normal curvature of the eyeball, best highlighted anteriorly in immersion, in high frequency (Fig. 12.65), but sometimes highlighted transocularly (Fig. 12.66).

## 12.5  Macula

### *12.5.1  Macular Holes (MH)*

Ultrasound at 10 or 20 MHz allows documentation of stage III and IV full-thickness macular holes (Figs. 12.67 and 12.68).

- **Presentation of the hole**

A serous detachment of the neuroepithelium ring results in a very echogenic macular protrusion with a small central depression that is weakly echogenic (by partial volume effect) corresponding to the retinal defect. This volume effect is less if the frequency is increased, which explains why the MH is better visualized with a 20 MHz probe [25].

- **Analysis of the vitreoretinal interface**

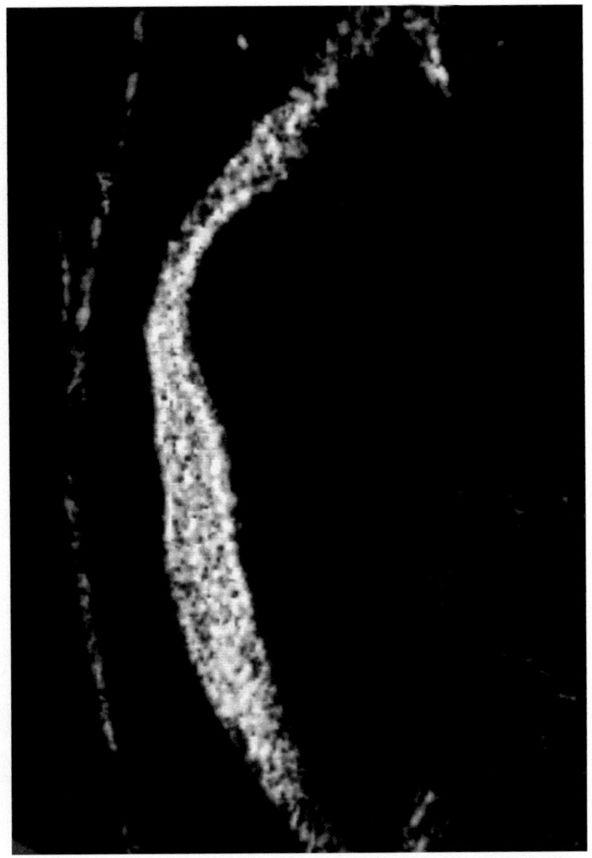

**Fig. 12.65  Congenital scleral ectasia**. Short-focal 20 MHz view of the inferior temporal quadrant, immediately behind the ciliary body, clearly showing the small localized deformation of the anterior ocular wall

Although PVD can readily be discerned by ultrasound, visualizing a localized detachment of the posterior hyaloid membrane can be difficult or even impossible. Indeed, at maximum gain, artifacts are observed due to the interface between the eye (anechoic) and the orbit (hyperechoic), whereas at reduced gain, the reflectivity of the hyaloid is insufficient. However, a retinal operculum always results in a small hyperechoic nodule next to the hole. Stage II MHs are difficult to detect and stage I MHs do not result in an ultrasound signal.

One must assess the vitreous status of the contralateral eye, which will allow for determining a high-risk group in the absence of detachment of the vitreous or intermediate risk group with a vitreous-foveolar separation. With a 20 MHz probe, at moderate gain, detailed analysis of the MH is much better, although a small posterior localized detachment of the hyaloid is often difficult to affirm.

Presently, optical coherence tomography remains the reference examination for assessing the vitreomacular interface [26, 27]. However, ultrasound has the advantage of providing an overall configuration of the vitreous, and it is the only examination that can be carried out in case of opacity of the media.

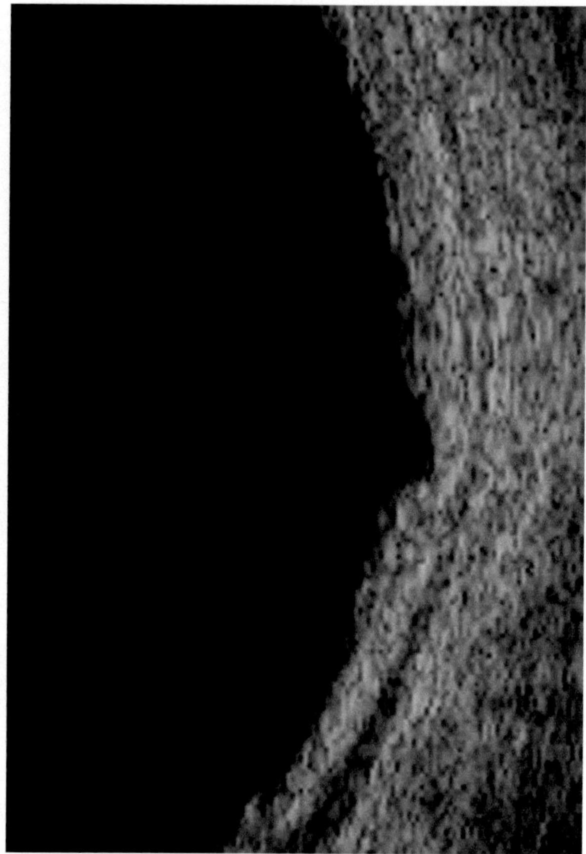

**Fig. 12.66 Scleral thinning.** Section at 20 MHz, transocularly, showing a parietal defect due to significant thinning of the sclera (more pronounced than a chorioretinal coloboma)

## 12.5.2 Epiretinal Membranes

Idiopathic epimacular membranes (EMMs) have well-codified surgical indications for significant functional improvement. These are self-limited fibrocellular proliferations that cover the macula and posterior pole and cause macular distortion when they contract. The characteristics of these membranes are currently well documented. However, EMMs can develop before the constitution of the PVD. This calls into question many theories accepted by many authors.

Ultrasound in B-mode is an excellent examination for assessing the vitreous as well as an excellent visualization of the characteristics of the EMMs with a 20-MHz probe [64] (Fig. 12.69).

This is an additional examination that must be carried out systematically because it provides the surgeon with useful information for the performance of the surgical procedure.

**Fig. 12.67  Stage III macular hole**. Section at 10 MHz showing the operculum supported by the posterior hyaloid, clearly visible in front of the thickening of the macular region. M = macula; NO = optic nerve

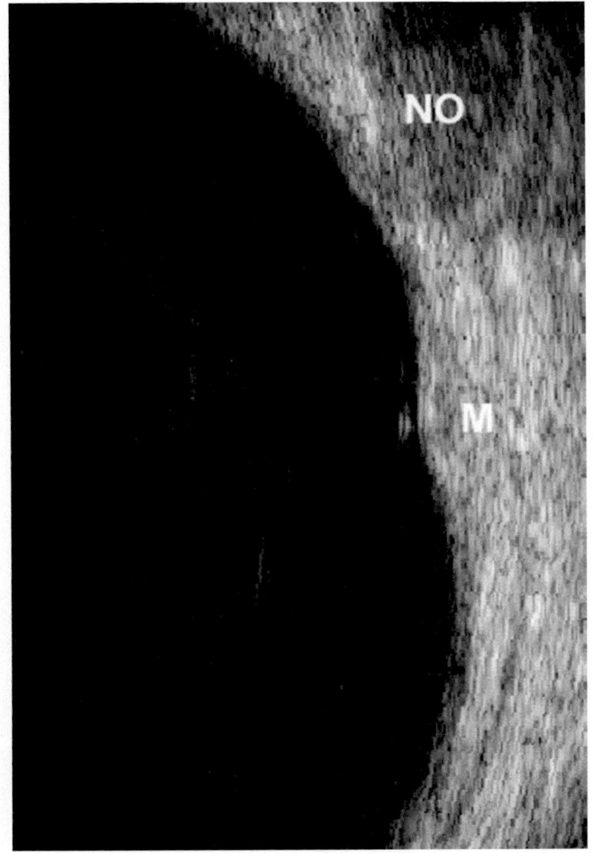


## *12.5.3  Vitreous Macular Traction (VMT)*

Confirming the diagnosis of VMT is easy with ultrasound examination [7]. Parietal thickening of the macular region is seen. The posterior hyaloid is clearly visible and is hyperreflective and thicker than normal (Fig. 12.70). It is partially detached from the posterior pole, but it remains adherent and stretched between the optic disc and the temporal part of the posterior pole, and it adheres to the top of the macula, on which it exerts traction (Fig. 12.71).

**Fig. 12.68 Stage IV macular hole**. Section at 20 MHz: macular protrusion with a small central depression corresponding to the defect of the neuroepithelium (→ arrow)

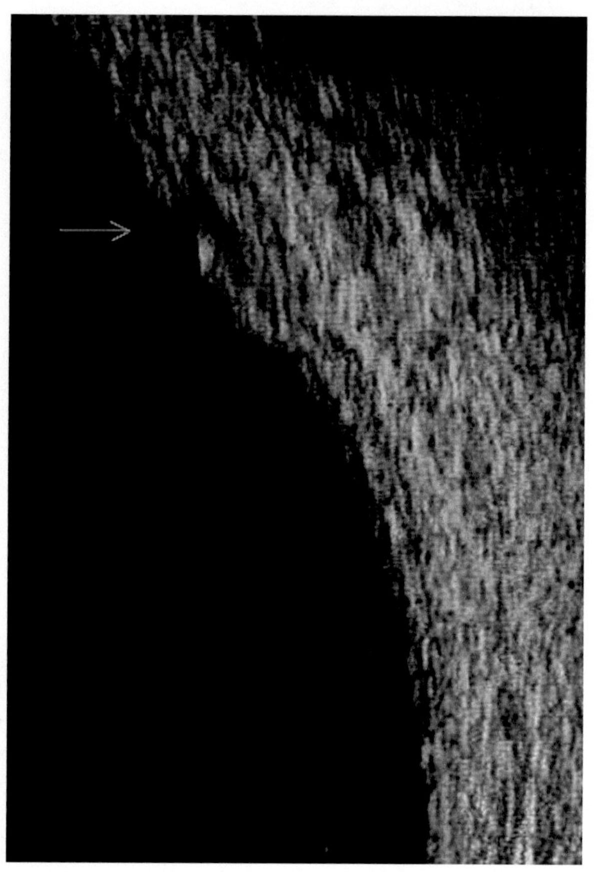

**Fig. 12.69  Epiretinal membrane**. Para-axial section showing a discreet irregular thickening of the macular region. M: macula; NO: optic nerve

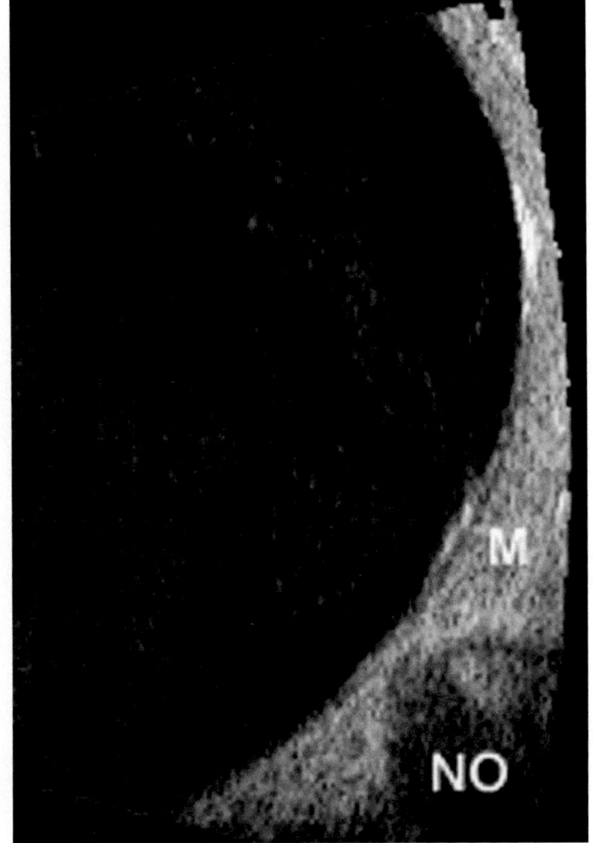

**Fig. 12.70  Vitreous macular traction**. Section at 20 MHz of the posterior pole. Discrete thickening can be seen and slight hyperreflectivity of the posterior hyaloid membrane, attached to the optic disc and to the macula, which is prominent, site of a cystoid macular edema. NO: optic nerve

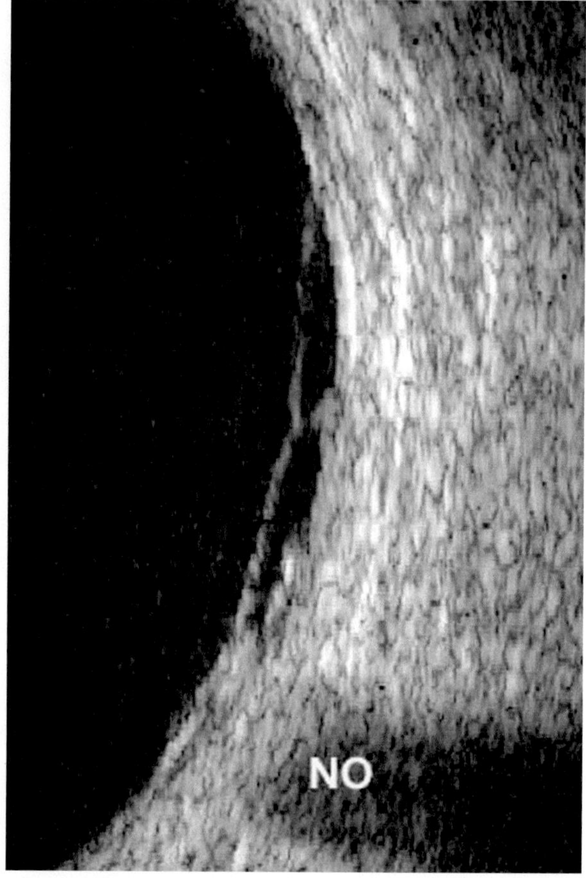


**Fig. 12.71  Vitreous macular traction and asteroid hyalosis**. Section at 10 MHz: Partial PVD, with papillary and macular attachment, clearly visible within the hypoechoic corona behind the hyperreflective asteroid bodies

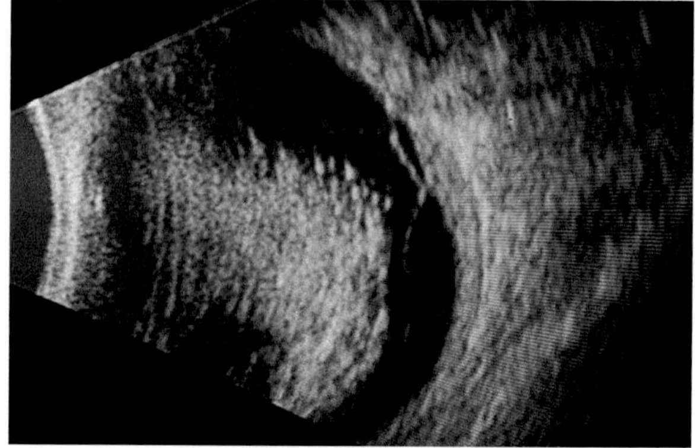

# References


1. Ryan SJ. Retina, vol. 3. 5th ed. Elsevier; 2013. p. 1640.
2. Rouberol F, Chiquet C. Proliferative vitreoretinopathy: pathophysiology and clinical diagnosis. J Fr Ophtalmol. 2014;37(7):557–65.
3. Wickham L, Ho-Yen GO, Bunce C, Wong D, Charteris DG. Surgical failure following primary retinal detachment surgery by vitrectomy: risk factors and functional outcomes. Br J Ophthalmol. 2011;95:1234–8.
4. Bergès O, Torrent M. Échographie de l'œil et de l'orbite. Paris: Vigot; 1986.
5. Atta HR. Ophthalmic ultrasound—a practical guide. Churchill Livingstone; 1996.
6. Frazier-Byrne S, Green RL. Ultrasound of the eye an orbit, 2nd ed. Mosby; 2002.
7. Perichon JY, Brasseur G, Uzzan J. Etude échographique du décollement postérieur du vitré chez l'emmétrope. J Fr Ophtalmol. 1993;16:538–44.
8. Brasseur G, Siahmed K. Examen du vitré Elsevier. Encycl Méd Chir Ophtalmol. 2008. [21-245-A-20—in French]
9. Arzabe CW, Akiba J, Jalkh AE, et al. Comparative study of vitreoretinal relationships using biomicroscopy and ultrasound. Graefes Arch Clin Exp Ophthalmol. 1991;229(1):66–8.
10. Fisher YL, Slakter JS, Friedman RA, Yannuzzi LA. Kinetic ultrasound evaluation of the posterior vitreoretinal interface. Ophthalmology. 1991;98(7):1135–8.
11. Bergès O, Siahmed K. Echographie de l'œil et de l'orbite. Elsevier. Encycl Méd Chir Ophtalmol. 2004. [21-062-A-10—in French]
12. Dibernardo C, Blodi B, Byrne SF. Echographic evaluation of retinal tears in patients with spontaneous vitreous hemorrhage. Arch Ophthalmol. 1992;110:511–4.
13. Nischal KK, James JN, Mcallister J. The use of dynamic ultrasound B-scan to detect retinal tears in spontaneous vitreous hemorrhage. Eye. 1995;9:502–6.
14. Machemer R, Blankenship G. Vitrectomy for proliferative diabetic retinopathy associated with vitreous hemorrhage. Ophthalmology. 1981;88(7):643–6.
15. Mcleod D, Restori M. Ultrasonic examination in severe diabetic eye disease. Br J Ophthalmol. 1979;63(8):533–8.
16. Haik GM, Breffeilh LA, Harrington MR. The differential diagnosis of diabetic retinopathy. New Orleans Med Surg J. 1950;103(4):151–5.
17. Ilim O, Akkin C, Degirmenci C, Mentes J, et al. The role of posterior vitreous detachment and vitreomacular adhesion in patients with age-related macular degeneration. Ophthalmic Surg Lasers Imaging Retina. 2017;48(3):223–9.
18. Verbeek AM. Differential diagnosis of intraocular neoplasms with ultrasonography. Ultrasound Med Biol. 1985;11(1):163–70.
19. Czorlich P, Burkhardt T, Regelsberger J, Skevas C, et al. Ocular ultrasound as an easy applicable tool for detection of Terson's syndrome after aneurysmal subarachnoid hemorrhage. PLoS ONE. 2014;9(12): e114907.
20. Ossoinig KC. Quantitative echography—the basis of tissue differentiation. J Clin Ultrasound. 1974;2(1):33–46.
21. Ossoinig KC, Islas G, Tamayo GE, Tamburelli C. Detached retina versus dense fibrovascular membrane (standardized A-scan and B-scan criteria). In: Ophtalmic echography (SIDUO 1984); Docum Ophthal Proc Series. 48:275–84.
22. Ossoinig KC. Standardized ophthalmic echography of the eye, orbit and periorbital region. A comprehensive slide set and study guide, 3rd ed. p. 44. Goodfellow Co., Iowa City.
23. Fledelius HC. Ultrasound in ophthalmology. Ultrasound Med Biol. 1997;23(3):365–75.
24. Wasano T, Hirokawa H, Trempe CL, Buzney SM, et al. Asteroid hyalosis: posterior vitreous detachment and diabetic retinopathy. Ann Ophthalmol. 1987;19(7):255–8.
25. Greven CM, Collins AS, Slusher MM, Weaver RG. Visual results, prognostic indicators, and posterior segment findings following surgery for cataract/lens subluxation-dislocation secondary to ocular contusion injuries. Retina. 2002;22(5):575–80.
26. Youssri AI, Young LH. Closed-globe contusion injuries of the posterior segment. Int Ophthalmol Clin. 2002;42(3):79–86.

27. Xia T, Bauza A, Langer PD, Bhagat N, et al. Surgical management and outcome of open globe injuries with posterior segment complications: a 10-year review. Semin Ophthalmol. 2018;33(3):351–6.
28. Tonini M, Krainik A, Chiquet C, Le Bas JF, et al. How helical CT helps the surgeon in oculo-orbital trauma. J Neuroradiol. 2009;36(4):185–98.
29. Ehlers JP, Kunimoto DY, Ho AC, Regillo CD, et al. Metallic intraocular foreign bodies: characteristics, interventions, and prognostic factors for visual outcome and globe survival. Am J Ophthalmol. 2008;146(3):427–33.
30. Sharma S, Thapa R, Pradhan E, Poudyal G, et al. Clinical characteristics and visual outcome, prognostic factor, visual acuity and globe survival in posterior segment intraocular foreign body at Tilganga Institute of Ophthalmology. Nepal J Ophthalmol. 2018;10(19):66–72.
31. Ossoinig KC, Bigar F, Kaefring SL, Mcnutt L. Echographic detection and localization of BB shots in the eye and orbit. Bibl Ophthalmol. 1975;83:109–18.
32. Newman TL, Russo PA. Ocular sequelae of BB injuries to the eye and surrounding adnexa. J Am Optom Assoc. 1998;69(9):583–90.
33. Lee R, Fredrick D. Pediatric eye injuries due to nonpowder guns in the United States, 2002–2012. J AAPOS. 2015;19(2):163-8.e1.
34. Bhavsar AR, Fong DS, Kerman B, Yoshizumi MO. Intraorbital air simulating an intraocular foreign body. Am J Ophthalmol. 1997;123(6):835–7.
35. Kiliç A, Avcu S, Cïnal A, Yasar T, et al. MRI-induced migration of retained metallic foreign body in the eye. Ophthalmic Surg Lasers Imaging. 2010;9:1–3.
36. Lawrence DA, Lipman AT, Gupta SK, Nacey NC. Undetected intraocular metallic foreign body causing hyphema in a patient undergoing MRI: a rare occurrence demonstrating the limitations of pre-MRI safety screening. Magn Reson Imaging. 2015;33(3):358–61.
37. Williams S, Char DH, Lincoff N, Moseley M, et al. Ferrous intraocular foreign bodies and magnetic resonance imaging. Am J Ophthalmol. 1988;105(4):398–401.
38. Otto PM, Otto RA, Kaude JV, Staab EV, et al. Screening test for detection of metallic foreign objects in the orbit before magnetic resonance imaging. Invest Radiol. 1992;27(4):308–11.
39. Kremmer S, Schiefer U, Wilhelm H, Zrenner E. [Mobilization of intraocular foreign bodies by magnetic resonance tomography]. [Article in German] Klin Monbl Augenheilkd. 1996;208(3):201–2.
40. Li J, Zhou LP, Jin J, Yuan HF. Clinical diagnosis and treatment of intraorbital wooden foreign bodies. Chin J Traumatol. 2016;19(6):322–5.
41. Machemer R, Aaberg TM, Lean JS, Michels RM. An updated classification of retinal detachment with proliferative vitreoretinopathy. Am J Ophthalmol. 1991;112(2):159–65.
42. Takkar B, Temkar S, Chawla R, Kumar A, et al. Retinal shortening: Ultrasonic evaluation of proliferative vitreoretinopathy. Indian J Ophthalmol. 2017;65(11):1172–7.
43. Wong AD, Cooperberg PL, Ross WH, Araki DN. Differentiation of detached retina and vitreous membrane with colorflow Doppler. Radiology. 1991;178(2):429–31.
44. Ido M, Osawa S, Fukukita M, Sasoh M, Uji Y et al. The use of colour Doppler imaging in the diagnosis of retinal detachment. Eye (Lond). 2007;21(11):1375–8.
45. Han SS, Chang SK, Yoon JH, Lee YJ. The use of contrast-enhanced colour Doppler ultrasound in the differentiation of retinal detachment from vitreous membrane. Korean J Radiol. 2001;2(4):197–203.
46. Lecler A, Chiaroni PM, Bergès O. Color doppler flow imaging helps to differentiate persistent fetal vasculature from retinal detachment. Acta Ophthalmol. 2021.
47. Bergès O, Nau E, Lafitte F, Caputo G, et al. Prognostic value of CDI of CRA for the surgery of retinal detachment. Oral Presentation to the SIDUO XXI meeting. Los Angeles; 1998.
48. Roldán-Pallarès M, Musa AS, Bravo-Llatassc C, Fernández-Durango R, et al. Retinal detachment and proliferative vitreoretinopathy: central retinalartery blood velocities, intraocular pressure, and endothelin 1. Retina. 2013;33(8):1528–39.
49. Bergès O, Le Mer Y, Caputo G, Lecler A et al. Etude CRADORED (Prognostic Value of the hemodynamic perturbations of Central Retinal Artery with Color Doppler Imaging of rhegmatogenous retinl detachment)—in progress.

50. Ghazza A, Bakhsh M, Hajji I, Moutaouki A. Traitement du décollement de rétine du pseudophake : vitrectomie sans indentation versus chirurgie ab externo [Article in French] Pan Afr Med J. 2019;32:44.
51. O'keefe GA, Rao NA. Vogt-Koyanagi-Harada disease. Surv Ophthalmol. 2017;62(1):1–25.
52. Wing GL, Schepens CL, Trempe CL, Weiter JJ. Serous choroidal detachment and the thickened-choroid sign detected by ultrasonography. Am J Ophthalmol. 1982;94(4):499–505.
53. Andreoli MT, Yiu G, Hart L, Andreoli CM. B-scan ultrasonography following open globe repair. Eye (Lond). 2014;28(4):381–5.
54. Kenney AH, Hafner JN. Ultrasonic evidence of inflammatory thickening and fluid collection within the retrobulbar fascia: the T sign. Ann Ophthalmol. 1977;9(12):1557–63.
55. Tabbut M, Bates A, Marple G, Gramer D, et al. Point-of-care ultrasound in the evaluation of the acutely painful red eye. J Emerg Med. 2019;57(5):705–9.
56. Agrawal R, Lavric A, Restori M, Pavesio C, et al. Nodular posterior scleritis: clinico-sonographic characteristics and proposed diagnostic criteria. Retina. 2016;36(2):392–401.
57. Shields JA, Shields CL. CME review: sclerochoroidal calcification: the 2001 Harold Gifford Lecture. Retina. 2002;22(3):251–61.
58. Shields CL, Hasanreisoglu M, Saktanasate J, Seibel I, Shields JA. Sclerochoroidal calcification: clinical features, outcomes, and relationship with hypercalcemia and parathyroid adenoma in 179 eyes. Retina. 2015;35(3):547–54.
59. Brahma VL, Shah SP, Chaudry NA, Prenner JL. Bilateral idiopathic sclerochoroidal calcifications. Open Ophthalmol J. 2017;27(11):76–9.
60. Slean GR, Kalevar A, Chen J, Johnson R. Enlargement of sclerochoroidal calcifications: multimodal imaging update. Retin Cases Brief Rep. 2018;12(Suppl. 1):S122–4.
61. Dedes W, Schmid MK, Becht C. [Sclerochoroidal calcifications with vision-threatening choroidal neovascularisation]. [Article in German] Klin. Monbl. Augenheilkd. 2008;225(5):473–5.
62. Siahmed K, Bergès O, Brasseur G. Evaluation des trous maculaires en échographie à 10 MHz et 20 MHz et par OCT. [article in French] J Fr Ophtalmol. 2005;28(7):733–6.
63. Mirza RG, Johnson MW, Jampol LM. Optical coherence tomography use in evaluation of the vitreo-retinal interface: a review. Surv Ophthalmol. 2007;52(4):397–421.
64. Hewick SA, Fairhead AC, Culy JC, Atta HR. A comparison of 10 MHz and 20 MHz ultrasound probes in imaging the eye and orbit. Br J Ophthalmol. 2004;88(4):551–5.

# Chapter 13
# Adult Eye Masses

**Olivier Bergès, Pierre Pégourié, and François Perrenoud**

**Abstract** This chapter deals with adult tumors of the uvea, and therefore essentially melanomas. Melanoma is the most frequently symptomatic eye tumor in adults. Positive diagnosis includes a morphometric study in B-mode, a study of the echotexture, best evaluated with standardized A-mode and the evaluation of the vascularization, which is the most characteristic sign, by color Doppler imaging (CDI). Successively are studied choroidal masses, iris tumors and tumors with ciliary body involvement. Ultrasound is of great help for differential diagnosis: metastases, angiomas, nevi, osteomas, melanocytomas, leiomyomas, adenomas; among pseudo-tumors: hematomas, granulomas, a serous pigment epithelial detachment in ARMD, a posterior nodular scleritis, and among the false masses: a subluxation of the crystalline nucleus, a voluminous, intumescent lens, a peristaphylomatous bulge related to high myopia, an anterior scleromalacia and a dilation of a vortex vein ampulla. Then the value of tissue characterization is highlighted, as well as 3D/4D imaging. Finally, extension of melanomas as well as post-conservative treatment follow-up are studied in detail.

## Introduction

In this chapter, we discuss adult tumors of the uvea, and therefore essentially melanomas, both their positive diagnosis as well as their differential diagnosis. Indeed, tumors of the adult retina only warrant an ultrasound when they are very large and pose a diagnostic problem. Tumors of the bulbar conjunctiva may benefit from very high-frequency ultrasound (VHFU) [1]; we have already discussed this

O. Bergès (✉)
Rothschild Foundation Hospital, Paris, France
e-mail: oberges@for.paris

P. Pégourié
University Hospital of Grenoble, Grenoble, France

F. Perrenoud
Explore Vision Ophthalmic Diagnostic Center Paris, Paris, France


O. Bergès (ed.), *Echography of the Eye and Orbit*,
https://doi.org/10.1007/978-3-031-41467-1_13

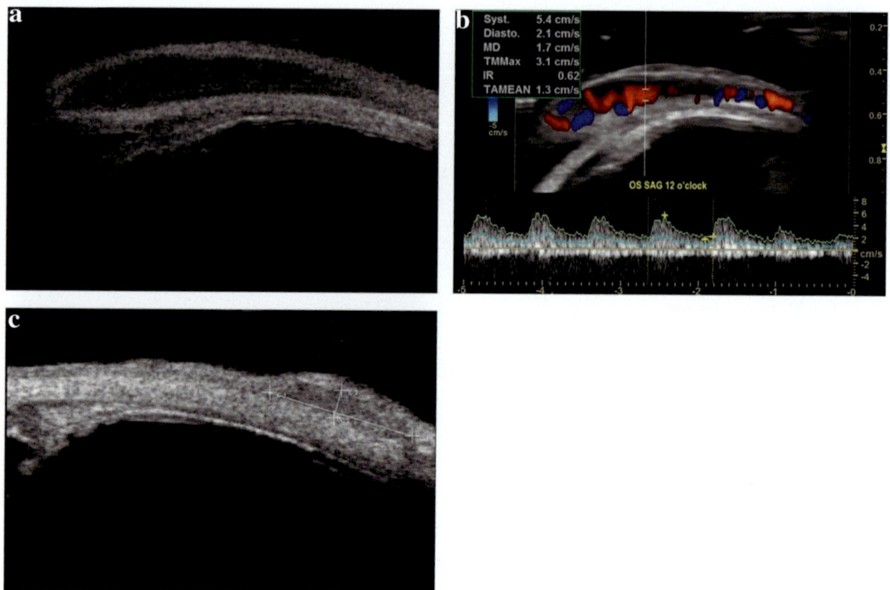



**Fig. 13.1 Conjunctival lymphoma a** and **b**: At the time of diagnosis; **c**: 9 months later after treatment with Rituximab (a chimeric monoclonal antibody). **a** and **c**: VHFU at 50 MHz; **b**: CDI with a frequency of 18 MHz for B-mode and 9 MHz for Doppler. The lesion is poorly echogenic, measuring 8.5 mm × 1.5 mm, and clearly vascularized by relatively slow and not very resistive vessels. After treatment, there is only a very small nodule, measuring 3.2 mm × 0.6 mm, which has become quite echogenic and without intrinsic flow in Doppler. Persistent remission has been observed more than three years after the end of treatment

subject in Chap. 11 (see Fig. 11.52), VHFU in particular assists in the diagnosis and monitoring of these small lesions (Fig. 13.1).

## 13.1 Uveal Melanoma

This is the most frequently *symptomatic* tumor in adults, especially adults over 50 years of age, although melanomas are sometimes also seen in young adults or even children. They affect the choroid in 80% of cases, the ciliary body in 17% of cases, and the iris in 3% of cases [2]. The warning sign is clinical: a pigmented mass of the fundus, with or without retinal detachment, with or without vitreous hemorrhage—fundus assessment most often performed for a decrease in visual acuity, but it is sometimes systematically discovered during a consultation for a refractive disorder. Ultrasound then plays an important role in affirming the diagnosis, with analysis of the pigmented mass itself (protrusion, presence of orange pigment), and angiography (presence of pinpoints, double circulation pattern). Histologically, there are fusiform forms (A, B), epithelioid forms, and more aggressive mixed forms [3].

Ultrasound has many roles to play:

- it must confirm the occurrence, and assess the location, shape, and dimensions,
- it provides an etiological orientation (approach to tissue characterization, differential diagnosis, and comparison with histological data)
- it must analyze possible extension
- it must monitor and evaluate the action of the treatment

On the other hand, there is no reason for routine ultrasound screening of pigmented lesions of the uvea, bearing in mind that a small choroidal lesion should not be disregarded if ultrasound was requested for another reason, in particular in case of intravitreal hemorrhage. The minimum thickness to detect a small parietal lesion in ultrasound is 0.2 mm. When the lesion is this small, most often only a discrete curvature anomaly is noted at 10 MHz, while (long focal length) 20 MHz allows better analysis of the characteristics of the lesion (Fig. 13.2).

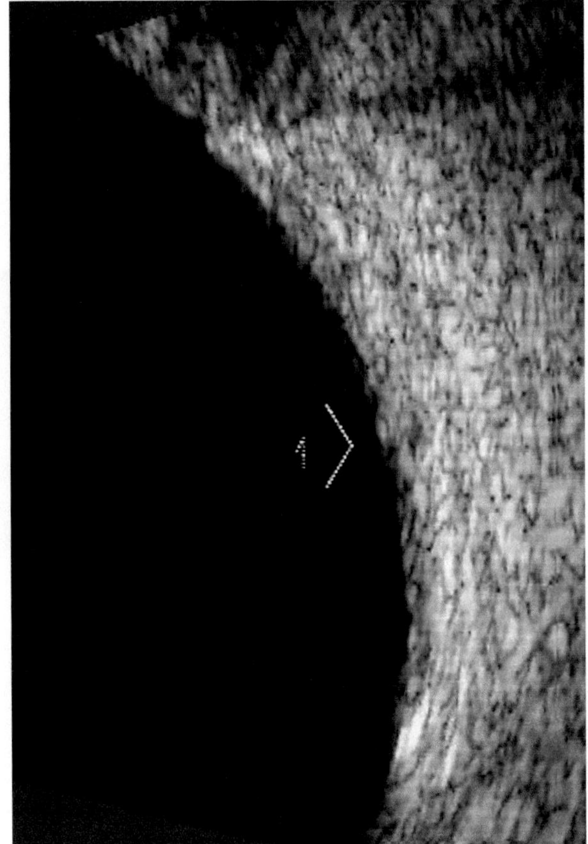

**Fig. 13.2  Temporomacular micro nevus**. Ultrasound with a long focal 20 MHz probe. The small lesion, less echogenic than the adjacent choroid, is really only measurable with this high-frequency probe: 1.3 mm in diameter and 0.3 mm thick

### *13.1.1  Choroidal Melanoma—Positive Diagnosis*

#### 13.1.1.1  The Morphometry

**The morphometry** of choroidal tumors can already be analyzed very well at 10 MHz; but when the lesion is not too protruding, a long-focal 20 MHz probe provides an advantage. It is sometimes difficult to assess small tumors using ultrasound, in the far and especially inferior periphery. Similarly, for peripheral lesions, the diameter according to the corresponding meridian is often measured by approximation, and it is often useful to associate a high-frequency study in immersion, using an anterior route.

When the lesion is small, it is most often lenticular (as a dome) and hypoechoic. The two diameters at the base and the maximum thickness should be measured (see Fig. 7.11). When more voluminous, it often has a mushroom or collar-button shape (Fig. 13.3). In this case, it is necessary to measure the two diameters of the base and the head as well as the thickness of the head and the base, and the total thickness. A small retinal detachment satellite to the tumor may be discerned, often inferior to it. A small serous retinal detachment (SRD) may also be seen at the apex of the tumor. In this case, the thickness should be measured with and without taking into account this small SRD; the whole lesion, tumor + SRD must be taken into account in the volume to be treated by brachytherapy/proton beam therapy. For each measurement, three successive measurements should be made, as consistent as possible, and the

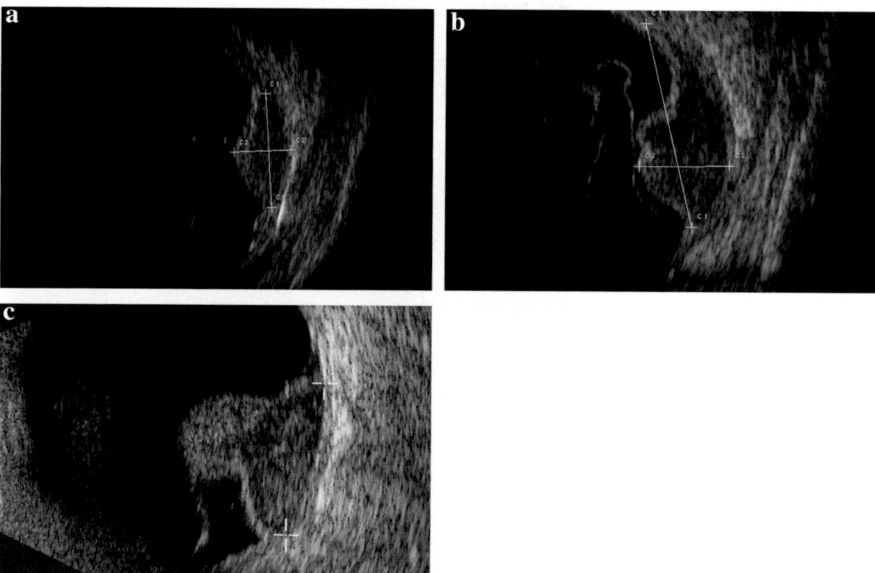

**Fig. 13.3  Choroidal melanoma**, 10 MHz B-mode. Different shapes. **a**: Dome shape (biconvex lens); **b**: mushroom shape; **c**: collar-button shape. Only the collar-button shape is characteristic, almost pathognomonic

maximum value and the average value should be stated in the report. A collar-button shape is very characteristic of uveal melanomas and corresponds to rupture of the Bruch's membrane by the tumor, and therefore to aggressive tumors. With this form, the tumor base is poorly echogenic, and the head is echogenic, because of the presence of many non-circulating vessels packed against each other [4]. The angle of connection with the wall tends to be at a gentle slope or at an obtuse angle in small dome tumors and at an acute angle in larger tumors with a collar-button or a mushroom shape. In addition to these three conventional forms, there is also a so-called diffuse form, with a reduced thickness, less than 3 mm, and large diameters, of 14 mm on average, with high metastatic potentials [5]. This form is rare, occurring in less than 3% of subjects.

### 13.1.1.2   The Echotexture

**The echotexture** of the lesion is best assessed in standardized A-mode, but it can also be visualized quite well in B-mode: melanomas are hyporeflective and attenuating lesions, due to the high density of small cells packed against each other, as for orbital lymphomas (Fig. 13.4).

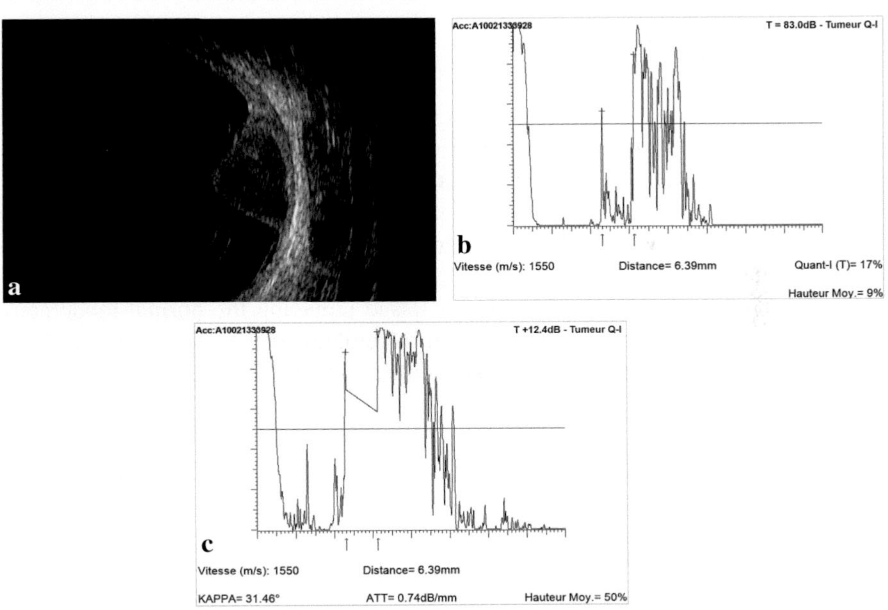


**Fig. 13.4  Hypoechoic and attenuating choroidal melanoma a**: section with a long focal 20 MHz probe; **b**: standardized A-mode at tissue sensitivity (T = 83 dB) for assessment of the reflectivity; **c**: standardized A-mode, the average peak height being equal to 50% (= T + 12.4 dB) to assess the attenuation. The lesion is not very echogenic, low reflective: 17% of the scleral peak in Quantification I and attenuating with a kappa angle at 31°. Attenuation is evident in A-mode but not in B-mode

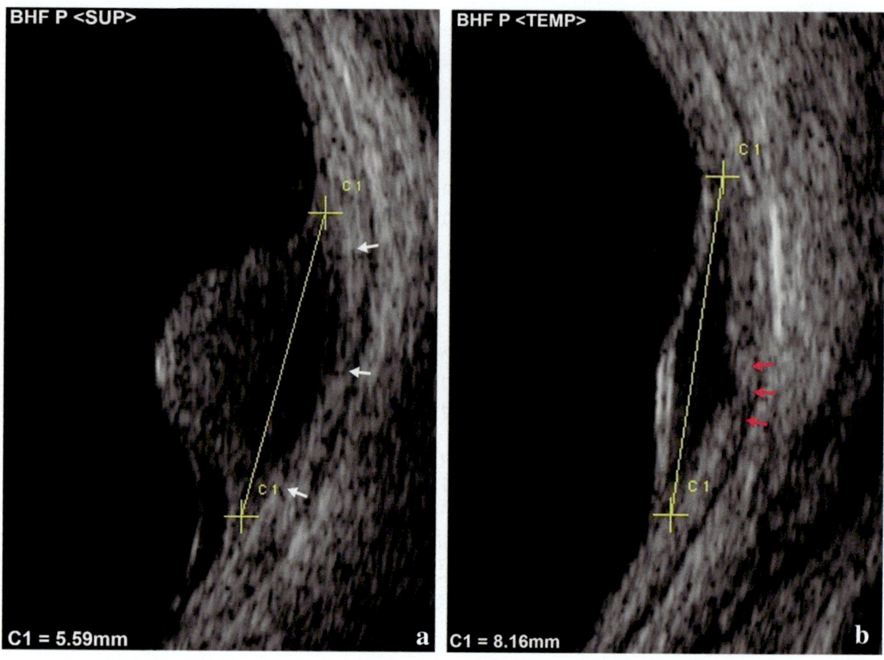


**Fig. 13.5 Choroidal excavation. a**: Extended to the entire base (→ white arrows) of a tumor of 7.6 mm in diameter; **b**: partial (⟶ red arrows) on a wider lesion, 8.2 mm in diameter, but less thick

The lesions are most often homogeneous, except for large lesions with hemorrhagic and/or necrotic rearrangements. It is exceptional to see intratumoral calcifications. Unusually, the tumor may appear mainly cystic, especially those with ciliary body involvement; however, a cystic tumor of the ciliary body tends to point to a medulloepithelioma.

The hyporeflective nature of the tumor tissue replacing the normal moderately reflective choroid gives rise to a characteristic semiological criterion: choroidal excavation. This sign sometimes extends to the entire base of the tumor or is more often localized (Fig. 13.5).

This sign is to be distinguished from the scleral bowing that is seen in melanomas with scleral infiltration [6], typical with aggressive lesions in young subjects.

### 13.1.1.3 Vascularization

**Vascularization:** melanomas are highly vascularized. In 80% of cases, A-mode allows visualization of pulsed oscillations of intrinsic tumor peaks [7]. This feature is also found (shiny appearance of the tumor) in 70% of cases in B-mode. Color Doppler Imaging (CDI) is, however, currently the best way to qualitatively and quantitatively evaluate the vascular nature of these tumors, found in more than 95%

of cases with this technique. CDI can identify five different types of vascularization [8].

- Type 1, the most common type, occurring in almost 70% of cases, is seen mainly in small choroidal tumors as domes of the posterior pole, with visible vessels on the surface of the tumor, and, once the tumor has a thickness greater than 4 mm, as perforating vessels, centripetal towards the center of the tumor, from the posterior short ciliary arteries. All these vessels have a fairly low PSV, not exceeding 15 cm/s, and a RI between 0.55 and 0.75 (Fig. 13.6).

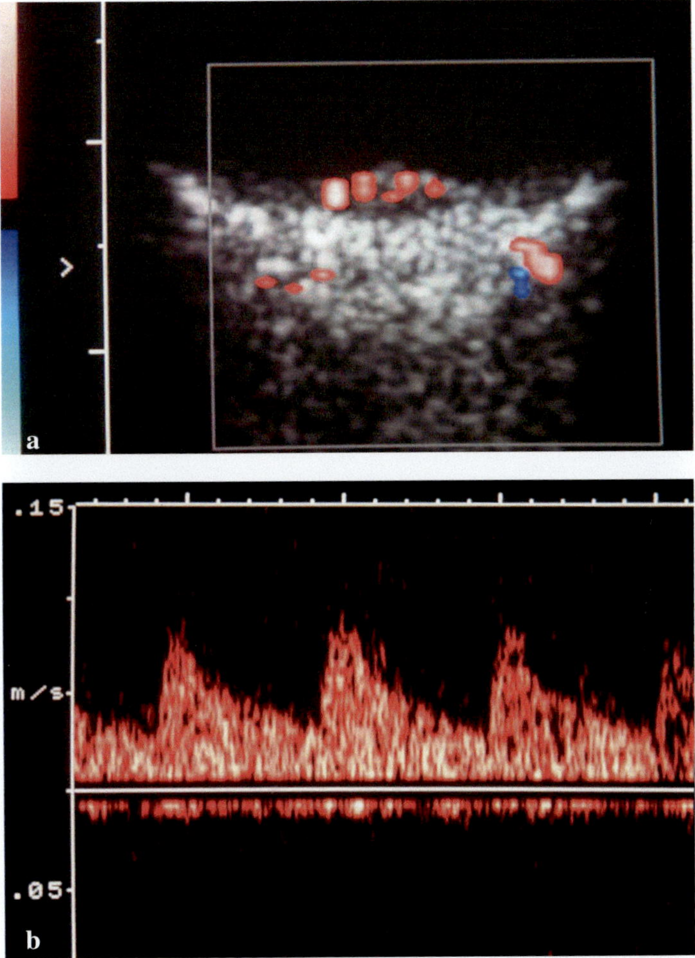

**Fig. 13.6  Type 1 vascularization** of a small melanoma of the posterior pole, 2.2 mm thick. **a:** Color mode; **b:** spectral mode. In color mode, small flows on the surface of the tumor. In spectral mode, the PSV is measured at 9.2 cm/s (without angle correction) and the RI calculated to be 0.64

- Type 2 is seen in larger choroidal tumors with a thickness between 5 and 9 mm. These are also quite common, being observed in 21% of cases. The arteries are visible at the tumor pole located near the optic nerve, with a higher PSV, between 15 cm/s and 40 cm/s. The RI is between 0.55 and 0.75. Veins are visible at the opposite pole (Fig. 13.7).

The other types are rare, each one being observed in only 3% of cases.

- Type 3a is found in very large tumors of more than 15 mm in thickness, to be enucleated. The mass appears to be hypervascular, with arteries that have a

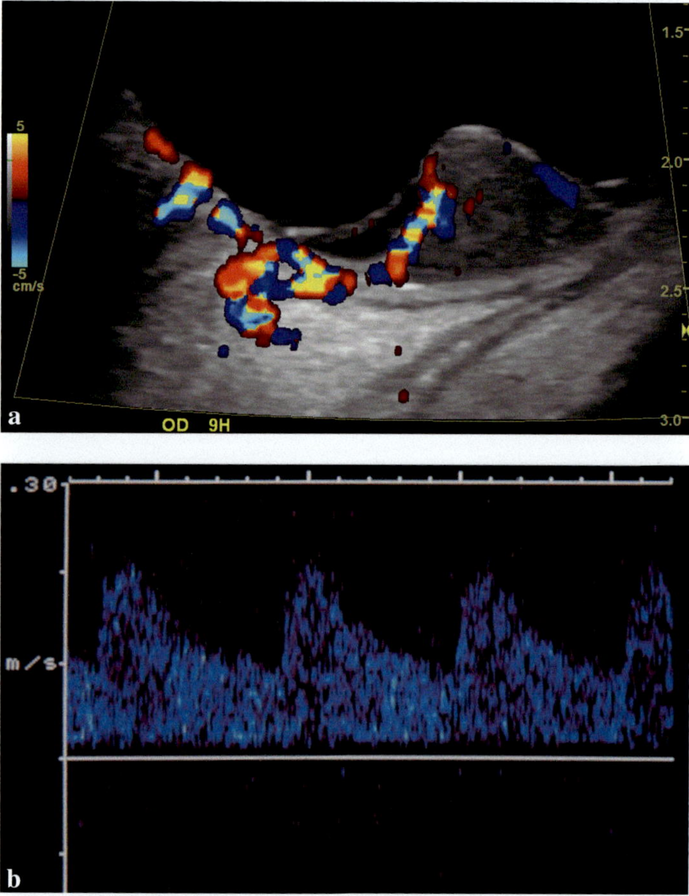

**Fig. 13.7  Type 2 vascularization** of a mushroom shaped melanoma located nasally to the optic disc; 8.6 mm thick. **a**: Color mode; **b**: spectral mode. In color mode, small arteries are visualized, encoded in red, at the pole of the tumor located near the optic nerve, and veins, encoded in blue, at the opposite pole. In spectral mode, the PSV is measured at 22 cm/s and the RI calculated to be 0.56

PSV between 15 and 40 cm/s and a rather low RI, between 0.50 and 0.60, and voluminous veins at the periphery (Fig. 13.8).

- Type 3b is also found in voluminous tumors that have a thickness greater than 10 mm. The PSV is between 15 and 40 cm/s and RI is high, greater than 0.80, correlated with associated ocular hypertension (Fig. 13.9). Large drainage veins that cross the sclera can also be seen.
- Type 0 corresponds to an absence of individualizable flow in CDI (Fig. 13.10). This absence of vascularization is seen in case of:

  - massive intratumoral hemorrhage (with or without thrombosis of a vorticose vein),
  - ocular hypertension greater than 40 mmHg [9],
  - very small lesions (less than 2.5 mm thick).

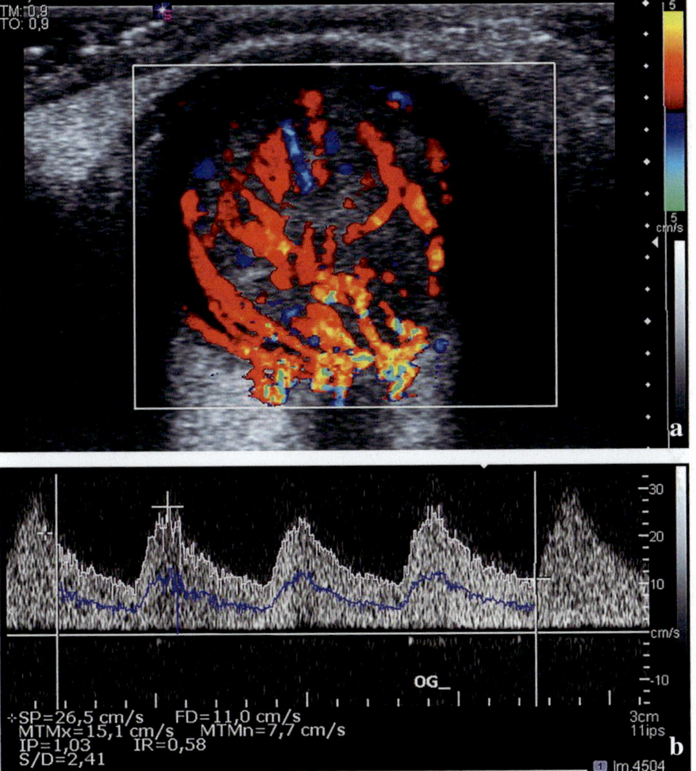

**Fig. 13.8  Type 3a vascularization** of a large melanoma, with diameters of 19 mm × 21 mm and a thickness of 16 mm. **a**: Color mode; **b**: spectral mode. In color mode, the large lesion appears to be hypervascularized. In spectral mode, the PSV is measured at 26.5 cm/s and the RI is rather low, calculated to be 0.58

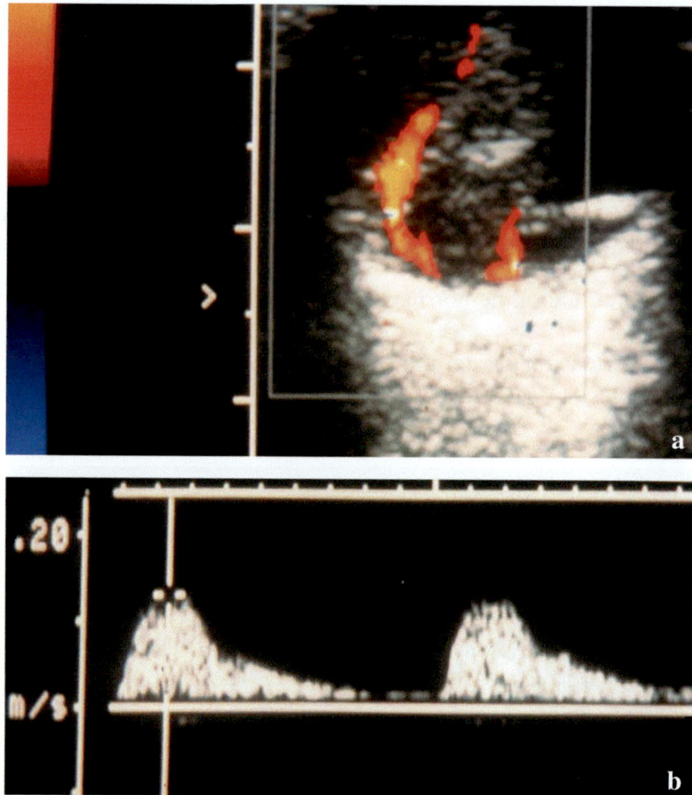

Fig. 13.9 **Type 3b vascularization of** a large mushroom shaped melanoma with a thickness of 14 mm, associated with ocular hypertension at 30 mmHg. **a**: Color mode; **b**: spectral mode. In color mode, large perforating arteries are seen, coded in red. In spectral mode, the PSV is measured at 17 cm/s and the RI is calculated to be 0.90 due to the almost complete disappearance of the diastolic flow

Fig. 13.10 **Type 0 vascularization** of a large choroidal and ciliary body melanoma. Color mode; no detectable vessels in relation to ocular hypertension at 45 mm Hg, with neovascular glaucoma

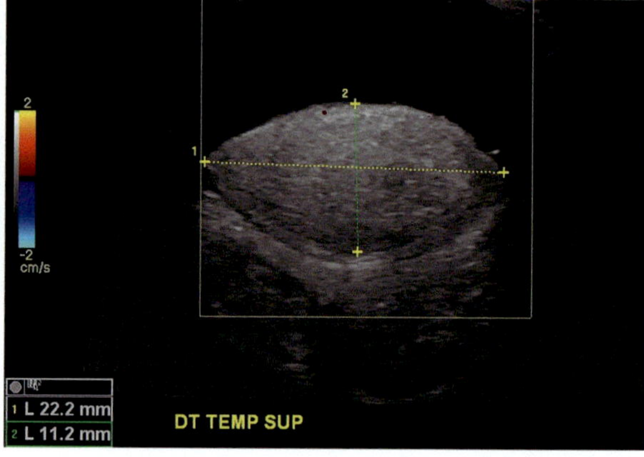

### 13.1.2   Iris Tumors

These require assessment by immersion, with a very high-frequency (VHFU) probe, at least equal to 50 MHz. Masses of the iris, regardless of their nature, are generally more frequent in the inferior regions.

- **A cyst of the posterior epithelium of the iris** is most frequently responsible for a localized bulge of the iris. VHFU is the gold standard for differentiating an epithelial cyst from a solid tumor, on the one hand, and other cysts of the iris, primary or secondary, in particular a cyst of the iris stroma, on the other hand [10]. A cyst of the posterior epithelium of the iris is rarely isolated and is most often associated with other cysts, smaller, iridociliary, non-symptomatic, achieving a true polycystic iridociliary dysplasia, without generally falling within the framework of other organic polycystic diseases, in particular hepato-renal or thyroid. Their contents are transonic and their walls are thin (Fig. 13.11).
- It is not necessary to institute ultrasound controls. On the other hand, an annual clinical check-up is desirable, with measurement of intraocular pressure (IOP) [11]. In rare cases, they may be associated with nevi or iridociliary melanomas

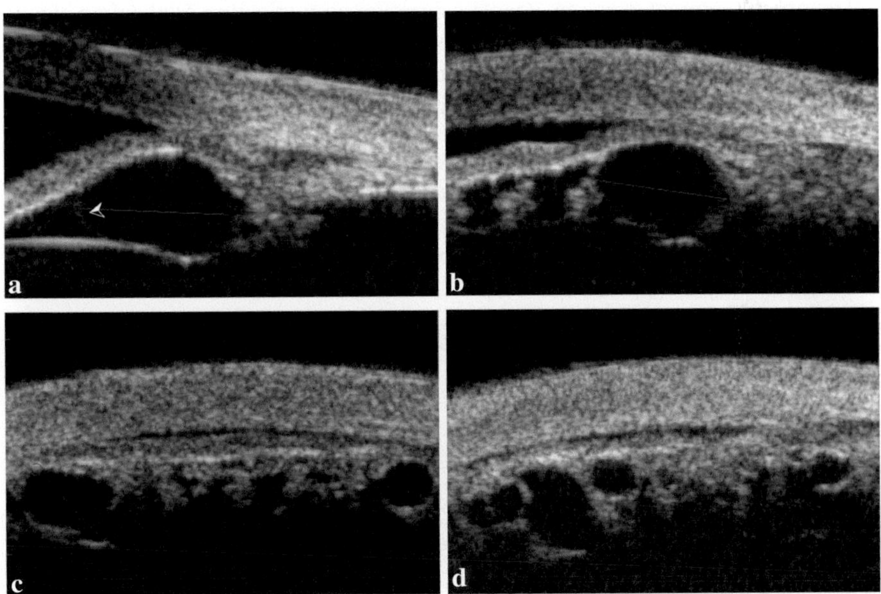

**Fig. 13.11  Iridociliary polycystic dysplasia**. Ultrasound BioMicroscopy at 50 MHz. **a**: OS, section along the 9 o'clock meridian; **b**: OS orthogonal nasal section; **c**: OS, inferior section; **d**: OD, temporal section. The nasal cyst of the left eye, symptomatic, measures 1.5 mm × 1.3 mm in diameter, × 1.1 mm in thickness and causes a localized closure of the anterior chamber angle. The iris next to the cyst is bulging and thinned. Note the thin wall of the cyst (➤) in contact with the posterior chamber. Evidence in all quadrants, in both eyes, of smaller asymptomatic ciliary cysts, measuring between 0.5 mm and 1 mm in diameter

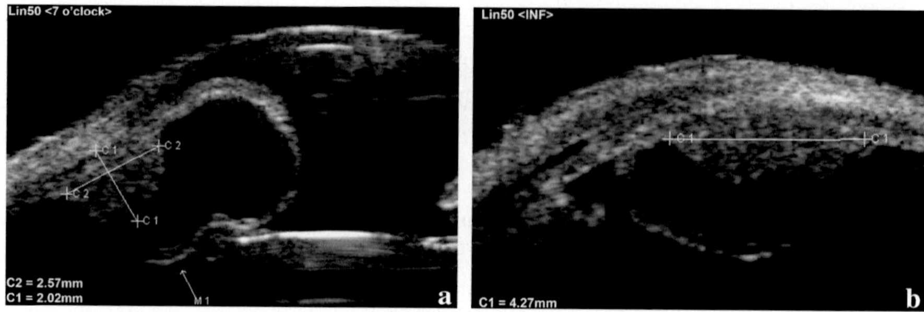



**Fig. 13.12 Large iris cyst** revealing a small hypoechoic melanoma, 4.27 mm in its maximum diameter × 2.02 mm in thickness: VHFU at 50 MHz. **a**: Section along the 7 o'clock meridian; **b**: transverse view of the inferior quadrant. The cyst extends to the corneal endothelium and pushes back the zonule (→)

(Fig. 13.12), which then require a very close follow-up or oncological care. Pigmented cysts floating in the anterior chamber may also be seen [12].

- **Iris stromal cysts** occur mainly in small children. They have more pronounced walls and may have a discreetly echogenic content (Fig. 13.13, see Fig. 4.1). Treatment (surgical excision, needle aspiration with injection of absolute alcohol or antimitotic) is necessary if they are troublesome due to their volume or due to the complications (cataract, rupture) that they can cause [13].
- **Nevi** of the iris present as an echogenic localized bulging of the iris,

  - when small in size, they are more echogenic than the adjacent iris stroma (Fig. 13.14), or sometimes, rarely less echogenic (Fig. 13.15);
  - when larger in size, they are often slightly less echogenic than the adjacent iris. The exact positioning of the calipers to measure the diameters of the lesion is

**Fig. 13.13 Iris stromal cyst.** UBM at 50 MHz. Horizontal section exploring the inferior field. The cyst is large, measuring 4.2 mm in diameter, coming into contact with the corneal endothelium and has a very discreetly echogenic content

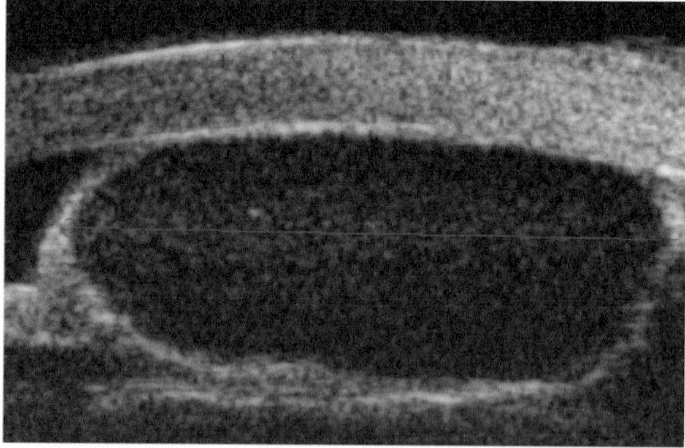

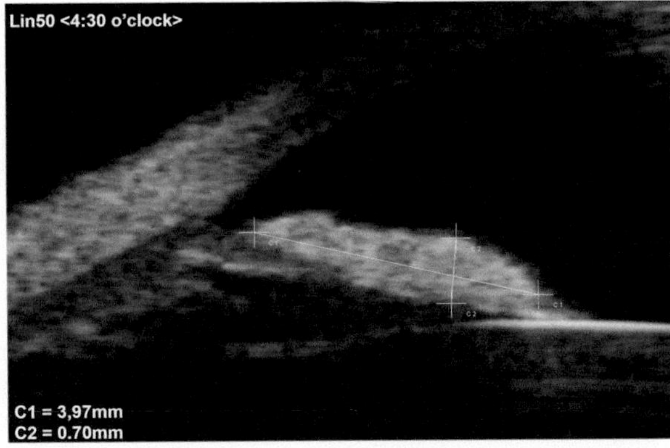



**Fig. 13.14  Small and very echogenic nevus of the iris.** VHFU at 50 MHz along the 4 o'clock meridian. The lesion is very echogenic, more than the adjacent iris stroma, and relatively thin: 0.7 mm

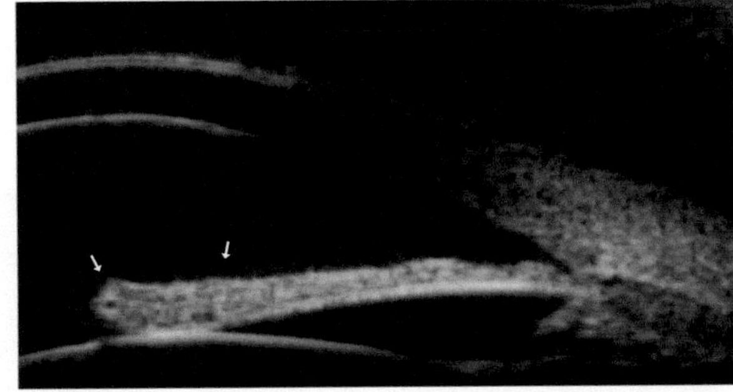

**Fig. 13.15  Very small nevus of the pupillary border of the iris.** VHFU at 50 MHz according to the 7 o'clock meridian. Slightly less echogenic than the adjacent iris stroma, and without localized thickening

sometimes difficult. On the other hand, accurate measurement of the thickness is easy. A hypoechoic plaque, indicative that the echogenic mass of the iris is benign, is often found on the surface of the nevus (Fig. 13.16) [14]. But this criterion of benignity has since been questioned. In our experience, we have also observed this sign with melanomas of the iris after proton beam therapy.

- **Melanomas** of the iris [14] are larger, often multilobulated, and have a heterogeneous and attenuating echotexture (Fig. 13.17a), often coming into contact with the cornea, with frequent deformation of the posterior epithelium of the iris, and sometimes a characteristic collar button appearance. Cystic areas are frequently found within or around them that may correspond to genuine associated iridociliary cysts, intratumoral vessels, or areas of necrosis. When they have a thickness greater than 2 mm, in 75% of cases, intrinsic vascular activity is apparent by CDI (Fig. 13.17b), while benign nevi of the same size are perfectly avascular.

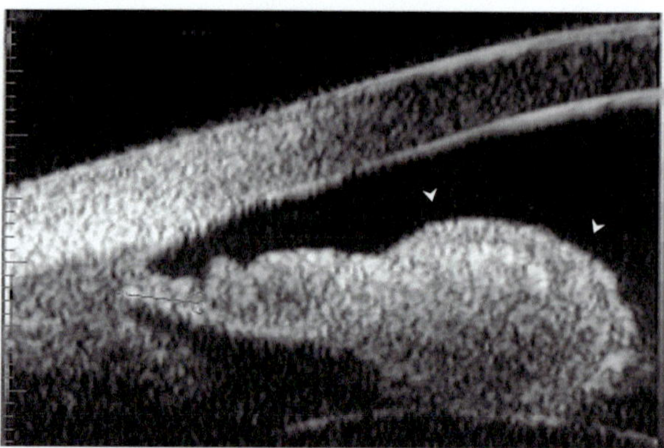

**Fig. 13.16 Nevus of the iris with surface plaque**. Ultrasound biomicroscopy at 50 MHz. Section according to the 6 o'clock meridian. Bell-shaped, perfectly even, the nevus extends to the pupil and remains at a distance from the angle (480 μm), which has a normal appearance. It is moderately attenuating and has a maximum thickness of 1.4 mm. The hypoechoic surface plaque (➤ arrowheads) is quite indicative of the benign nature of the lesion

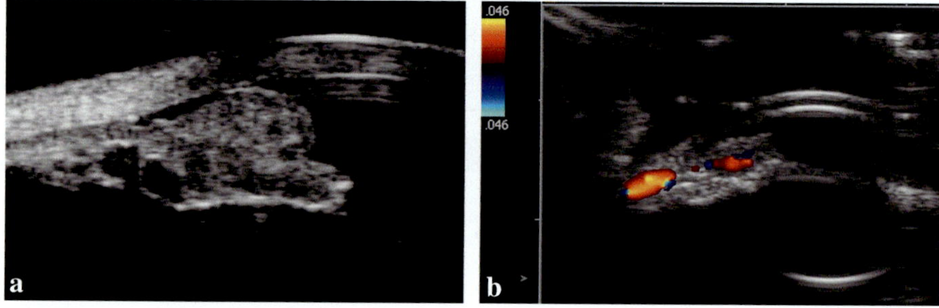

**Fig. 13.17 Iris melanoma**. **a**: VHFU at 50 MHz along the 4 o'clock meridian; **b**: CDI, same section with an 18 MHz probe for the B-mode and 9 MHz for the Doppler. The mass is multilobulated and comes into contact with the corneal endothelium; Note its heterogeneous nature, deformation of the posterior iris epithelium, attenuation, and the presence of cysts. It measures 5 mm × 6.6 mm in diameter × 2.2 mm in thickness, and intrinsic Doppler flows are highlighted; all signs in favor of a malignant lesion

### 13.1.3  *Tumors with Ciliary Body Involvement*

- VHFU at 50 MHz, on the other hand, is not very suitable for assessment of iridociliary or ciliochoroidal tumors, because they are often large at the time of their diagnosis, and, on the other hand, they strongly attenuate the ultrasound beam, making even the measurement of their thickness often impossible at this frequency. It is, therefore, necessary to use a lower frequency, close to 20 MHz, at which the tumor is very well visualized while the spatial resolution is still satisfactory (Fig. 13.18, see Fig. 4.5).

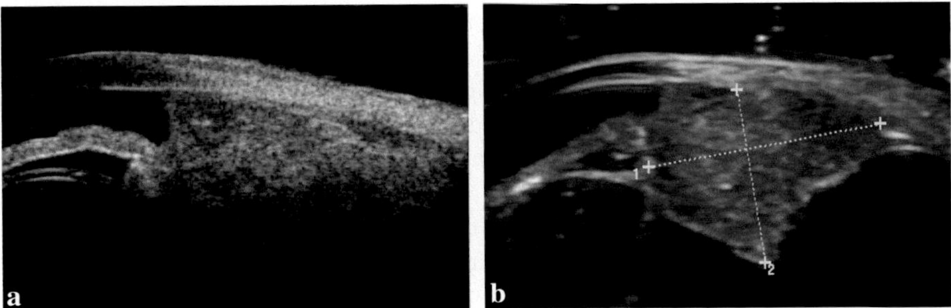

**Fig. 13.18 Ciliary body melanoma invading the root of the iris. a**: VHFU at 50 MHz, section along the 4 o'clock meridian; **b**: same section with an 18 MHz probe. The tumor is large, measuring 5.2 mm × 4.8 mm in diameter and 6.2 mm of thickness. Its size and significant attenuation mean that it can only be viewed in its entirety at high frequency and not at 50 MHz. But the integrity of the sclera in relation to the tumor is best appreciated at 50 MHz. The displacement of the lens and the sectorial contact cataract are also better visualized at 18 MHz

- Visualization at 50 MHz is, however, essential for detailed assessment of the sclera in relation to the tumor (risk of scleromalacia see Fig. 13.40, scleral effraction see Fig. 13.43) and, for ciliochoroidal tumors, measurement of the distance between the periphery of the tumor and the anterior chamber angle (/scleral spur). VHFU at 50 MHz is also very useful for monitoring small tumors that are less than 3 mm thick, which have a low tendency to progress [15].

With the most recent devices, working in immersion with 12 MHz probes, the vascular nature of melanomas of the ciliary body is found as frequently as for choroidal melanomas: 93% for any tumor size, and with good flows in 80% of cases if the thickness is greater than 5 mm (Fig. 13.20), but in less than 5% of cases

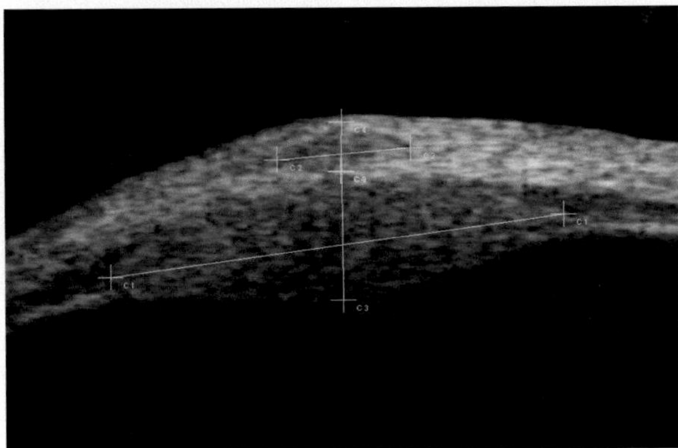

**Fig. 13.19 Ciliochoroidal melanoma with scleral effraction and small subconjunctival extension.** Section at 50 MHz. The ultrasound requested for the small subconjunctival lesion discovered the underlying hourglass ciliochoroidal lesion, with a characteristic echotexture: poorly echogenic, homogeneous, and attenuating

if the thickness is less than 3 mm. At the usual settings, the arteries are most often coded in blue, since they come from the arterial circle of the iris and move away from the probe. The PSV is most often slightly less than 10 cm/s, and the RI, in the absence of ocular hypertension, is just under 0.60.

As a corollary, it can be said that the absence of flow in CDI within a tumor of the ciliary body tends to indicate a lesion associated with a high IOP (> 40 mmHg), a melanoma after conservative treatment, or a benign tumor, such as an adenoma.

Although the most likely diagnosis of a partially cystic tumor of the ciliary body is medulloepithelioma (see Chap. 14) , melanomas of the ciliary body can also be cystic (Fig. 13.21).

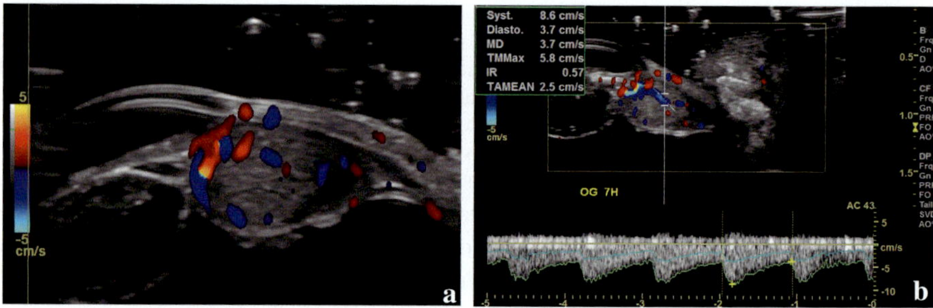

**Fig. 13.20 Highly vascularized ciliary body melanoma**. Color Doppler Imaging. The lesion is large: 7.4 mm × 9.1 mm in diameter × 5.1 mm thick. **a**: Color mode; **b**: spectral mode. At the usual settings, arteries coming from the arterial circle of the iris are coded in blue and have a negative spectrum in spectral mode because their flow moves away from the probe. The velocimetric constants are very much in concordance with the diagnosis: PSV = 8.6 cm/s, RI = 0.57

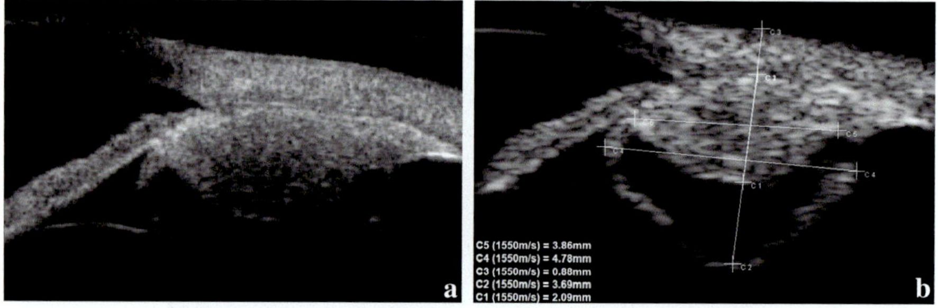

**Fig. 13.21 Cystic melanoma of the ciliary body**. Sections along the 7:30 meridian. **a**: VHFU at 50 MHz; **b**: HFU at 25 MHz. Even partially cystic, the tumor is fully visible only at 25 MHz. But at 50 MHz, the attenuation of its solid part is better evaluated. Strictly normal appearance of the sclera by high and very high-frequency ultrasound

## 13.1.4   Differential Ultrasound Diagnosis: Etiological Orientation

The diagnosis of uveal melanoma is based on a collection of considerations taking into account the clinical and fundus findings, angiography, ultrasound, and—for delicate or difficult cases—an MRI, or even close follow-up of the progression. Since the late 1960s, ultrasound, as a complementary examination, has played an important role in the etiological orientation of ocular parietal masses, first in standardized A-mode, then in A-mode and B-mode, and more recently, in A-mode, B-mode and CDI. Currently, with conservative treatments, the percentage of difficult cases is close to the 5% that Poujol reported as the percentage of diagnostic errors in 1986 [16]. Hence the usefulness of taking into consideration all possible arguments before making this diagnosis.

Many lesions can simulate melanoma at the clinical or ultrasound level [17], and here we will only consider the most troublesome and frequent. For tumors, these comprise metastases, choroidal hemangiomas, choroidal osteomas and other calcified parietal ocular lesions, leiomyomas, and nevi, and for non-tumorous lesions, these are subretinal hematomas, granulomas, posterior nodular scleritis, nucleus dislocations of the lens, intumescent lenses, varices of a vortex vein ampulla, and wall thickness irregularities in the vicinity of staphylomas.

### 13.1.4.1   Metastases

These are undoubtedly the **most frequent** tumors of the uvea [18], but they are sometimes unexplored because they occur in terminally ill patients. In approximately 20% of cases, they reveal the primary cancer. They are mainly associated with breast cancer in women, and lung and prostate cancer in men. At fundoscopy, the lesion is not pigmented, but yellowish. In ultrasound, the lesion is mainly localized at the posterior pole, **wider than elevated**, and frequently associated with serous retinal detachment. The lesion appears quite echogenic (medium to high) and especially uneven and non-attenuating. In A-mode, the vascularity is less obvious than for melanomas, while in CDI, the lesion discloses many small vessels, without arborization, and without their characteristic velocimetric constants (Fig. 13.22). It is essential to carry out a careful bilateral examination because the discovery of another lesion, sometimes discreet, is an element that further supports the diagnosis.

### 13.1.4.2   Choroidal Angioma

Two forms can be discerned:

- A circumscribed, lenticular shape at the posterior pole (Fig. 13.23), appearing as an orange-red lesion at fundoscopy and homogeneous hyperechoic in ultrasound for which ultrasound is very useful for the differential diagnosis with achromic

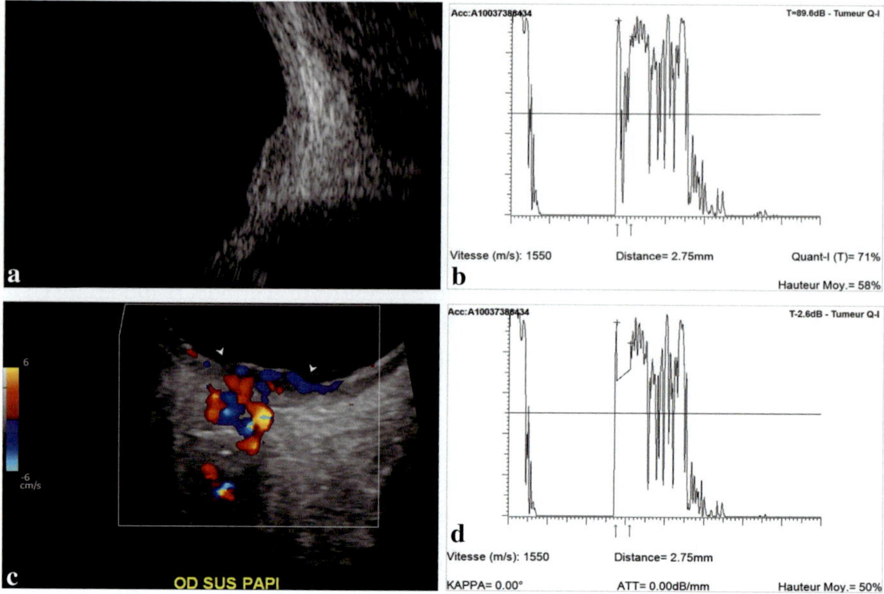



**Fig. 13.22** **Metastasis indicative** of lung cancer, as well as bone metastases, at the time of diagnosis in a 56-year-old man. **a**: B-mode at 10 MHz of the 12 o'clock meridian; **c**: CDI, suprapapillary axial section; **b**: standardized A-mode at tissue snsitivity (T = 89.6 dB) to assess the reflectivity, and **d**: standardized A-mode, the average peak height being equal to 50% (at T-2.6 dB) to assess the attenuation. The lesion, located above the optic disc, is associated with a small serous retinal detachment (SRD) that extends to the macula, giving rise to a decrease in visual acuity. It is bilobed, wider (6.8 mm × 6.4 mm in diameter) than high (2 mm). Note the small area of SRD in the center and around the lesion, its high reflectivity, and its very heterogeneous echotexture (very uneven height of the peaks), the absence of attenuation in A-mode; Furthermore, its vascularization is very different (many vessels, without arborization) from that of melanoma in CDI

melanoma [19]. In CDI, flows are only found at the tumor pole located close to the optic nerve by perforating vessels from the posterior short ciliary arteries, with a RI close to that of the nutrient arteries, lower than that of melanomas. It should be noted, however, that in case of associated glaucoma, the RI may be higher, or even equal to 1.00 by abolition of the end-diastolic flow.

- A more diffuse form, more frequently associated than the circumscribed form to Sturge–Weber syndrome, with diffuse hyperechoic choroidal thickening of both the nasal and temporal quadrants (see Fig. 14.33).

Calcifications can be seen on their surface. Both forms can be complicated by exudative retinal detachment. A conservative treatment, TTT or proton beam therapy, aims at fighting against these retinal detachments.

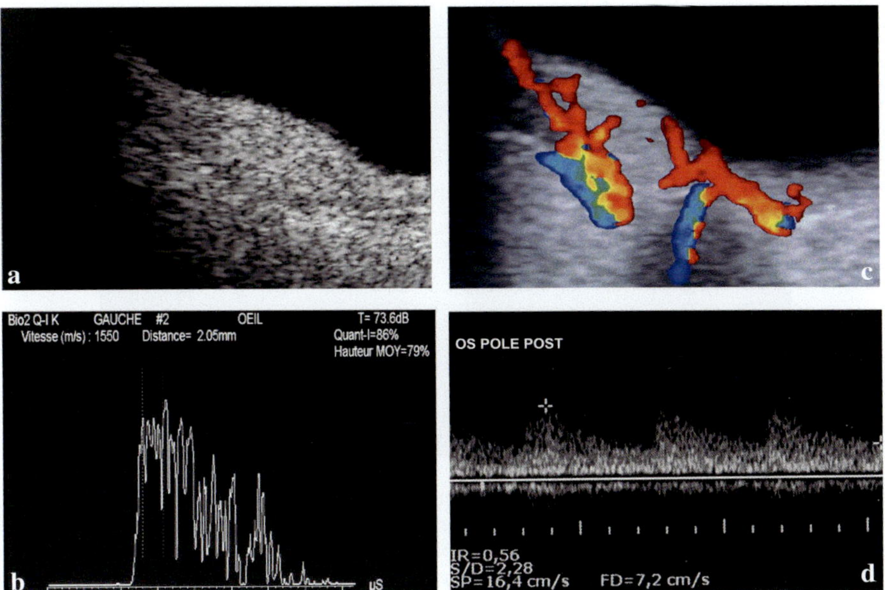

**Fig. 13.23  Choroidal angioma located at the posterior pole. a**: B-mode with a 20 MHz long-focal probe; **b**: standardized A-mode; **c**: CDI, color mode; **d**: CDI, spectral mode. Small dome-shaped tumor, located at the posterior pole, 2 mm thick, hyperechoic (86% in standardized A-mode), vascularized by the Short Posterior Ciliary Arteries (with a relatively low RI, identical to that of its nutrient arteries: 0.56)

### 13.1.4.3   Nevus

- **Flat**, they may not exhibit any ultrasound translation, even with a 20 MHz probe.
- **Thin / small in size**, with a 20 MHz probe, a very discreetly hypoechoic lesion can be seen once the height reaches 0.3 mm (see Fig. 13.2).
- **Purely benign**, they are small, with diameters inferior to 7 mm and a thickness inferior to 2 mm; they appear either entirely highly echogenic (Fig. 13.24), or more echogenic than melanoma with a very echogenic anterior part, not leading to any sign of choroidal excavation and without flows in CDI (Fig. 13.25).
- **with suspicious features**: This is **the** real differential diagnosis with melanoma of the choroid, which can sometimes be tricky or difficult, and possibly even requires close clinical ultrasound monitoring every 3 to 6 months [20]. They pose a problem when they are large, with a diameter superior to 7 mm and prominent, with an ultrasound thickness of about 2 mm. Clinically, the existence of orange pigment and/or of serous retinal detachment is worrying. In ultrasound, the presence of choroidal excavation in B-mode, strong attenuation in standardized A-mode and/ or of intrinsic flows in CDI (Fig. 13.26) must lead to a very close follow-up or to a treatment, taking into account the clinic, and in particular the situation in relation to the optic disc and the macula.

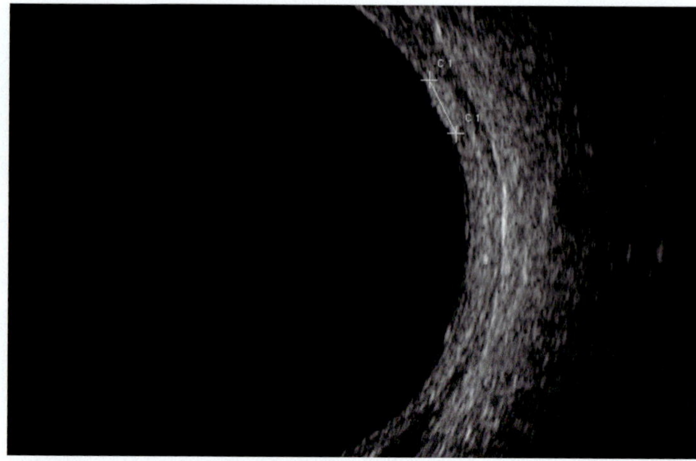

**Fig. 13.24 Small benign nevus.** Section of the temporal quadrant with a 20 MHz long-focal probe. The supramacular and quite echogenic nevus is very small, measuring 2.8 mm × 2.4 mm in diameter × 1.1 mm thick, resulting in only a minimal protrusion on the curvature of the ocular wall. It is associated with a thin epimacular membrane, detected by OCT.

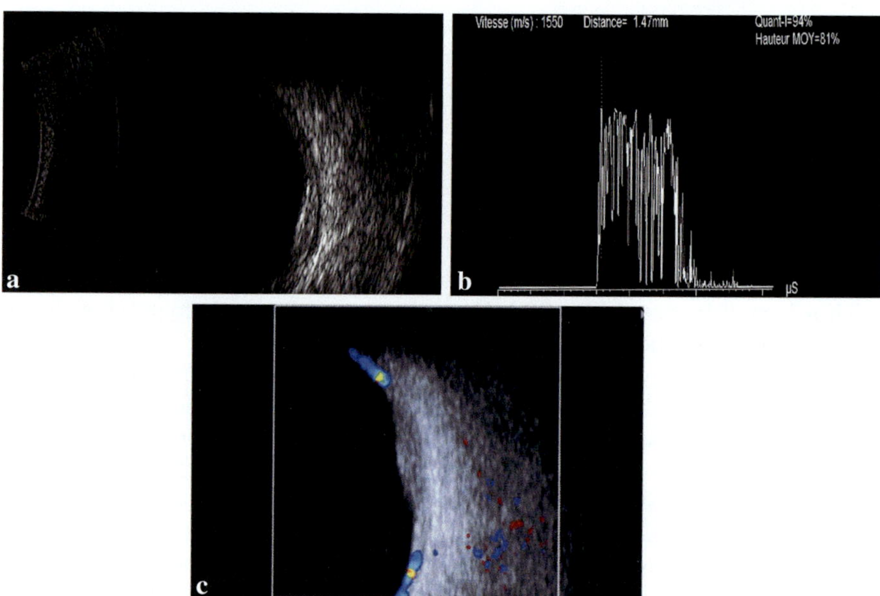


**Fig. 13.25 Benign choroidal nevus** centered on the 4 o'clock meridian in the left eye. **a**: B-mode at 10 MHz; **b**: standardized A-mode; **c**: CDI, color mode. The small lenticular lesion measures 6.6 mm × 6.8 mm in diameter × 1.5 mm thick. It is hyperechoic (94%) with an irregular echotexture and has no intrinsic flow, while the adjacent vortex veins can be clearly seen

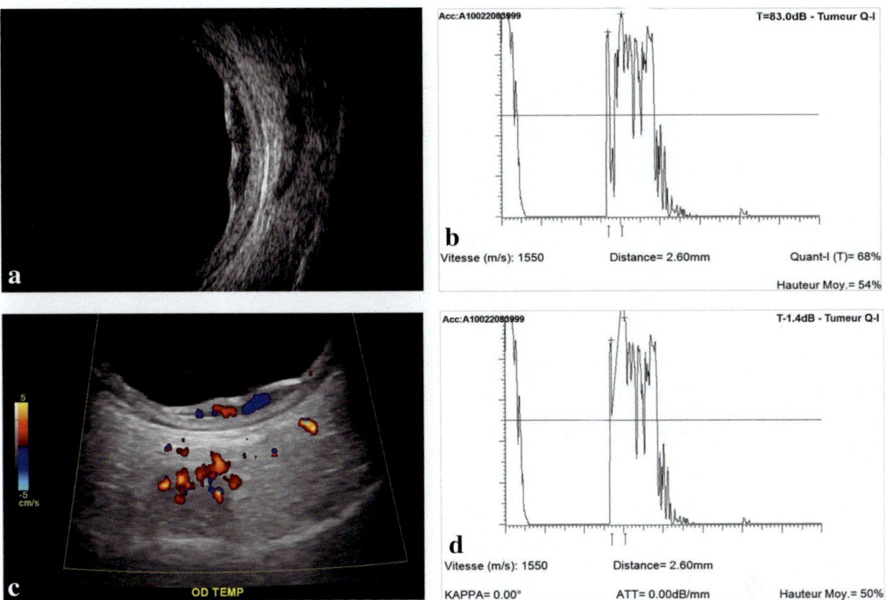

**Fig. 13.26 Suspicious nevus** based on its size and vascularization. **a**: Section of the temporal quadrant at 20 MHz; **c**: section of the same temporal quadrant in CDI, color mode; **b**: standardized A-mode at tissue sensitivity (T = 83 dB) assessing the reflectivity, and **d**: standardized A-mode, the average peak height being equal to 50% (at T-1.4 dB) to assess the attenuation. The nevus is large, measuring 13.4 mm × 10.8 mm × 2.4 mm, which makes it already suspicious, with a bilobed surface. Even if in standardized A-mode, it has the characteristics of a benign nevus (reflectivity > 60% and kappa angle = 0) and not those of melanoma, the presence of intrinsic flows in Color Doppler Imaging makes it doubly suspicious: Frequent clinical-ultrasound monitoring should be carried out because the risk of transformation into choroidal melanoma is high

### 13.1.4.4    Choroidal Osteoma

Ranging from yellowish-white to orange-red, these unilateral peripapillary lesions in young women have a characteristic ultrasound appearance: with a more or less even surface and calcified, thus resulting in a total shadowing on the posterior structures, the sclera and the orbit (Fig. 13.27).

**Idiopathic sclerochoroidal calcifications** [21] are more frequent, often bilateral, and symmetrical; and especially discovered fortuitously in subjects over 50 years of age in the superior temporal quadrant of the macular area, or sometimes in the superior nasal quadrant. Smaller than osteomas (see Fig. 12.63), there is very often a thin retinal layer in front of the calcification (Fig. 13.28); they do not usually pose a differential diagnostic problem with an ocular parietal tumor. Such parietal calcifications may be associated with disorders of phospho-calcium metabolism.

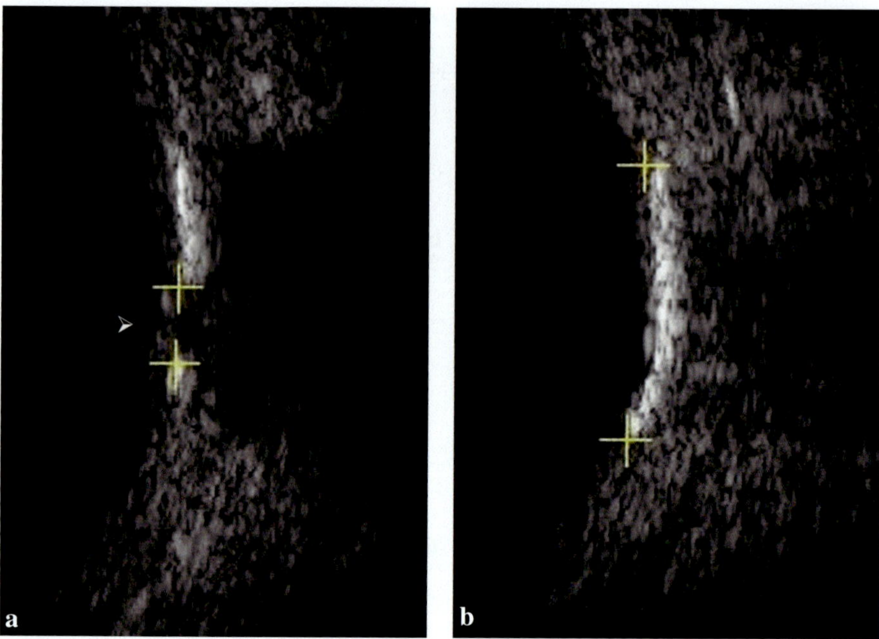

**Fig. 13.27** **Choroidal osteoma in a 28-year-old woman**. B-mode at 10 MHz. **a**: Para-axial section of the right eye; **b**: vertical section of the right eye passing through the macula. Hyperechoic with posterior shadowing, the lesion surrounds the optic disc (➤ white arrowhead), but is more developed on the temporal side. Its maximum vertical diameter measures 6.1 mm

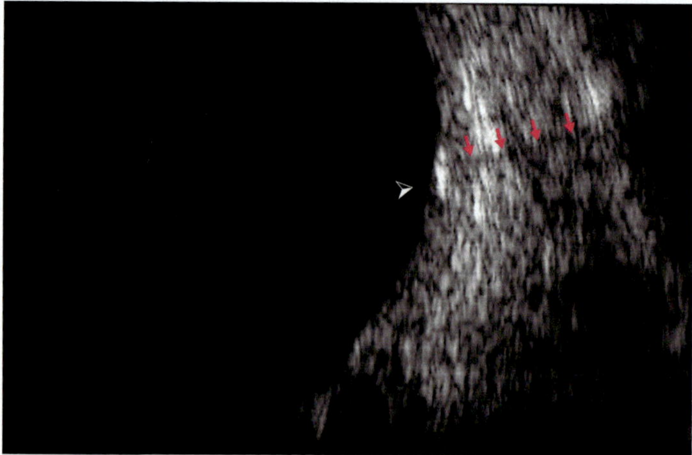

**Fig. 13.28** **Idiopathic sclerochoroidal calcification** in a 55-year-old woman. OD section along the 10:30 o'clock meridian at 10 MHz. The small calcified area (➤), in the superior temporal area of the macula, is preceded by a thin retinal layer and leads to a discreet shadowing (→ red arrows) on the retrobulbar space

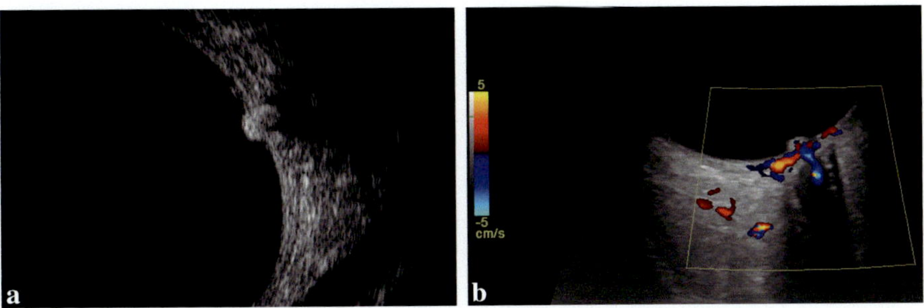

**Fig. 13.29  Optic disc melanocytoma. a**: B-mode para-axial section with a 20 MHz long-focal probe; **b**: CDI, color mode with a B-mode frequency of 18 MHz and a Doppler frequency of 9 MHz. The resolution allows measurements of the papillary elevation and the entire mass (2.1 mm in diameter by 3.2 mm deep), quite echogenic, occupying the entire optic nerve head and invaginating at the level of the lamina cribosa. The appearance is very different from drusen. In particular, naturally, there is no posterior shadowing because this mass is not calcified. There are some small vessels within the lesion that circulate much slower than the central retinal artery

### 13.1.4.5  Melanocytoma

Also called magnocellular nevus [22], these are highly pigmented benign tumors, composed of large cells, selectively located on the surface of the optic disc (Fig. 13.29), but they can also involve the iridociliary complex. Ultrasound reveals a very echogenic lesion, with little vascularization which is purely localized to the optic disc, thus helping in the differential diagnosis with a parapapillary melanoma invading the disc or a primary melanoma of the optic disc, with or without extension to the optic nerve. When localized to the anterior segment, the mass is difficult to differentiate from a melanoma in A-mode or B-mode, but it is more echogenic, heterogeneous, and poorly vascularized in CDI (Fig. 13.30).

### 13.1.4.6  Leiomyoma

These benign, non-pigmented tumors are rare [23] and, as they develop from smooth muscle cells; they are most often peripheral, with involvement of the ciliary body (in more than 70% of published cases). The difference with melanoma or another peripheral parietal tumor can be impossible by ultrasound (Fig. 13.31). The diagnosis is anatomopathological on excisional specimen after special staining showing the characteristic myofibrils.

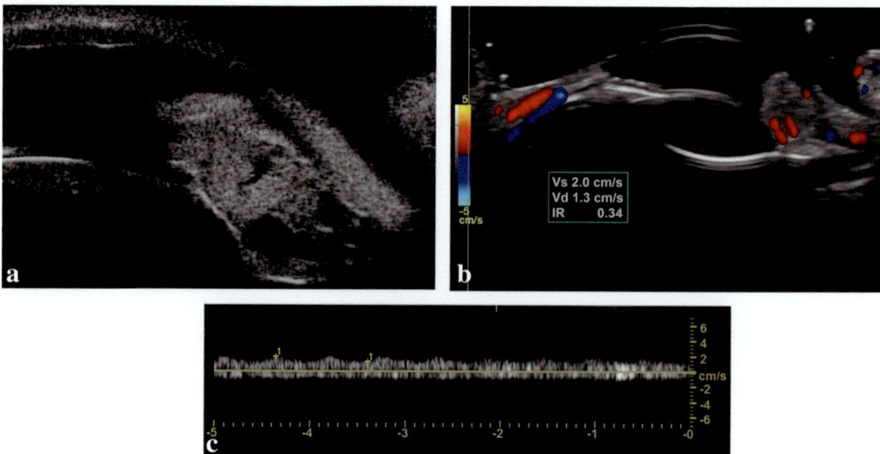

**Fig. 13.30 Iridociliary melanocytoma. a:** B-mode with a 25 MHz short-focal probe along the 7:30 o'clock meridian; **b:** CDI, color mode, cross section according to 1:30–7:30; **c:** CDI, spectral mode. The lesion was not visualized at 50 MHz. In high frequency (**a**), it is correctly visualized, with a moderately echogenic, and above all a very heterogeneous echotexture. In color mode (**b**), some vessels are seen within the posterior part of the lesion, which circulate very slowly in spectral mode (**c**)

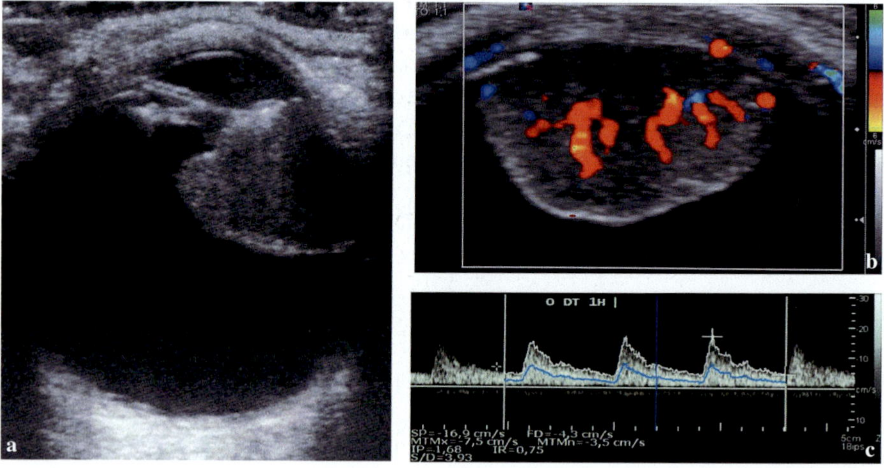

**Fig. 13.31 Ciliochoroidal leiomyoma** in a 22-year-old man. **a:** B-mode, para-axial section in immersion; **b:** CDI, color mode; **c:** CDI, spectral mode. The mass developed from the ciliary body and extending onto the choroid is voluminous, multilobed, moderately echogenic, homogeneous, and highly vascularized, with slightly more resistive flows (RI = 0.75) than what is usually seen in melanoma (apart from associated ocular hypertension). Note the presence of an intraocular implant following an eye trauma two years previously. The non-pigmented appearance of the mass, its position, and its occurrence in a young patient led to tumor excision, thereby providing an exact histological diagnosis and ensuring a good prognosis

### 13.1.4.7   Adenomas

Belonging to acquired tumors developed from the ciliary epithelium, pigmented (PCE) or non-pigmented (NPCE) [24], adenomas exhibit ultrasound signs that are very different from melanomas of the ciliary body with which they are often clinically confused when the latter are poorly pigmented. Adenomas are oval or round, homogeneous, and not very attenuating, displacing the lens without sectorial cataracts, and above all remain stable for a long period of time (Fig. 13.32).

### 13.1.4.8   Pseudotumors

#### a)   Hematomas

These were among the most troublesome problems before modern ultrasound, and being able to detect subretinal hematomas (especially in the context of ARMD) is

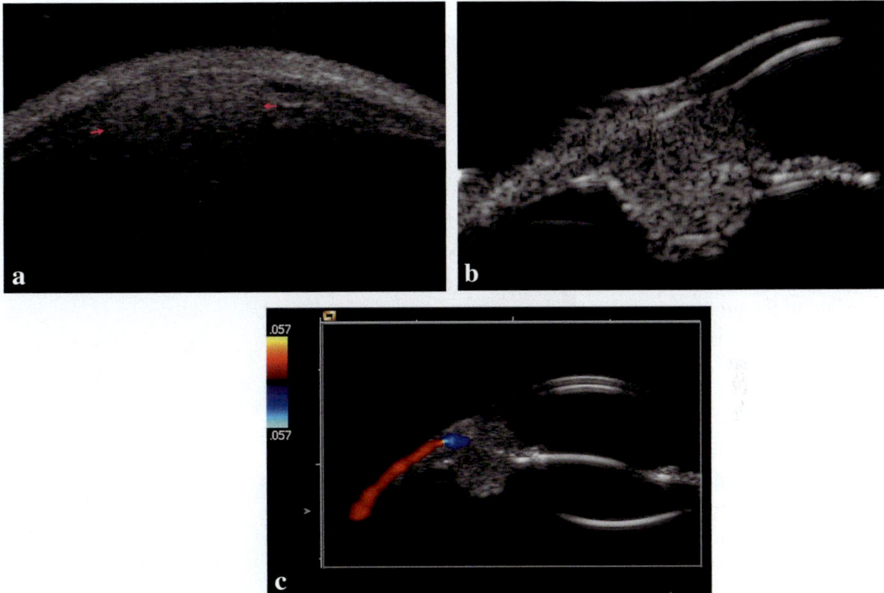

**Fig. 13.32   Adenoma of pigmented epithelium of the ciliary body. a:** Cross-section of the ciliary body, temporal field at 50 MHz; **b:** section of the ciliary body according to the 3 o'clock meridian at 25 MHz; **c:** CDI, color mode. At 50 MHz (**a**), the lesion can barely be discerned (→ pink arrows), but it cannot be measured or evaluated. With high frequency (**b**), the lesion presents as a round, moderately echogenic, homogeneous, and moderately attenuating mass. It invades the iris root and represses the lens without causing cataract, even sectorial. In color mode (**c**), one of the vessels from the arterial circle of the iris can readily be seen, abutting the mass that is not vascularized. This vessel changes color, first anterograde coded in red, then finally with a posterior direction and appearing blue

one of the most decisive contributions provided by CDI. The diagnosis can certainly be guided by the clinical findings, but it is sometimes very difficult, especially when the hematoma is the consequence of peripheral neovessels. It is an echogenic and heterogeneous lesion in B-mode (sometimes even calcifications can be visualized), with an uneven surface, often with bubbles of serous retinal detachment, without signs of choroidal excavation and without any detectable flow in CDI. It is frequently associated with velocimetric disorders of the vessels of the optic nerve head (Fig. 13.33).

b)  **Granulomas** [tuberculosis, sarcoidosis, toxocariasis (see Chap. 14)] are also heterogeneous, but quite echogenic and often located near the posterior pole; they are typically vascularized, however, without characteristic velocimetric constants (Fig. 13.34).

c)  **A serous pigment epithelial detachment in age-related macular degeneration** may present as a small melanoma at the posterior pole. However, choroidal excavation is not usually seen (Fig. 13.35, see Fig. 12.54), and the echotexture is often heterogeneous or even stratified.

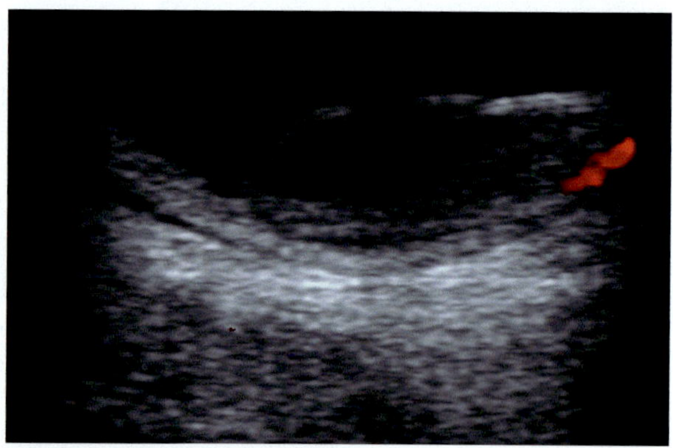

**Fig. 13.33  Subretinal hematoma complicating peripheral neovessels**. CDI inferior temporal field section in the median periphery. The parietal mass is hypoechoic and heterogeneous without centripetal vascularization. The choroidal neovessel at the origin of the process, circulating slowly, is visible for a short distance

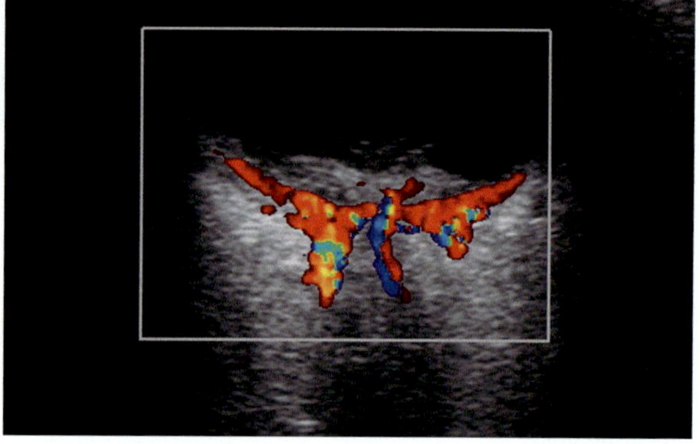

**Fig. 13.34  Sarcoidosis granuloma**. CDI, color mode, axial section. The prepapillary lesion is rather spread out, hyperechoic, weakly vascularized, and associated with some small inflammatory vitreous echoes. (Compare this with Fig. 13.26)

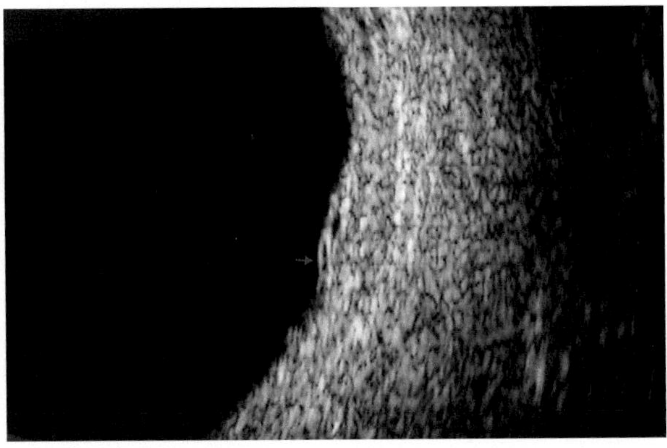

**Fig. 13.35  Macular retinal pigment epithelial detachment.** Parasagittal section passing through the macula at 10 MHz. The small macular protrusion is clearly hypoechoic, but there is no choroidal base (absence of choroidal excavation). Also, note the small underlying serous retinal detachment (→ red arrow). (Compare this with Fig. 12.31)

### d)  Pseudotumoral posterior nodular scleritis

Posterior scleritis appears as a hyperechoic parietal thickening with a sub-tenon episcleral reaction (see Chap. 12). The diagnosis is more difficult when it involves a localized nodular form which can suggest, clinically, an eye tumor. Ultrasound clearly shows the scleral or episcleral situation of the inflammatory or infectious lesion. Moreover, the reflectivity, which varies according to the etiology, is always very different from the hypoechoic and homogeneous reflectivity of a melanoma. (see Fig. 12.62).

In the same way, an anterior scleral granuloma can present as a tumor, but its exact scleral localization is well demonstrated in VHFU, and its heterogeneous echotexture helps to rectify the diagnosis (Fig. 13.36).

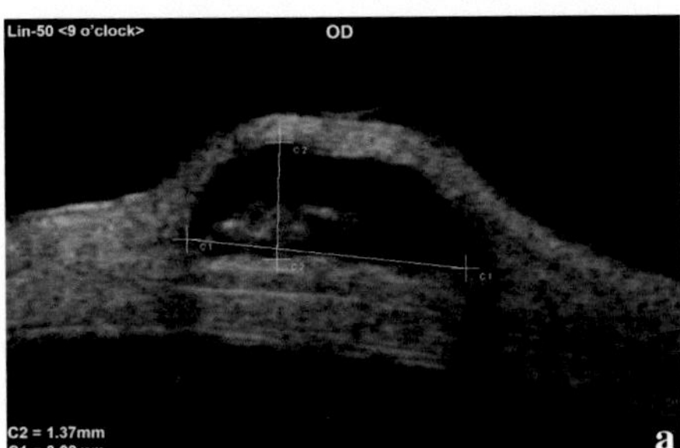

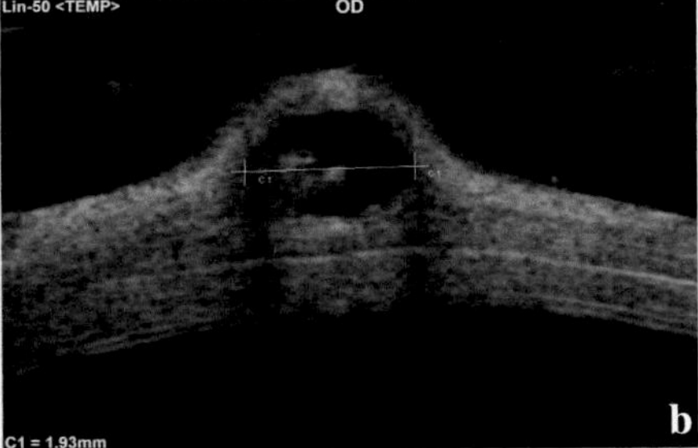


**Fig. 13.36  Anterior scleral granuloma** of the right eye by VHFU at 50 MHz. **a:** Section along the 9 o'clock meridian; **b:** orthogonal section according to the temporal quadrant. The lesion is located 8 mm from the scleral spur. It is not very echogenic and very heterogeneous. The lack of attenuation and, on the contrary, a discreet posterior (acoustic) enhancement as well as the funnel-shaped edge artifacts lateral to the mass are not indicative of a tumoral lesion

**Fig. 13.37 Posterior dislocation of the lens.** B-Mode exploring the inferior quadrant. The nucleus of the lens, placed on the vitreoretinal interface is large, echogenic, heterogeneous, and cataractous, resulting in a posterior shadowing; it is associated with hemorrhagic echoes in the vitreous

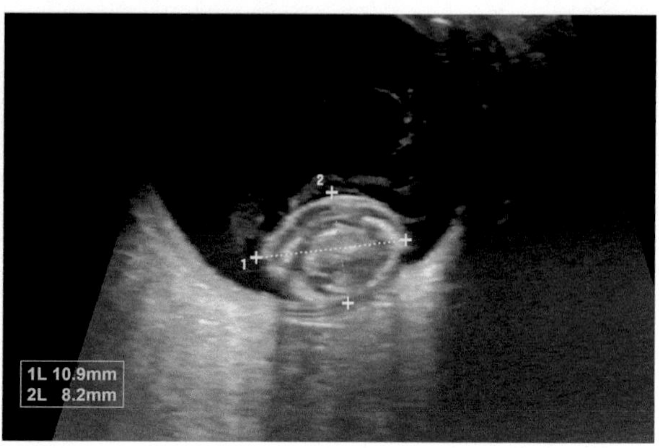


### 13.1.4.9   False Masses

#### a)  Lens dislocation

Differential diagnoses of melanomas typically include dislocations of the nucleus of the lens in the posterior segment [17] (Fig. 13.37). A good semiological analysis readily reveals that the lesion is not hypoechoic, but echogenic and heterogeneous, often, but not always with calcifications resulting in a significant posterior shadowing. In addition, the lesion is frequently mobile, always declive, with the movements of the eyes or the head of the patient.

#### b)  A voluminous, intumescent lens

In the same vein, a voluminous, intumescent, moderately echogenic lens can resemble a parietal mass on very oblique sections approaching the ciliary body and the lens (Fig. 13.38). Naturally, a suitable technique, using a 20 MHz probe in immersion, corrects the diagnosis by revealing such a voluminous lens and invalidating the existence of a ciliary body mass.

#### c)  A peristaphylomatous bulge with high myopia

When prominent (Fig. 13.39), it can sometimes impose for a mass. The location on the periphery of staphyloma, a thickness identical to that of a normal wall, and the absence of choroidal excavation help to the diagnosis.

#### f)  Anterior scleromalacia

Particularly in the vicinity of a previously treated tumor, the appearance can sometimes impose for an externalization or a tumor recurrence (Fig. 13.40). Here again, a suitable technique, in immersion, with a high-frequency probe allows a correct diagnosis to be made.

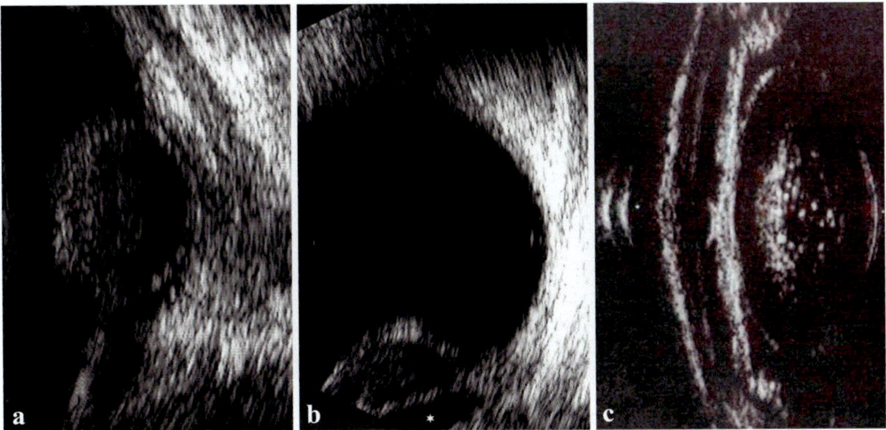

**Fig. 13.38  Intumescent lens.** Patient referred from overseas for a parietal mass (melanoma?) discovered on ultrasound. But no mass was found on clinical examination. **a**: 10 MHz B-mode section of the nasal quadrant in the extreme periphery; **b**: 10 MHz B-mode section OD along the 3 o'clock meridian in the extreme periphery. **c**: 20 MHz short-focal B mode axial section. The section exploring the nasal area in the extreme periphery gives the impression of a parietal mass (of the ciliary body). The section exploring the corresponding meridian already provides a straightforward diagnosis by revealing the anterior chamber (★) and an echogenic lens, due to a cataract. The axial section at 20 MHz clearly shows the intumescent lens, 5.2 mm thick, with its voluminous and echogenic nucleus. Naturally, no mass of the ciliary body is visible in **b** and **c**

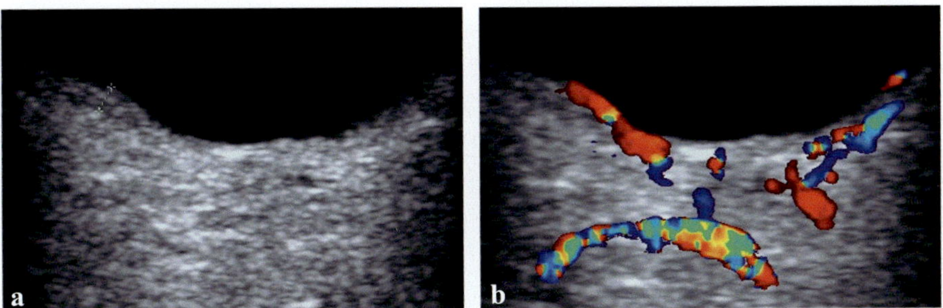

**Fig. 13.39  Peristaphylomatous bulge in a myopic eye**. **a**: B-mode at 20 MHz; **b**: CDI, color mode. On the periphery of the staphyloma, the wall appears thickened when compared to the parietal thickness at the bottom of the staphyloma, which is very thin but in fact has a normal value, measured here as 1.2 mm. Note the retinal vessel, inferior temporal, that perfectly follows the ocular wall, and is very different from a tumor vessel with a centripetal direction

### e)  **Dilation of a vortex vein ampulla**

This should be a consideration when the lesion is small and changes in size during the examination, especially if the probe presses on the eye or after a Valsalva maneuver.

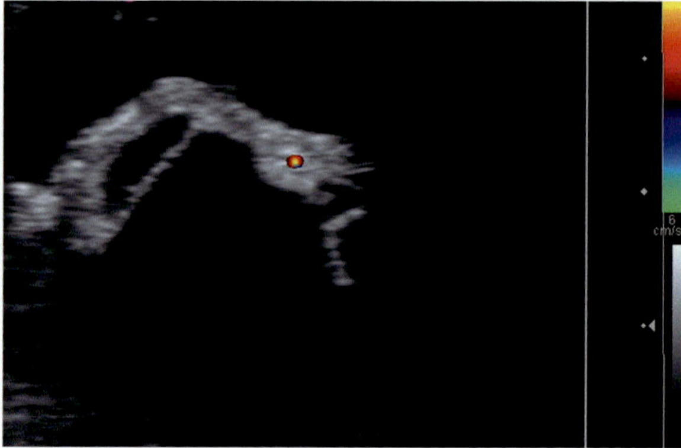

**Fig. 13.40  Scleromalacia behind the ciliary body** following treatment with a $^{125}$I disc for cilio-choroidal melanoma. CDI, color mode, section along the 3 o'clock meridian. The parietal protrusion, which is quite wide and clinically pigmented, is not due to a mass but weakening of the sclera, in contact with the hyperechoic treated tumor, where a very low flow persists. Also, note a small retinal detachment in the concavity of the scleral outgrowth

A characteristic situation involving the emergence of one of the four vortex veins and the venous flows on the periphery of the lesion in CDI in the vicinity of the small protrusion that is anechoic and non-hypoechoic are the diagnostic criteria (Fig. 13.41).

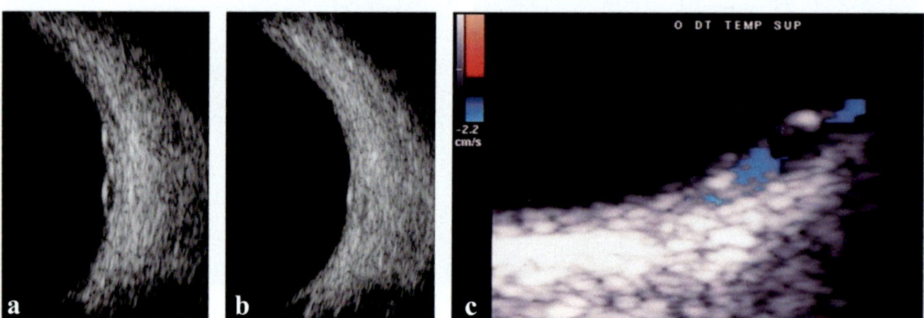


**Fig. 13.41  Varix of a superior temporal vortex vein ampulla. a:** Superior temporal section; **b:** identical section after slight pressure on the globe by the probe; **c:** CDI, color mode. The lesion is bilobed and hypoechoic. It almost disappears with slight pressure. CDI clearly shows the vortex vein flow, coded in blue, on both sides of the small protrusion and emanating from it

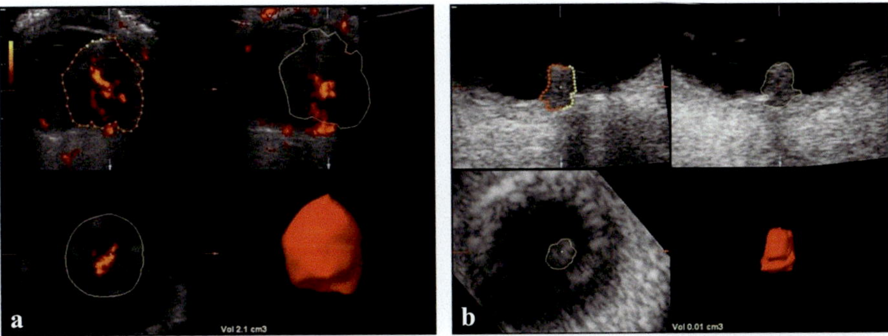



**Fig. 13.42  4D acquisition** of two melanomas with very different volumes. **a**: A rather large cilio-choroidal melanoma of 2.1 cm³; **b**: a small melanoma of the posterior pole of 0.1 cm³. For each case, representation of the lesion in the three dimensions of space, horizontal, sagittal, and azimuthal, as well as a volume reconstruction

### *13.1.5  Tissue Characterization*

The theory for this has already been presented in Chap. 1. Tissue characterization methods focus on estimation of the backscatter coefficient as a function of frequency. The two main teams that have studied tissue characterization of melanomas are those of Han Thijssen in Nijmegen [25] and Jackson Coleman in New York [26]. Both focused on characterization of the different histological types of melanomas and their associated prognosis. We have shown [27] that these same backscatter parameters can also be applied to the changes observed in these tumors after proton beam therapy.

Unfortunately, all these studies require processing of data acquired in the laboratory, and this processing takes a lot of time. It can, therefore, not be routinely used through a simple program.

### *13.1.6  3D/4D Imaging*

It is rarely available in France, and yet deserves to be developed. Indeed, it is not a gadget, but it is a really useful technique for evaluation of the exact volume of lesions (Fig. 13.42), the occurrence of metastases being parallel to the volume of the primary tumor; for monitoring of small tumors by studying the convexity of their surface; and for undertaking tissue characterization.

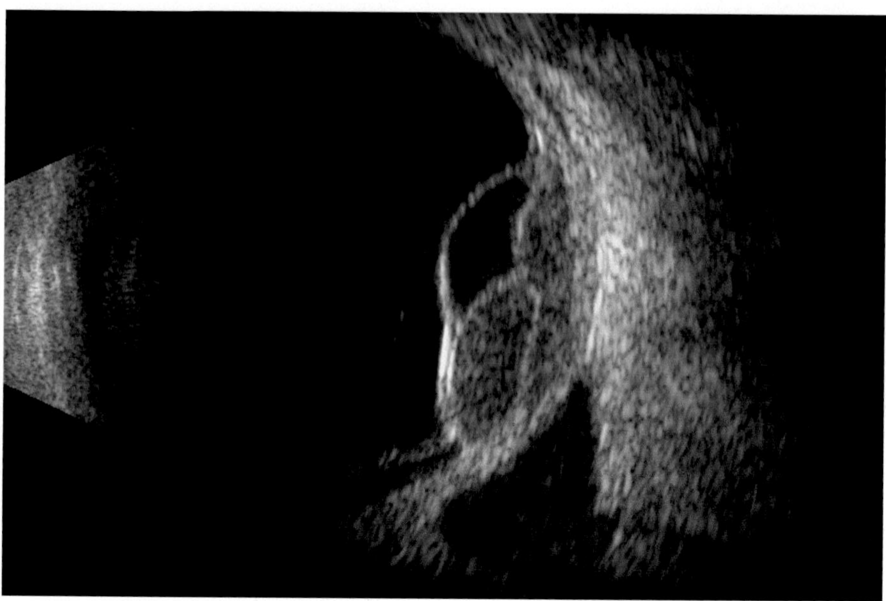

**Fig. 13.43** **Transscleral extension of a melanoma associated with retinal detachment.** Section at 10 MHz according to the 12 o'clock meridian. The nodular orbital lesion is molded to the sclera and remains limited by the Tenon capsule. The different attenuation and contrast with the vitreous, on the one hand, and with the orbit, on the other hand, make the sub-tenonian extension appear less echogenic than the intraocular lesion

### 13.1.7 Extension

This can be **transscleral** (Fig. 13.43), limited by the Tenon capsule. A classic pitfall [17] is to consider the tendon of an oblique muscle passing behind the ocular wall next to the tumor as an extension of a inferior temporal or superior temporal melanoma (Fig. 13.44).

An extension **to the optic nerve** of a parapapillary melanoma is difficult to visualize by ultrasound if the affected optic nerve is not very large (see Fig. 18.16). It is best revealed with MRI after gadolinium injection.

Finally, it may consist of **a large orbital mass**. Ultrasound is able to reveal a hypoechoic and vascularized retrobulbar lesion, although again, MRI is superior for a more detailed study, especially at the orbital apex.

### 13.1.8 Post-Treatment Follow-Up

When the tumor is not too large, it is eligible for conservative treatment, either brachytherapy with a disc of radioactive cobalt, ruthenium, or iodine, or by proton beam therapy. Along with clinical examination, ultrasound naturally plays a role in the follow-up of tumors after conservative treatment. After proton beam therapy, the

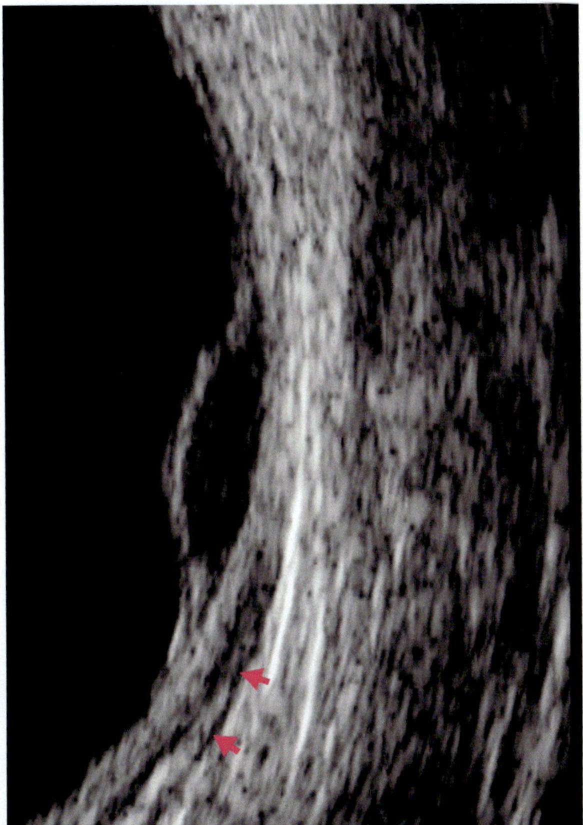

**Fig. 13.44  False extension of a superior temporal melanoma**. B-mode with a 20 MHz long-focal probe. The small episcleral hypoechoic area (➤ thick red arrows) corresponds to the tendon of the inferior oblique muscle, which is easily identified by its moderately echogenic fibers

tantalum clips can be seen that were placed on the sclera around the tumor to guide the proton beam (Fig. 13.45).

During the first month, in connection with inflammatory phenomena, the tumor may temporarily increase in volume. From the sixth month after treatment, and often only a year later, the tumor starts to decrease in thickness and gradually assumes an echogenic and heterogeneous echotexture, sometimes with hypoechoic areas of necrosis (Fig. 13.46) in relation to fibro-hemorrhagic changes. This volume reduction is slow and rarely results in a flat scar.

At the healing stage, the lesion has the appearance of a small hyperechoic lesion.

Similarly, in CDI there are changes at the end of the treatment. Very early on, at approximately 6 months before the decrease in size of the tumor, a decrease in tumor vascularization can be observed: in color mode, fewer vessels are seen, and in spectral mode, a decrease can be detected in the PSV of the intratumoral vessels (Fig. 13.46). While lacking certainty, one can wonder if a too rapid disappearance of

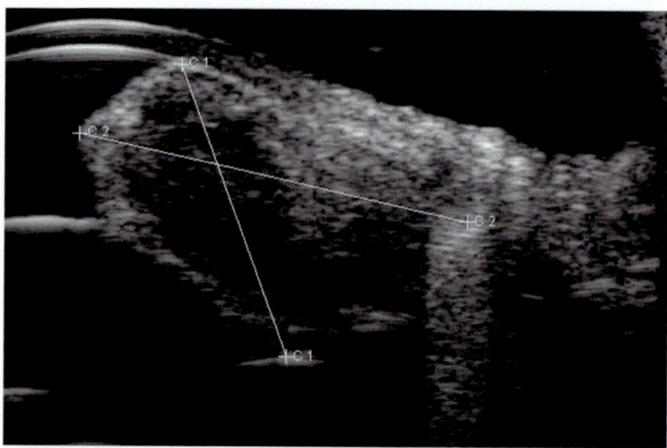

**Fig. 13.45 Quite large iridociliary melanoma explored after placement of clips for proton beam therapy**. Section at 50 MHz along the 8 o'clock meridian. The clip, which is readily recognized because of the comet-tail artifact that it causes, is located at the posterior edge of the tumor, which is, even not yet treated, slightly to moderately echogenic and heterogeneous

**Fig. 13.46 Melanoma of the ciliary body assessed four years after proton therapy**. CDI, color mode. The lesion is still voluminous and very heterogeneous, with areas of necrosis that are poorly echogenic. It is entirely avascular

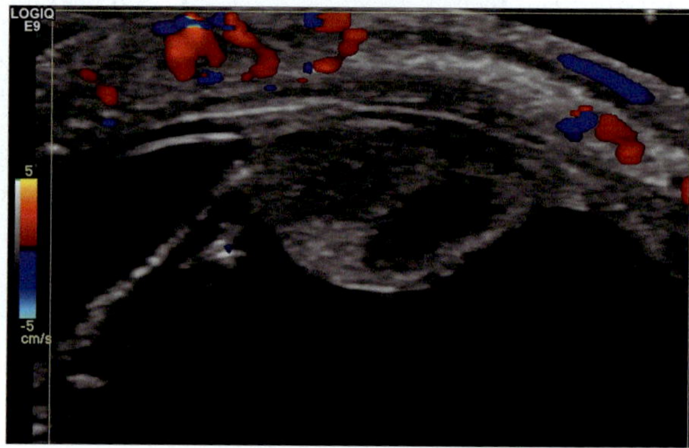

intratumoral vascular activity (less than 9 months after treatment) could be a pejorative development, as this corresponds with tumors with very fast tumor doubling times. On the other hand, visualization of vessels a long time (more than 18 months) after conservative treatment is often related to recurrence of the tumor (Fig. 13.47).

However, in some cases, we have observed the same vascular activity for many (up to 15) years. It is, therefore, important not to assume that a recurrence may have occurred based on a single examination. Rather, the measured dimensions and the echotexture of the lesion should also be taken into account.

There are many other eye tumors in adults, of the uvea or retina [23], such as capillary, cavernous, and racemose hemangiomas of the retina, vasoproliferative tumors of the retina; neuroglial tumors, astrocytic hamartomas, progressive solitary astrocytomas and glioneuromas; benign and malignant intraocular lymphoid tumors (Fig. 13.48), and phakomatoses.

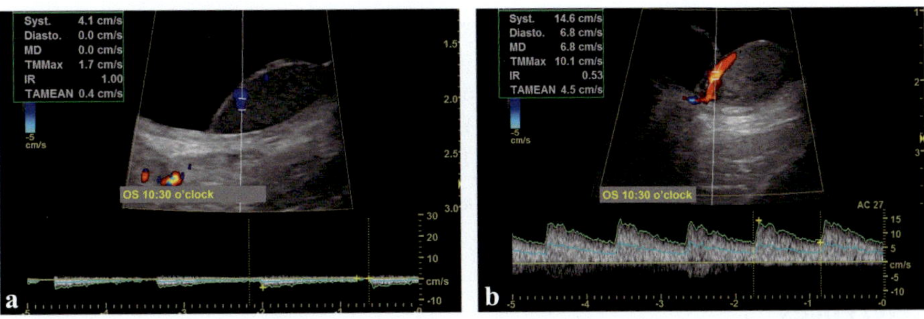

**Fig. 13.47 Progressive recurrence of a choroidal melanoma treated with proton beam therapy**. CDI color mode section according to the 11 o'clock meridian. **a**: Six months after proton therapy; **b**: eighteen months after proton therapy. In **a**, the lesion is weakly vascularized by small centripetal vessels from superficial vessels with a low PSV of 4 cm/s. In **b**, the mass has increased in thickness (7.4 mm vs. 4.9 mm) and a superficial vessel appears that has quite fast circulation, with a PSV of 14.6 cm/s. In addition, total retinal detachment is also seen

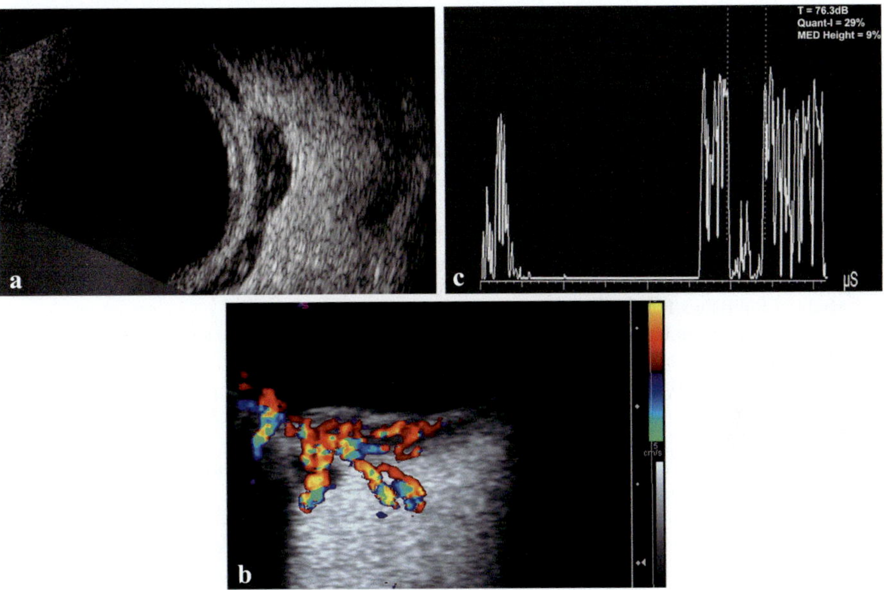

**Fig. 13.48 Slowly progressing parietal lymphoma of the left eye**. **a**: Temporal field section at 10 MHz with intermediate gain (86 dB); **b**: CDI color mode along the 9 o'clock meridian; **c**: standardized A-mode at tissue sensitivity (T = 76.3 dB). The most obvious lesion is **episcleral, subtenonian**, thick, from 2 to 3.5 mm, scalloped outwards (orbital intraconal space), poorly echogenic, heterogeneous, and highly vascularized, but there is also a less voluminous and thinner **retinochoroidal** lesion, with similar characteristics. Follow-up over several years did not reveal any progression of this lymphoid lesion

In all cases, along with clinical assessment and angiography, ultrasound helps in the diagnostic work-up, with MRI, to assess the extension, and, with clinical assessment, to follow the tumor after treatment. For posterior segment lesions, it is always useful to combine B-mode, at 10 (or15) MHz and 20 MHz, standardized A-mode and Color Doppler Imaging, and for the anterior segment VHFU at 50 MHz, HFU at 25 MHz, and Color Doppler Imaging.

# References


1. Shields CL, Shields JA. Tumors of the conjunctiva and cornea. Surv Ophthalmol. 2004;49(1):3–24.
2. Dorval T, Dendale R, Desjardins L. Mélanome Oculaire. Rev Prat. 2004;54(19):2093–101.
3. Zimmerman LE. Melanoma of uvea in Spencer WH: ophthalmic pathology, an atlas and textbook. 3rd ed. Philadelphia:WB Saunders Company; 1986, pp. 2072–2139.
4. Berges O, Cerezal L, Sterkers M, Mimoun G, Piekarski JD. Mélanome choroïdien en bouton de col. Corrélations anatomo-radiologiques. J Neuroradiol. 1994;21(1):50–5.
5. Shields CL, Shields JA, De Potter P, Cater J, Tardio D, Barrett J. Diffuse Choroidal melanoma. clinical features predictive of metastasis. Arch Ophthalmol. 1996;114(8):956–63.
6. Cham MC, Pavlin CJ. Ultrasound detection of posterior scleral bowing in young patients with choroidal melanoma. Can J Ophthalmol. 2000;35(5):263–6.
7. Verbeek AM. Ultrasonography as a diagnostic tool in Ophthalmology—atlas and diagnostic strategies. Oosterbeek: Veress Publishing; 2000.
8. Tranquart F, Berges O, Koskas P, Arsene S, Rossazza C, Pisella PJ, Pourcelot L. Color doppler imaging of orbital vessels: personal experience and literature review. J Clin Ultrasound. 2003;31(5):258–73.
9. Guthoff R. Ultrasound in ophthalmologic diagnosis—a practical guide. New York: Thieme Medical Publishes Inc.; 1991.
10. Georgalas I, Petrou P, Papaconstantinou D, Brouzas D, et al. Iris cysts: a comprehensive review on diagnosis and treatment. Surv Ophthalmol. 2018;63(3):347–364.
11. Krema H, Santiago RA, Gonzalez JE, Pavlin CJ. Spectral-domain optical coherence tomography versus ultrasound biomicroscopy for imaging of nonpigmented iris tumors. Am J Ophthalmol. 2013;156(4):806–12.
12. Maslin JS, Teng CC, Materin M. Free-floating, pigmented cysts in the anterior chamber causing ocular hypertension. Ocul Oncol Pathol. 2016;2(4):239–41.
13. Shields JA, Shields CL, Lois N, Mercado G. Iris cysts in children: classification, incidence, and management. The 1998 Torrence A Makley Jr Lecture. Br J Ophthalmol. 1999;83(3):334–8.
14. Giuliari GP, Krema H, McGowan HD, Pavlin CJ, Simpson ER. Clinical and ultrasound biomicroscopy features associated with growth in iris melanocytic lesions. Am J Ophthalmol. 2012;153(6):1043–9.
15. Weisbrod DJ, Pavlin CJ, Emara K, Mandell MA, McWhae J, Simpson ER. Small ciliary body tumors: ultrasound biomicroscopic assessment and follow-up of 42 patients. Am J Ophthalmol. 2006;141(4):622–8.
16. Poujol J, Chaintron M-C. Analysis of a recent series (254 cases) of choroidal tumours in Documenta Ophthalmologica Proceedings Series 51—Ultrasonography in Ophthalmology 11. In: Thijssen JM, Hillman J-S, Gallenga PE, Cennamo G, editors. Dordrecht: Jluwer Academic Publishers;1988. pp 157–164.
17. Frazier Byrne S, Green RL. Ultrasound of the eye and orbit. 2nd ed. Mosby, St. Louis; 2002.
18. Mathis T, Jardel P, Loria O, Delaunay B, Nguyen AM, Lanza F, Mosci C, Caujolle JP, Kodjikian L, Thariat J. New concepts in the diagnosis and management of choroidal metastases. Prog Retin Eye Res. 2019;68:144–76.

19. Campagnoli TR, Medina CA, Singh AD. Choroidal melanoma initially treated as hemangioma: diagnostic and therapeutic considerations. Retin Cases Brief Rep. 2016;10(2):175–82.
20. Farguette F, Bonnin N, Nezzar H, Chiambarretta F, Bacin F. Mélanome choroïdien et tumeur mélanocytaire à potentiel évolutif » controlatérale chez un patient de 45 ans, à propos d'un cas. J Fr Ophtalmol. 2012;35(8):635–41.
21. Honavar SG, Shields CL, Demirci H, Shields JA. Sclerochoroidal calcification: clinical manifestations and systemic associations. Arch Ophthalmol. 2001;119(6):833–40.
22. Cogan DG. Discussion of pigmented ocular tumors. In: Boniuk M, editors. Ocular and adnexal tumors : new and controversial aspects. Mosby, St. Louis; 1964. p. 385.
23. Zografos L. Tumeurs intra-oculaires—rapport de la Société Française d'Ophtalmologie. Paris: Masson; 2002.
24. Green WR. Neuroepithelial tumors of ciliary body in spencer WH: ophthalmic pathology, an atlas and textbook. 3rd ed. Philadelphia: WB Saunders Company; 1986. pp. 1246–1292.
25. Thijssen JM, Verbeek AM, Romijn RL, De Wolffrouendaal D, Oosterhuis JA. Echographic differentiation of histologic types of intraocular melanomas. Ultrasound Med Biol. 1991;17:127–38.
26. Coleman DJ, Lizzi FL. Computerized ultrasonic tissue characterization of ocular tumors. Am J Ophthalmol. 1983;96(2):165–75.
27. Boudinet M, Bergès O, Le Huerou JY, Lumbroso-Le Rouic L, Desjardins L, Laugier P. Quantitative echography in the follow-up of patients treated with proton-beam irradiation for primary choroidal melanomas. Ultrasound Med Biol. 2007;33(7):1046–56.

# Chapter 14
# Eye Masses in Children

Olivier Bergès and Monique Elmaleh-Bergès

**Abstract** This chapter deals with the eye masses in children, emphasizing first the diagnostic issues of retinoblastoma (RB), which is the most common eye tumor in children, with three anatomical clinical forms: endophytic, exophytic and diffuse infiltrative. Ultrasound, that has to be exhaustive and bilateral, is essential to disclose calcifications which are characteristic of the disease. Color Doppler imaging (CDI) can show a non-characteristic vascularization. Usually, RB occurs on a normal axial length eye. The extension of the tumor can be seen in ultrasound, but is the responsability of MRI. Among the long list of differential diagnoses known as pseudogliomas, only the most frequent are detailed: persistent fetal vasculature and vitreo-retinal dysplasia, Coats' disease, toxocariasis, colobomas and morning glory disc anomaly, retinal detachments and congenital retinal folds. Finally, other tumors and masses in children are considered: diffuse choroidal angioma and Sturge–Weber syndrome, medulloepithelioma, juvenile nevoxanthoendothelioma or xanthogranuloma, cavernous angioma of the retina and prepapillary capillary angioma.

## 14.1   Introduction

Ultrasound is the foremost medical imaging technique for exploration of an eye lesion, especially in children [1]. Before the child is able to cooperate (approximately 4–5 years of age), sedation is necessary to perform the examination. Before 4 months, a baby bottle after a period of fasting is most often sufficient. In infants and small children, different sedation protocols can be used, in a hospital setting. In case of failure, it is necessary to resort to general anesthesia (GA), which will be more or less essential depending on the information to be obtained. For example, Chap. 11

O. Bergès (✉)
Rothschild Foundation Hospital, Paris, France
e-mail: oberges@for.paris

M. Elmaleh-Bergès
Robert Debré University Hospital, Paris, France

    327
O. Bergès (ed.), *Echography of the Eye and Orbit,*
https://doi.org/10.1007/978-3-031-41467-1_14

provides examples whereby ultrasound under general anesthesia was coupled with a clinical examination for exploration of neonatal corneal opacities. In addition to VHFU at 50 MHz, a detailed study of vessels by Color Doppler Imaging (CDI) also often benefits from GA in small children. In the absence of anesthesia, it is advisable to work through the eyelids, without topical corneal anesthesia but using ophthalmic contact gel warmed to body temperature [2]. In this chapter, we not only discuss eye masses in children but also the various conditions of the posterior segment in children, for which ultrasound can provide useful information for diagnosis and management.

## 14.2   Leukocoria and Retinoblastoma

Leukocoria (a white appearance of the pupil with no red reflection of the fundus upon illumination) or visual disturbances (absence of pursuit, strabismus, nystagmus, etc.) are the most frequent warning signs for requesting eye imaging. Leukocoria can be indicative of a congenital cataract or a lesion of the posterior segment, which in half of cases is related to retinoblastoma, which is a malignant tumor, and in the other half of cases with a multitude of congenital malformations or vascular entities. The latter are benign conditions that are not life-threatening, albeit often with a rather poor visual prognosis. In order to guide the diagnosis, an initial ultrasound, without general anesthesia (GA), should be performed very rapidly, allowing a retinoblastoma (a most often calcified lesion) or another cause to be identified and thus determine the urgency of the explorations to be followed.

### *14.2.1   Retinoblastoma (RB)*

This is the most common eye tumor in children [3], with an incidence of 1/20,000 births. In more than 98% of cases, they occur before three years of age. Sixty percent of cases are unilateral, with a median age at diagnosis of two years. In 40% of cases, retinoblastoma is bilateral, with a median age of onset of one year. All bilateral and unilateral multifocal forms are hereditary with a syndrome of genetic predisposition to cancer, the subject having a constitutional mutation of the *RB1* gene, resulting in a more than 90% risk of developing retinoblastoma as well as a risk of secondary tumors [4].

The first procedure to be performed is a fundus examination under general anesthesia. In typical cases, this reveals a white eye mass with vessels on the surface. This fundus examination also allows establishment of the stage of the tumor according to the ABC classification [5]. Differential diagnosis with other pathologies is most often easy.

When the fundus examination under GA has confirmed the diagnosis of retinoblastoma, it is advisable to perform an MRI and an ultrasound, preferably carried out during the same GA.

Ultrasound:

- allows precise axial length measurements of both eyes (B-mode guided biometry)
- confirms the diagnosis, or refers to another pathology
- locates the mass as accurately as possible and evaluates its size
- identifies and characterizes calcifications
- looks for extension to the optic disc and the retrolaminar portion of the optic nerve, depending on the situation and the morphology of the calcifications.

Local and distal extension can **only** be determined by MRI, which is **essential**: to the optic nerve, to the orbit, to the CNS (and in particular the search for trilateral retinoblastoma). However, at present, no imaging modality is able to properly assess extension to the choroid.

### 14.2.1.1  Positive Diagnosis

(a) **This is established** based on the presence of a calcified ocular parietal mass associated with retinal detachment occurring in a small child with normal-sized eyes [6]. The lesion(s) must be measured as accurately as possible in all three dimensions, and should be located according to the meridians where it is/they are detected.

(b) **The three anatomical clinical forms** [7] to be discerned by imaging are: the endophytic form (with development towards the vitreous) and the exophytic form (with subretinal development), which are the most frequent, involving a calcified mass (Fig. 14.1a, b)); and the diffuse infiltrative form, which is rare and difficult to diagnose because the clinical presentation is often atypical (inflammatory), and which can occur in older children, with a delay in diagnosis (on average five months); ultrasound is essential for the diagnosis as it reveals a thick and bloated retinal detachment [8], often without calcifications (Fig. 14.1c).

(c) **The calcifications** can be voluminous, or on the contrary very fine and punctiform (in which case without an obvious posterior shadowing). The three imaging techniques, ultrasound, CT, and MRI reveal the voluminous calcifications quite well. For discrete microcalcifications, it appears that the performance of scanners, even the most recent ones, is not actually better than the latest generation of ultrasound devices [9] (Fig. 14.2). **And a CT scan is absolutely contraindicated** to reveal these calcifications, since it is irradiating and it could, therefore, promote the occurrence of secondary tumors in carriers of the mutated *RB1* gene, even in the long run.

(d) **Vascularization.** This type of lesion is vascularized, but less than melanoma in adults, and without arborization. In spectral Doppler, the resistivity index (RI) is close to 0.50, which is close to that of the central retinal artery (Fig. 14.3). It can

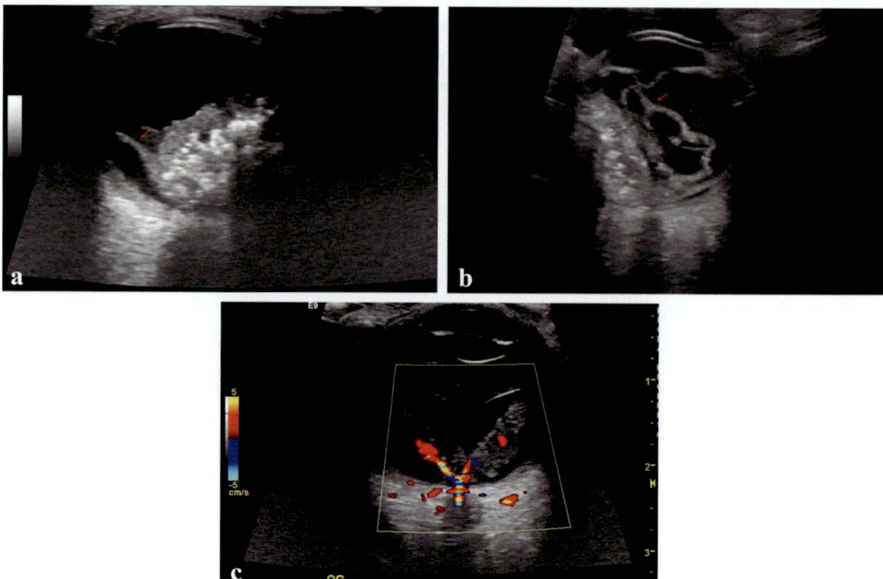

**Fig. 14.1  Retinoblastomas: anatomical ultrasound forms. a: Endophytic form,** group IV and D: the calcified mass is located in front of the retinal detachment (→); **b: exophytic form** group V and E: the calcified mass is located under the detachment (→;), associated with inferior dislocation of the lens, which is not seen on this axial section, and extension to the anterior chamber; **c: diffuse infiltrative form:** total retinal detachment, without visible calcification, with a very significant moderately echogenic thickening of the detached retina, weakly vascularized

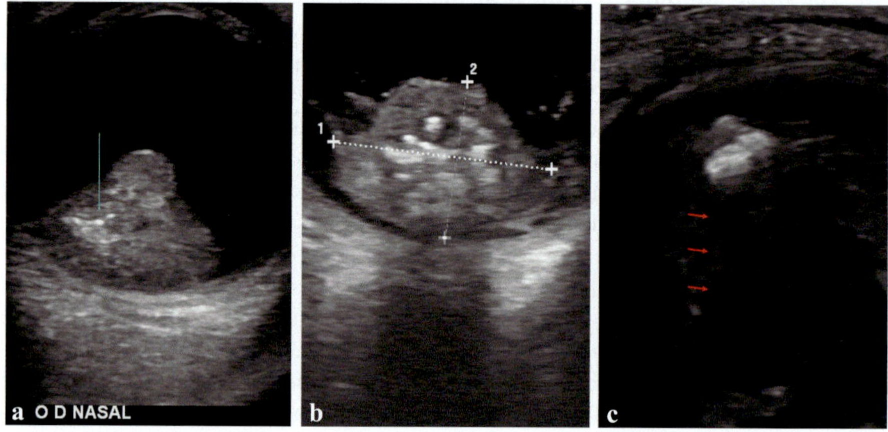

**Fig. 14.2  Retinoblastoma—calcifications. a: Punctiform,** without posterior shadowing; **b: small in size,** but with posterior shadowing; **c: unique, and macroscopic,** with posterior shadowing (→ red arrows)

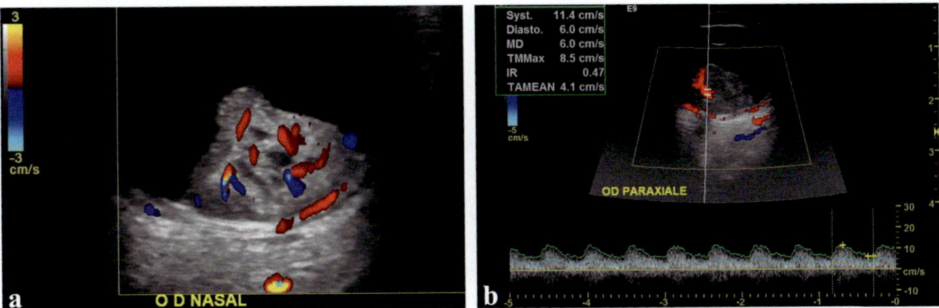

**Fig. 14.3  Retinoblastoma—vascularization. a: Color mode; b: spectral mode.** Quite characteristic: present, but poorly developed and without arborization, with a RI = 0.47

be useful to assess the degree of vascularization of the lesion, the different orbital arteries, and muscles before and during treatment with intra-arterial injections of alkylating agent. In addition, any colored dot in color Doppler is not necessarily a vessel but can be caused by calcification (twinkling artifact) (Fig. 14.4).

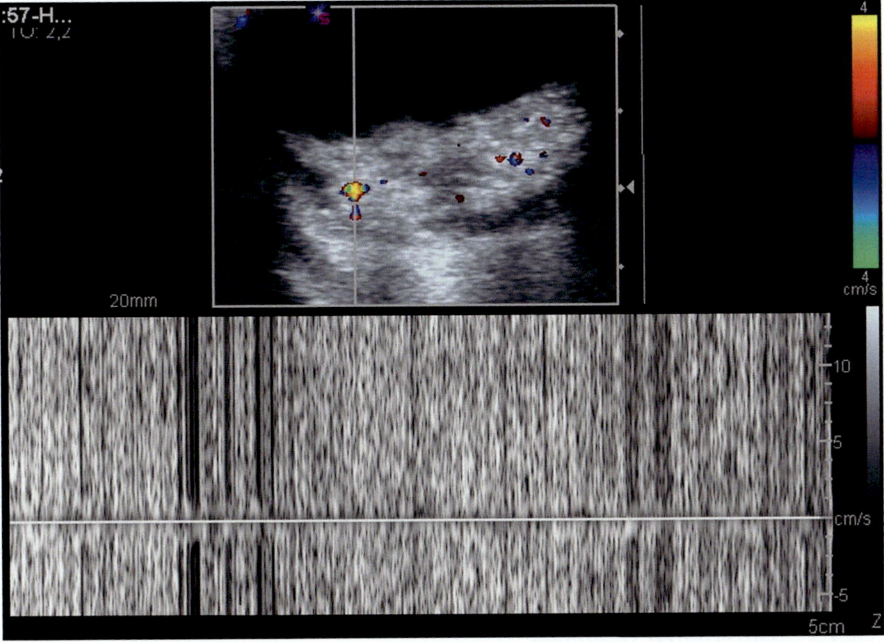

**Fig. 14.4  Twinkling artifact** disclosing a calcification within an echogenic mass, that was not visible in B-mode; CDI, color and spectral modes. In color mode, the colored spot is coarser and lighter than that of a vessel. In spectral mode, no flow can be discerned, but there are high bidirectional frequency disturbances

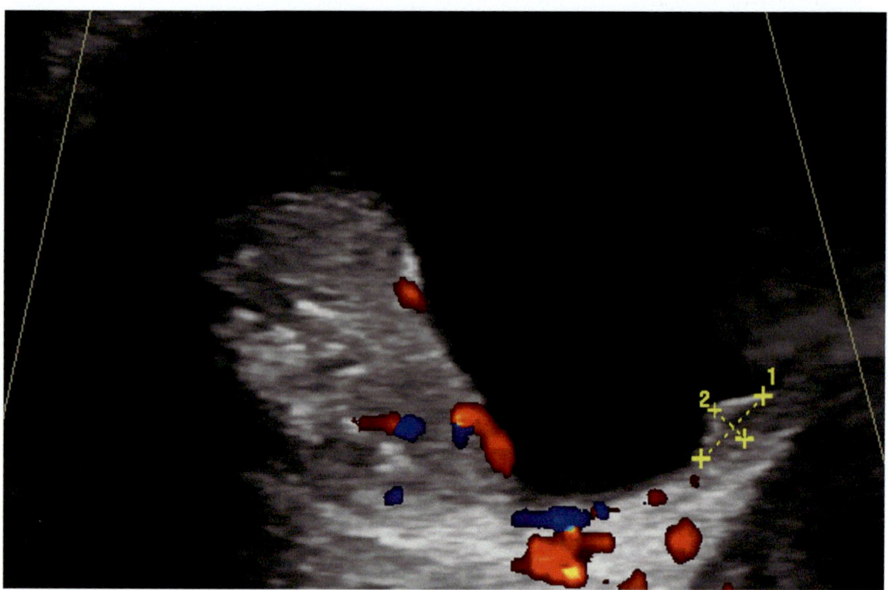

**Fig. 14.5 Multifocal retinoblastoma of the left eye**. CDI cross-section ranging from approximately 5 o'clock to 11 o'clock. The larger of the two lesions, inferior temporal, endophytic, with calcifications and vessels measured 13 mm long × 7 mm thick. The smaller one, superior nasal, without calcification or vessel is measured at 3 mm long × 1.5 mm thick

(e) **The axial length** of the two eyes should be measured (in relation to the age of the child). With some exceptions, the affected eye is not microphthalmic.

(f) **Bilaterality, or multifocality** (Fig. 14.5), should always be checked, and it is associated with hereditary forms in subjects carrying the mutated *RB1* gene.

(g) **Assessment of extensions** is typically performed using MRI [10], with a well-established protocol [11]. However, as in 3 T MRI, ultrasound can also reveal extension to the optic disc (Fig. 14.6) or choroid (Fig. 14.7). It should always assess the impact on the anterior segment, the anterior chamber (Fig. 14.8), and the lens. It must also look for spreading into the vitreous (see Fig. 12.31) and into the subretinal space.

(h) **The diffuse anterior form** [12]. This is rare, accounting for 1–2% of cases, occurring in older children, affecting the iris and/or the ciliary body (Fig. 14.9), the lesions typically being less calcified (Fig. 14.10).

### 14.2.1.2 Differential Diagnosis

This relates to lesions formerly referred to as pseudogliomas, or pseudoretinoblastomas. They form a long list [13], including: persistent fetal vasculature (PFV), Coats' disease, retrolental fibroplasia, the last stage of retinopathy of prematurity (ROP), chorioretinal colobomas, morning glory syndrome, myelin fibers, toxocarosis, other

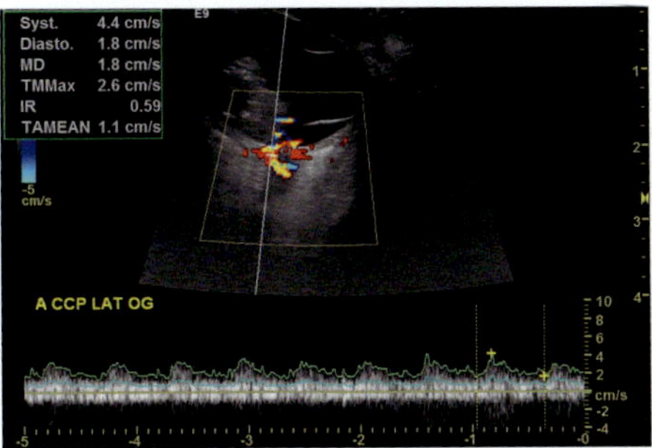

**Fig. 14.6** **Microinvasion to the optic disc by a group V or D retinoblastoma**. CDI, color and spectral modes, of vessels of the optic nerve head. No visualization of the normal central retinal vessels, the ocular flow being taken over by a large short posterior lateral ciliary artery. As the invasion was microscopic and not confirmed by MRI, a conservative treatment, triple chemotherapy + laser and cryotherapy was undertaken, with a favorable outcome at four years

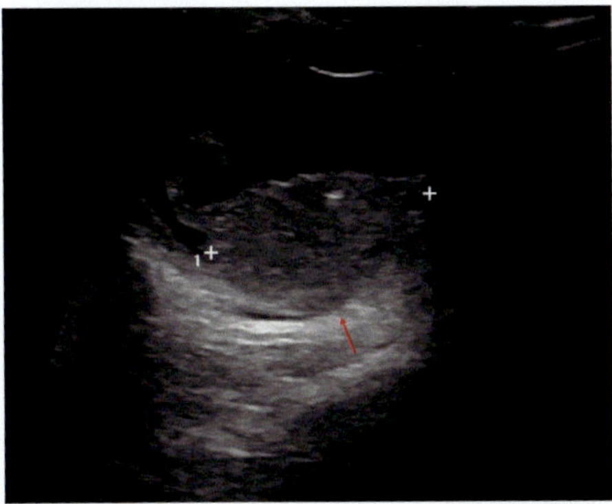

**Fig. 14.7** **Probable extension of a Group D exophytic retinoblastoma to the choroid**. Large moderately echogenic mass of 14 mm in diameter × 8 mm in thickness with areas of necrosis and a small calcification without shadowing. There appears to be a choroidal excavation (→ red arrow), as in melanoma, leading to the diagnosis of a possible extension to the choroid

pediatric tumors and intraocular masses, uveitis, X-linked retinoschisis, congenital retinal folds, retinal detachments, familial exudative vitreoretinopathy (FEVR), vitreoretinal dysplasia, incontinentia pigmenti, and tunica vasculosa lentis.

We will only detail the most frequently encountered:

For all these conditions, the first differential diagnostic criterion is the axial length, to be related to the age of the child [14]: normal in case of retinoblastoma and decreased (microphthalmia) in congenital anomalies such as persistent fetal vasculature.

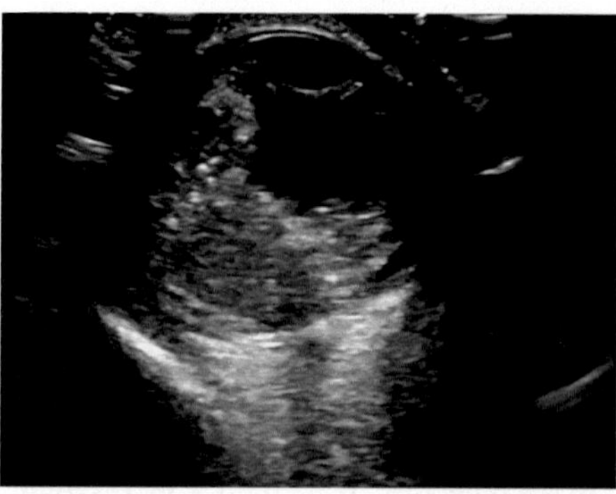

**Fig. 14.8** **Impact on the anterior segment of a huge retinoblastoma of group V or E**. Athalamia and ocular hypertension led the clinicians believe for a time that it was a congenital glaucoma. Ultrasound corrected this impression. Enucleation was the only possible treatment because of the size of the lesion and the impact on the anterior segment

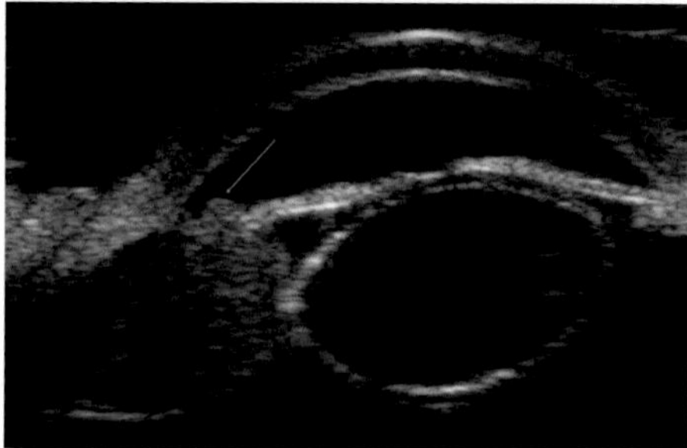

**Fig. 14.9** **Diffuse anterior retinoblastoma**. HFU at 25 MHz. The ultrasound revealed the large mass of the ciliary body, the submerged part of the iceberg of the small iris nodule that was clinically visible (→ green arrow). Neither lesion exhibits calcification. Densification of the capsules of the voluminous lens can be seen, related to cataract

## Persistent Fetal Vasculature (PFV)

This is a bona fide syndrome, exhibiting multiple abnormalities of the anterior segment, the posterior segment, or both, or even abnormalities of the optic nerve, and even malformations of the size and shape of the eyes [15]. For a time, the forms interesting the posterior segment were called persistent hyperplastic primary vitreous (PHPV) [16], but this term is too restrictive and should no longer be used. The damage is always unilateral; otherwise, vitreoretinal dysplasia (VRD) is considered. It appears to affect boys slightly more than girls, and microphthalmia is very common. It is found in 75% of cases, and it is moderate to severe in almost half of cases [17].

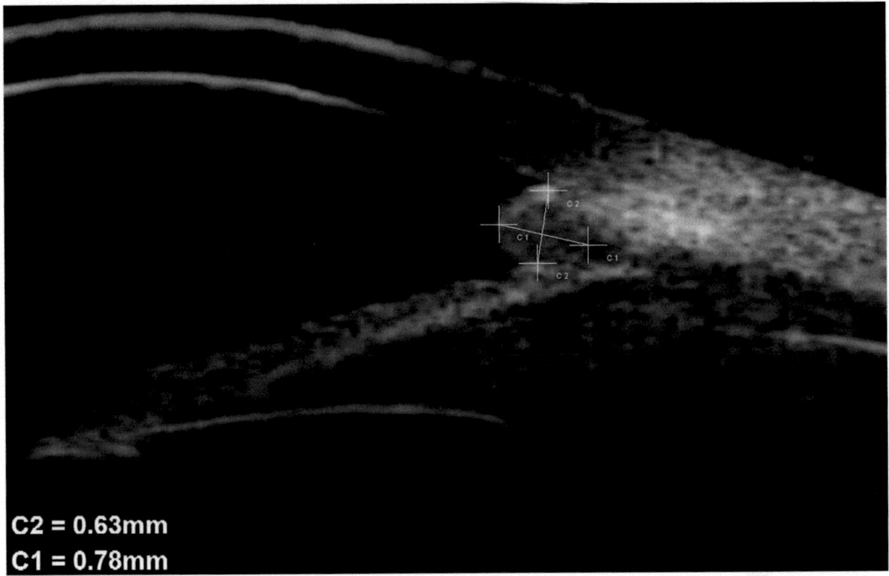


**Fig. 14.10  Diffuse anterior retinoblastoma**. VHFU at 50 MHz: small iris nodule in the angle, isolated, moderately echogenic, without calcification, appeared after lesions of the posterior segment that were successfully treated by triple chemotherapy. The small iris lesion disappeared after intravitreal and intracameral injections of an alkylating agent. The outcome at 5 years was favorable

In terms of the purely anterior forms, ultrasound usually recapitulates the clinical findings, namely perilental opacity (Fig. 14.11) and less often purely of the lens, as in a congenital cataract.

It can, however, sometimes be associated with a cataract. Stretching of the ciliary processes is a very good clinical sign indicative of PFV, which is not to be confused with ectropion of the uvea. It can be visualized in ultrasound (Fig. 14.12, *see* Fig. 14.30), with or without posterior subluxation of the lens.

In color Doppler, vascular activity can be seen at the level of a Mittendorf dot (Fig. 14.13) or iridohyaloid vessels (Fig. 14.14).

Purely posterior forms are rare. On the other hand, abnormalities of the posterior segment are common in combined forms. One can readily discern a rather thin membrane corresponding either to a persistently permeable hyaloid artery (Fig. 14.15) or to an avascular Cloquet's canal (Fig. 14.16).

When the membrane is thicker, or even in a very tight V or Y shape, it is naturally necessary to consider a retinal detachment or a retinal fold (Fig. 14.17).

Color Doppler Imaging is a good way to differentiate a hyaloid artery from retinal vessels [18]: the resistivity index (RI) being close to that of the central retinal vessels in retinal detachments, and equal to 1.00 when it is a persistent hyaloid artery (Fig. 14.18). CDI localized prepapillary vascularization can be seen in case of

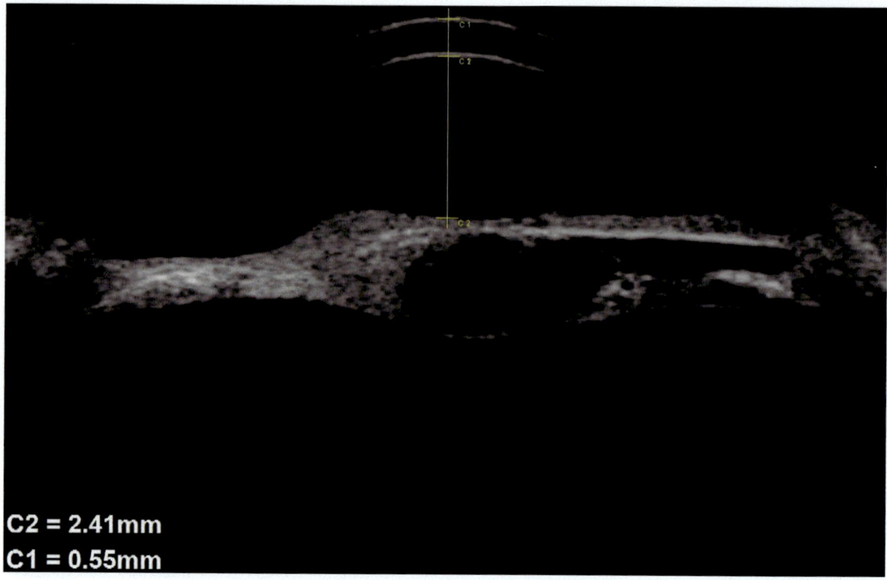



**Fig. 14.11 Anterior PFV OS**. VHFU at 50 MHz, axial section of the left eye. Normal appearance of the cornea, anterior chamber, and lens. A perilental mass was particularly developed in the temporal quadrant

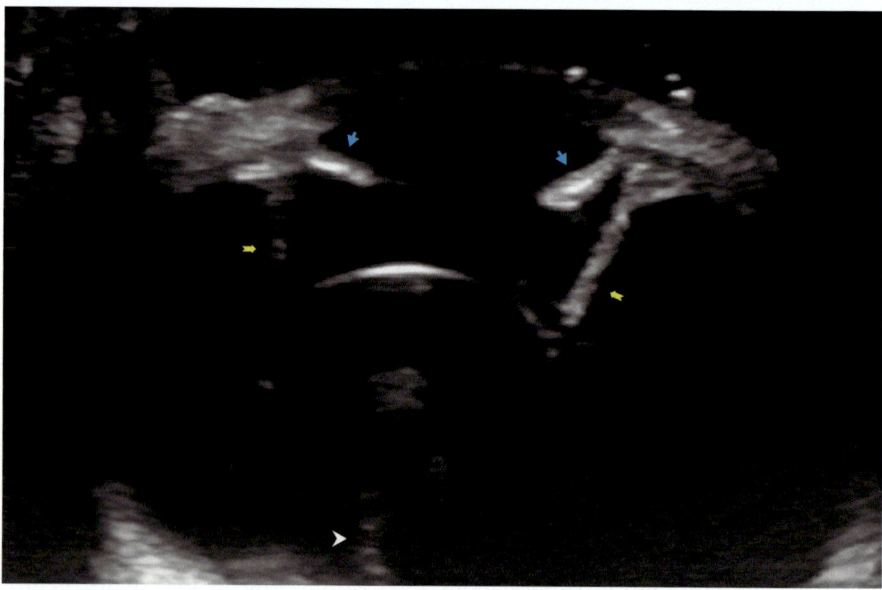

**Fig. 14.12 Stretching of ciliary processes**. HFU at 18 MHz. Particularly obvious (➡ yellow arrows) due to the posterior dislocation of the echogenic cataractous lens. It should not be confused with the iris (➡ blue arrows). One can also guess the departure of a membrane connecting the lens to the optic disc (➤ white arrowhead), which proved to be a total retinal detachment

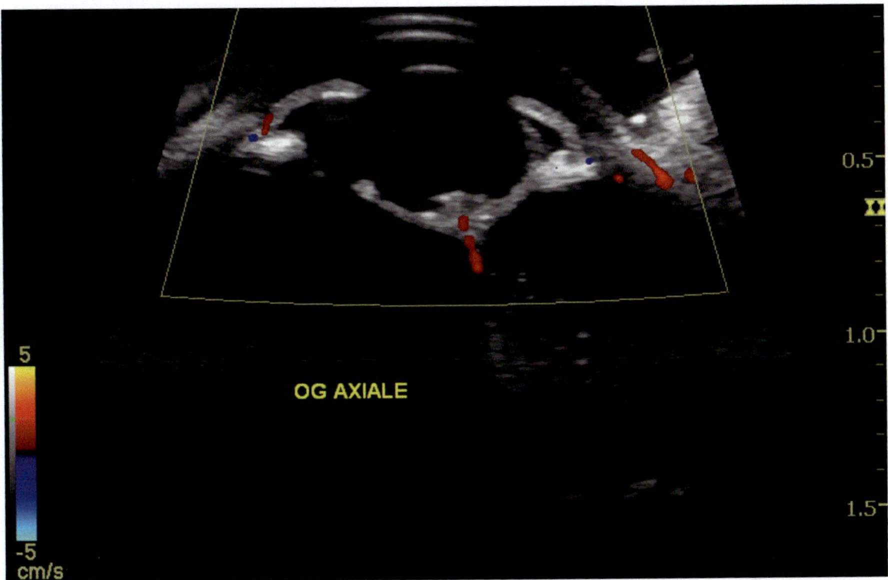



**Fig. 14.13 Vascularized Mittendorf dot.** Small localized condensation of the posterior crystalline lens next to the attachment of the persistent hyaloid artery on the lens, with a small colored dot at its level

Bergmeister papilla. Finally, associations with other pathologies: glaucoma, abnormalities of the optic nerve, colobomas, and many others, and even intraocular tumors have been described.

## Vitreoretinal Dysplasia

These abnormalities in the development of the retina and the vitreous can be isolated or become part of a polymalformative syndrome. They are characterized by congenital retinal detachment associated with the presence of a retrolental fibrovascular organization. Among the associated syndromes are Walker–Warburg syndrome (brain MRI disclosing lissencephaly, hydrocephalus, and severe hypoplasia of the brain stem and cerebellum) and Norrie's disease in boys, because of X-linked transmission (search for mutations in the *NDP* gene) [19].

The ultrasound signs resemble the most advanced combined forms of PFV, but most often bilaterally with total retinal detachment and retrolental fibrovascular proliferation (Fig. 14.19). The subretinal fluid is often slightly echogenic, serohemorrhagic.

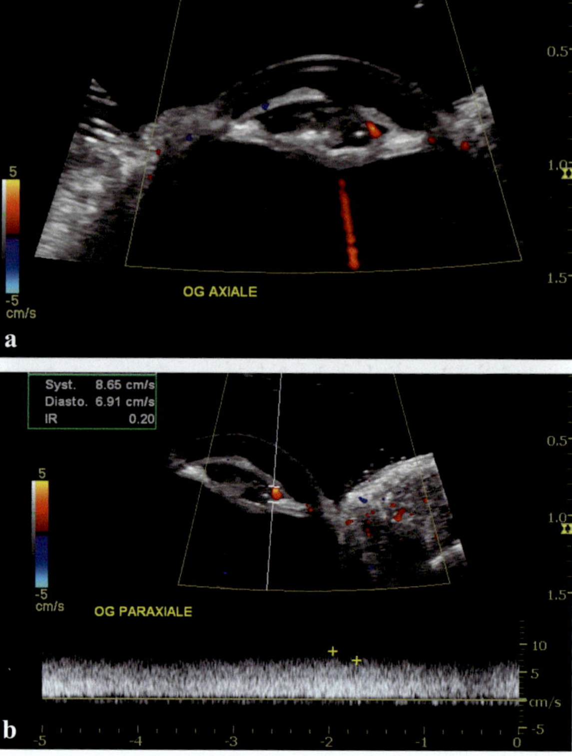

**Fig. 14.14 Small iridohyaloid vessel**, lateral to the echogenic cataractous lens and behind the iris. High Frequency CDI with a frequency of 22 MHz for the B-mode and 14.3 MHz for the Doppler. **a**: Color mode; **b**: spectral mode. Spectral analysis shows that it is a vein. In **a**, a persistently permeable hyaloid artery can be seen

## Coats' Disease

Coats disease is a rare idiopathic disease, with less than 1/1,000,000 births in the UK. It is characterized by retinal telangiectasiae with deposition of intra- or subretinal exudates, without vitreous or retinal traction, occurring in 80% of cases in boys, most often between 6 and 8 years of age at diagnosis, in a unilateral manner [20]. Younger children have more severe and advanced forms with a less favorable prognosis [21]. Early stages are often asymptomatic, and ultrasound is only useful in advanced stages or in the presence of complications.

### (a) **Exudative masses**

Quite often, it can be an ultrasound problem, but fortunately clinical assessment is available, revealing a yellowish exudate which resolves the doubt. In B-mode, they show up as a small moderately echogenic dome mass (Fig. 14.20a), often located at the posterior pole. It is not uncommon, however, in older children, and this can make  the ultrasound diagnosis difficult, to observe calcifications within the mass. In CDI, there is no intrinsic flow, but the underlying parietal flows are clearly visible (Fig. 14.20b).

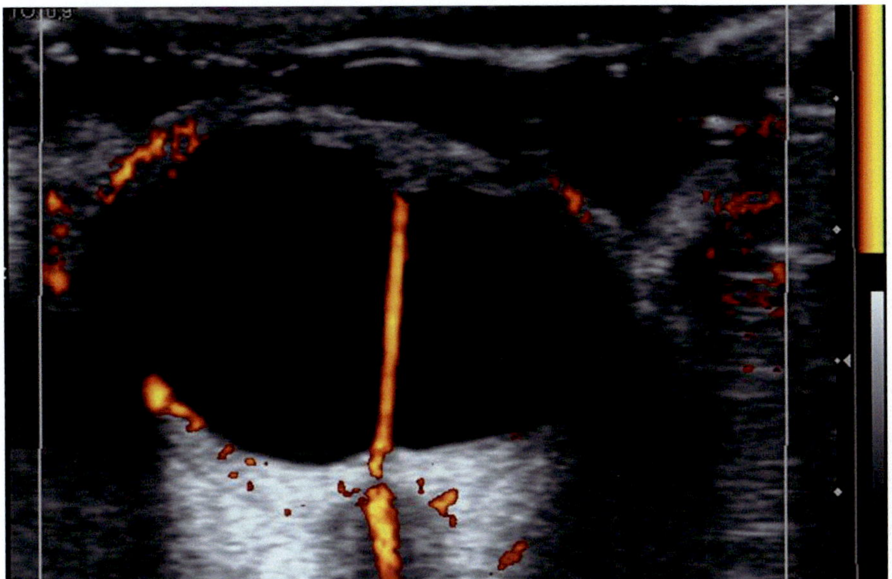

**Fig. 14.15  Persistent hyaloid artery**—CDI, power mode. Occurring on a microphthalmic eye of 16.2 mm, the artery is visible all the way from the optic disc to the lens, with a small, echogenic, cataractous lens, with blurred margins

### (b)  Retinal detachment

Associated with a vitreous disorder, retinal detachment (RD) is often total, of the exudative type, with thick retinal leaflets (Fig. 14.21a) and a subretinal space filled with small punctiform very low reflective echoes (Fig. 14.21b).

The subretinal fluid is sometimes hemorrhagic, with an appearance identical to that of a retrohyaloid hemorrhage, discreetly more echogenic than for a pure exudative fluid. When the detachment is total with hemorrhage in the vitreous and subretinal, it may appear in negative (Fig. 14.22).

In CDI, the micromovements of the red blood cells that fall downwards into the sub-retinal space are responsible for a puddle coded in blue (Fig. 14.23). This type of RD is often hypervascularized (Fig. 14.24).

### (c)  Microphthalmia

Rarely severe, it is nonetheless frequent, which is one of the good diagnostic arguments (Fig. 14.25).

### (d)  Vascular disorders

CDI can reveal velocimetric disturbances on the affected side versus the normal opposite side [22].

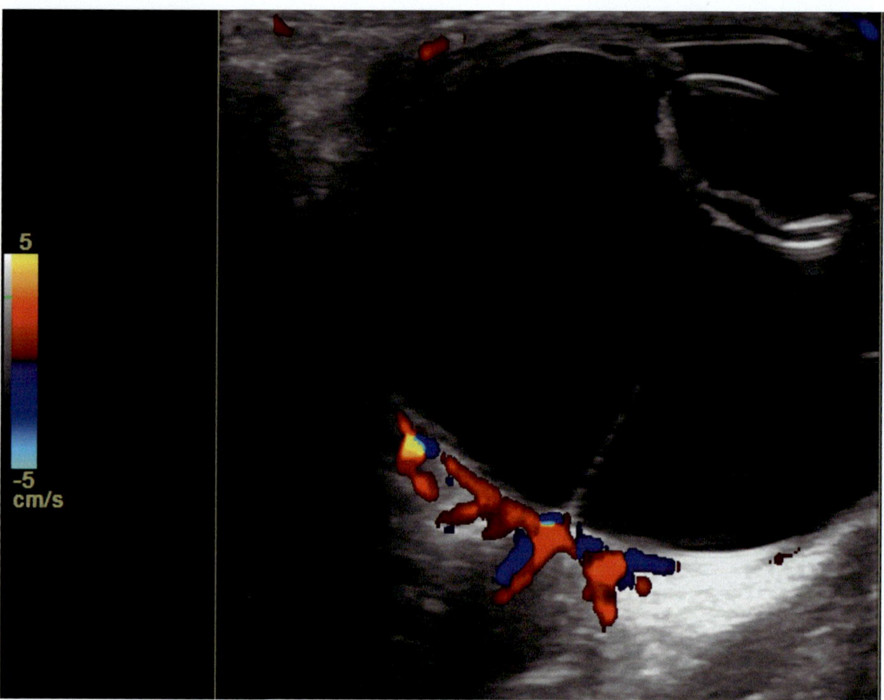

**Fig. 14.16 Avascular Cloquet's canal**—CDI, color mode. Normal appearance of the vessels of the optic nerve head. Absence of flow on the membrane. The lens is thick with subcapsular opacity

### (e)  Differential diagnosis

This can be extremely difficult with retinoblastoma when the fundus is not accessible, and when telangiectasiae are not visible. Indeed, it has been noted that for parietal masses, there can be calcifications in the progression of subretinal exudates, and it is known that some retinoblastomas, when they are small, may not exhibit calcification. In addition, when there is a total retinal detachment, the detached retinal leaflets are generally thick in both cases and calcifications are uncommon in diffuse infiltrating retinoblastomas.

The arguments for either diagnosis are:

- The existence or not of microphthalmia, present in Coats' disease and absent in retinoblastoma. Of course, cases of spontaneously cured retinoblastoma associated with microphthalmia have been described, but these are exceptional cases.
- Assessment of the subretinal fluid, anechoic in diffuse infiltrating retinoblastoma and finely hypoechoic (exudative or hemorrhagic) in Coats' disease. This difference can also be found by MRI.
- Finally, of course, a bilateral lesion will tend to indicate retinoblastoma or other abnormalities that are, most often, bilateral – FEVR, von Hippel-Lindau disease,

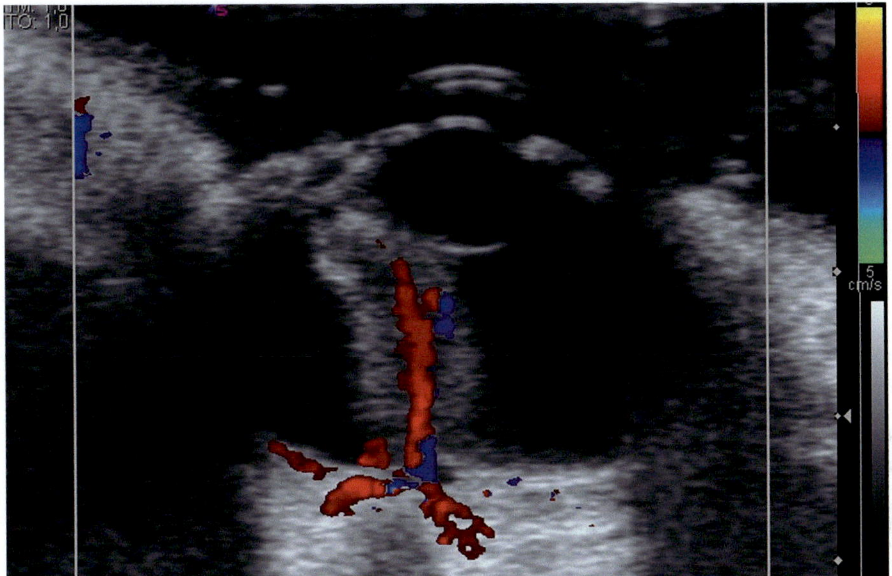

**Fig. 14.17  Retinal fold**, thick and vascularized, slightly lateralized—CDI, color mode

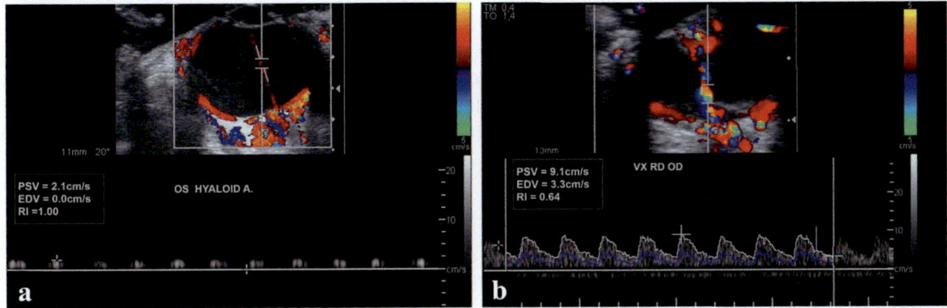



**Fig. 14.18  Velocimetric constants within intraocular membranes**—CDI, color and spectral modes. **a**: Hyaloid artery; **b**: total retinal detachment. The PSV of the hyaloid artery, = 2.1 cm/s, is much lower than in the retinal vessels, = 9.1 cm/s. The RI of the hyaloid artery = 1.00. The RI of the retinal vessel = 0.64

and incontinentia pigmenti. However, autosomal recessive bilateral forms of Coats' disease have been described, particularly in the context of Coats-plus syndrome, which is the systemic version of Coats' disease [23], associating cerebroretinal microangiopathy with calcifications and cysts, secondary to a mutation in the CTC1 gene, with signs suggestive of Coats' disease.

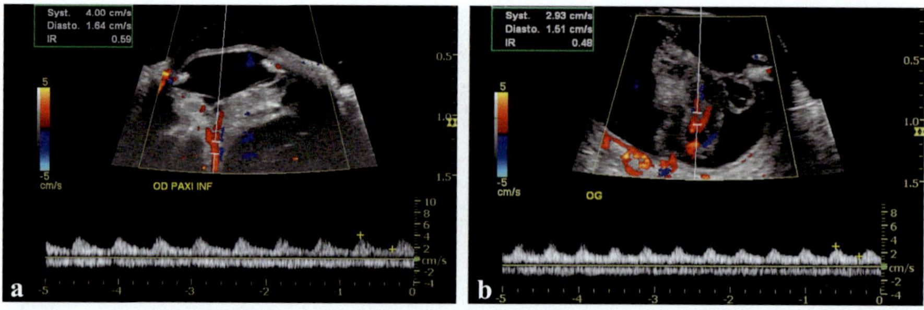

**Fig. 14.19** **Vitreoretinal dysplasia**—CDI, color and spectral modes. **a**: Right eye; **b**: left eye. On both sides there is moderate microphthalmia, total retinal detachment with massive fibrovascular proliferation behind a large crystalline lens, anteriorly subluxated, with a narrow anterior chamber

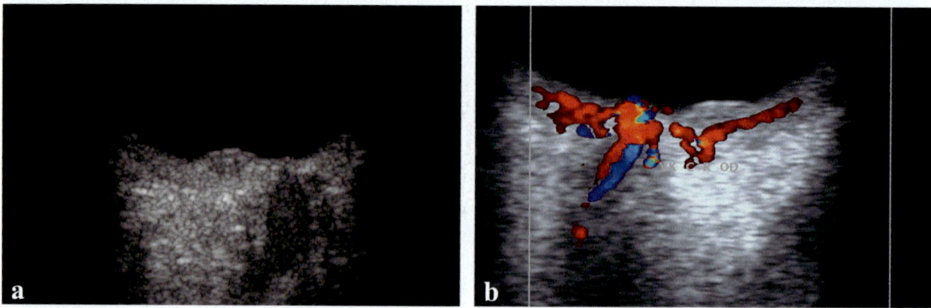

**Fig. 14.20** **Coats' disease, subretinal exudative mass located at the posterior pole**. **a**: In a left eye in B-mode; **b**: in a right eye in another child in color Doppler. The lesions are moderately echogenic, very discreetly less echogenic than the adjacent choroid, heterogeneous and have no intrinsic flow. No choroidal excavation. Presence of underlying choroidal flows

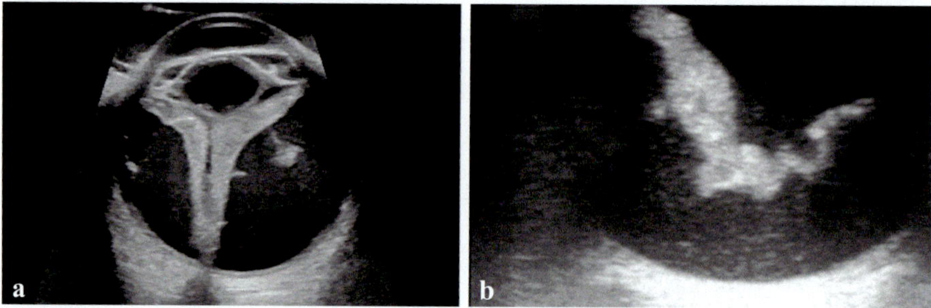

**Fig. 14.21** **Coats' disease, retinal detachment—B-mode**. **a**: Axial section; **b**: section exploring a quadrant. In both cases, the thickness of the detached retinal leaflets can be seen, and, particularly in **b**, the subretinal space is discreetly hypoechoic, in relation to the exudative nature of the detachment

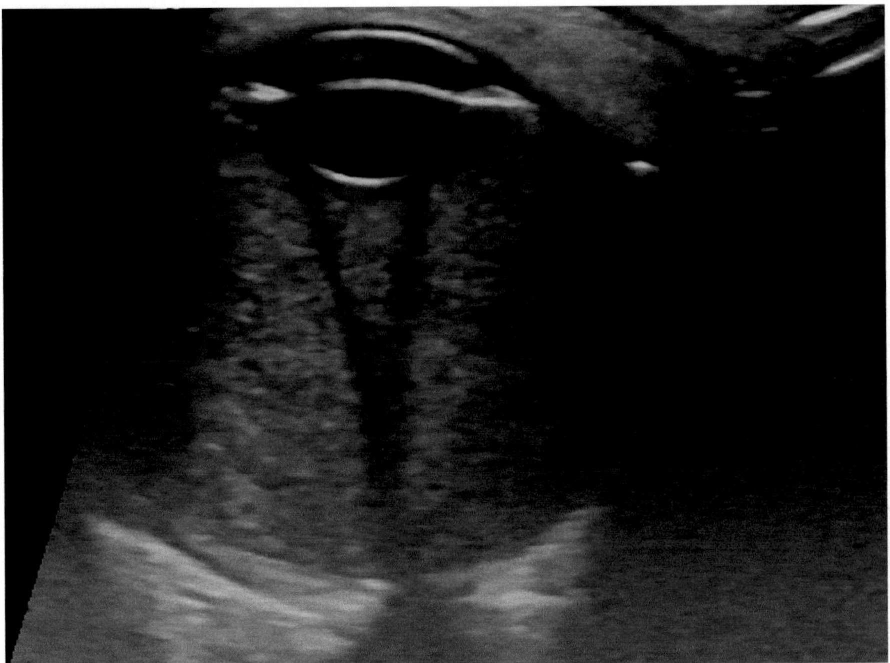

**Fig. 14.22 Coats' disease, "phantom" retinal detachment**. When there is an intravitreal **and** subretinal hemorrhage, the detached retinal leaflets appear as negative, especially since the ultrasound beam is not perpendicular to the different interfaces

## Toxocariasis

This is due to infestation of humans by larvae of a parasitic nematode of Canidae (*Toxocara canis*) or Felidae (*Toxocara cati*). It is the ground soiled by animal droppings that is responsible for the contamination, not the direct contact with the dogs (puppies excepted) or cats. Toxocariasis often occurs in people who have infected dogs in their environment, or in children, who tend to put their hands in their mouths after touching the ground or disturbing the soil.

Clinically, different syndromes can be observed.

**Visceral larva migrans** (hepatic granuloma in adults).

**Covert Toxocariasis**

**Allergies**

And finally, **ocular toxocariasis, which to varying degrees associates**:

- **posterior retinal granuloma:** a parapapillary mass that can be neovascularized.

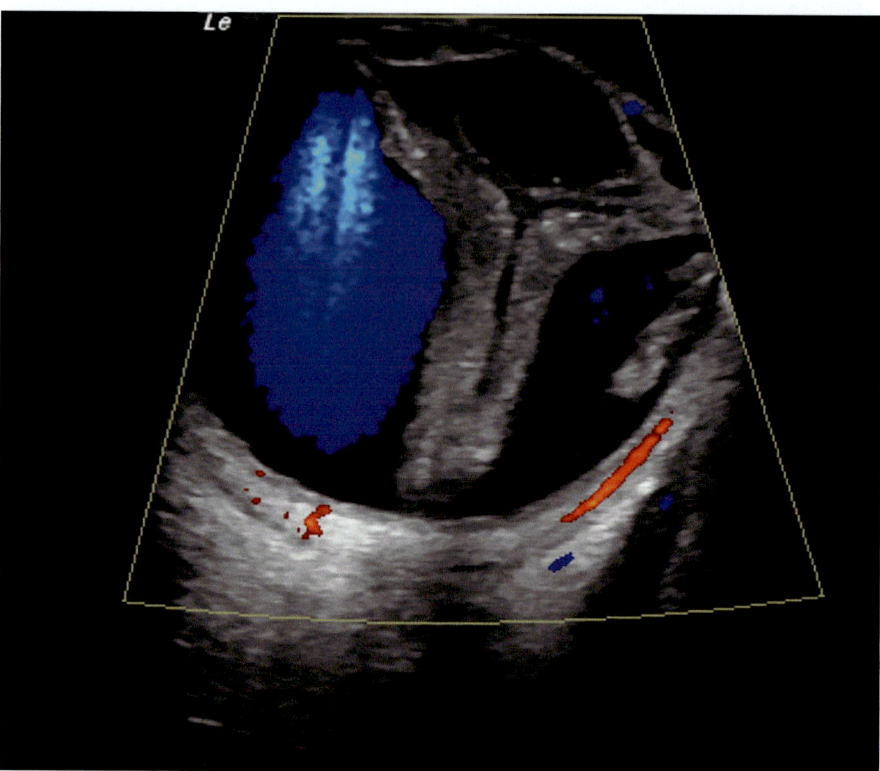

**Fig. 14.23 Coats' disease, hemorrhagic retinal detachment**, CDI, color mode. The red blood cells of the subretinal space fall in the sloping position, and their movement is coded blue in color mode

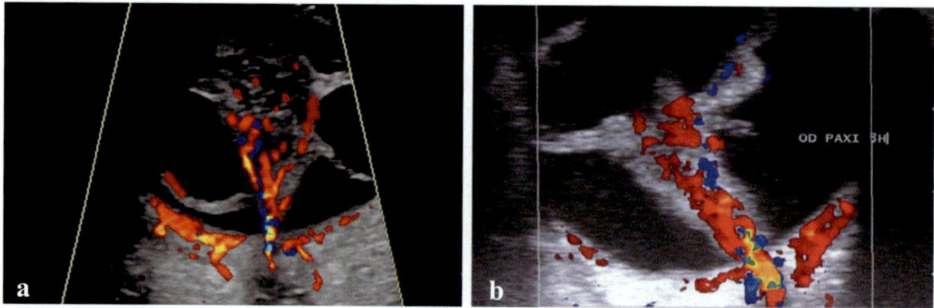

**Fig. 14.24 Coats' disease, hypervascular retinal detachment**. In color mode, the RD is much more "colored" than other retinal detachments. This aspect is quite characteristic of the RD in this vascular retinopathy. But in spectral mode, the flows are not accelerated, the PSV being 5.6 cm/s and the RI 0.71

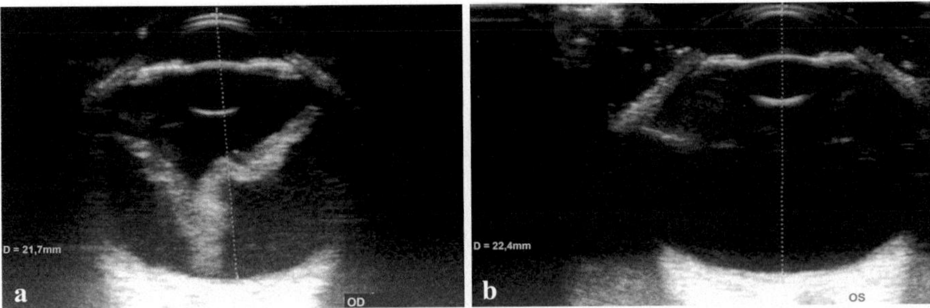

**Fig. 14.25   Coats' disease of the right eye with microphthalmos.** B-mode guided biometry. The right microphthalmic eye is immediately noticeable, affecting the antero-posterior axis and the equatorial diameter. The difference in axial length does not differ much but corresponds to a volume of 10% less than on the normal side

- **leukocoria, which** is not too difficult to differentiate from retinoblastoma. Moreover, retinoblastoma is typically observed before two years of age and toxocariasis after this age, but this is not a general rule.
- **hypopyon uveitis**
- **inflammation of the retinal periphery**: the presence of small granulomas near the ora serrata associated with a distinct fibrosis that extends to the optic disc or the vitreous.

**Ultrasound** can visualize these different signs, in particular pre- or parapapillary granuloma, which is often vascularized, and vitreous membranes (Fig. 14.26), which can lead to traction retinal detachments. On the other hand, small peripheral granulomas are more difficult to disclose. Blood eosinophilia, sometimes considerable, can be seen, but it can be lacking in pure ocular forms; a clear increase in the level of total IgE is as well helpful. The positive diagnosis is based on serology, essentially ELISA, the results of which must be confirmed by immunoassay (western blot), but there is a lack of specificity.

Colobomas

These are the consequence of a defect or improper closure of the embryonal fissure, and they are, therefore, mainly localized in the inferonasal quadrant, associating to varying degrees the iris (Fig. 14.27), the chorioretina, and the optic disc.

Ultrasound of the posterior segment may reveal localized deformation of the ocular wall, an associated retinal detachment, or other intraocular abnormalities (Fig. 14.28), but is often unsatisfactory.

On the other hand, coloboma of the optic disc is readily visualized and differs quite clearly from a glaucomatous excavation even of the bean-pot cupping type (Fig. 14.29). A coloboma of the optic disc can be associated with a more or less large orbital cyst (Fig. 14.30).

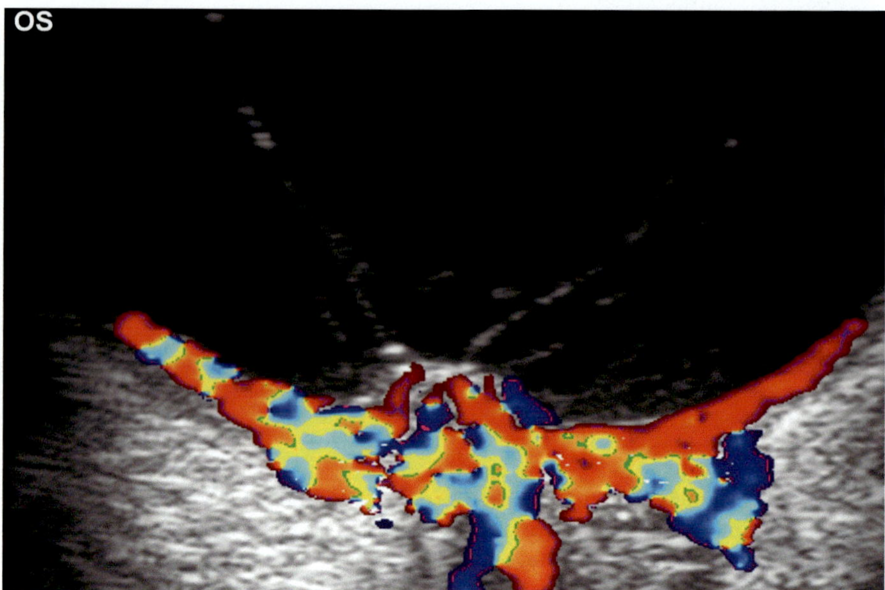


**Fig. 14.26 Toxocara canis toxocariasis in a 12-year-old child**. The granuloma of the posterior pole is vascularized, associated with many vitreal membranes emanating from the mass

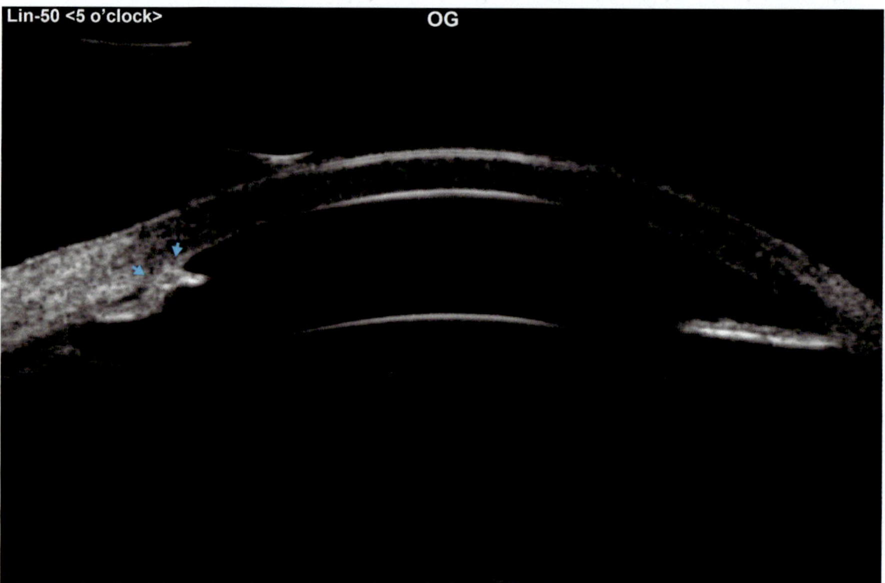


**Fig. 14.27 Inferior iris coloboma, sagittal section of the anterior segment at 50 MHz.** Compared to clinical coloboma, the iris is very short, with peripheral synechia related to Axenfeld–Rieger syndrome (➤ blue arrows)

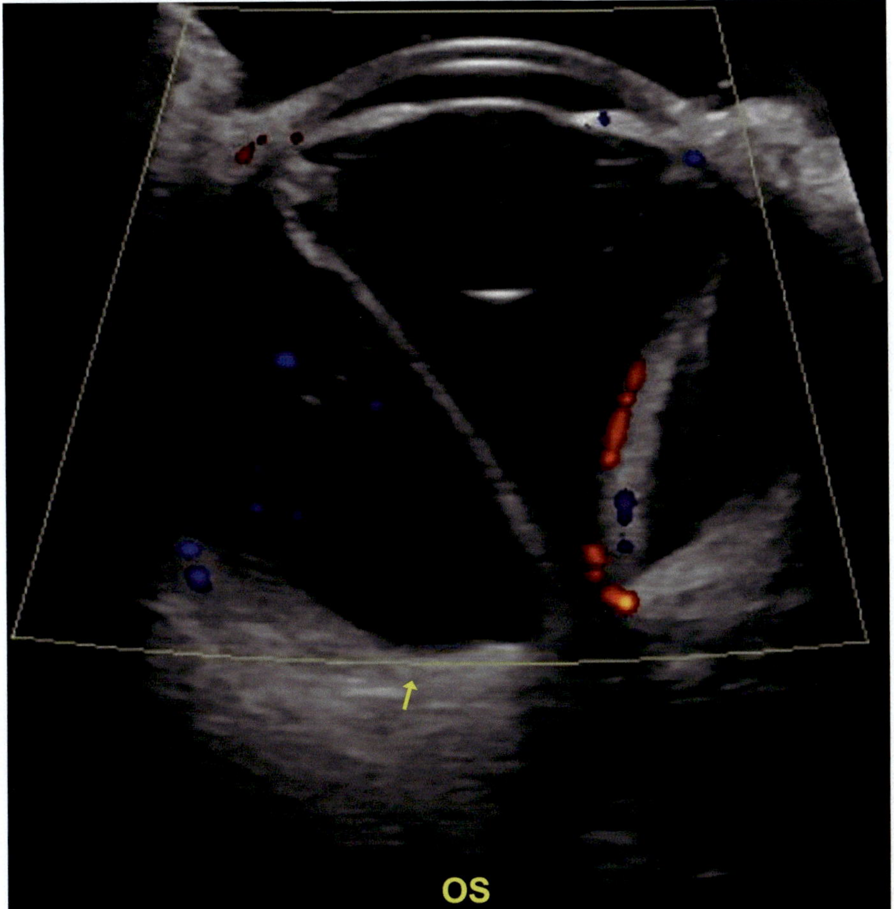



**Fig. 14.28  Chorioretinal coloboma and total retinal detachment of the right eye in an 8 ½ month-old child**. CDI, section from 5 o'clock to 11 o'clock. The parietal deformation, although subtle, is clearly visible (→ yellow arrow) however, as well as the retinal detachment and a voluminous lens, measuring 4.8 mm in thickness. The eye was microphthalmic, with an axial length of 14.3 mm (up to the pigmentary epithelium since there is a total RD)

Morning glory disc anomaly (MGDA)

This is a rare (2.6/100,000) congenital malformation of the optic disc [24], the name of which reflects the clinical presentation of the optic disc as a flower (hence the term 'morning glory'), which can be associated with abnormalities of the central nervous system. Ultrasound reveals a large, cup-shaped optic disc surrounded by more or less developed echogenic material where the short posterior ciliary arteries are recorded in Doppler. In CDI, a possible retinal detachment at the bottom of the defect is better seen than in B mode (Fig. 14.31). MRI is essential, as it allows detailed analysis of

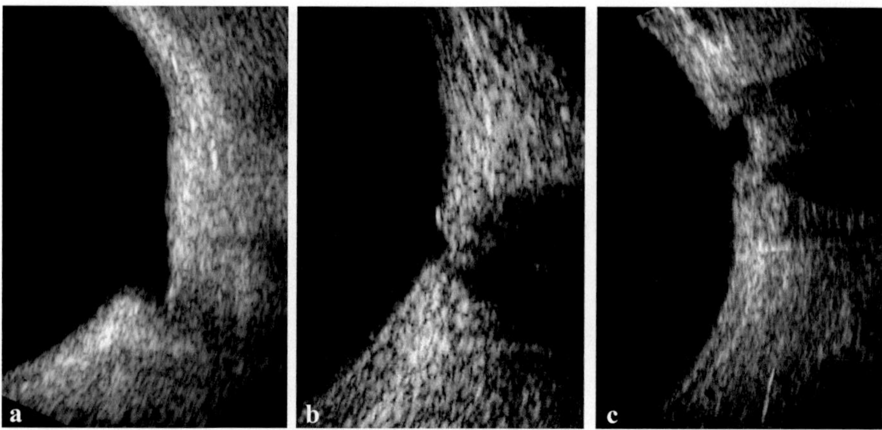

**Fig. 14.29** **Optic disc coloboma (a), large excavation of 0.9 with abnormal neuroretinal rim (b), and bean-pot optic disc cupping (c).** The optic disc coloboma is deeper and has softer connection angles with the wall

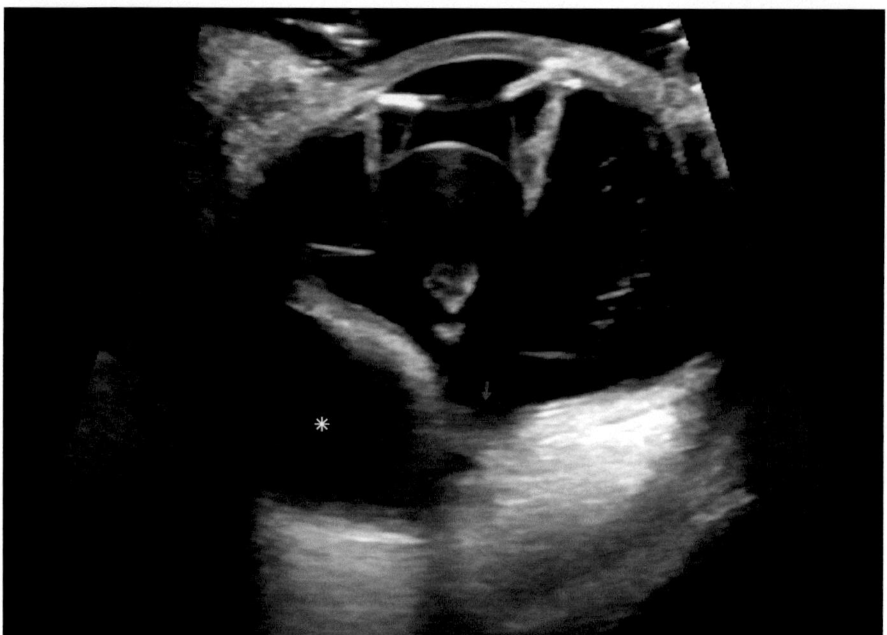

**Fig. 14.30** **Complex, coloboma, chorioretinal and of the optic disc** with severe microphthalmia of 13.6 mm, optic disc coloboma (→ red arrow) and optic atrophy, and combined form of PFV. There is also a voluminous colobomatous cyst (∗) of the optic nerve in the inferior nasal area of the nerve, indenting the ocular wall and masking the usual parietal deformation of chorioretinal colobomas

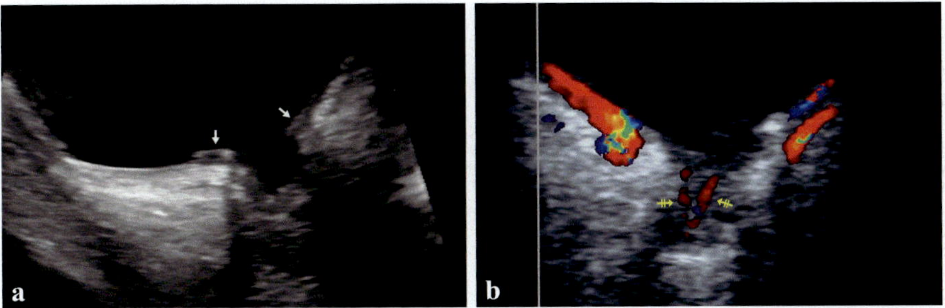

**Fig. 14.31  Morning glory anomaly. a**: B-mode; **b**: CDI. The optic disc is hollowed out, very deeply. A partial volume artifact causes the contents of this malformed, liquid-like, optic disc to appear hypoechoic. The edges of the disc are prominent and echogenic (→ straight arrows). In Doppler, the vascularized nature of the small retinal detachment localized at the malformation makes it visible (↕ yellow barred arrows), while it was not discernible in B-mode

the optic nerve (which is often enlarged) and detection of possible associated brain abnormalities.

Retinal Detachments and Congenital Retinal Folds in Children

RD in children child is rare, accounting for 2–12% of all RDs [25]. They have etiological, therapeutic, and prognostic specificities differentiating them from those of adults (see Chap. 12). Falciform retinal folds reflect displacement of the retina [26] and are observed in vitreoretinal dysplasia, familial exudative vitreoretinopathy, retinopathy of prematurity, and PFV. They appear as a stretched and rather thick fold from the optic disc to the extreme retinal periphery (Fig. 14.32). The flows circulating at their level have constants identical to those of RD, which may pose a problem for their ultrasound diagnosis.

## 14.3  Other Tumors and Eye Masses

Their clinical symptomatology is variable. They rarely manifest as leukocoria, and there is rarely an issue differentiating them from retinoblastoma.

### 14.3.1  Diffuse Choroidal Angioma and Sturge–Weber Syndrome

The circumscribed form of choroidal angiomas has already been discussed in Chap. 13. In children, the diffuse form, associated with Sturge–Weber syndrome

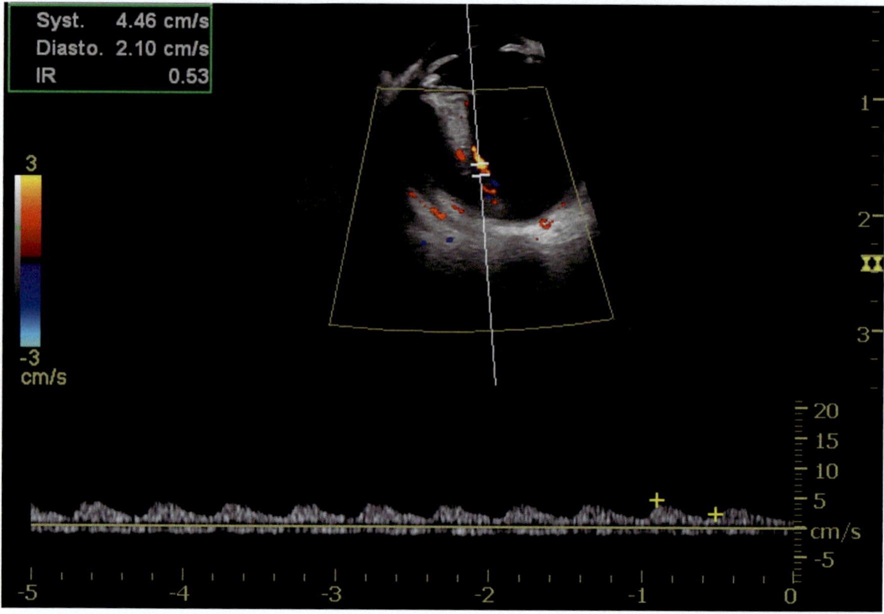


**Fig. 14.32 Congenital retinal fold—CDI, color and spectral modes**. A thick fold stretching from the optic disc to the ciliary body over the 4:30 o'clock meridian and vascularized with retinal velocimetric constants: PSV = 4.5 cm/s and RI = 0.53

is the most common [27]. This form can lead to decreased vision, induced hyperopia, macular edema, retinal detachment, or amblyopia. In ultrasound, the angioma is hyperechoic and hypervascularized in CDI. Low-dose proton beam therapy allows reapplication of even substantial exudative retinal detachment (Fig. 14.33). In spectral Doppler, these involve high flows that are not very resistive (RI < 0.60), except when glaucoma complicates this angioma. On an axial section, diffuse angioma can give the impression that the eye is diamond-shaped. MRI, which is essential to screen for the presence of leptomeningeal angioma, can be very suitable for assessment of ocular angioma [28].

## 14.3.2 Medulloepithelioma

Belonging to the congenital neuroectodermal tumors of the ciliary body, medulloepithelioma is a rare embryonic tumor that develops from the non-pigmented ciliary medullary epithelium. There are benign and malignant forms, as well as teratoid forms that are benign and malignant. Microcystic forms are also observed. It occurs mainly in young children, the average age being 3.8 years at the appearance of the first clinical sign and 5 years at treatment. Ultrasound (Fig. 14.34) reveals lesion of the ciliary body enclosing the lens and giving rise to a cataract.

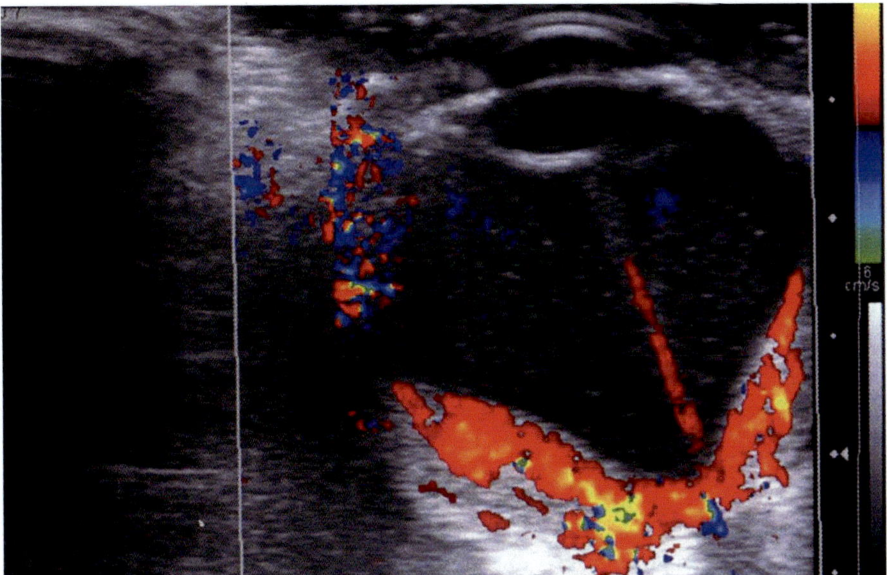

**Fig. 14.33 Diffuse choroidal angioma associated with Sturge–Weber syndrome—CDI, color mode**. One can readily see the hypervascularization of the diffuse angioma, the T-shape total retinal detachment, going up to the lens, and a subretinal space that is discreetly hypoechoic due to the exudative nature of the detachment

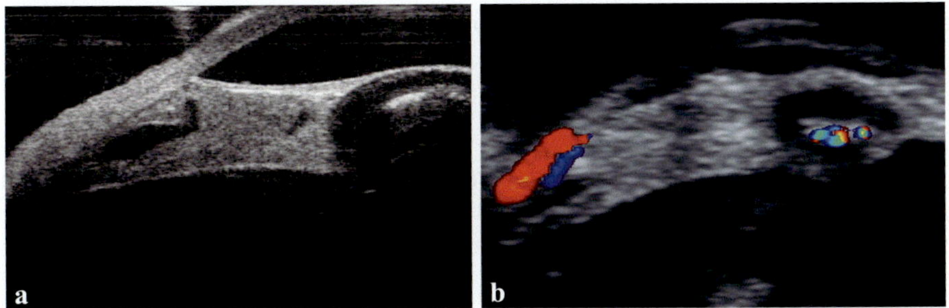

**Fig. 14.34 Medulloepithelioma of the ciliary body. a**: VHFU at 50 MHz; **b**: CDI at 10 MHz. The lesion reaches the lens, which it encloses, with a calcified cataract (note the hyperechoic nodule in B-mode and the small twinkling artifact in Doppler). It is moderately echogenic and even, crossed by small vessels that circulate very slowly, as they are not found in Doppler

Histological diagnosis with retinoblastoma can be difficult, as there can be rosettes [29].

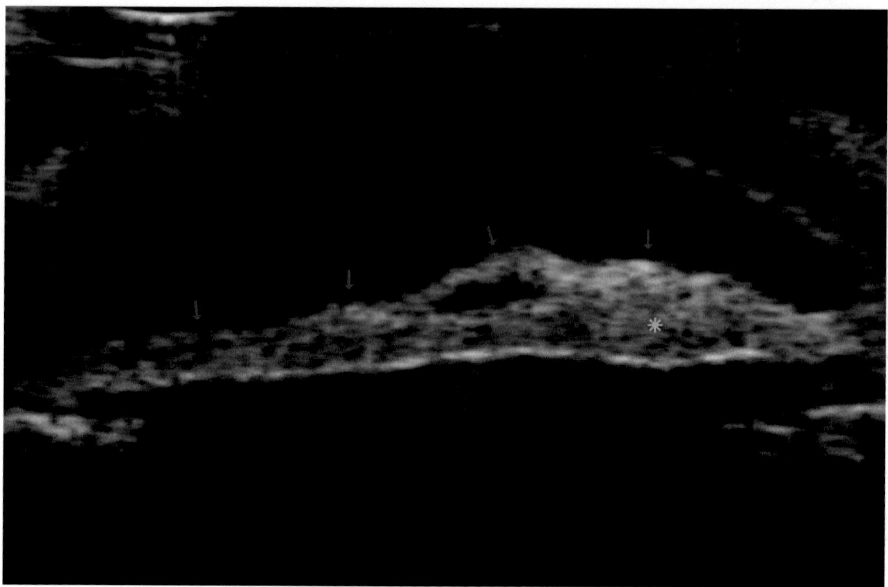

**Fig. 14.35** **Nevoxanthoendothelioma of the iris**. VHFU at 50 MHz; temporal parasagittal section, showing an unevenly thickened iris that is moderately echogenic (✳ green star), covered with a fairly irregular echogenic blade corresponding to the recurrent sedimented hyphema (→ red arrows), a clinical sign resulting in the lesion being discovered

### 14.3.3  *Juvenile Nevoxanthoendothelioma or Xanthogranuloma*

Occurring in children, from a few weeks to two years of age [30], a very suggestive clinical sign is the existence of a recurrent spontaneous hyphema, revealing a mass of the iris corresponding to histiocytic infiltration. Ultrasound reveals a rather poorly delineated iris lesion, less echogenic than the adjacent stroma and even less echogenic than the sedimented hyphema that covers the lesion (Fig. 14.35). The lesion is sensitive to corticosteroids, and it is often necessary to add eye drops to treat the glaucoma that frequently complicates this lesion.

### 14.3.4  *Cavernous Angioma of the Retina*

This is a rare vascular hamartoma of the retina [31], most often unilateral, which can contain phleboliths and can be associated with cerebral involvement, especially for bilateral cases. Ultrasound reveals an entirely non-characteristic lesion with Doppler, slow venous flows like those that can be seen in orbital cavernous angiomas (Fig. 14.36). A family study should also be carried out in case of bilateral cases.

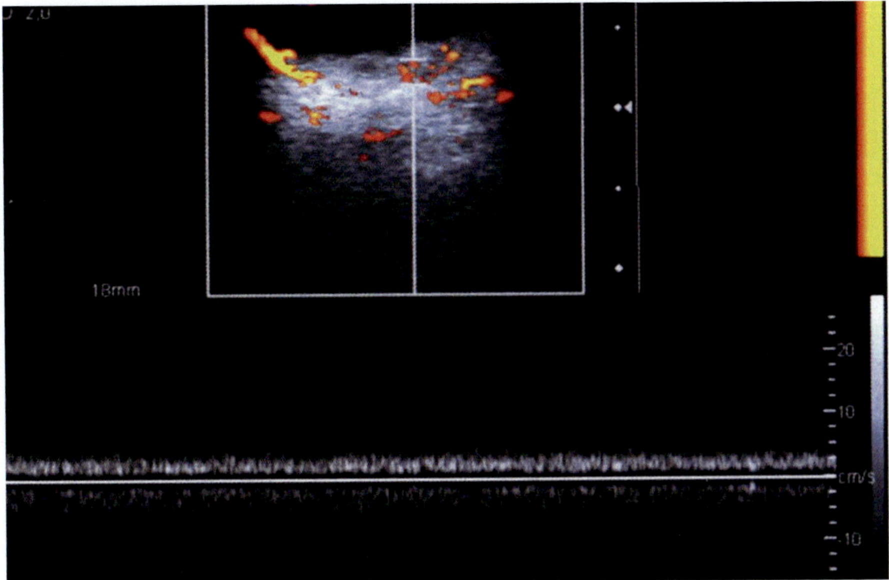

**Fig. 14.36 Cavernous angioma of the retina**. CDI, Power and spectral modes. Small parietal lesion of moderately echogenic echotexture without choroidal excavation, with small typically venous flows

## 14.3.5 Prepapillary Capillary Angioma

Associated or not with von Hippel-Lindau disease [32], they are vascular hamartomas. They can be pre- or juxtapapillary, isolated, or associated with macular edema, intravitreal hemorrhage, or epiretinal membrane. In B-mode, they tend to be poorly echogenic, and in Doppler, they are vascularized to a certain degree (Fig. 14.37).

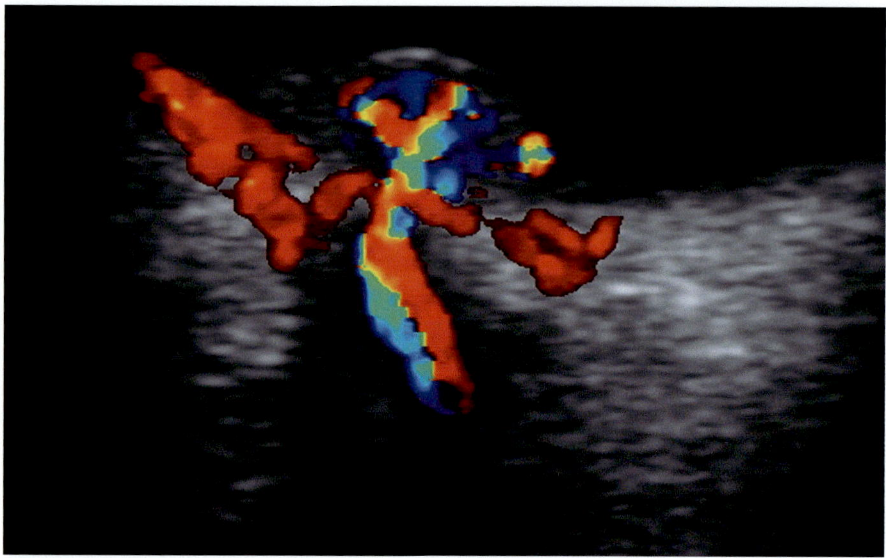

**Fig. 14.37 Von Hippel–Lindau disease prepapillary capillary angioma**. CDI, color mode. Usually not imaged, the indication here was the large volume of the lesion in front of the optic disc and extending laterally, slightly to moderately echogenic and highly vascularized. In spectral doppler, PSV = 21.9 cm/s and RI = 0.59. Compared to the central retinal artery, where PSV = 16.9 cm/s and RI = 0.63

# References


1. Glasier CM, Brodsky MC, Leithiser RE Jr, et al. High resolution ultrasound with Doppler: a diagnostic adjunct in orbital and ocular lesions in children. Pediatr Radiol. 1992;22(3):174–8.
2. Elmaleh-Bergès M, Bergès O. Pathologie Ophtalmologique in Imagerie pédiatrique et fœtale In: Adamsbaum C, editor. Flammarion Paris; 2007. p. 172–86.
3. Desjardins L. Les tumeurs en ophtalmo-pédiatrie: diagnostic et stratégie thérapeutique. J Fr Ophtalmol. 2000;23(9):926–39.
4. Aerts I, Lumbroso-Le Rouic L, Gauthier-Villars M, Brisse H, Doz F. Actualités du rétinoblastome. Arch Pediatr. 2016;23(1):112–6.
5. Murphree AL. Intraocular retinoblastoma: the case for a new group classification. Ophthalmol Clin N Am. 2005;18:41–53.
6. Kaste SC, Jenkins JJ III, Pratt CB, Langston JW, Haik BG. Retinoblastoma: sonographic findings with pathologic correlation in pediatric patients. Am J Roentgenol. 2000;175:495–501.
7. Zimmerman LE. Retinoblastoma and retinocytoma in Spencer WH. Ophthalmic Pathology, an atlas and textbook. WB Saunders Company (Philadelphia), 3rd ed. 1985. p. 1292–1351.
8. Brisse HJ, Lumbroso L, Freneaux PC, et al. Sonographic, CT, and MR imaging findings in diffuse infiltrative retinoblastoma: report of two cases with histologic comparison. AJNR Am J Neuroradiol. 2001;22:499–504.
9. Galluzzi P, Hadjistilianou T, Cerase A, De Francesco S, Toti P, Venturi C. Is CT still useful in the study protocol of retinoblastoma? AJNR Am J Neuroradiol. 2009;30(9):1760–5.
10. Brisse HJ, de Graaf P, Galluzzi P, European Retinoblastoma Imaging Collaboration (ERIC), et al. Assessment of early-stage optic nerve invasion in retinoblastoma using high-resolution 1.5 Tesla MRI with surface coils: a multicentre, prospective accuracy study with histopathological correlation. Eur Radiol. 2015;25(5):1443–52.

11. de Graaf P, Göricke S, Brisse HJ, European Retinoblastoma Imaging Collaboration (ERIC) et al. Guidelines for imaging retinoblastoma: imaging principles and MRI standardization. Pediatr Radiol. 2012;42(1):2–14.

12. Yang J, Dang Y, Zhu Y, Zhang C. Diffuse anterior retinoblastoma: current concepts. Onco Targets Ther. 2015;22(8):1815–21.

13. Apushkin MA, Shapiro MJ, Mafee MF. Retinoblastoma and simulating lesions: role of imaging. Neuroimaging Clin N Am. 2005;15:49–67.

14. Fledelius HC, Christensen AC. Reappraisal of the human ocular growth curve in fetal life, infancy, and early childhood. Br J Ophthalmol. 1996;80(10):918–21.

15. Goldberg MF. Persistent fetal vasculature (PFV): an integrated interpretation of signs and symptoms associated with persistent hyperplastic primary vitreous (PHPV). LIV Edward Jackson Memorial Lecture. Am J Ophthalmol. 1997;124(5):587–626.

16. Reese AB. Persistent hyperplastic primary vitreous. Am J Ophthalmol. 1955;40(3):317–31.

17. Bergès O, Dureau P, Caputo G, Lecler A, Chiaroni PM, Persistent fetal vasculature (PFV) in the light of color doppler imaging (CDI). In: Presentation at the XVII SIDUO meeting, Puerto Varas, Chile November 20–24th 2018

18. Chiaroni PM, Lecler A, Bergès O, et al. Diagnostic accuracy of quantitative color doppler flow imaging in distinguishing persistent fetal vasculature from retinal detachment. Acta Ophthalmol. 2021.

19. Amouyal F, Butet, B, Landré, C, Matonti F, Metge-Galatoire F, Gastaud P. Dysplasies Vitréorétiniennes in Ophtalmologie Pédiatrique, rapport de la société française d'Ophtalmologie. In: Denis D, editor. Elsevier Paris; 2017. p. 380–5.

20. Sen M, Shields CL, Honavar SG, Shields JA. Coats disease: An overview of classification, management and outcomes. Indian J Ophthalmol. 2019;67(6):763–71.

21. Mrejen S, Metge F, Denion E, Dureau P, Edelson C, Caputo G. Management of retinal detachment in Coats disease. Study of 15 cases. Retina. 2008;28(3 Suppl):S26–32.

22. Zhao Q, Peng XY, Yang WL, Li DJ, You QS, Jonas JB. Coats' disease and retrobulbar haemodynamics. Acta Ophthalmol. 2016;94(4):397–400.

23. Troumani Y, Ackermann F, Cohen S, Touhami S, Nasser G, Denier C, Labetoulle M, Rousseau A. Coats Plus: la version systémique de la maladie de Coats. J Fr Ophtalmo. 2016;39(7):e167–70.

24. Ceynowa DJ, Wickström R, Olsson M, et al. Morning glory disc anomaly in childhood—a population-based study. Acta Ophthalmol. 2015;93(7):626–34.

25. Bourges JL, Dureau P, Uteza Y, Roche O, Dufier JL. Particularités du décollement de rétine chez l'enfant. J Fr Ophtalmol. 2001;24(4):371–7.

26. Denion E, Metge F, Dureau P, Caputo G. Plis rétiniens pédiatriques J Fr Ophtalmol. 2010;33(3):222–4.

27. Singh AD, Kaiser PK, Sears JE. Choroidal hemangioma. Ophthalmol Clin North Am. 2005;18(1):151–61.

28. Lewis GD, Li HK, Quan EM, Scarboro SB, Teh BS. The role of eye plaque brachytherapy and MR Imaging in the management of diffuse choroidal hemangioma: an illustrative case report and literature review. Pract Radiat Oncol. 2019;9(5):e452e456.

29. Green WR. Neuroepithelial tumors of ciliary body in ophthalmic pathology an atlas and textbook. 3rd ed. Spencer WH, editor. Philadelphia: WB Saunders Co; 1986. p. 1246–92.

30. Sanders TE. Intraocular juvenile xanthogranuloma (nevoxanthogranuloma): a survey of 20 cases. Trans Am Ophthalmol Soc. 1960;58:59–74.

31. Wang W, Chen L. Cavernous Hemangioma of the retina: a comprehensive review of the literature (1934–2015). Retina. 2017;37(4):611–21.

32. Magee MA, Kroll AJ, Lou PL, Ryan EA. Retinal capillary hemangiomas and von Hippel-Lindau disease. Semin Ophthalmol. 2006;21(3):143–50.

# Chapter 15
# Ultrasound and Orbital Disorders

Olivier Bergès

**Abstract** This represents an introduction to all the 11 chapters dedicated to the orbit. The role of ultrasound versus MRI and CT scan is developed, mainly useful for detection, localization, and characterization, but of little help to study the extension of an orbital lesion. A diagnostic algorithm is proposed in case of exophthalmos with or without dystopia. Also, special cases are discussed, such as the anterior palpable masses in children, lesions of the lacrimal fossa, and vascular exophthalmos (orbital varix and arteriovenous fistulae) for which color Doppler imaging plays a major role. Finally, fine-needle biopsy under ultrasound control is presented, mainly useful for posteriorly located malignant lesions (and hence treatable with chemo- or radiotherapy).

## 15.1 Introduction

These chapters 15 to 26 constitute a paradox: it will be one of the longest sections of this book because the etiologies are many and varied, but at the same time, ophthalmology sonographers rarely have to undertake evaluation of an orbital lesion. Hopefully, this will arouse their interest in a relatively unknown area. Moreover, as Mario de La Torre likes to say, the orbit is the "Cinderella" of ophthalmology, a princess hidden behind ashes.

And yet, more than elsewhere, a rigorous and exhaustive approach relying on all possible techniques, B-mode, naturally, but also standardized A-mode and color Doppler imaging (CDI), combined with a flawless semiological analysis, allow for obtaining useful and often sufficient information to diagnose and monitor such orbital lesions, based on a morphological and quantitative approach. I had the good fortune that Mario de La Torre from Lima, Peru, the secretary of SIDUO, the Societas Internationalis pro Diagnostica Ultrasonica in Ophthalmologia, helped me to demonstrate the importance of standardized A-mode ultrasound for these various orbital pathologies. I thank him very warmly for this.

O. Bergès (✉)
Rothschild Foundation Hospital, Paris, France
e-mail: oberges@for.paris



O. Bergès (ed.), *Echography of the Eye and Orbit*,
https://doi.org/10.1007/978-3-031-41467-1_15

Ultrasound along with CT and MRI are the three techniques for exploring orbital pathologies. However, first of all, one should note that:

- **Ultrasound** examination highly depends on the sonographer's experience and the equipment that is used. In addition to A-mode and color Doppler imaging, B-mode images can be generated with a single-purpose device, with a conventional probe and an annular probe, as well as with a multipurpose ultrasound device with an electronic scanning probe. However, for the orbit, very high-frequency ultrasound, at 50 MHz, is rarely useful.
- A **CT scan** is an irradiating technique that must be used appropriately, especially in children, and for monitoring.
- **MRI** requires good cooperation from the patient, with sometimes long acquisition sequences; moreover, it is expensive.

The challenge of medical imaging is to progress from a clinical sign (exo/enophthalmos, visualization/palpation of an anterior mass) to a diagnosis, with its four stages: **detection, localization, characterization, and extension**, as well as appropriate therapeutic management: surgical excision (and deciding on the approach), medical treatment, or merely monitoring but without treatment.

Finally, if a diagnostic decision tree is to be devised for a particular clinical sign suggesting an orbital lesion, one needs to account for the technical platform available (properties and age of item used) but also the delay in scheduling an appointment to perform a specific examination.

## *15.1.1   Detection of a Lesion*

CT, MRI and ultrasound have approximately equivalent performances. First, one should rule out pseudoexophthalmos: ultrasound can confirm unilateral myopia, sometimes unknown or underappreciated by the patient, and by CT scan, with preferably 3D study, to reveal a decrease in the size of the orbital cavity. For detecting space-occupying lesions (SOLs), in France today, it is rare for an easily accessible CT scan not to be performed as first-line. Additionally, MRI can rapidly, and should preferably, replace CT scans.

However, ultrasound can also entirely fulfill this role, except with small lesions of the posterior orbit (Fig. 15.1).

In contrast, with a visible or palpable anterior (palpebral) lesion, even (and above all) if small, ultrasound is certainly the first examination to be performed.

## *15.1.2   The Location of the Lesion*

This should be as accurate as possible, to allow the surgeon to decide on the procedure and the surgical approach:

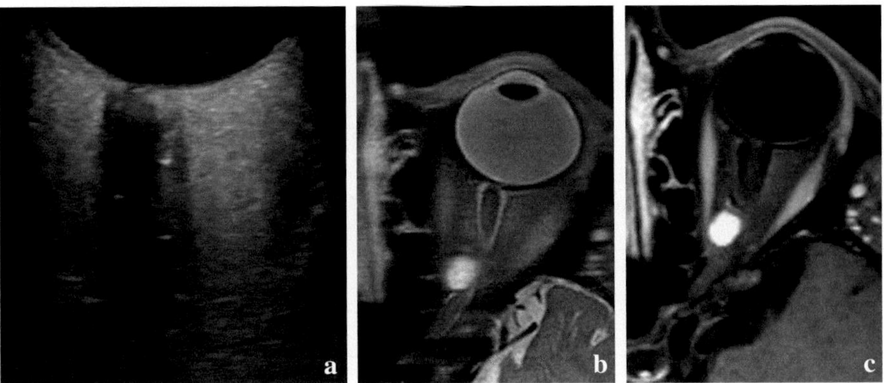

**Fig. 15.1  Failed ultrasound detection of a small, cavernous angioma of the posterior orbit.**
**a**: B-mode axial section; **b**: MRI, T2-weighted axial section; **c**: MRI, T1-weighted axial section
after gadolinium chelate injection. The small lesion, hyperintense in T2 weighted and very intense
after contrast injection, is characteristic of a cavernous hemangioma measuring 5 mm in diameter
× 8 mm in length. It is readily visible by MRI and is not detectable by ultrasound, despite the latter
being performed after the MRI, probably due to its small size and posterior location

- first of all in relation to the muscle cone for retrobulbar lesions and in relation to
  the septum for an eyelid lesion;
- then according to four quadrants (superomedial, superolateral, inferomedial, and
  inferolateral), and three areas (anterior orbit, middle orbit, and posterior orbit/
  apex) [1], to allow the surgeon to decided on the approach (Table 15.1).

However, ultrasound is less efficient than CT and MRI in precisely establishing
this localization, especially if the lesion is large, because in this case, assessing the
lateral edges is often difficult.

### 15.1.3  Characterization of the Lesion

This is based on quantitative elements that are mainly provided by ultrasound (reflectivity, attenuation, and echotexture) but also by MRI (signal intensity [T1, T2, $\rho$]
texture, diffusion characteristics, contrast enhancement, and the T1 dynamic contrast-
enhanced perfusion curve). Assessment of density by CT scan is generally far from
satisfactory, aside from the detection of fatty lesions and small calcifications (e.g.,
phleboliths), which can also be visualized by ultrasound.

This is also based on kinetic elements (e.g., detection of Brownian movements
within a vascular malformation, compressibility of a cavernous hemangioma by the
probe, variability in the volume of an orbital varicose vein). These kinetic criteria
can be assessed even better if CDI is performed together with standard ultrasound,
by studying the vascularization of these different SOLs.

**Table 15.1** Choice of surgical approach for orbital tumors based on [1]

| **Anterior orbit** | |
| --- | --- |
| Superomedial lesions | Central eyebrow incision or in the palpebral crease |
| Superolateral lesions | Incision in the eyebrow or upper eyelid crease by shifting lateraly |
| Anterior and inferior lesions | Either subciliary cutaneous approach or in a fold or conjunctival approach to the inferior fornix |
| Anterolateral lesions | External canthal pathway ± conjonctival pathway |
| Anteromedial lesions | Internal canthal cutaneous approach or conjunctival route |
| **Medium orbit** | Same as anterior orbit ± lateral or inferior osteotomy (Kronlein …) |
| **Orbital apex** | |
| Medial lesions | Conjunctival approach ± lateral route |
| Lesions above the optic nerve | Neurosurgical approach (removal of the orbital roof) |
| Superolateral lesions | Lateral or coronal approach (removal of the lateral wall or roof of the orbit) |
| Inferior lesions, under the optic nerve | Lateral approach or inferior marginotomy |

It should also be clear that the demonstration of such tumor vascularization, with the visualization of small arteries and/or veins, is a semiological element that differs greatly from contrast enhancement of a SOL (iodinated contrast medium for CT, gadolinium chelate for MRI, microbubbles for ultrasound), which reflects the quality and density of microvessels, especially capillaries at the tissue level [2].

## *15.1.4 Extent of the Lesion*

Especially when the lesion is small, ultrasound can visualize the entire lesion and confirm whether a lesion is entirely located in one of the orbital compartments and distinguish it from the normal adjacent structures (optic nerve, muscles). For example, this is the case for small cavernous hemangiomas systematically discovered on CT scan or MRI performed for another indication that can be outlined very well by ultrasound. In this case, ultrasound is also the examination of choice for monitoring this type of small lesion (Fig. 15.2).

When the lesion is larger, and in particular, whether it comes into contact with a bone wall, a high-resolution CT scan with bone windows and filters should be used to assess the exact nature of the bone damage (simple deformation, thinning, erosion, lysis, permeation, condensation, etc.). Ultrasound can, in fact, only reveal

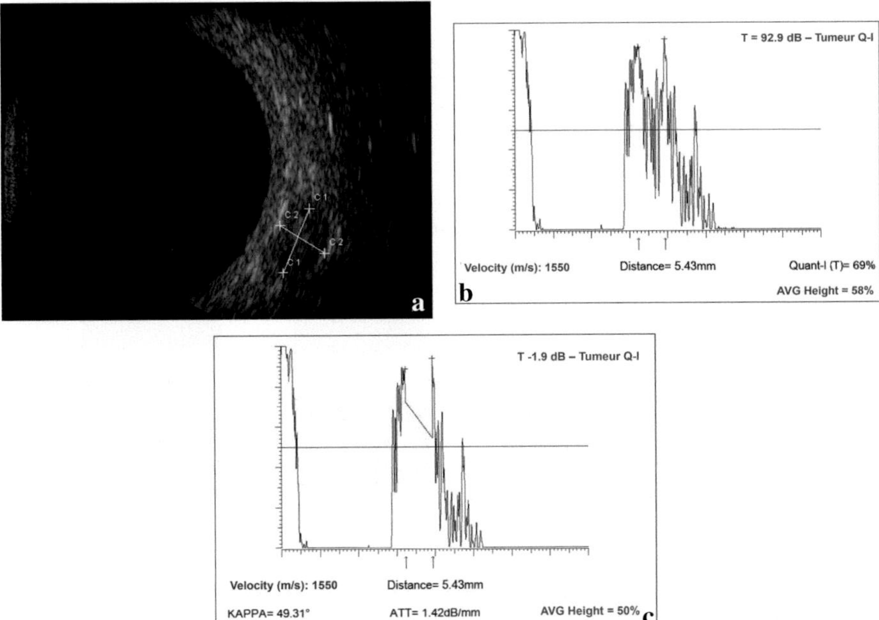

**Fig. 15.2  Microscopic cavernous hemangioma that is readily seen in ultrasound**. a: B-mode section of the temporal quadrant: a small inferior temporal mass discovered fortuitously on a CT scan performed for sinusitis; not far from the eyeball and not distorting its parietal wall, measuring 5.8 mm × 4.3 mm; **b**: standardized A-mode at tissue sensitivity, T = 92.9 dB, to assess the reflectivity of the lesion; **c**: standardized A-mode at T −1.9 dB so that the mean height of the peaks is equal to 50%, to assess the attenuation. The lesion is quite reflective, 69% in Quantification I, and attenuating, with a kappa angle = 49°. Because the lesion is very small and asymptomatic, there is no surgical indication, and annual monitoring by ultrasound is recommended

extensive bone lyses (see Fig. 23.7). MRI is particularly well suited for detecting and assessing orbital SOL extension to the spaces surrounding the orbit (endocranium, paranasal sinuses, pterygomaxillary fossa) as well as for detecting other associated lesions in the various spaces of the head and neck.

Thus, ultrasound plays an important role because it is used at all stages of the diagnosis of an orbital pathology: its detection (even though this step is generally entrusted to CT or MRI), its location and extension, and **especially its characterization**, by assessing the reflectivity, attenuation, texture, and vascularization (by CDI). Therefore, we propose the following algorithm for assessing exophthalmos (Fig. 15.3).

However, the other modalities (CT and MRI) have indications which must be understood and known and that depend on careful analysis of clinical signs:

- **In case of an anterior mass**, when visible and palpable, ultrasound, as the first examination, can detect the lesion and locate it in relation to the septum. It is an adequate examination to characterize the lesion: a dermoid cyst, vascular mass, lymphoid lesion, or another malignant lesion. If the lesion appears to be in contact

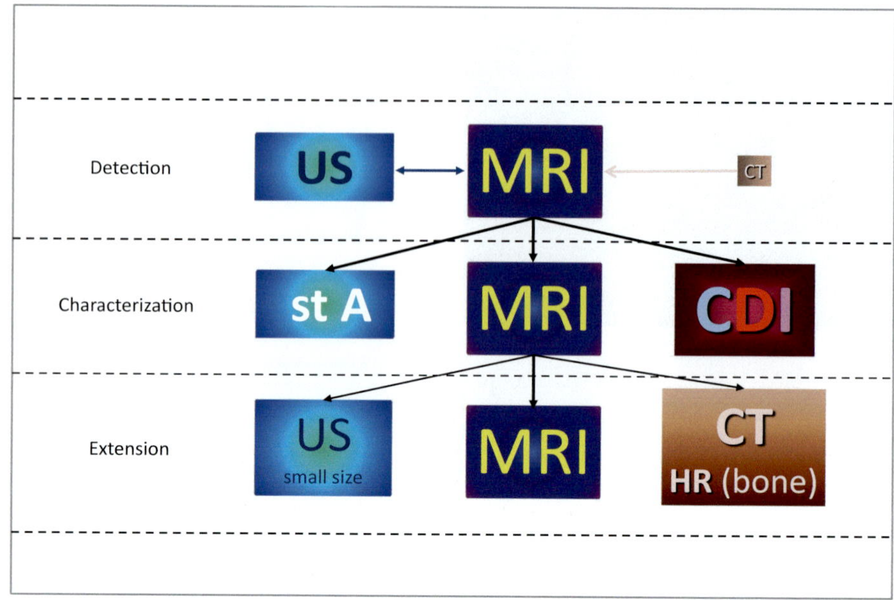



**Fig. 15.3** **Diagnostic algorithm for exophthalmos**

with the bone surface, or if it is a mass of the lacrimal gland, a CT scan allows for assessing the bone in contact with the mass. Ultrasound (and CDI) is sufficient in this case to consider the subsequent diagnostic steps (see Chap. 21).

- **In case of suspected retrobulbar mass**, mainly resulting in exophthalmos, the characteristics of exophthalmos can already point to a particular diagnosis: its axial nature or, by contrast, association with an eyeball displacement, its isolated nature, or in association with anomalies of visual acuity or the visual field, oculomotor disorders, ptosis, the existence or absence of associated pain, the age of the patient, the nature of the onset: sudden, fast, pseudoinflammatory, or slow, not noticed by the patient but noted by those around them (in this case, old photographs can be useful).

In all of these cases, imaging (and therefore ultrasound) allows for diagnosis of:

- damage to the optic nerve (see Chaps. 18 and 19);
- dysthyroid orbitopathy (see Chap. 16);
- a retrobulbar SOL separate from the optic nerve (see Chap. 20);

  - vascular masses;
  - fibrous tumors;
  - nerve tumors;

- orbital inflammation, lymphoma (see Chaps. 17, 22 and 24);
- a malignant, primary, metastatic, or spreading tumor (see Chap. 24);
- a granuloma, an abscess (see Chap. 23).

Ultrasound is rarely used to evaluate the orbital damage of general diseases.

- **In case of suspected varicose vein**, in which the main symptom is exophthalmos that varies according to the position (standing/head tilted forward, decubitus/procubitus) or circumstances (at rest/exertion/Valsalva). The exophthalmos can even be absent at rest and replaced by enophthalmos, with the diagnosis based on the appearance or increase in the volume of the lesion in these triggering circumstances. Regardless of the method used, one must generate sections at rest in decubitus, then in procubitus (in ultrasound, a position preferentially replaced by hyperdecubitus, with the head tilted back in hyperextension) (see Chap. 20).
- **In case of suspected arteriovenous fistula**, in which exophthalmos is associated with conjunctival redness and chemosis, CDI is a necessary and adequate examination, followed by an interventional neuroradiological procedure. In a traumatic context, a CT scan of the base of the skull can provide assessment of any bone lesions (see Chap. 20).
- **Fine-needle biopsy under ultrasound control.** This also still involves a role for ultrasound [3]. However, the indications are relatively infrequent because they involve a mass with a mostly posterior localization (therefore, a tricky surgical approach), quite voluminous (at least 20 mm in diameter), clearly visible on ultrasound, and presumed to be malignant (and hence treatable with chemo- or radiotherapy), not hypervascularized, and accessible using a 16G or 18G needle without risk to the eyeball. The sampling is more informative if it can provide tissue rather than just cells. Finally, the ability to perform an extemporaneous examination is useful. Such a puncture with a fine needle can also be used to evacuate a hematoma (see Chap. 25).

The following chapters follow an order that appears logical to us, but we are also cognizant that certain etiologies can be encountered in different sections, especially for vascular, malignant, childhood, and lacrimal fossa tumors. In these instances, the most illustrative image is placed in the most logical place, and to avoid redundancies, we refer the reader to this figure when we address this etiology a second time.

Nonetheless, we hope that these chapters will help you find the "glass slipper" to discover the "orbit" princess.

# References


1. Morax S. Chirurgie orbitaire (chap 21). In: Pathologie Orbito-Palpébrale Adenis JP et Morax S, editors. Rapport de la Société Française d'Ophtalmologie, Masson, Paris; 1998. p. 765–818
2. Ibrahim MA, Hazhirkarzar B, Dublin AB. Gadolinium magnetic resonance imaging. In: StatPearls [Internet]. Treasure Island (FL): StatPearls Publishing; 2021.
3. Timmis A, Touska P, Uddin J, Pilcher J. The role of ultrasound-guided tissue sampling techniques in the management of extra-ocular orbital lesions. Ultrasound. 2018;26(3):145–52.

# Chapter 16
# Dysthyroid Orbitopathy

François Lafitte, Mario de La Torre, and Olivier Bergès

**Abstract** Dysthyroid orbitopathy is frequent: it is responsible for 15% to 30% of all unilateral exophthalmos and 80% of all bilateral exophthalmos. Although CT scan is frequently thought to be the best technique, ultrasound is useful for the diagnosis: showing hyperreflective muscles, with normal tendons. Color Doppler imaging is as efficient as MRI to evaluate the degree of inflammation of the muscles: hypervascularization of the affected muscles. It is also useful to look for damage to the optic nerve: decrease in the peak systolic velocities of the central retinal artery, with a high resistive index or dark signal of the spectral analysis curve, and dilation and reverse flow in the superior ophthalmic vein. In standardized A-mode, validated muscle indices allow for grading the severity of the disease. Differential diagnosis of large extraocular muscles includes orbital inflammation, and tumoral or vascular causes (fistulae, ischemia or traumatism).

In 90% of cases, the dysthyroid pathology is due to autoimmune hyperthyroidism (mainly Graves' disease, sometimes toxic adenoma); in 5% of cases it is due to Hashimoto's thyroiditis, and in the remaining 5%, it is due to isolated biological autoimmune abnormalities [1]. It comprises an inflammatory phase, followed secondarily by progression to fibrosis.

It is the most common orbitopathy, affecting approximately 0.5% of the population in the United States, and it is responsible for 15% to 30% of all unilateral exophthalmos and 80% of all bilateral exophthalmos [2]. However, atypical forms, such as involving simple retraction of the upper eyelid, should not be ignored. A thyroid and autoimmune biological assessment should be performed, which is sometimes normal in 5% to 10% of patients with orbitopathy, resulting in Means or Saint-Yves' syndrome [3].

F. Lafitte · O. Bergès (✉)
Rothschild Foundation Hospital, Paris, France
e-mail: oberges@for.paris

M. de La Torre
Universidad Nacional Mayor de San Marcos, Lima, Perú

© The Author(s), under exclusive license to Springer Nature Switzerland AG 2024   365
O. Bergès (ed.), *Echography of the Eye and Orbit*,
https://doi.org/10.1007/978-3-031-41467-1_16

Proponents of standardized echography affirm the effectiveness of this technique for the diagnosis and management of this disease [4]. However, aside from expert hands and experience in this technique, an orbital CT scanner **without injection** is the first examination to be performed. It allows for reliable measurement of the degree of exophthalmos [5, 6] and reveals varying extents of bilateral increase in the volume of the orbital fat (especially retrobulbar) and several extraocular muscles (in order of frequency: inferior rectus, medial rectus, and superior muscular complex). However, the damage can be unilateral or limited to fat hypertrophy or a single muscle. In these unusual forms, a differential diagnosis can arise with orbital myositis, a muscle tumor, or even a dural fistula. It also allows for assessing orbital bone walls and adjacent paranasal sinuses. MRI is mainly useful for assessing the degree of inflammation of the muscles or to look for damage to the optic nerve, especially by muscle compression at the apex.

**B-mode ultrasound and color Doppler imaging (CDI)** is usually not performed as first-line, but it nonetheless provides very useful information. B-mode shows the increase in volume of the affected muscle(s) in the muscle belly, but especially sparing the tendon (Fig. 16.1). It also shows the hyperreflective nature of the muscle, especially at its anterior part and less at the level of the muscle belly, where it is thickest (Fig. 16.2). **standardized A-mode** can reveal these signs and allows for evaluating the severity of the disease based on validated muscle indices for grading the orbitopathy [7, 8] (Table 16.1). The first index is the muscle index (M.I.), equal, for each orbit, to the sum of the maximum thicknesses of each muscle divided by 6. Another muscle index, useful for severe forms, is the supero nasal index (S.N.I.), equal, again for each orbit, to the sum of the maximum thicknesses of the superior rectus, the medial rectus, and the superior oblique muscle, divided by 3. The curves of the different muscles in A-mode and the index constitute the Muscle Profile (Fig. 16.3). Also, the optic nerve and lacrimal gland can be measured and orbital edema in B-mode searched for.

According to de La Torre [9], depending on these grades, the following approach can be proposed:

Grade 0: No ultrasound monitoring or monitoring according to clinical symptoms.

Grade 1: Annual ultrasound monitoring.

Grade 2: Half-yearly ultrasound monitoring (with assessment based on the S.N.I.).

Grade 3: Ultrasound monitoring at 3 months (with optic nerve evaluation).

Grade 4: Ultrasound monitoring at 1 month (with evaluation of visual function++ and an indication of orbital decompression.

CDI provides important signs regarding the vascular factor associated with orbitopathy and is particularly useful for monitoring the effectiveness of treatment [10]. In case of compression at the orbital apex or excessive stretching of the optic nerve in pronounced exophthalmos, it may reveal possible vascular damage to the optic nerve head.

**With CDI**, inflammatory muscles are hypervascularized, with intrinsic capillary-arterial flows (Fig. 16.4). In addition, orbital inflammation results in increased flow in the ophthalmic artery and the central retinal vessels (an increase in the peak systolic and diastolic velocities).

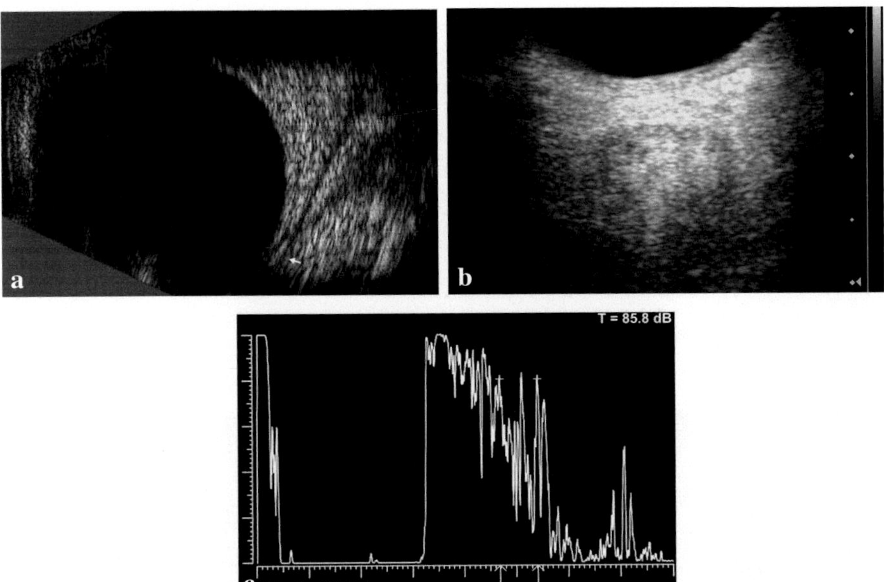



**Fig. 16.1 Graves' disease: inferior rectus muscle. a**: Longitudinal section of the muscle:10 MHz B-mode probe, with an ophthalmic dedicated unit; **b**: Coronal section of the muscle: B-mode wide band probe centered on 10 MHz with a multipurpose unit. **c**: standardized A-mode at the level of the muscle belly, along the red dotted line generated in **a**. The muscle has a significantly increased volume; its diameter (at the level of the belly) is 5.62 mm. Whatever the ultrasound unit and mode, its belly is hyperechoic, its echotexture is heterogeneous; outlines are blurry, with a thickened hyperechoic fibrous envelope. The tendon is thin (white arrow in **a**)

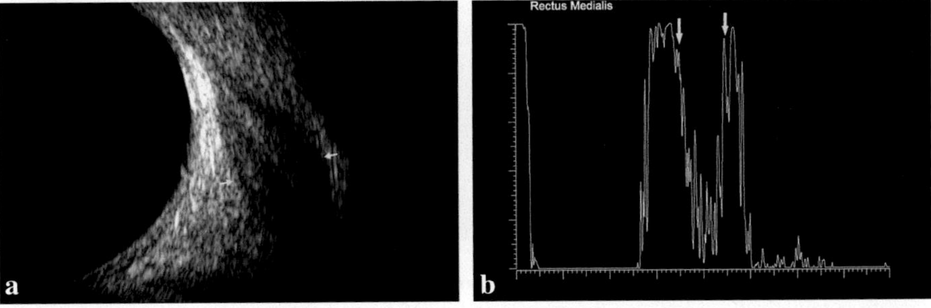



**Fig. 16.2 Graves' disease: medial rectus muscle. a**: Longitudinal muscle section: 10-MHz B-mode probe with a dedicated ophthalmic device; **b**: standardized A-mode at the level of the muscle belly, where it is thickest. The muscle is very large (measured diameter = 7.08 mm) at the level of its belly (→ yellow arrows), whereas the tendon is normal (→ red arrow). The echotexture is only moderately echogenic (compare with Fig. 16.1c) because the section passes through the muscle belly, which is slightly less echogenic than its anterior part, especially because the ultrasound beam is slightly more oblique to the muscle belly and a little more perpendicular to the tendon

**Table 16.1** Severity of dysthyroid orbitopathy according to the muscle index (M.I.) and supero nasal index (S.N.I.)

| Muscle profile and severity of dysthyroid orbitopathy | Thickness (mm) | Grade |
|---|---|---|
| *Muscle index* | | |
| Normal | 3.5–4.5 | 0 |
| Slight | 4.5–5.4 | 1 |
| Moderate | 5.5–6.4 | 2 |
| Severe | > 6.5 | 3 |
| *Supero nasal index* | | |
| Risk of optic nerve compression at orbital apex | > 7 | 4 |

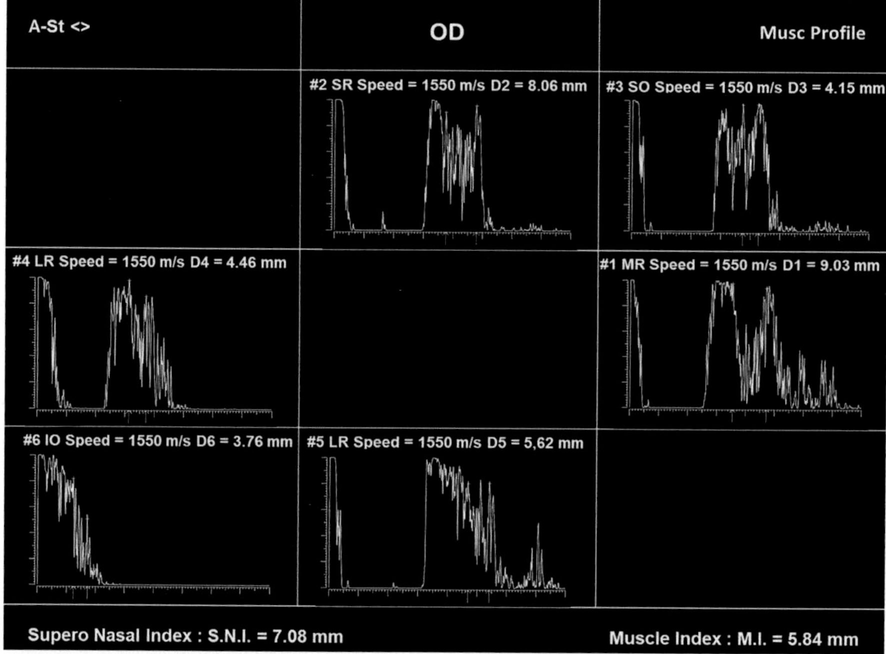


**Fig. 16.3 Muscle profile in standardized A-mode.** All muscles are recorded and measured. The program automatically calculates the muscle index (M.I.) and the superior nasal index (S.N.I.). This is a severe form, with an M.I. of 5.84 mm and an SNI of 7.08 mm, which indicates a risk of compression of the optic nerve at the orbital apex; corticoid eyedrops and/or orbital decompression are indicated

Quantifying fat hypertrophy is usually more difficult with ultrasound than with CT and MRI. In addition, significant fat hypertrophy can perturb the homogeneity and energy of the ultrasound beam. One should also look for fatty infiltration (especially in the vicinity of affected muscles) or thickening of the optic nerve meninges.

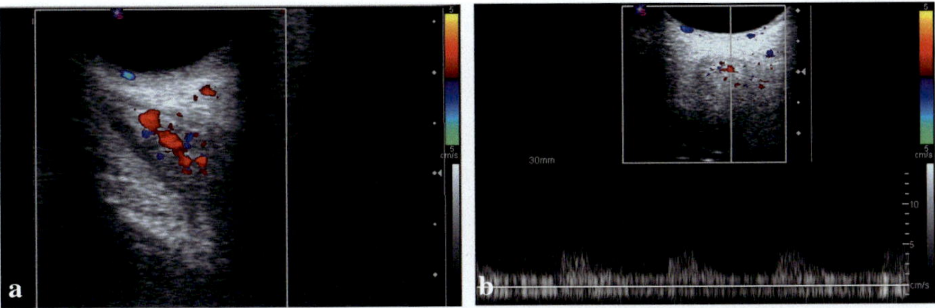

**Fig. 16.4 Graves' disease: medial rectus muscle. Color Doppler imaging. a**: Longitudinal section of the muscle: color mode; **b**: Muscle cross-section: color and spectral modes. The anterior part of the very echogenic muscle is vascularized. The flows are capillary-arterial, rather resistive, with no characteristic value

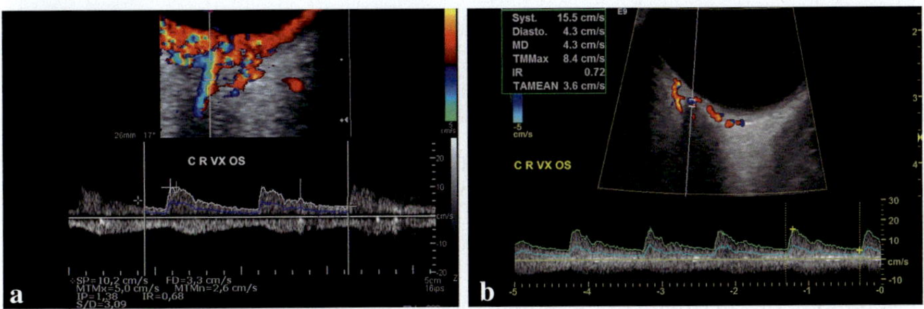

**Fig. 16.5 Graves' disease.** Color Doppler imaging of the central retinal vessels. **a**: Dilated appearance of the vessels of the optic nerve head in an inflammatory form, with rather weak flows (peak systolic velocity = 10.2 cm/s) but with a normal resistive index (0.68); **b**: thin appearance of the vessels of the optic nerve head and slight elevation of the resistive index of the central retinal artery in a form with compression of the optic nerve at the orbital apex

In case of optic nerve compression at the orbital apex, which is more frequent in cases of involvement of the medial rectus, superior rectus, and superior oblique muscles, one can visualize dilation of the perioptic subarachnoid spaces, papilledema, or, even in CDI, signs of vascular damage to the vessels of the optic nerve head: decrease in the peak systolic velocities of the arteries, with an increase in the resistive index or a decrease in the signal of the spectral analysis curve (Fig. 16.5), dilation and reverse flow in the superior ophthalmic vein (Fig. 16.6), the latter sign being well correlated with the abnormalities observed in the visual field [11].

At the fibrous phase, the muscles are reduced in volume, remaining hyperechoic, but they are sometimes even filiform and no longer appear hypervascularized.

In ultrasound, the differential diagnosis of one or more large muscle(s) includes the following:

- A specific or idiopathic inflammatory origin, but typically the muscle(s) concerned appear hypoechoic, with thickening of the tendon (see Chap. 17).

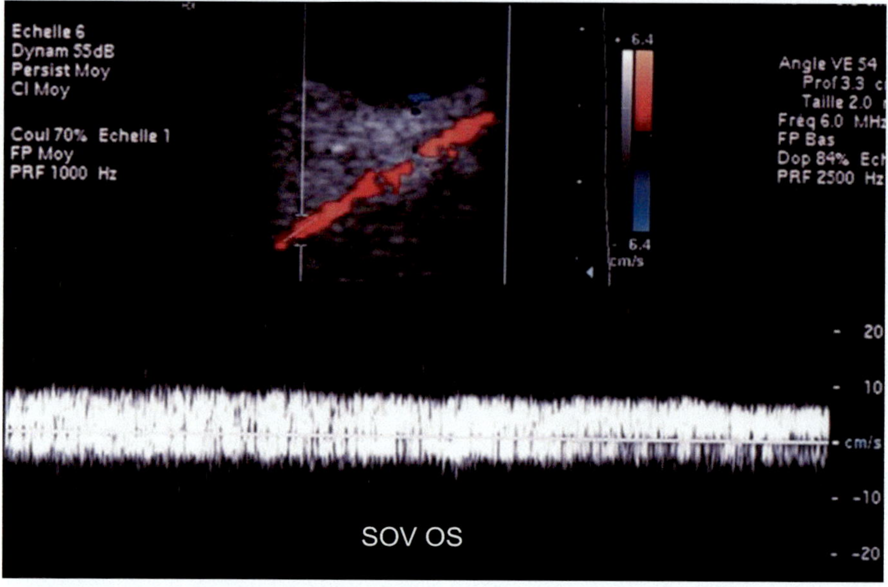


**Fig. 16.6  Graves' disease with compression of the optic nerve at the orbital apex.** Color and spectral Doppler of the superior ophthalmic vein (SOV). The SOV appears linear, red in color mode, with an inverted flow that remains venous: linear and positive in spectral mode

- A tumoral origin (mainly lymphoma, metastasis, of a known or unknown primary tumor, or infiltrated by an adjacent tumor) (see Chaps. 22 and 24)
- A vascular origin: carotid-cavernous fistula, dural fistula, ischemia, or traumatic hemorrhage (see Chaps. 20 and 25).

# References


1. Bourjat P. Pathologie inflammatoire et infectieuse de l'orbite *in* Imagerie oculo-orbitaire. Paris: Masson; 2000. p. 51.
2. Weber AL, Dallow RL, Sabates NR. Grave's disease of the orbit. Neuroimaging Clin N Am. 1996;6(1):61–72.
3. Hornez N, Morell-Dubois J, Wemau JL, Hatron PY, et al. Le syndrome de means : à propos d'une observation. Rev Med Interne. 2009;30(11):988–90.
4. Ossoinig KC. [A new echographic sign for the reliable diagnosis of Grave's disease (author's transl) [Article in German] Klin Monbl Augenheilkd. 1982;180(3):189–97.
5. Guo J, Qian J, Yuan Y. Two-dimensional versus three-dimensional techniques. Curr Eye Res. 2018;43(5):647–653.
6. Delmas J, Loustau JM, Martin S, Bourmault L, Adenis JP, Robert PY. Comparative study of 3 exophthalmometers and computed tomographic biometry. Eur J Ophthalmol. 2018;28(2):144–9.
7. Ossoinig KC. The role of standardized ophthalmic echography in the management of Grave's ophthalmopathy. In: Pickardt CR, Boergen KP editors. graves opthalmopathy—developments

in diagnostic methods and therapeutical procedures. International workshop. Homburg/Saar, October 7, 1987 Dev Ophthalmol. 1989;20:28–37.

8. Ossoinig KC. The diagnosis and differential diagnosis of neoplastic lesions of the extraocular muscles with standardized echography. In: Thijssen JM, Fledelius HC, Tane S, editors. Ultrasonography in Ophthalmology 14 Proceedings of the 14th SIDUO Congress, Tokyo, Japan; 1992. pp. xxxiii-lvi. Documenta Ophthalmologica Proceedings Series, vol 58. Springer Science + Business Media Dordrecht 1995.

9. de La Torre M. The role of Standardized echography for diagnosis and management of Grave's orbitopathy. Presentation at the pre SIDUO meeting standardized Course, SIDUO XXIII Edimburgh (Scotland) September 10, 2010.

10. Numan Alp M, Ozgen A, Gunalp I, et al. Colour Doppler imaging of the orbital vasculature in Grave's disease with computed tomographic correlation. Br J Ophthalmol. 2000;84:1027–30.

11. Berges O, Lafitte F, Koskas P. The orbit in Grainger and Allison's, diagnostic radiology, vol. 3, 4th ed. London:Churchill Livingstone;2001. p. 2530.

# Chapter 17
# Inflammatory Lesions

**François Lafitte, Augustin Lecler, Mario de La Torre, and Olivier Bergès**

**Abstract** Formerly called pseudotumors, these frequent lesions are presented rather according to their location: myositis (with involvement of the tendon), dacryoadenitis (with involvement of the two lobes), optic nerve perineuritis, posterior scleritis, blepharitis, or sometimes a true pseudotumor mass. They may be idiopathic or related to a systemic disease. The lesions are firm, low to moderately echogenic, often heterogeneous when chronic due to fibrosis and consistently vascularized, with a resistive index inferior to 0.70.

These are frequent lesions, often with a histologic appearance that is not specific: polyclonal lymphoplasmacytic infiltration, except in the case of IgG4-related disease. Idiopathic orbital inflammation (IOI) is often a diagnosis of exclusion, which needs to be differentiated from infections, systemic inflammatory disease, or even neoplasms. An etiology is found in only approximately 50% of cases, even after a careful general assessment.

The main etiologies are represented by local causes (adjacent infectious foci, especially sinus or dental) and by specific systemic diseases (sarcoidosis, Sjögren syndrome, etc.) (Table 17.1).

Dysthyroid orbitopathy is discussed in a separate chapter (Chap. 16).

Clinically, there is pain, a certain degree of exophthalmos [1] and often ocular motricity or vision disorders. The eye is red with anterior involvement (conjunctiva, sclera) but may appear normal with isolated posterior involvement.

The affected structures are, in order of decreasing frequency, the lacrimal gland, muscles, wall of the globe (sclera and episclera), optic nerve sheaths, and fat. These lesions can sometimes extend intracranially and are then related to Tolosa-Hunt syndrome [2].

F. Lafitte · A. Lecler · O. Bergès (✉)
Rothschild Foundation Hospital, Paris, France
e-mail: oberges@for.paris

M. de La Torre
Universidad Nacional Mayor de San Marcos, Lima, Perú


O. Bergès (ed.), *Echography of the Eye and Orbit*,
https://doi.org/10.1007/978-3-031-41467-1_17

                                                                  

**Table 17.1** The main systemic causes of inflammatory lesions

| Common causes | Rare causes |
| --- | --- |
| Sarcoidosis | Polyarterisis nodosa |
| Wegener granulomatosis | Lupus |
| Sjögren syndrome | Anti-neutrophil cytoplasmic autoantibody vasculitis |
| IgG4 | Atrophying polychondritis |
| | Xanthogranulomatosis |
| | Myelin oligodendrocyte glycoprotein vasculitis |

The affliction can occur in two ways:

- Either poorly delineated infiltrating lesions without real mass: cellulitis can then be an issue, although in this case, the infectious presentation would be more pronounced, the progression more rapid, with a tendency to abscess, and there is often a suggestive context (trauma, recent intervention).
- Or it is a true pseudotumor compact mass (formerly called "inflammatory pseudotumor"). A differential diagnosis then arises with a tumor, particularly a lymphoma, especially because these two entities can switch from one to the other. Also, the term inflammatory pseudotumor should no longer be used but rather, a word associating the precise localization with the suffix, itis for inflammation: myositis for inflammation of a muscle, dacryoadenitis for inflammation of the lacrimal gland, etc.

## 17.1  Orbital Inflammation: Positive Diagnosis

**In ultrasound,** all these lesions present as slightly echogenic and firm upon pressure from the probe [3]. This firmness is even more pronounced when the lesions have progressed to fibrosis. They are not altered during positional maneuvers.

- Myositis generally involves the entire muscle **with involvement of the tendon** (Fig. 17.1) (unlike Graves' disease).
- Dacryoadenitis results in a hypoechoic lacrimal gland with regular contours, discreetly hypoechoic, sometimes bilateral.

  - In the acute stage, the enlarged gland is swollen and well delineated, with cellular infiltration resulting in a low echogenic background on which moderate echogenic areas corresponding to edema are noted (Fig. 17.2).
  - In the chronic stage, the lesion appears overall a little less hypoechoic, with more considerably echogenic areas corresponding to fibrosis. Because the two lobes of the gland (palpebral and orbital) are generally affected, the anterior part of the lesion is usually evaluated paraocularly and its posterior part transocularly (Fig. 17.3).

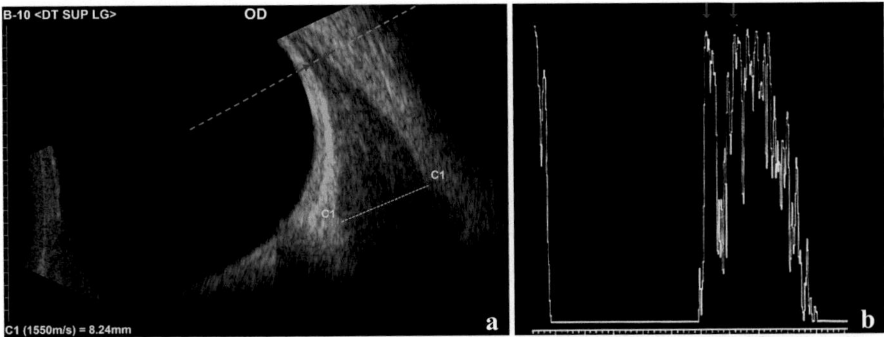

**Fig. 17.1 Inflammatory myositis** associated with Lyme disease. **a**: B-mode, longitudinal section of the superior rectus muscle; **b**: standardized A-mode at the tendon (muscle insertion). The inflammatory infiltration is not very echogenic; it thickens the muscle, not only in its lower third, in the muscle belly, where it measures 8.24 mm (yellow dotted line), but also at the level of its insertion tendon (→ red arrows)

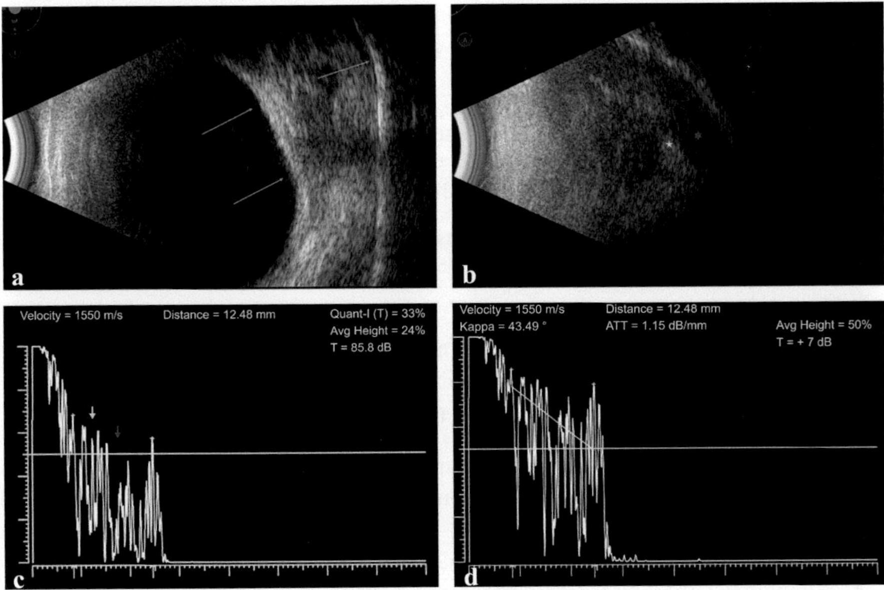

**Fig. 17.2 Acute dacryoadenitis due to herpes simplex virus infection.** **a**: B-mode, transocular section; **b**: B-mode, paraocular section; **c**: standardized A-mode at tissue sensitivity (T = 85.8 dB), for assessing reflectivity; **d**: standardized A-mode at T + 7.0 dB, the average height of the peaks being 50%, for assessing the attenuation. The lesion, which appeared rapidly, is voluminous. The transocular section (**a**) shows the deformation of the eye wall (→ blue arrows) and the bony wall opposite (→ green arrow). Via the paraocular approach (**b**), and in A-mode, the lesion is clearly visible on both lobes of the gland. Its echotexture is moderately echogenic, with a slightly echogenic background (✪ and → red star and arrow) with many patches of relatively reflective edema (★ and → yellow star and arrow)

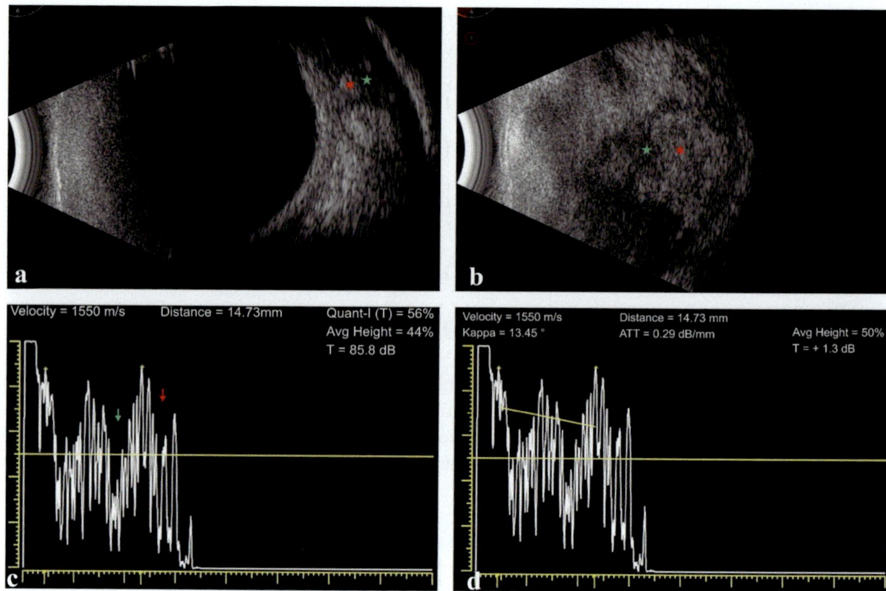

**Fig. 17.3 Chronic dacryoadenitis. a**: B-mode, transocular approach; **b**: B-mode, paraocular approach; **c**: standardized A-mode at tissue sensitivity (T = 85.8 dB), for assessing the reflectivity; **d**: standardized A-mode at T + 1.3 dB, the average height of the peaks being 50%, for assessing the attenuation. The gland is overall more echogenic than in the acute stage, already discernible in B-mode, but quantifiable in standardized A-mode, with reflectivity of 56% versus 33% mainly because of the appearance of areas of fibrosis (★ and → red stars and arrow) surrounding less echogenic inflammatory areas (★ and → green stars and arrow)

- Perineuritis is seen as an echogenic inflammatory thickening around the optic nerve fibers (see Fig. 18.15), associated with optic disc protrusion and inflammatory signs surrounding it (in the vitreous) (Fig. 17.4).

  - Posterior scleritis results in thickening of the posterior wall, with often an associated effusion in the sub-Tenon space (Fig. 17.5), sometimes associated with significant masses, which can sometimes present a diagnostic problem with a genuine tumor (see Fig. 12.62).
  - Blepharitis: imaging is rarely requested, except when the damage is substantial and bilateral, suggesting Morbihan syndrome, a syndrome associating recurrent, cortico-resistant palpebral edema, progressing by flares, in a chronic manner and in a context of rosacea, for which a lymphoma should be ruled out (Fig. 17.6).

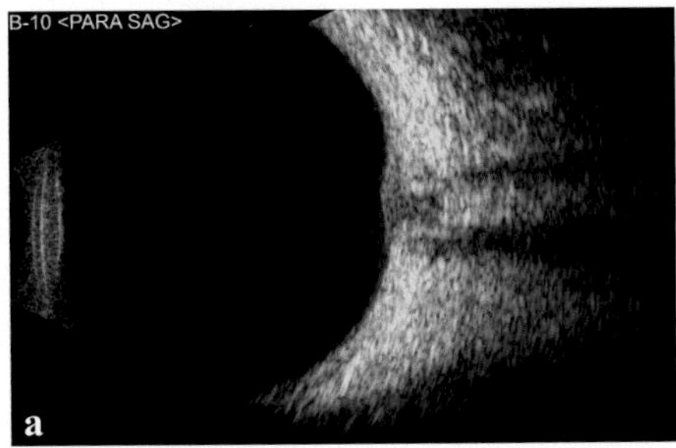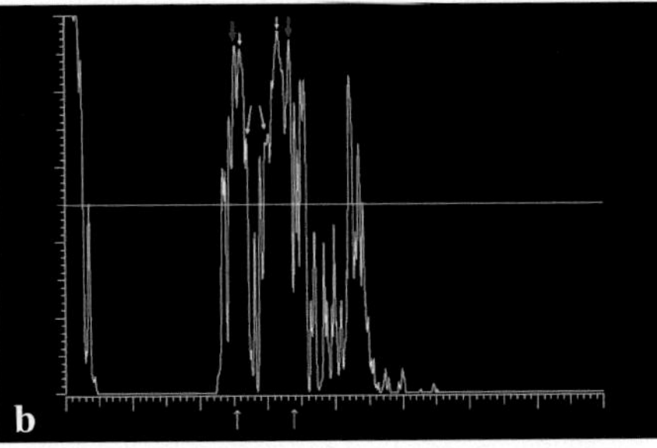

**Fig. 17.4  Optic perineuritis. a**: B-mode; **b**: standardized A-mode. The protrusion of the optic disc is clearly visible in B-mode, but the alterations of the optical complex are better evaluated in A-mode. The diameter of the optical fibers, from pia mater to pia mater (→ yellow arrows), is normal. There is discreet enlargement of the diameter from arachnoid to arachnoid (→ white arrows) and discreet enlargement from dura mater to dura mater (→ red arrows), albeit remaining within the normal range because it measures 5.84 mm. The diagnosis in this case is established by comparison with the contralateral side

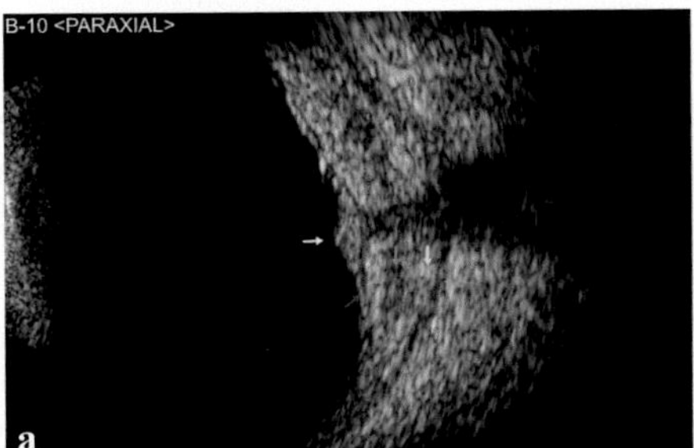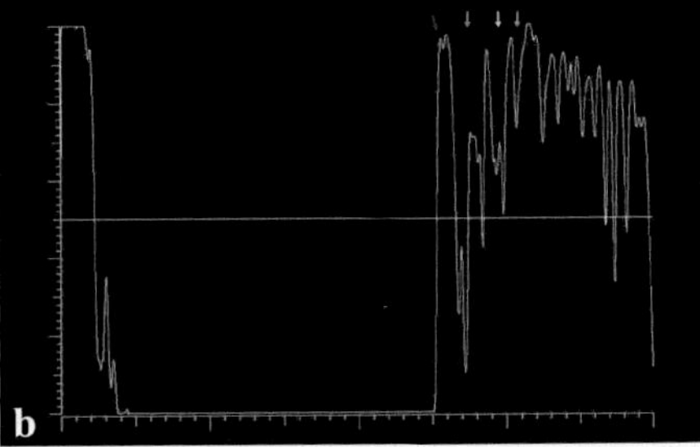

**Fig. 17.5  Granulomatous uveoscleral inflammation with papillitis. a**: B-mode; **b**: standardized A-mode. Pronounced parietal thickening affecting all tunics, the sclera (→yellow arrow), the choroid (→blue arrow) with hypo- and moderately echogenic areas. Note also papillitis (→ white arrow), and a peripapillary SRD (→red arrow). Finally, there is also episcleritis (→green arrow)

## 17.2  Diagnostic Guidance

- When the lesion is bilateral (especially in the lacrimal region), it preferentially suggests sarcoidosis or Mikulicz syndrome, but tumor involvement should be ruled out (especially lymphoma or Erdheim–Chester disease: non-Langerhans histiocytosis, with multisystemic involvement, although rare).
- Aggressive lesions can result in destruction of the orbital walls, better visible by CT [6]. In this case, Wegener's granulomatosis or mycosis is the first consideration.
- Extensive involvement with infiltration and hypertrophy of the V2 nerves in the infraorbital canal++ suggests IgG4-related disease [7].

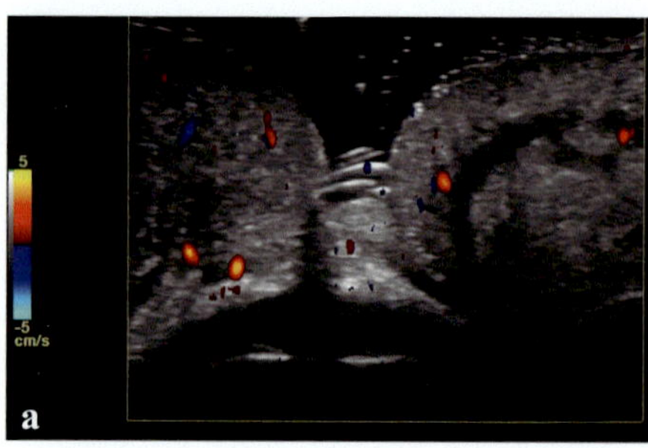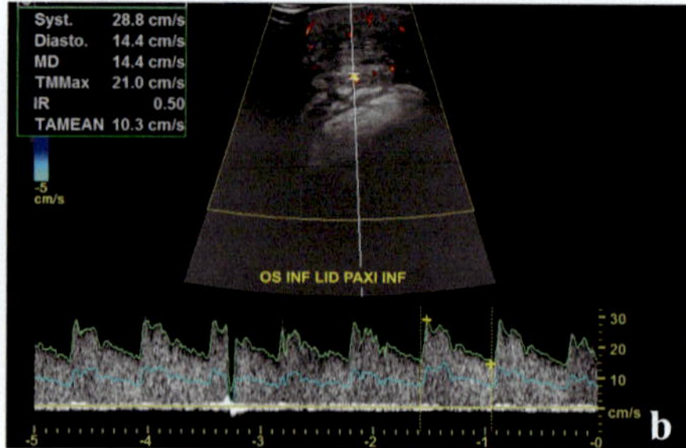


**Fig. 17.6 Morbihan syndrome. a**: Color Doppler imaging (CDI), color mode, sagittal section of both inferior and superior eyelids; **b**: CDI, color and spectral modes at the level of the lower eyelid, para-axial section. The appearance is bilateral and symmetrical, with a greatly increased eyelid volume, 1.5 mm thick, moderately echogenic, with hypoechoic and vascularized trabeculae, reflecting inflammatory edema. Like all lesions in this chapter, the flows are not very resistive (resistivity index [RI] = 0.50)

## 17.3 Contribution of MRI

This is often performed as a complementary procedure to assess extension of the lesions (++ to the posterior part of the orbit), to measure exophthalmos, to look for a cause (sinusitis++), and possibly to look for other locations including the cavernous sinus or meninges.

The main differential diagnoses are represented by tumor infiltrations (especially hematological malignancies such as lymphoma or leukemia, and metastases), cellulitis (infectious context) and fistulas of the cavernous sinus (through venous stasis).

However, the main interest is to assess the apparent diffusion coefficient (ADC). For this, the lesion has to be sufficiently large: cellulitis has a high ADC, inflammatory lesions an intermediate ADC, and lymphomas a low ADC [8].

## 17.4 Progression

The practical attitude (after imaging examinations and general assessment) consists of rapid treatment with systemic corticosteroids, which generally leads to a noticeable and rapid improvement. A biopsy sample is only taken during the first or second recurrence in case of corticosteroid resistance or in case of doubt with lymphoma or a cause requiring appropriate immunosuppressive treatment (Wegener granulomatosis, IgG4-related disease, etc.).

Follow-up monitoring reveals total regression of the lesions (with a risk of relapse) or chronic persistence with general progression to fibrosis (Figs. 17.7, 17.8, 17.9 and 17.10).

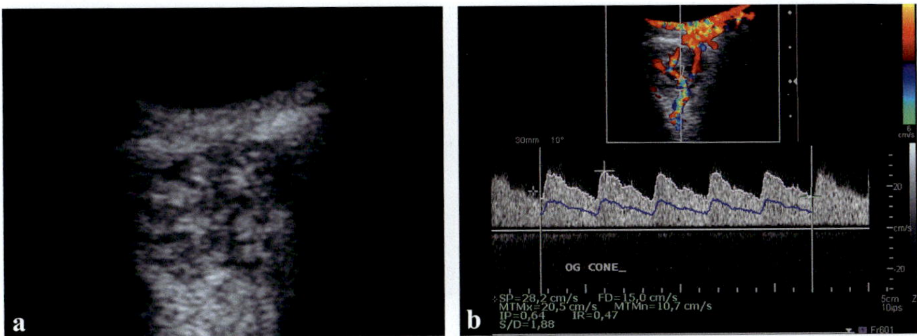

**Fig. 17.7 Retrobulbar inflammatory mass, "inflammatory pseudotumor" a**: B-mode; **b**: CDI, color and spectral modes. The retrobulbar, rounded, slightly echogenic, and heterogeneous mass does not affect the walls of the eyeball. It is vascularized with low resistive flows (RI = 0.54)

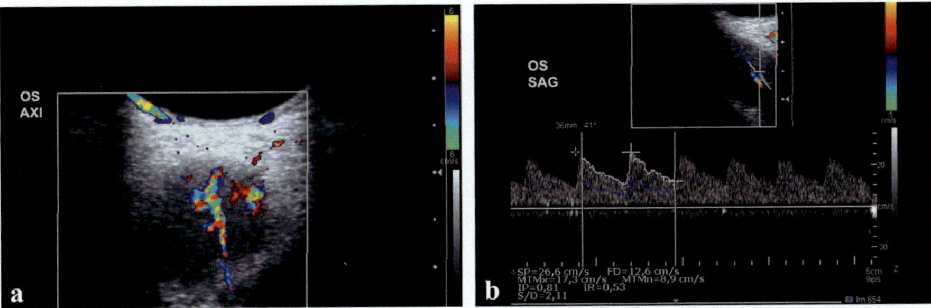

**Fig. 17.8 Inflammatory myositis of the inferior rectus muscle**. CDI. **a**: Color mode, cross-section; **b**: spectral mode, section along the 6 o'clock meridian. The muscle, which is significantly increased in size and hypoechoic, is quite vascularized with large vessels and low resistive flows (RI = 0.53)

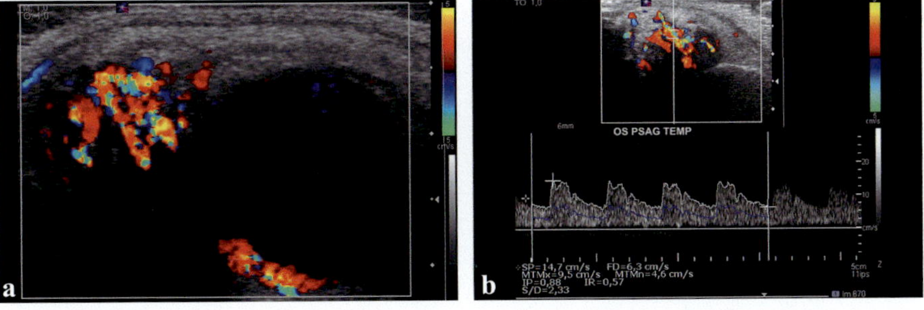

**Fig. 17.9 Acute dacryoadenitis**. CDI. **a**: Color mode, paraocular section; **b**: spectral mode. The lacrimal gland, slightly enlarged in size and hypoechoic, appears highly vascularized, with relatively non-resistive flows (RI = 0.57)

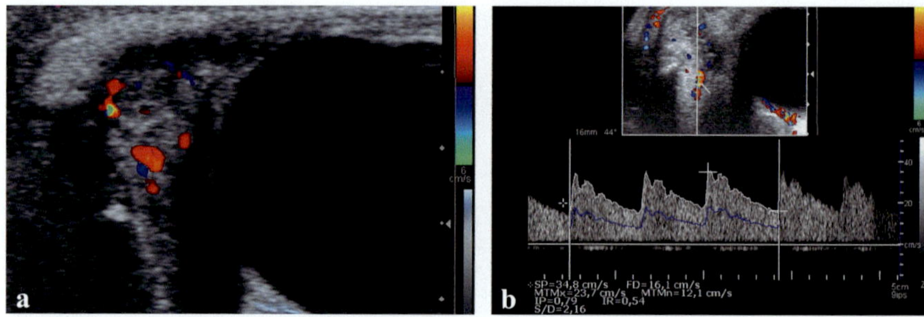

**Fig. 17.10  Chronic dacryoadenitis**. CDI. **a**: Color mode; **b**: spectral mode. The lacrimal gland, moderately increased in size, is quite echogenic and heterogeneous; it is vascularized, with low resistive flows (RI = 0.54)

# References


1. Weber AL, Romo LV, Sabates NR. Pseudotumor of the orbit. Clinical, pathologic, and radiologic evaluation. Radiol Clin North Am. 1999;37(1):151–68, xi.
2. Tedeschi E, Ugga L, Califano F, Brunetti A et al. Intracranial extension of orbital inflammatory pseudotumor: a case report and literature review. BMC Neurol. 2016;16:29.
3. Harr DL, Quencer RM, Abrams GW. Computed tomography and ultrasound in the evaluation of orbital infection and pseudotumor. Radiology. 1982;142(2):395–401.
4. Le L, Galatoire O, Jacomet PV, Morax S et al. Le syndrome du Morbihan. J Fr Ophtalmol. 2009;32(S1):1S183.
5. Lecler A, Morax S, Putterman M, Bergès O, et al. Usefulness of colour Doppler flow imaging in the management of lacrimal gland lesions Eur Radiol. 2017;27(2):779–789.
6. Frohman LP, Kupersmith MH, Lang J, et al. Intracranial extension and bone destruction in orbital pseudotumor. Arch Ophthalmol. 1986;104:380.
7. Lecler A, Puttermann M, Heran F, Galatoire O, et al. Infraorbital nerve involvement on magnetic resonance imaging in European patients with IgG4-related ophthalmic disease: a specific sign. Eur Radiol. 2017;27(4):1335–43.
8. Kapur R, Saran N, French A, Mafee MF. MRI of orbital cellulitis and orbital abscess: the role of diffusion-weighted imaging. AJR Am J Roentgenol. 2009;193(3):W244–50.

# Chapter 18
# Tumors and Masses of the Optic and Perioptic Nerve Fibers

Olivier Bergès and Mario de La Torre

**Abstract** Although MRI plays a major role in the diagnosis of these lesions of the optic nerve, ultrasound is useful too, especially combining B-mode, standardized A-mode and color-Doppler imaging (CDI). Optic pathway gliomas occur mainly in children and are frequently associated with neurofibromatosis type 1. When involving the orbital optic nerve, there is an enlarged fusiform optic nerve, with a possible angulation when posteriorly located and a subsequent dilation of the subarachnoid spaces around the anterior optic fibers. The lesion is well delineated, homogeneous, with sometimes small cystic areas; on CDI, the lesion is most often weakly vascularized. Meningiomas affect especially women from 40 to 60 years of age. On ultrasound, the optic nerve may be coarse and uneven or fusiform, with the optic nerve fibers generally seen inside the mass, more or less eccentric, with an optic disc swelling, or a flattening of the posterior pole and the visibility of calcified nodules (psamomas). On CDI, the tumor is generally quite vascularized. Hemangioblastoma, associated with von Hippel-Lindau disease, most often involves the orbital optic nerve and is very vascularized, with low resistive flows. Lymphoid lesions may be related to optic nerve lymphomas or optic perineuritis; they appear as low reflective, well-limited lesions, which are vascularized with low resistive (RI < 0.70) vessels. The search for an extension of an ocular tumor to the optic nerve involves MRI. Ultrasound would only be able to reveal large lesions, fortunately rare. Cysts may be related to optic nerve coloboma or to pseudocysts, which are small, retrobulbar, superiorly located and incidentally discovered when exploring a normal tension glaucoma.

Ultrasound plays a minimal role in the diagnosis of these lesions of the optic nerve. Although they can certainly be analyzed using ultrasound, their diagnosis is based primarily on MRI. However, one must be aware of their semiology in ultrasound.

O. Bergès (✉)
Rothschild Foundation Hospital, Paris, France
e-mail: oberges@for.paris

M. de La Torre
Universidad Nacional Mayor de San Marcos, Lima, Perú

© The Author(s), under exclusive license to Springer Nature Switzerland AG 2024
O. Bergès (ed.), *Echography of the Eye and Orbit*,
https://doi.org/10.1007/978-3-031-41467-1_18

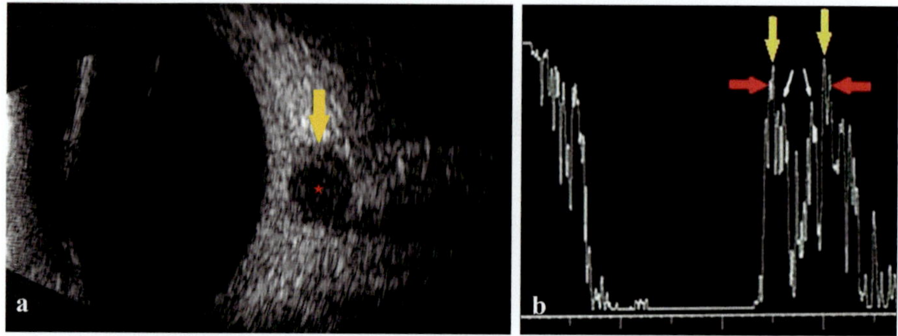

**Fig. 18.1 Normal optic nerve. a**: Presentation in B-mode; **b**: presentation in A-mode. In B-mode, the optic nerve, seen in cross-section, has a round shape in relation to the refraction of the US beam. One can clearly see the dura mater (➜ orange arrow) and, in the center, the optic nerve fibers (★ red star). The subarachnoid spaces can be discerned between the two. In A-mode, the highest peaks correspond to the arachnoid (➜ orange arrows); laterally, and almost as high, one can clearly see the peaks of the dura mater (➜ red horizontal arrows); in the center, the peaks of the pia mater (→ small white oblique arrows)

Standardized A-mode is considerably superior to B-mode for analysis of the normal, and *a fortiori* pathological, optic nerve (Fig. 18.1).

## 18.1 Glioma of the Optic Pathways

Histologically, gliomas of the optic/hypothalamic pathways are WHO Grade 1 juvenile pilocytic astrocytomas [1, 2]. They are the most common intraconal tumor in children. They occur before 30 years of age: 90% before the age of 20, and 75% before the age of 10. However, rare cases have been described in older adults.

More than 50% of patients have neurofibromatosis type 1 (NF1), and glioma of the optical pathways is the most frequent tumor of the central nervous system associated with NF1. The tumor can affect any site along the optic pathways; however, involvement of the optic chiasm and one or both optic nerves is more common than involvement of a single isolated optic nerve. Bilateral tumors are almost pathognomonic for NF1, and isolated optic nerve involvement is more common in patients with NF1.

The warning signs differ depending on whether it is an intraorbital or intracranial glioma. Decreased visual acuity is the most common sign in children; it can manifest as strabismus or amblyopia. A total loss of visual acuity is more common in sporadic cases than in those associated with NF1. Intraorbital gliomas rapidly lead to axile exophthalmos. Gliomas of the optic chiasm tend to lead to visual-field defects, hypothalamic-pituitary dysfunctions and signs of intracranial hypertension, with exophthalmos being rarer and occurring later.

Two architectural forms are generally recognized [3]: in the most frequent, the optic nerve (ON) is affected diffusely, voluminous, and fusiform and is limited by stretched and thinned but intact meninges; the other form, limited by the dura mater, is associated with infiltration of the meninges. Some tumors appear gelatinous or cystic. Microscopic foci of hemosiderin or microcalcifications are sometimes detected on histology in case of "chronic" tumors, but calcifications visible on imaging are rare [3, 4]. Histologically, the tumor consists of portions of compact bipolar cells and other, looser portions of multipolar cells.

From all this, it follows that ultrasound can be used to diagnose intraorbital glioma [5] but that this technique is rarely used because it does not allow analysis of extension of the lesion to the intracranial optical pathways. Therefore, MRI is the technique of choice to assess these lesions, by combining orbital sequences and sequences on the optic chiasm, retro-chiasmatic optic tracts, and the cerebral parenchyma. However, a patient with NF1 should only undergo imaging if there are clinical warning signs [6].

**In ultrasound,** when it is performed, the signs associate:

- A fusiform increase in volume of the ON, which can reach all the way to the orbital apex (Fig. 18.2), the lesion being well delineated, readily discernible in B-mode and with a double peak in A-mode. When the lesion is posteriorly located, there is often angulation of the optic nerve, with dilation of the subarachnoid spaces of the anterior ON behind the eyeball (Fig. 18.3).

When the lesion is small and retrobulbar, the thickening of the ON is clearly visible, well delineated in A-mode, with a homogeneous hypoechoic echotexture (Fig. 18.4).

- The lesion is most often homogeneous, although small cystic areas can often be detected (Fig. 18.2); calcifications remain rare (Fig. 18.5).
- On color Doppler imaging, the lesion is most often weakly or sometimes moderately vascularized, although occasionally an increase in the size of the central retinal artery can be seen (Fig. 18.6).


## 18.2  Optic Nerve Sheath Meningioma

These are especially common in adults between 40 and 60 years of age, and most occur in women (90%). However, they can also occur in children, before 10 years of age, as part of neurofibromatosis type 2 (NF2). The clinical signs combine exophthalmos and decreased visual acuity. A decrease in visual acuity leading to rapid optic atrophy can be a sign of intracanalicular involvement. Oculomotor nerve palsy and corneal sensitivity disorders are delayed: when the tumors are large with posterior extension. They can be bilateral, in young patients, with dense, numerous, and extensive calcifications in the context of NF2. As with all optic nerve masses, MRI is the examination of choice for their assessment.

**On ultrasound,** the ON may be coarse and uneven or fusiform (Figs. 18.7 and 18.8) and of variable size.

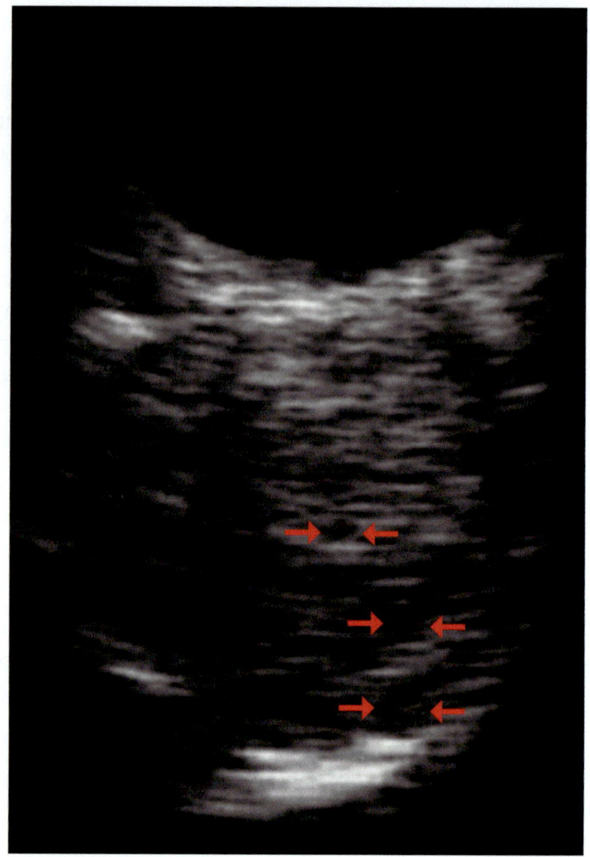

**Fig. 18.2  Large right intraorbital glioma**. B-mode, para-axial section. The mass occupies the entire intraconal space up to the apex. It cannot be separated from the optic nerve. It is slightly hypoechoic, generally homogeneous, and not very attenuating (the posterior wall of the orbit can be clearly seen). Note the presence of several small cystic entities (→ red arrows), these cysts being frequent

The ON fibers can generally be seen inside the mass, more or less eccentric (Figs. 18.8, 18.9, 18.10). On a coronal section, the diameter of these optic nerve fibers is usually less than 3 mm, less than that of a normal ON, but this is not a specific sign because it can also be found in some pseudotumors.

The reflectivity of the tumor is variable, often heterogeneous (Fig. 18.9a), and the attenuation medium to high (Fig. 18.9b), which often prevents the tumor from being seen at the orbital apex when the lesion is large.

Quite frequently there is a small hyperechoic optic disc swelling (Figs. 18.10 and 18.11) [7] and/or flattening of the entire posterior pole (Fig. 18.11).

Calcified nodules (psamommas) are visualized quite well as hyperechoic nodules, with a posterior shadowing if they are located in the anterior or middle part of the orbit (Fig. 18.12).

Finally, on color Doppler imaging, the tumor is generally quite vascularized [8] (Fig. 18.13). However, ultrasound cannot be used to visualize small meningiomas of the orbital apex (those that before the advent of high-resolution MRI were called "impossible meningiomas") nor to analyze optic canal or intracranial extension.

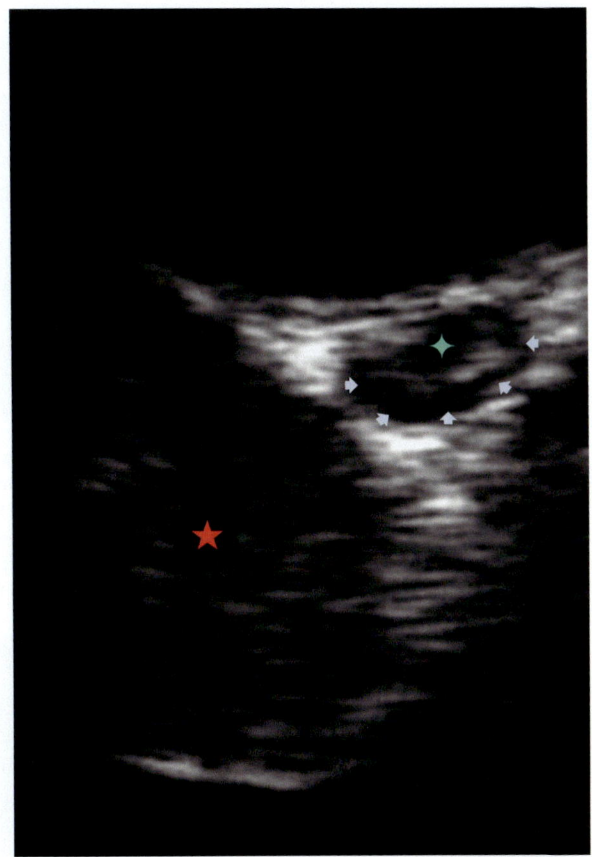

**Fig. 18.3  Glioma of the posterior orbital optic nerve** with dilation of the subarachnoid spaces of the immediately retrobulbar optic nerve, which forms an angle with the axis of the glioma. B-mode, parasagittal section. The tumor (★ red star) is located at the orbital apex and is directed toward the lower part of the orbit. Dilation of the subarachnoid spaces (✦ pale gray short arrows) surrounding the optic nerve fibers (✦ green star), of normal caliber, at the level of the immediately retrobulbar optic nerve, the axis of which is at an angle relative to that of the glioma

Therefore, ultrasound is rarely performed, in favor of MRI (with gadolinium injection) and CT scan (for detailed assessment of the optic canal, in high resolution with bony filters and windows): the canal can be enlarged or, in contrast, narrowed with condensed walls [9].

## 18.3  Hemangioblastoma

These are rare tumors, most often associated with von Hippel-Lindau disease, but they can be sporadic [10], most often involving the orbital ON (Fig. 18.14), but cases with an extension to the intracranial ON have been described.

The ultrasound appearance differs little from that of a meningioma in B-mode, but on color Doppler imaging, the lesion is naturally very vascularized, with low resistive flows, such as for intraocular capillary angiomas (see Fig. 14.37). They are excised surgically [11], but treatments with radiosurgery (linear accelerator radiotherapy) [12] are also effective.

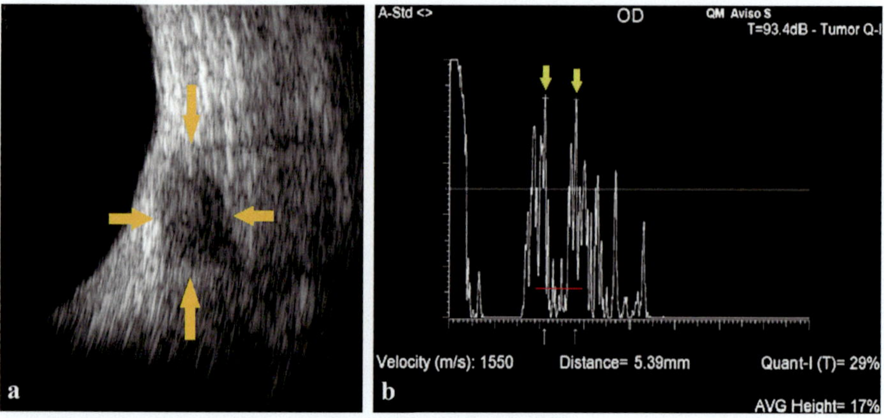

**Fig. 18.4  Small anterior glioma of the optic nerve. a**: B-mode, coronal section of the retrobulbar optic nerve; **b**: standardized A-mode—the arrows show the arachnoid. The thickening of optic nerve fibers stands out more in A-mode, the diameter of the thickened neural tissue being 5.39 mm. Very good delineation of the lesion (→ yellow arrows) is seen in A-mode and less so in B-mode. The lesion is not very reflective and had an even appearance. No attenuation can be evaluated on such a small lesion. In B-mode, one cannot specify which part of the nerve is thickened

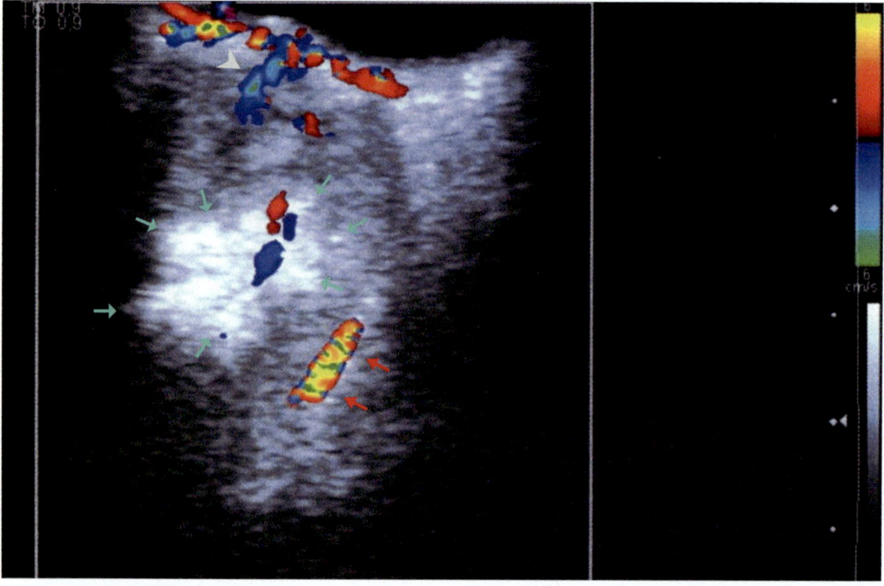

**Fig. 18.5  Optic nerve glioma with large central calcifications**. Color Doppler imaging, color mode, para-axial section. This type of calcification is rarely encountered in gliomas. Histological confirmation was required before undertaking excision surgery. The ophthalmic artery (→ red arrows) runs along the medial edge of the mass. In addition to the central retinal vessels (▷ pale gray arrowhead) behind the voluminous papillary protrusion, there are some flows in the vicinity of the large calcified area (→ green arrows)

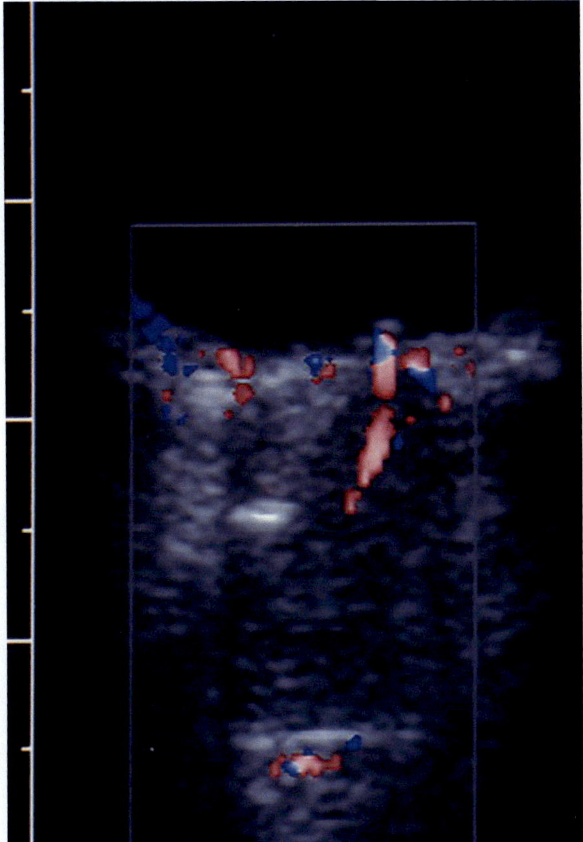

**Fig. 18.6  Glioma of the optic nerve.** Color Doppler imaging, color mode, para-axial section. The central retinal artery is enlarged. Its peak systolic velocity (PSV) is discreetly increased (18.7 cm/s) but remains within the normal range. The resistive index (RI) is normal (0.68)

## 18.4  Lymphoid Lesions

Like elsewhere in the orbit, these can be inflammatory lesions (optic perineuritis) or lymphomas. However, ultrasound has a limited role, in favor of MRI, and is rarely specific.

Lymphomatous infiltration of the ON is rare: occurring in 1.3% of lymphomas of the central nervous system [13]. Such ON lymphomas may be primary or a recurrence of systemic non-Hodgkin lymphoma [14], and they can be bilateral [15]. There is no characteristic appearance in imaging, and biopsy is often indicated to diagnose isolated ON lymphoma [16].

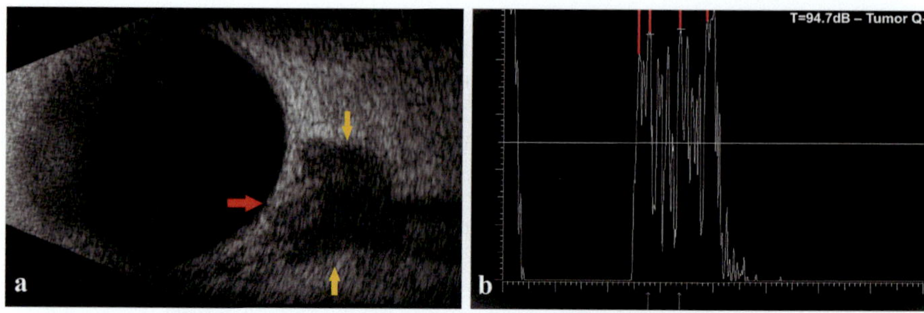

**Fig. 18.7  Small optic nerve sheath meningioma.a**: B-mode; **b**: standardized A-mode. In B-mode, the tumor that surrounds the optic nerve fibers takes on the appearance of a "cobra's head".
In A-mode, the red lines correspond to the boundaries of the tumor, on either side of the optic nerve fibers, eccentric but having retained a normal caliber. The tumor tissue has a medium to high reflectivity of 68% in Quantification I, an irregular structure, and is relatively poorly attenuating (angle kappa = 24°)

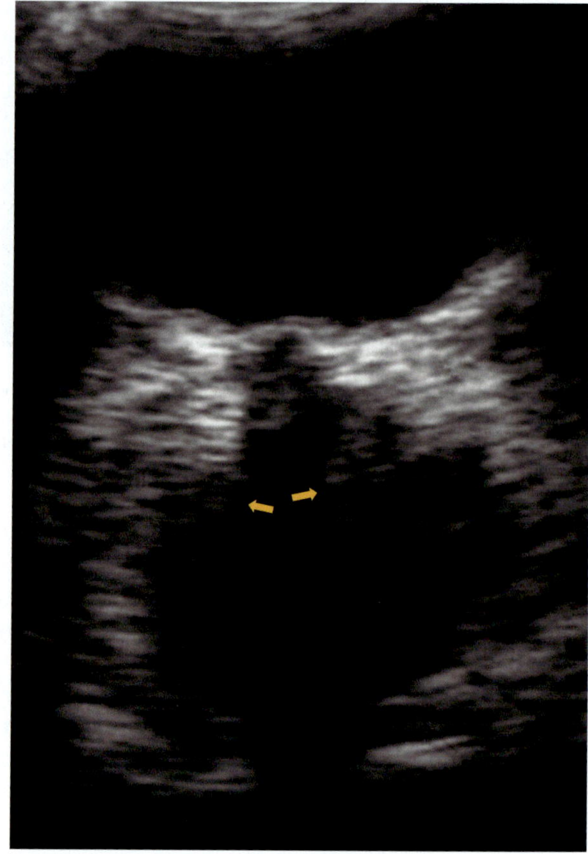

**Fig. 18.8  Large optic nerve sheath meningioma**. B-mode axial section. Large intraconal tumor, surrounding the optic nerve fibers and giving rise to a small protrusion of the optic disc. The mass has a heterogeneous echotexture, with hypoechoic areas and others that are moderately echogenic. It is attenuating, which does not allow the optic nerve fibers to be discerned within the mass, except at its anterior part (→ orange arrows)

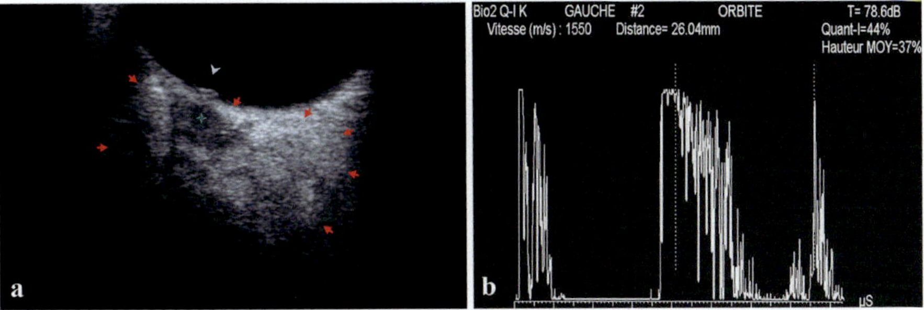

**Fig. 18.9   Optic nerve sheath meningioma. a**: B-mode para-axial section; **b**: standardized A-mode at tissue sensitivity. Large intraconal tumor, surrounding the optic nerve fibers and resulting in a small optic disc swelling (▷ pale gray arrowhead). The mass has a heterogeneous echotexture. In standardized A-mode, the reflectivity of the entire lesion is average (44% in Quantification I), but that of the first nasal centimeter of the mass is high (78%), and the attenuation is substantial (kappa angle = 57°). In B-mode, there is a sharp and thin border (➜ red arrows) between the mass and the orbital fat. Behind the globe, there is narrowing of the optic nerve fibers (✦ green star) in accordance with the recent decrease in the visual acuity of this patient whose lesion had been known for more than 10 years, having initially manifested itself as exophthalmos

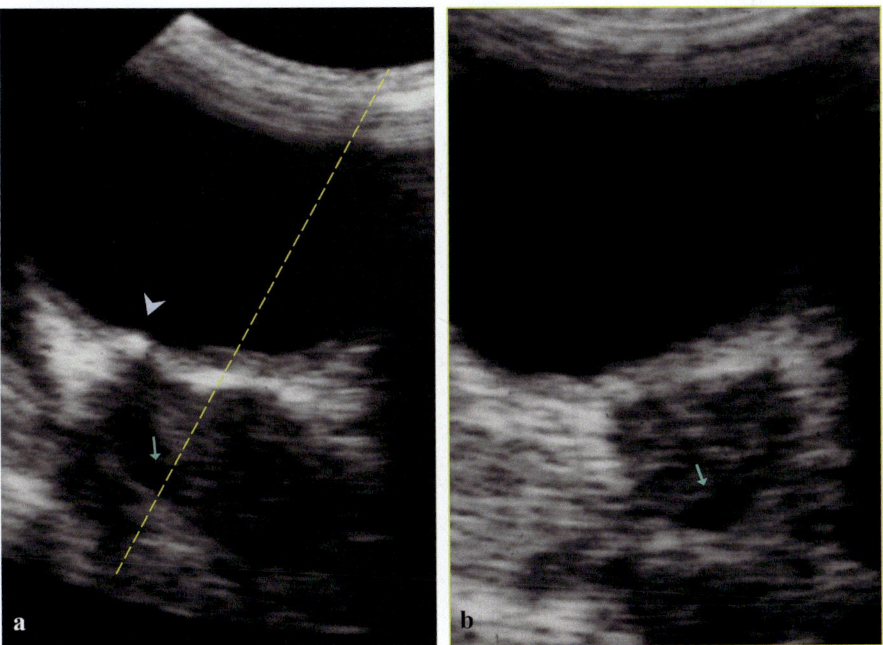

**Fig. 18.10   Meningioma of the left optic nerve. a**: B-mode para-axial section; **b**: B-mode, coronal section. The tumor has primarily formed on the medial side of the optic nerve fibers. The optic disc, which is slightly swollen, appears hyperechoic (▷ pale gray arrowhead). The optic nerve fibers are small (→ green arrows), with a diameter of 1.9 mm; they have been displaced to the temporal side of the hypoechoic mass measuring 11 mm in diameter. In **a**, the yellow dotted line indicates the section plane of Fig. 18.9**b**

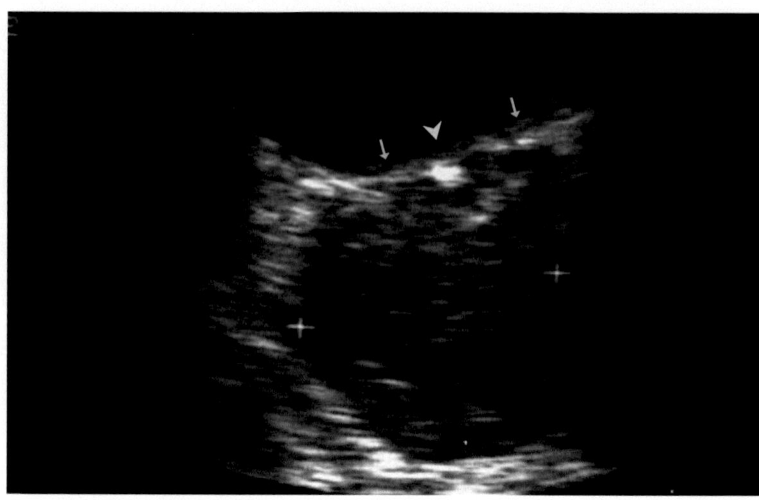

**Fig. 18.11  Optic nerve sheath meningioma**. B-mode para-axial section. Large hypoechoic intraconal mass, with a small hyperechoic optic disc (▷ gray arrowhead) and rectitude of the posterior pole (→ green arrows). The optic nerve fibers are not individualized on this section, as they are displaced downwards

**Fig. 18.12  Calcified optic nerve sheath meningioma in a 9-year-old child with NF2**. B-mode axial section. The optic nerve is slightly enlarged (the diameter of the mass is only 5.3 mm), although it has large calcifications (psammomas)

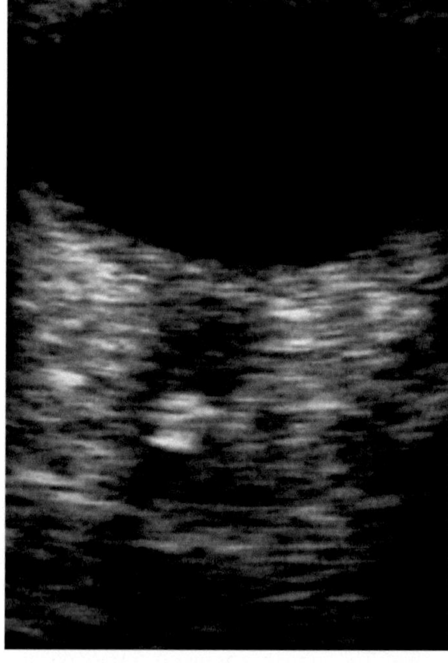

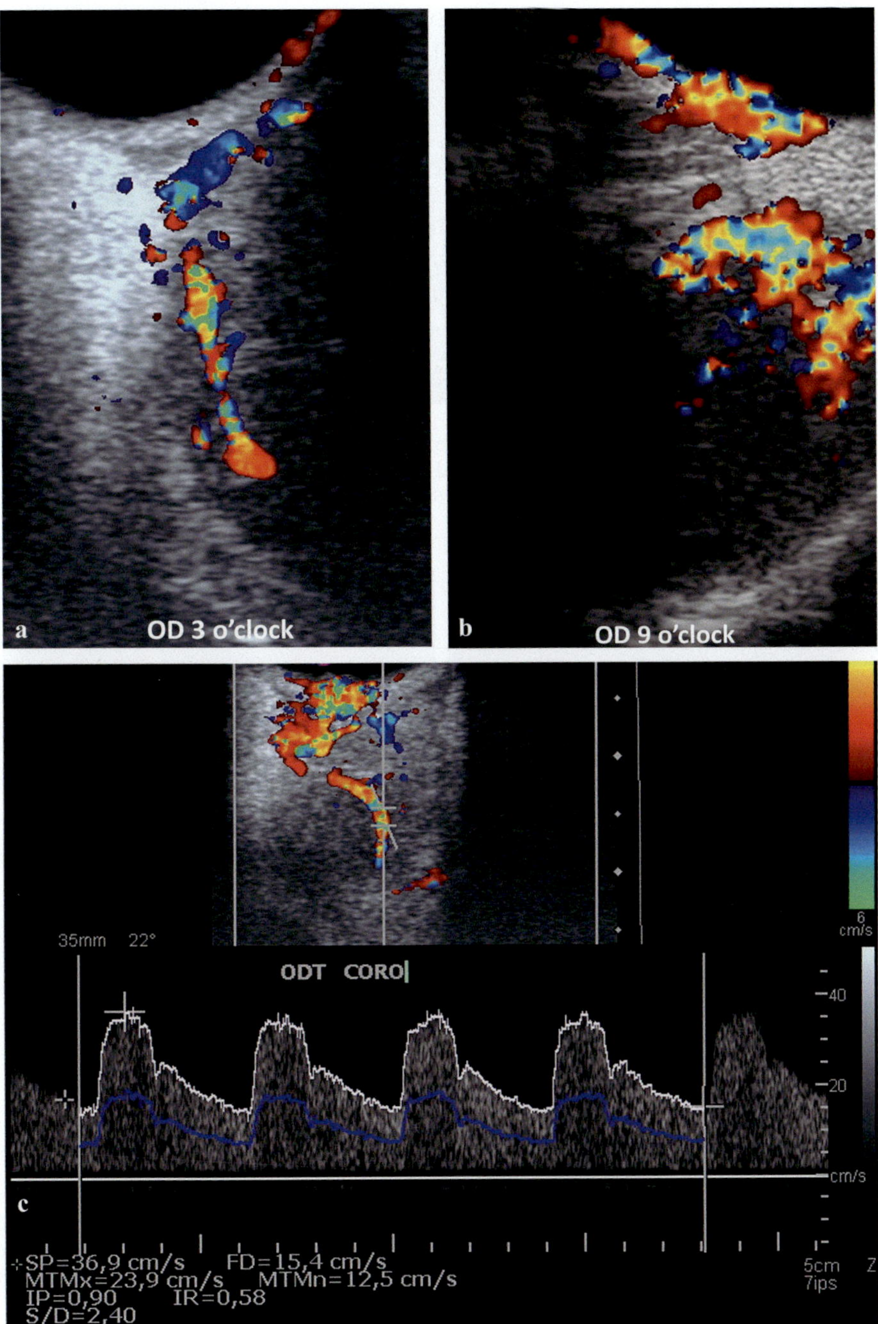


**Fig. 18.13  Optic nerve sheath meningioma**. Color Doppler imaging; **a**: color mode of the medial part of the mass; **b**: color mode of the temporal part of the mass; **c**: spectral mode. The tumor is highly vascularized, with fairly fast flows (PSV = 37 cm/s) that are moderately resistive (RI = 0.58). The flows in the central retinal artery are low.

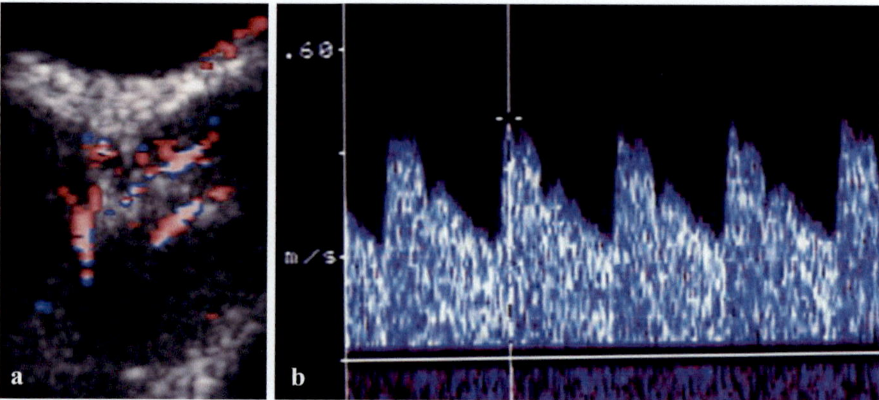

**Fig. 18.14 Optic nerve hemangioblastoma**. Color Doppler imaging. **a**: Color mode; **b**: spectral mode. The mass, which is large, hypoechoic, and heterogeneous, is highly vascularized, with fast flows (PSV = 44 cm/s), and it exhibits relatively low resistivity (RI = 0.54). The flows in the central retinal artery are normal

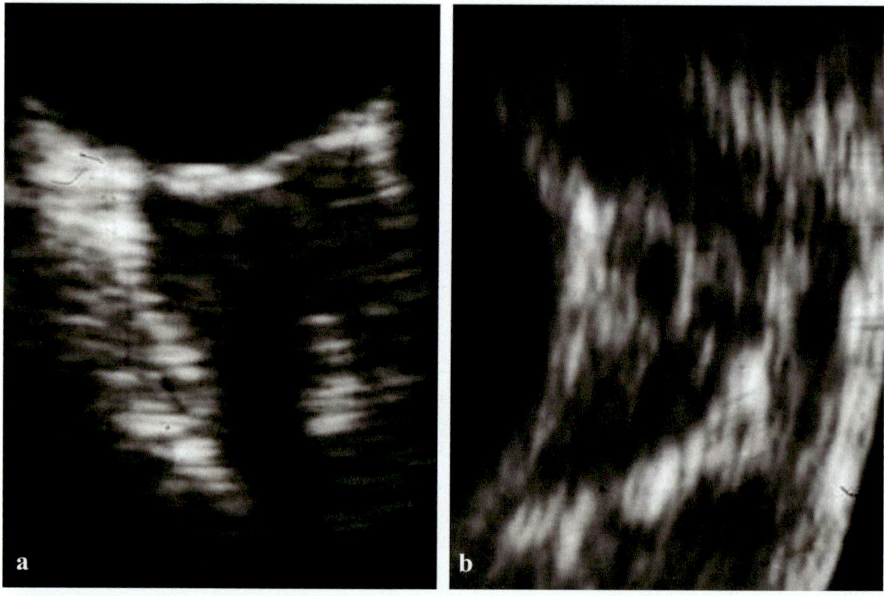

**Fig. 18.15 Idiopathic optic perineuritis**. B-mode. **a**: Axial section; **b**: coronal section. The lesion that surrounds the optic nerve fibers is clearly visible on the coronal section, and in particular the perioptic meninges. It is hypoechoic with irregular contours. The diagnosis was confirmed when the lesion completely disappeared after 2 months of non-steroidal anti-inflammatory drugs and without recurrence at 1 year without treatment

Idiopathic or specific inflammatory perineuritis can also be seen (Fig. 18.15) [17], and the rule is to systematically consider sarcoidosis in case of any diplopia or abnormality of the anterior visual pathways, which are frequent neuro-ophthalmological signs [18, 19]. Infiltrations of the optic nerve are also seen in Wegener's granulomatosis, although optic neuropathies are most often of the compressive type, at the orbital apex [20].

## 18.5  Extension of Ocular Tumors to the Optic Nerve (ON)

Their diagnosis was considered in Chap. 13. They are most often an extension of retinoblastoma, the diagnosis of which is ensured by MRI with gadolinium injection, especially if it is a retrolaminar extension. Ultrasound of the ON is indeed difficult behind calcified retinoblastoma. It can only show voluminous extensions of the entire retrobulbar ON, which have fortunately become rare. It can rarely be an extension of uveal melanoma (Fig. 18.16), most often parapapillary [21]. However, here again, ultrasound can only reveal a bulky extension, with significant widening of the ON, and is not performed in favor of MRI with Gadolinium injection. There is a very slight possibility of primary melanoma of the ON [22].

## 18.6  Optic Nerve (ON) Cysts

a) **Colobomatous cyst of the ON.** Colobomatous cysts are of malformative origin: colobomas are defects in the closure of the fetal optic vesicle; hereditary, most often autosomal dominant [23]. They present as purely cystic on ultrasound, are anechoic, and are accompanied by microphthalmia (see Fig. 26.1). The aphorism, a microphthalmic eye without enophthalmos hides a colobomatous cyst of the ON, is also very often true. Given the inferior position of the colobomic fissure, cysts are most often inferior and can even manifest as a bluish palpebral mass (Fig. 18.17).

   Ultrasound is sufficient to diagnose a microphthalmic eye and a retrobulbar cyst, but a CT scan is essential in deciding the surgical procedure [24], primarily for esthetic purposes, because the visual acuity is always poor [25].

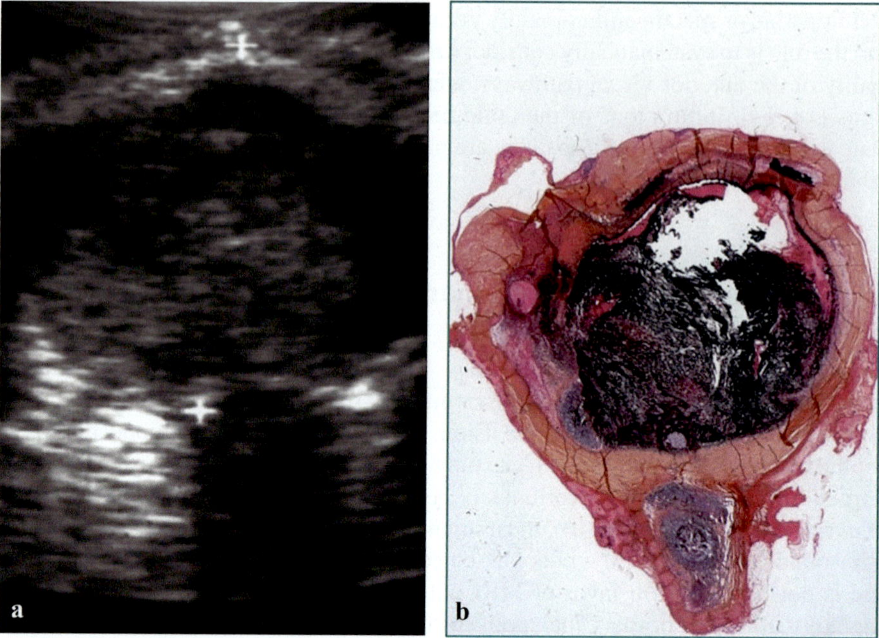

**Fig. 18.16  Extension of a large choroidal melanoma to the optic nerve. a**: B-mode, para-axial section; **b**: macroscopic anatomical section, hematoxylin and eosin × 3.5. In addition to the tumor and its extension to the optic nerve, there is ocular atrophy, with an axial length of 20.2 mm. *The anatomical section (**b**) was kindly provided by Dr. F. d'Hermies, Hôtel-Dieu de Paris, France*

b)  **Other cysts of the ON**. The other cysts (or pseudocysts) of the ON are much smaller and often located at the superior part of the ON immediately retrobulbar. In our experience, they are discovered during assessment of normal-tension glaucoma which fails to respond to treatment. On ultrasound, they are hyperechoic (indicating a protein-rich content?) (Fig. 18.18).

Their etiopathogeny is unknown. On color Doppler imaging, the compression they exert on the ON fibers results in a slight increase in the resistive index of the central retinal artery and surprisingly, also at the level of the short posterior ciliary arteries. On MRI, the ON behind the cyst and the optic chiasm appear normal [26].

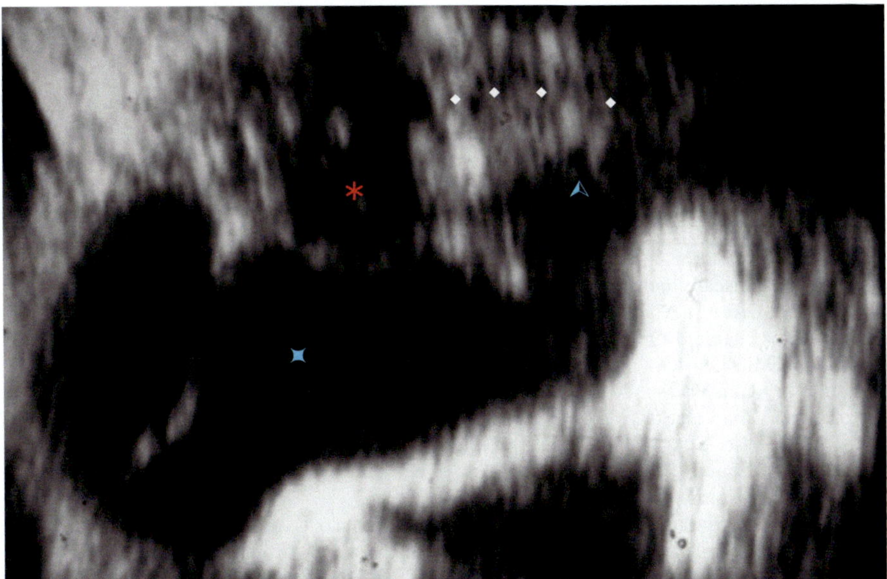

**Fig. 18.17   Large colobomatous cyst of the optic nerve**. B-mode, parasagittal section. The cyst, which is large and partitioned (blue star), protrudes under the lower eyelid and masks the microphthalmic eye (red star). It is located under the optic nerve (white diamonds), starting at the optic fissure (blue arrowhead)

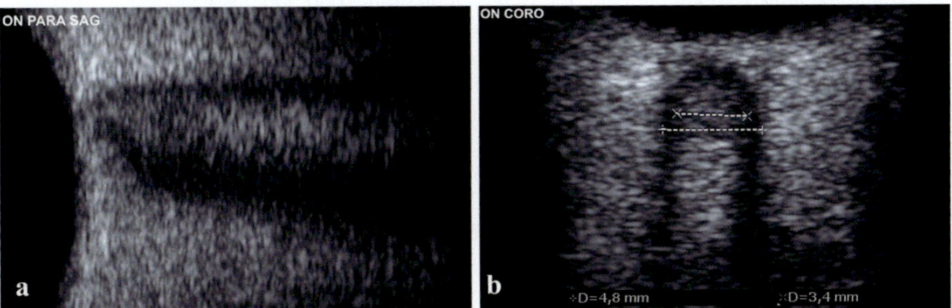


**Fig. 18.18   Pseudocyst of the optic nerve**. B-mode. **a**: Parasagittal section; **b**: coronal section of the optic nerve. Discovered during exploration of normal-tension glaucoma, the echogenic cyst is located at the superior part of the optic nerve; it compresses the optic nerve fibers, thus explaining the clinical symptoms

# References

1.  Font R, Croxatto J, Rao N. Tumors of the optic nerve and optic nerve head: juvenile pilocytic astrocytoma. In: Silverberg S, Sobin L, editors. AFIP atlas of tumor pathology: tumors of the eye and ocular adnexa. Washington, DC: American Registry of Pathology; 2006. p. 140–5.

2. Burger P. Pilocytic astrocytoma. In: Kleihues P, Cavanee W, editors. World Heath Organization classification of tumors, pathology and genetics: tumors of the nervous system. Lyon, France: IARC Press; 2000. p. 45–51.

3. Chung EM, Specht CS, Schroeder JW. from the archives of the **AFIP**: Pediatric orbit tumors and tumorlike lesions: neuroepithelial lesions of the ocular globe and optic nerve. Radiographics. 2007;27(4):1159–86.

4. Gupta V, Sabri K, Whelan KF, Viscardi V. Rare case of optic pathway glioma with extensive intra-ocular involvement in a child with neurofibromatosis type 1. Middle East Afr J Ophthalmol. 2015;22(1):117–8.

5. Berrocal T, de Orbe A, Prieto C, Izquierdo C, et al. US and color Doppler imaging of ocular and orbital disease in the pediatric age group. Radiographics. 1996;16(2):251–72.

6. Pinson S, Créange A, Stalder JF, Chaix Y, et al. Neurofibromatose 1 : recommandations pour la prise en charge. J Fr Ophtalmol. 2002;25(4):423–33.

7. Kyoung Min Lee KM, Hwang JM, Woo SJ. Optic disc drusen associated with optic nerve tumors. Optom Vis Sci. 2015;92(4 Suppl 1):S67–75.

8. Zhang W, Zhao H, Song G. [The value of color Doppler imaging ultrasound in diagnosis of orbital diseases]. [Article in Chinese]. Zhonghua Yan Ke Za Zhi. 2001;37(6):447–50.

9. Mafee MF, Goodwin J, Dorodi S. Optic nerve sheath meningiomas. Role of MR imaging. Radiol Clin North Am. 1999;37(1):37–58, ix.

10. McGrath LA, Mudhar HS, Salvi SM. Hemangioblastoma of the optic nerve. Surv Ophthalmol. 2019;64(2):175–84.

11. Raila FA, Zimmerman J, Fratkin J, Parent AD, et al. Successful surgical removal of an asymptomatic optic nerve hemangioblastoma in von Hippel-Lindau disease. J Neuroimaging. 1997;7(1):48–50.

12. Sims E, Doughty D, Darlison R, Plowman PN, et al. Stereotactically delivered cranial radiation therapy: a ten-year experience of linac-based radiosurgery in the UK. Clin Oncol (R Coll Radiol). 1999;11(5):303–20.

13. El Kettani A, Lamari H, Lahbil D, Rais L, Zaghloul K. Neuropathie optique bilatérale et lymphome non-Hodgkinien. Bull Soc Belge Ophtalmol. 2006;300:35–9.

14. Kim UR, Shah AD, Arora V, Solanki U. Isolated optic nerve infiltration in systemic lymphoma—a case report and review of literature. Ophthal Plast Reconstr Surg. 2010;26(4):291–3.

15. Millar MJ, Tumuluri K, Murali R, Ng T, Beaumont P, Maloof A. Bilateral primary optic nerve lymphoma. Ophthal Plast Reconstr Surg. 2008;24(1):71–3.

16. Behbehani RS, Vacarezza N, Sergott RC, Bilyk JR, Hochberg F, Savino PJ. Isolated optic nerve lymphoma diagnosed by optic nerve biopsy. Am J Ophthalmol. 2005;139(6):1128–30.

17. Purvin V, Kawasaki A. Optic perineuritis secondary to Wegener's granulomatosis. Clin Experim Ophthalmol. 2009;37(7):712–7.

18. Lamirel C, Badelon I, Gout O, Berthet K, Héran F, et al. Présentations initiales neuro-ophtalmologique de la sarcoïdose. J Fr Ophtalmol. 2006;29(3):241-9.

19. Phillips YL, Eggenberger ER. Neuro-ophthalmic sarcoidosis. Curr Opin Ophthalmol. 2010;21(6):423–9.

20. Shunmugam M, Morley AM, O'Sullivan E, Malhotra R, et al. Primary Wegener's granulomatosis of the orbital apex with initial optic nerve infiltration. Orbit. 2011;30(1):24–6.

21. Lindegaard J, Isager P, Prause JU, Heegaard S. Optic nerve invasion of uveal melanoma. APMIS. 2007;115(1):1–16.

22. Patel M, McNally L, McCormick SA, Abramson DH, et al. Primary melanoma of the optic nerve in a patient with 16-year follow up. Ophthal Plast Reconstr Surg. 2011;27(3):e69–71.

23. Pagon RA, Kalina RE, Lechner DJ. Possible autosomal-recessive ocular coloboma. Am J Med Genet 1981;9(3):189–93.

24. Mafee MF, Jampol LM, Langer BG, Tso M. Computed tomography of optic nerve colobomas, morning glory anomaly, and colobomatous cyst. Radiol Clin North Am. 1987;25(4):693–9.
25. Hornby SJ, Adolph S, Dandona L, Foster A, et al. Visual acuity in children with coloboma: clinical features and a new phenotypic classification system. Ophthalmology 2000;107(3):511–20.
26. Bertrand A, Vignal C, Bergès O, Héran F, et al. Open-angle glaucoma and paraoptic cyst: first description of a series of 11 patients. AJNR Am J Neuroradiol. 2015;36(4):779–82.

# Chapter 19
# Optic Neuropathies and Vascular Occlusions

Patricia Koskas, Jacques Laloum, Mario de La Torre, Violaine Caillaux, and Olivier Bergès

**Abstract** In evaluating the optic nerve, we first review the respective roles of B-mode, standardized A-mode and color Doppler imaging. Then we cover inflammatory lesions, such as papillitis and optic neuritis and then vascular optic neuropathies: arteritic and non-arteritic anterior ischemic optic neuropathy; central retinal artery occlusion, according to embolisms (with its B-mode translation as an hyperechoic spot sign), thrombosis, or bleeding disorders; and central retinal vein occlusion with the four distinct forms (edematous, ischemic, mixed, or regressive in young patients). After that, pseudopapilledema (optic disc drusen) and stasis papilledema are considered with a diagnostic decision tree in case of an optic disc elevation on ocular fundus displaying the major and initial role of ultrasound versus other imaging modalities. Finally, we discuss the role of color Doppler imaging in the evaluation of the glaucomatous neuropathy.

## Introduction

Optic nerve damage is clinically characterized by a constant decrease in visual acuity, albeit of varying intensity; and ophthalmoscopically translated only at the level of the optic disc; even if in the early stages of inflammatory disease, ophthalmoscopic signs may be lacking. In most cases, clinical data such as age, terrain, mode of appearance, and progression allow to diagnose neuropathy and suspect its etiology.

In the context of acute vascular neuropathy, fundus data, or even angiography, are sufficient for the diagnosis and assessing the degree of severity. In the context of a suspected inflammatory etiology, additional examinations are essential (initial

P. Koskas · J. Laloum · O. Bergès (✉)
Rothschild Foundation Hospital, Paris, France
e-mail: oberges@for.paris

M. de La Torre
Universidad Nacional Mayor de San Marcos, Lima, Perú

V. Caillaux
Explore Vision Ophthalmic Diagnostic Centers, Paris, Rueil, France

assessment and follow-up): head and optic nerve MRI, neuro-ophthalmological examinations, and paraclinical neurological assessment (including lumbar puncture).

The question then arises regarding the role of ultrasound in the assessment of these pathologies. In standard ultrasound textbooks, exploration in A-mode and B-mode is presented as an important element of the diagnosis, revealing abnormalities of optic disc and optic nerve (diameter, morphology, and reflectivity), but these abnormalities do not have specific features and are only useful when they are present.

The development of color Doppler [flow] imaging (CDI/CDFI) has allowed for assessing the small vessels of the posterior pole of the eye, as well as the orbital vessels, with increasing accuracy. Numerous articles on the contribution of oculo-orbital CDI to the diagnosis and monitoring of optic neuropathies have been published in recent years. In light of our experience and critical reading of the literature, here we show the contribution and limitations of the ultrasound techniques at our disposal.

## 19.1   Exploration Methods

### 19.1.1   B-Mode

This is undoubtedly the most commonly used mode, as a first-line option. It allows for evaluating the topography of the retrobulbar optic nerve, such as its relation with intraorbital components. It provides a clear view of changes in the optic disc, the posterior pole, and the wall of the globe. To properly visualize the optic nerve, a fairly low gain is used, as close as possible to the tissue sensitivity (T) used in standardized A-mode, and axial, longitudinal, and transverse sections are used.

In primary gaze, when the probe is placed on the cornea and passes through the lens, the optic nerve appears as an anechoic tubular area behind the globe. A vertical approach, which avoids the lens, provides a circular section of the optic nerve, just behind the globe. By being fully perpendicular to the optic nerve (when the nerve appears circular and not oval), one can obtain fairly reliable measurements of the optic nerve and subarachnoid spaces, allowing comparison from one eye to another.

### 19.1.2   Standardized A-Mode

This technique, the oldest, remains widely used and has retained all of its value for the accuracy of the morphological information concerning the optic nerve and subarachnoid spaces [1, 2].

The probe is placed on the globe temporally, next to the equator. The measurements of the optic nerve are precise, performed in primary gaze, then with the eye in abduction at 30°. When the ultrasound beam is perpendicular to the optic nerve, a well-defined defect can readily be found on A-scan ultrasound. This defect, which is the optic nerve itself, is hyporeflective and is bordered by the subarachnoid spaces, which are hyperreflective, and typically appears as a double peak. The innermost peak corresponds to the pia mater and the external peak corresponds to the dural envelope (see Fig. 18.1).

The diameter of the optic nerve should be measured toward the front (a few millimeters behind the wall of the globe) and toward the back (as close as possible to the orbital apex) using a velocity of 1550 cm/s.

The 30° abduction test allows for differentiating cases involving an increase in the diameter of the subarachnoid spaces from authentic thickenings of the optic nerve itself. This test is based on the following premise: when the eye is turned outward, the optic nerve and its envelopes are stretched, allowing distribution of the cerebrospinal fluid (CSF) over a larger area. This test can be even more sensitive by taking measurements after exercise (several movements to the right and left of both eyes; see below, Fig. 19.2). Thus, with an increase in the volume of the CSF (enlargement of the subarachnoid spaces), the test is said to be positive, as the diameter of the optic nerve complex–subarachnoid spaces decreases. The test is positive for intracranial hypertension (idiopathic or secondary), inflammatory or traumatic neuropathy [1, 2]. The test is negative with a tumor of the optic nerve (glioma, meningioma) [1]. Neither ischemic neuropathy nor venous occlusion alters the values of the optical diameter in the acute stage.

### 19.1.3  *Color Doppler Imaging (CDI) / Color Doppler Flow Imaging (CDFI)*

This mode, used in ophthalmology since the 1990s/2000s, has steadily undergone technical improvements, allowing for increasingly accurate assessment of low velocity flows (see Chap. 3). The flows of the following vessels [3] are assessed: the central retinal artery (CRA) and vein (CRV) as they run along the optic nerve, the medial and lateral short posterior ciliary arteries (sPCA), the ophthalmic artery (Opht A), and the superior ophthalmic vein (SOV). For each of these arteries, the peak systolic velocity, the end-diastolic velocity, and the resistivity index are determined, and for the veins, the peak velocity and the average velocity. Numerous articles have shown the contribution of CDI / CDFI to ocular hemodynamic assessment in diabetes, glaucoma, optic neuropathies, tumor lesions, orbital pathology, intracranial hypertension, and retinal detachments.

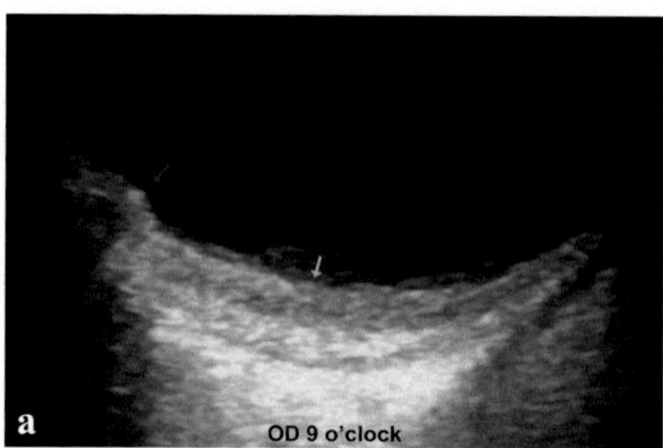
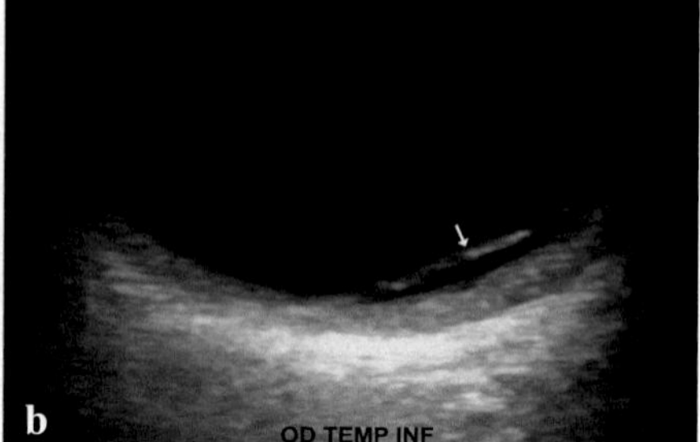



**Fig. 19.1 Vogt-Koyanagi-Harada disease**. B-mode with an 8–18 MHz probe. **a**: 9 o'clock meridian section of the right eye; **b**: mid-peripheral section of the inferotemporal quadrant. Papillitis (→ red arrow), and uveitis (→ blue arrow), with a wall thickness measuring 2.9 mm and partial retinal detachment (→ white arrow). Even at this reduced gain, some inflammatory echoes can be discerned in the vitreous

## 19.2  Inflammatory Pathology

### *19.2.1  Papillitis*

This is an inflammatory syndrome of the optic disc, primarily affecting young adults, resulting in an ophthalmoscopic picture that resembles the papilledema visible in intracranial hypertension. However, three signs allow it to be distinguished: the unilateral nature, the permanent and constant alteration of vision, and the characteristic angiographic appearance. This inflammatory syndrome can be isolated or associated with uveal or meningeal involvement. Papillitis can be the consequence of a focal disease (ENT) or systemic disorders [Behcet, Sarcoidosis, Vogt-Koyanagi-Harada (Fig. 19.1)].

The diagnosis is based on clinical considerations, ophthalmoscopy, and fluorescein angiography. In general, there is no point in using ultrasound or Doppler for the diagnosis. However, if ultrasound is performed, it reveals an increase in the size of the optic nerve, enlargement of the subarachnoid spaces surrounding the optic nerve, and optic disc elevation. In Doppler, hemodynamic alterations in the flows of the central retinal artery and ciliary arteries are rare or insignificant.

### *19.2.2  Optic Neuritis*

Inflammatory damage to the optic nerve is linked to several etiologies. Multiple sclerosis is the best-known etiology. Several articles [2–7] have studied the optic nerve (morphology, reflectivity, diameter) and the flows of cilioretinal vessels in the context of optic neuritis. However, the authors have reported conflicting results, especially when using Doppler data. Thus, numerous authors [2, 4, 5] have shown that

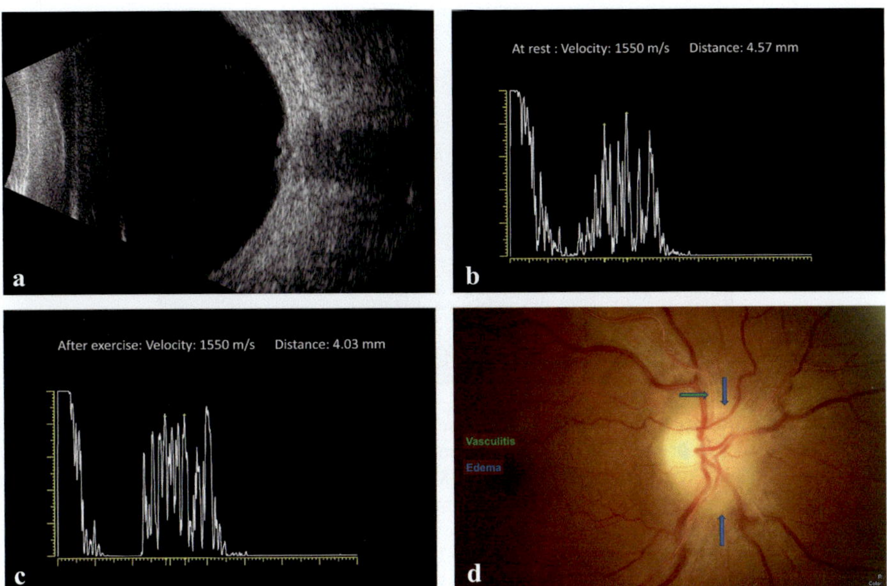


**Fig. 19.2  Acute optic neuritis related to multiple sclerosis. a**: Parasagittal section of the optic disc, 20 MHz annular probe; **b**: standardized A-mode of the optic nerve at rest; **c**: standardized A-mode of the optic nerve after exercise; **d**: fundus photograph of the posterior pole. Moderate optic disc protrusion is evident in B-mode (**a**). There is clear increase in the size of the optic nerve, the edges of which are indicated by the small yellow crosses; measured after exercise as 4.03 mm (**c**). Because the diameter at rest measures 4.57 mm (**b**), there is also a small amount of inflammatory fluid around the optic nerve fibers that have increased in volume, visible only at this acute stage, when ultrasound is rarely performed. Some signs of vasculitis (→ green arrow) (**d**) are seen on the photograph of the posterior pole

the diameter of the optic nerve is significantly increased when using, as a reference, the unaffected contralateral eye (A-mode, B-mode). Thus, according to Gerling et al. [4], the optic nerve affected by neuritis can reach a mean diameter of 5.4 ± 0.5 mm, with a healthy optic nerve measuring 3.0 ± 0.3 mm. In our experience [3], a normal optic nerve measures a mean of 3.3 ± 0.3 mm, whereas an optic nerve with neuritis tends to be 4.5 ± 0.5 mm (Fig. 19.2).

In contrast, the results obtained from Doppler data are more heterogeneous in the literature and not particularly in line with our experience. Some authors [5–7] claim that there are changes in the cilioretinal hemodynamic parameters, with an increase in the resistive index (RI) and a decrease in the peak systolic velocity (PSV). In our experience, in the absence of papilledema and compression at the optic nerve head, the cilioretinal hemodynamic parameters are not commonly altered (Fig. 19.3), which is a differential sign with ischemic optic neuropathy (ION).

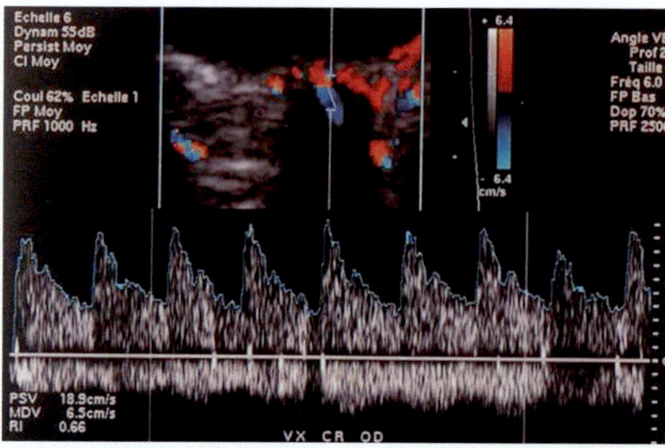

**Fig. 19.3** **Retrobulbar optic neuritis at the acute stage**; color Doppler imaging (CDI), color and spectral modes. Normal velocimetric constants of the central retinal artery, with a significant aliasing artifact: peak systolic velocity (PSV) = 18.9 cm/s and resistive index (RI) = 0.66. Although not measured accurately on this section in color mode, one can discern an enlarged optic nerve

## 19.3 Vascular Optic Neuropathies

Acute anterior ischemic optic neuropathy (ION) is the consequence of ischemia of the optic disc by occlusion of the short posterior ciliary arteries.

### 19.3.1 Arteritic Anterior Ischemic Optic Neuropathy (ArteriticAION/AAION)

Horton disease is a classic etiology of AION. Horton's disease has several presentations in its ophthalmological form: AAION, central retinal artery occlusion (CRAO), and oculomotor disorder by ischemic involvement of the ocular motor (III, IV, VI) nerves. It is often the first diagnosis that comes to mind with a decrease in visual acuity with papilledema, true ischemic edema in the acute stage with microhemorrhages, progressing toward optical atrophy with sharp edges. The first test to order is a biological one: sedimentation rate and C-reactive protein levels. The assessment includes cervicocephalic MRI, Doppler assessment of the cervicocephalic and temporal vessels, and temporal artery biopsy (TAB). The purpose of an MRI performed in emergency is to detect other sites of encephalic ischemia that are small, or in "mute" neurological territories. It also helps to fully visualize the vessels from the aortic arch and, using complex sequences with injection, to assess the wall of the arteries and in particular the superficial temporal artery in search of thickening enhanced by the gadolinium, which supports the diagnosis of Horton disease and can thus limit the use of TAB. Ultrasound and Doppler assessment of the temporal artery should be performed by experienced physicians. The specific sign in B-scan ultrasound is the dark halo visible around the lumen of the temporal artery [8]. It is useful when present and provides an excellent correlation with the histological results of TAB (Fig. 19.4).

However, its absence does not rule out the diagnosis. At the level of the vessels of the optic nerve head, the CDI signs vary according to the clinical presentation. Spectral Doppler reveals a pronounced decrease in the PSV of the central retinal artery and short posterior ciliary arteries in the acute phase as well as an increase in the RI (Fig. 19.5).

A spectral analysis curve with little signal for the artery and perturbation of the central retinal vein can occur. The magnitude of Doppler signs correlates with the severity of the decrease in visual acuity. In total, 2% of Giant cell arteritis cases are complicated by CRAO (see below).

In advanced stages, severe atrophy of the optic nerve manifests as a decrease in the caliber of the optic nerve (in comparison with the contralateral side) and persistent alteration of the flows recorded at the cilioretinal level and in less severe forms, a near normalization of the parameters of the ciliary vessels but a persistent decrease in the PSV and/or an increase in the RI at the level of the central retinal artery.

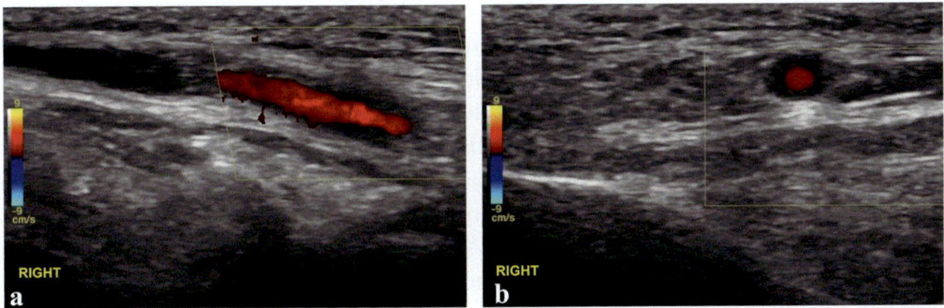


**Fig. 19.4** **Horton disease**, superficial temporal artery. CDI, color mode. **a**: Longitudinal section; **b**: cross-section. Moderate thickening (dark halo) resulting in discrete narrowing of the lumen without focal acceleration of the flow

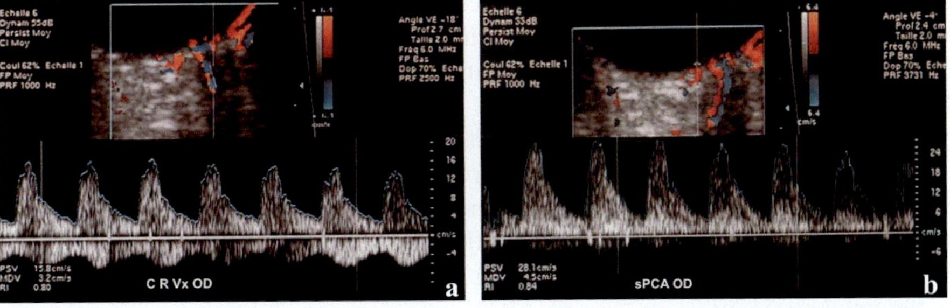


**Fig. 19.5** **Anterior ischemic optic neuropathy (AION)**. CDI. **a**: Of the central retinal vessels; **b**: of the medial posterior short ciliary artery. It is mainly RI that is highly pathological, calculated at 0.84 for the medial short posterior ciliary arteries and 0.80 for the central retinal artery

## *19.3.2 Non-arteritic AION*

The diagnostic approach is often the same because the spectrum of Horton disease remains the first diagnosis to rule out, in the presence of reduced visual acuity. The conditions are also often the same, namely an elderly person. However, the clinical picture suggesting AION can also occur in a younger individual, with typical vascular risk factors (high blood pressure, diabetes, hypercholesterolemia, blood hyperviscosity, etc.). When the terrain is highly suggestive and the clinical presentation typical, neuroradiological examinations (CT, MRI) are rarely required. However, biological and cardiovascular assessments, as well as cervico cephalic Doppler, remain essential.

Doppler assessment of cilioretinal and orbital vessels has its place, especially when the condition (age, gender, absence of risk factors) is not as usual. A specific anatomical conformation called "small crowded optic disc" is an important risk factor [9]; a small optic disc is defined by a particular anatomical conformation, usually occurring on a "short" hyperopic eye, with the optic fibers crowded within the optic disc, which has a small surface area. There may be worsening of this congestion by the presence of drusen. In some cases, the diagnosis between AION and optic neuritis may not be obvious, especially a considerable time after the initial episode or during a reassessment (especially when there can be some uncertainty in regard to inflammatory neuropathy versus posterior ischemic neuropathy (rarer, in less than 10%, and which does not include papilledema).

In the acute phase, neuro-ophthalmic MRI is of great value. When it shows damage to the optic nerve (changes in size, signal and enhancement in posterior or even cisternal topography), a diagnosis of inflammation (optic neuritis) is more likely. Its negativity often leads to the diagnosis of AION, even even if the patient's condition and clinical symptoms are atypical. In such casesoculo-orbital CDI then comes to the fore. On ultrasound, in our experience, and in accordance with the literature [2–4, 9], there is an increase in the size of the optic nerve in case of inflammatory involvement (in the acute stage), whereas in case of AION, the size of the affected optic nerve remains within the normal range, comparable to that of the contralateral eye. For Doppler, several authors have published results similar to ours [9]. Thus, in the acute phase, an optic disc edema results in altered flow of the central retinal artery (increase in the RI and decrease in the PSV) as well as altered flows (elevation of the RI) of the short posterior ciliary arteries. However, in the acute phase, and even more so in the subacute or chronic phase, signs of hemodynamic alteration of ciliochoroidal vascularization can be lacking [9]. This can be explained by the fact that only the ciliary branches, responsible for the vascularization of the optic disc, are affected, and that it is very difficult to differentiate and record them safely and discriminately, given their size and the tangle of the ciliochoroidal vessels at the posterior pole. The authors point out the absence of modification of the flow of the ophthalmic artery in case of AION-type damage. All insist on the value of modification of the hemodynamics of the central retinal artery, even more so than the inconstant alteration of ciliary flows, the nasal artery being affected more often than the temporal artery. This is probably related to the nasal vascularization being less abundant and less anastomosed and the collection of Doppler information being easier to obtain in contact with the optic disc.

## *19.3.3  Central Retinal Artery Occlusion (CRAO)*

CRAO is a rare pathology; CRAOs most often afflict people in their 60s. It is bilateral in only 1–2% of cases. It manifests as a sudden decrease in visual acuity, sometimes preceded by one or more previous episodes of transient amaurosis, with a white, calm eye.

On fundoscopic examination, there is diffuse narrowing of the arterial caliber with sometimes a granular flow. In the hours that follow, an ischemic retinal white edema appears, reflecting the ischemic damage to the inner layers of the retina. The foveola, which is vascularized only by the choroid, retains its normal coloration and appears redder by contrast, as a "cherry-red spot of the macula".

The etiological assessment is all the more exhaustive the younger the individual. The causes can be classified into several main classes according to the mechanism involved: (1) embolisms, (2) thrombosis, (3) bleeding disorders.

1. **Embolisms**: Even when an embolic mechanism is strongly suspected, the embolus is not necessarily visible on the fundus. The most frequent emboligenic pathologies are:

   - carotid atheroma, the most common cause,
   - emboligenic heart disease.

   Finally, rarely, lipid emboli (fat embolism due to fracture of the long bones) or tumor emboli (myxoma of the atrium) should be considered.

2. **Thrombosis**: These include Horton disease and systemic diseases.

   - Horton disease is an emergency: it must be systematically sought in individuals over 50 years of age, although only 2% of Horton cases present CRAO (see above).
   - Systemic diseases: less common, these include systemic lupus erythematosus, Wegener's granulomatosis, Takayasu's arteritis, Kawasaki disease, and Churg–Strauss syndrome.

3. **Bleeding disorders** are the same as for central retinal vein occlusion (see below).

**If requested, ultrasound, and oculo-orbital ultrasound and CDI, and not as an emergency procedure, are not intended to establish the diagnosis but can be useful as an initial reference work-up.** One can see the absence of flow within the CRA, with only the central vein visible, encoded in blue (Fig. 19.6).

However, this examination is mainly useful for looking for an embolus when it is not visible at the fundus [10]. Such an embolus results in a small hyperechoic nodule

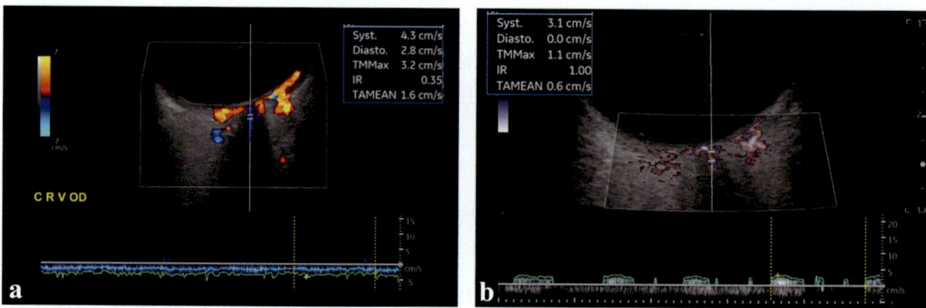

Fig. 19.6 **Central retinal artery occlusion (CRAO)**. CDI. **a**: Color and spectral mode in a 39-year-old man with acute retinal necrosis for 6 days. Total absence of flow within the central retinal artery and persistent flow in the central vein, with a rather low mean velocity of 3.2 cm/s; **b**: B-flow and spectral mode, in a 76-year-old man, 4 h after a sharp decline in visual acuity. Because there is no blooming artifact, the two flows together seem very thin behind the spot sign; some systolic microflows persist in the central retinal artery, and the central vein, fully permeable, has a mean velocity of 3.4 cm/s

(spot sign) within the optic nerve, distinctly behind the lamina cribrosa, more or less echogenic depending on its nature, cholesterol or calcium (Figs. 19.6b and 19.7), the image regressing quite slowly within the first week. Its recognition is ultimately useful for obtaining an indication of the effectiveness of intra-arterial thrombolysis [11].

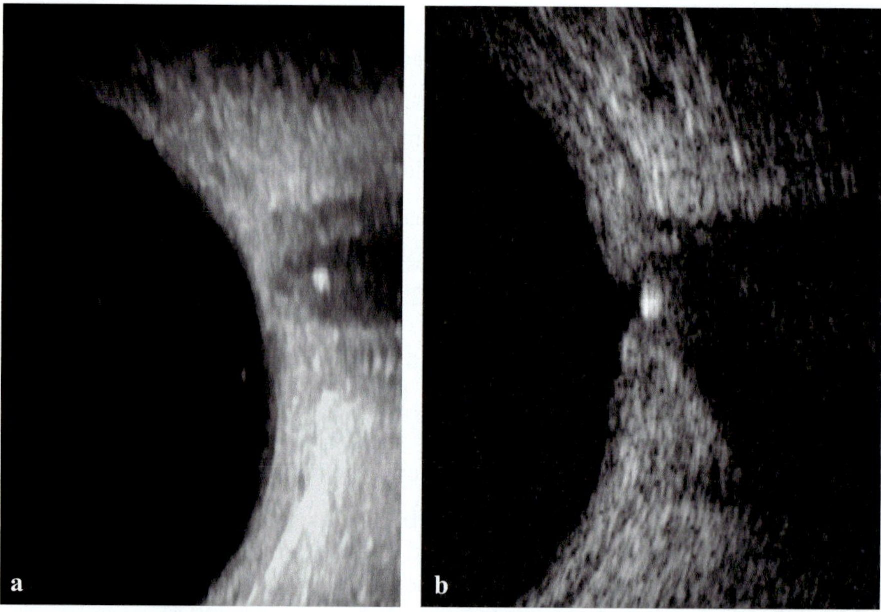

Fig. 19.7 **CRAO, embolic origin: spot sign**. B-mode at 10 MHz. In **a**, the embolus is located behind the lamina cribrosa and is very echogenic. Although not visible at the fundus, it was visible in **b**, because it is more anterior and because of the optic disc excavation

CRAO is an emergency. Etiological assessment and treatment of the arterial occlusion should be urgently carried out at the same time.

1. **Etiological assessment**: This is in particular the search for carotid atheroma and emboligenic heart disease:
2. **Treatment of CRAOs**: The treatment of CRAOs remains disappointing. **Intravenous fibrinolytic treatment**, or better yet intra-arterial treatment by catheterization of the ophthalmic artery, is intended to achieve arterial repermeabilization. To be effective, it must be introduced very early (less than 6 h, similar to the delay for a stroke), which is rarely feasible in practice.

   **Hypotonic** medications, **vasodilators** and **anticoagulant** treatments are only adjuvant treatments.

   In all cases, occlusion of the central retinal artery should alert to the risk of emboligenic recurrences in the cerebral area.

## 19.3.4 *Central Retinal Vein Occlusion (CRVO)*

CRVO is a frequent pathology, the consequence of acute circulatory slowdown in the venous compartment, usually caused by abnormal compression of the vein by the artery within the inextensible common sheath that surrounds them. The increase in size of the artery wall causing compression may be related to an underlying vascular pathology (hypertension, diabetes, hyperlipidemia, etc.) or aging.

Exudation related to venous vascular stasis (edema, hemorrhages, etc.) can disrupt retinal function and be the cause of a decrease in visual acuity of varying intensity. Examination of the fundus allows for the diagnosis and to determine whether it is an occlusion of the central vein (CRVO) or a branch (BRVO); it can also estimate the age of the problem. One can see the following:

- venous dilatations, the veins being dark and tortuous;
- papilloretinal edema, due to venous stasis;
- retinal hemorrhages, often as streaks, following the direction of the optic nerve fibers;
- cotton-wool spots, corresponding to the retinal insult.

The intensity of the signs is variable; many signs can be associated with retinal vein occlusion: papilledema, macular edema, and vitreous hemorrhage.

Fluorescein retinal angiography is essential, confirming the diagnosis by highlighting venous circulatory delay and allowing the assessment of its severity by analysis of the capillary bed.

Schematically, **four clinical forms of CRVO are described**:

- **Edematous form**, the most common (60% of cases). Edema dominates the clinical picture, there is hyperemia or edema of the optic disc, cotton-wool spots are rare, and hemorrhages are visible at the periphery. Macular cystoid edema is sometimes described. Visual acuity evolution is usually good. Overall, 20% of these forms evolve into an ischemic form.

- **Ischemic form**, the most feared (20% of cases). The retinal edema is mild; the arteries are narrow and rigid, with deep hemorrhages. A key sign is the presence of ischemic retinal areas characterized by numerous and confluent cotton-wool spots, realizing true dysoric nodules. The capillary bed is not perfused. This ischemia will lead to local production of angiogenic factors, with the appearance of dreaded neovessels that can progress into neovascular glaucoma, vitreous hemorrhage, or even retinal detachment with proliferative vitreoretinopathy. The ischemic maculopathy that may be present is accompanied by very poor vision and an unfavorable prognosis. The outcome of this form is often poor, and the visual acuity does not improve.
- **Mixed edematous ischemic form**. This combines the signs of the previous two and can progress to a severe ischemic form.
- **Regressive form in young people**. Described in the 1960s, these are generally **young** patients, between 30 and 40 years of age, who exhibit CRVO with **good prognosis**, with full recovery of visual acuity. Once the visual disorder is noted, the vision is found to be fairly well preserved, the veins are dilated, and there are few hemorrhages, with significant papilledema.

In the acute stage, **Color Doppler imaging** mainly reveals the arterial abnormalities responsible for venous occlusion in connection with the central retinal vein but also on all homo- and contralateral orbital arteries [12]. This mainly involves a decrease in the PSV and an increase in the RI (Fig. 19.8).

These abnormalities appear to be more severe in ischemic forms [13]. It can also be used to monitor the progress of cases undergoing treatment [14].

**Management of the patient in the acute phase** consists in rapidly identifying the etiological factors, mainly arteriosclerosis, but which are sometimes interrelated; with a somewhat lesser degree of urgency; one has to consider the medical treatment

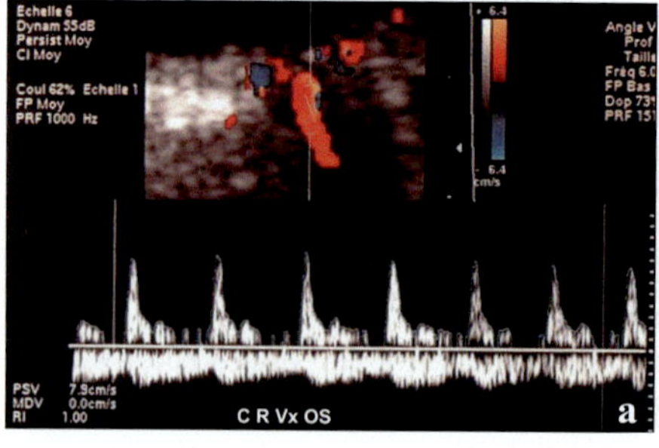
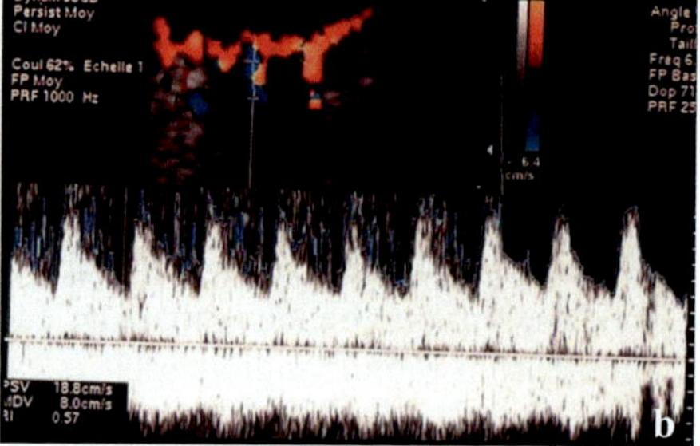

**Fig. 19.8 Central retinal vein occlusion (CRVO)**. CDI. In the acute stage (**a**), hemodynamic disturbances predominate in the central retinal artery: the PSV is low, recorded at 7.9 cm/s. The protodiastolic flow is low and there is no end-diastolic flow, resulting in an RI of 1.00. The central vein circulates, albeit slowly, with an average speed of 2.7 cm/s. Six months after treatment of vascular risk factors (**b**), clear improvement in the flow of the vein, with an average speed of 4.6 cm/s. and it is less pulsated by the beating of the adjacent artery but also on the artery, with a PSV of 18.8 cm/s and an RI of 0.57

options, which aim to improve the circulatory conditions in the retinal vessels, to restore vision as well as possible; and to at least limit the risks of secondary worsening.


## 19.4  Pseudopapilledema: Optic Disc Drusen

Optic disc drusen are small congenital developmental anomalies located in the optic nerve head. They are most often discovered during a routine examination in a child or adolescent, and they can be mistaken for papilledema [15]; they more rarely are discovered during visual field disorders. They are relatively common, with a prevalence of 2% [16].

However, suspicion of papilledema requires a rigorous course of action, especially in children (Table 19.1, decision tree).

The most likely pathogenic hypothesis today is deposition of axonal material related to an interruption of axoplasmic transport, probably caused by a particular anatomical configuration (an optic nerve that is too small and with too many axons) and a localized vascular deficit responsible for a decrease in perfusion of the optic disc.

Their appearance is, in general, noted in adolescence or childhood.

Ultrasound is the best way to detect optic disc drusen. Indeed, whether or not they are small, calcified, buried, single or multiple, B-mode ultrasound remains the best diagnostic means, far ahead than CT scan (even at high resolution) and sometimes even ahead of a fundus examination and even assessment by autofluorescence.

The best way to assess the optic nerve head and visualize optic disc drusen is to use a long focal 20-MHz probe, or an annular one with the retina setting, providing more resolution to the posterior pole. At 20 MHz, small calcified clusters can be seen,

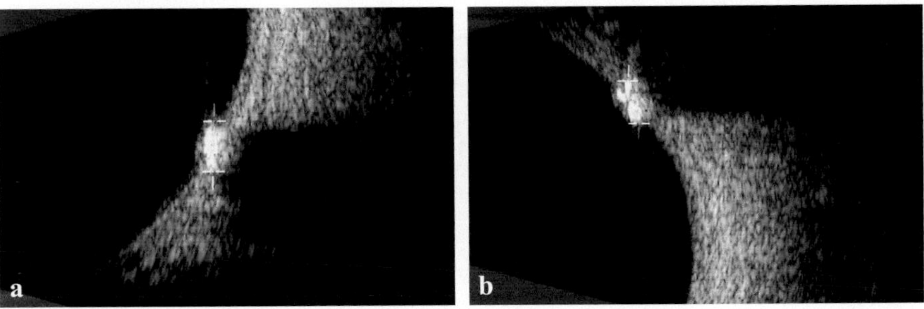

**Fig. 19.9  Optic disc drusen**. B-mode. At 10 MHz (**a**), only one nodule is seen, which is voluminous, measured as 2.4 mm in diameter, whereas at 20 MHz (**b**), three hyperechoic nodules of smaller size can be discerned

**Table 19.1** Diagnostic decision tree for optic disc elevation on ocular fundus

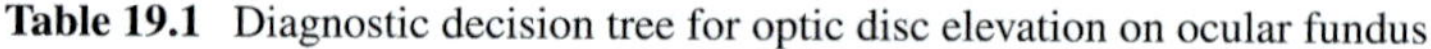

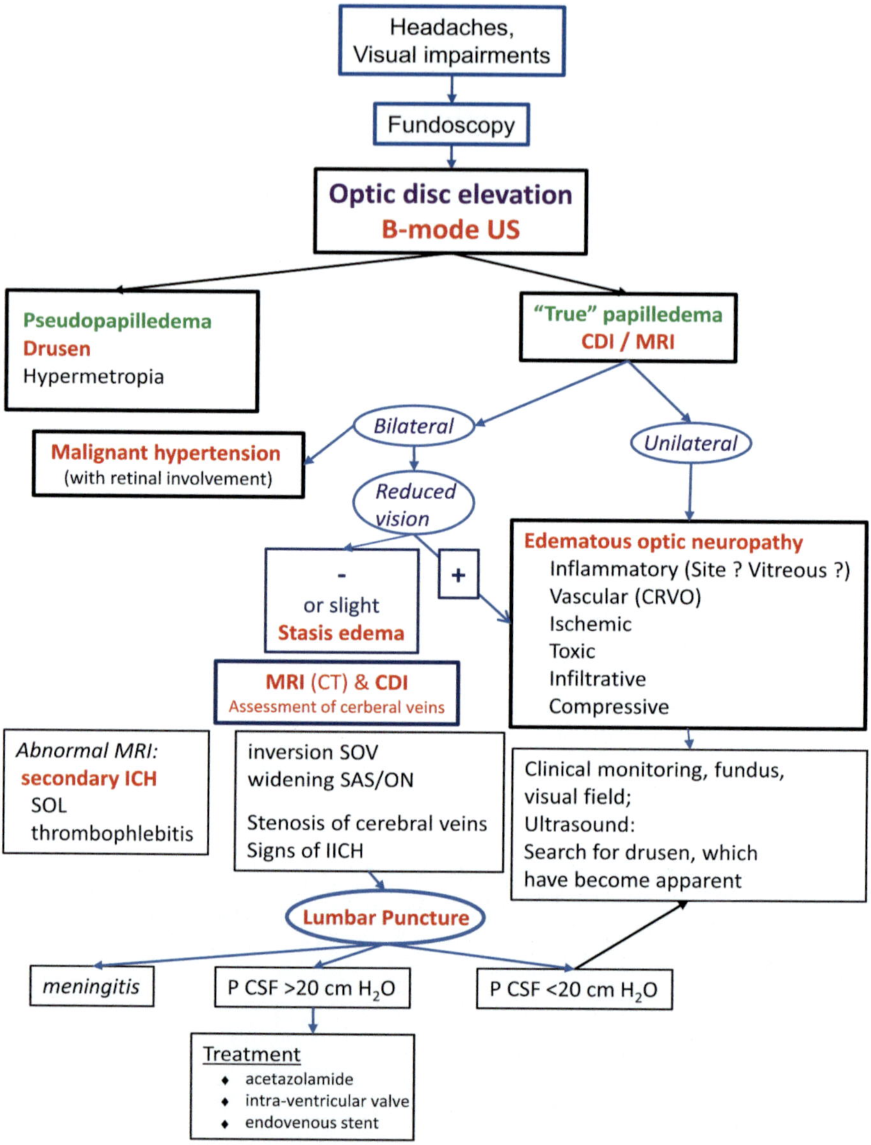

whereas at 10 MHz, these different foci are represented by a single large nodule (Fig. 19.9).

They are round, oval, or multilobulated, protruding or buried within the optic nerve head [17, 18]. Moving the eye is useful to distinguish the shadow of the optic nerve from the posterior shadowing linked to the calcified drusen (Fig. 19.10).

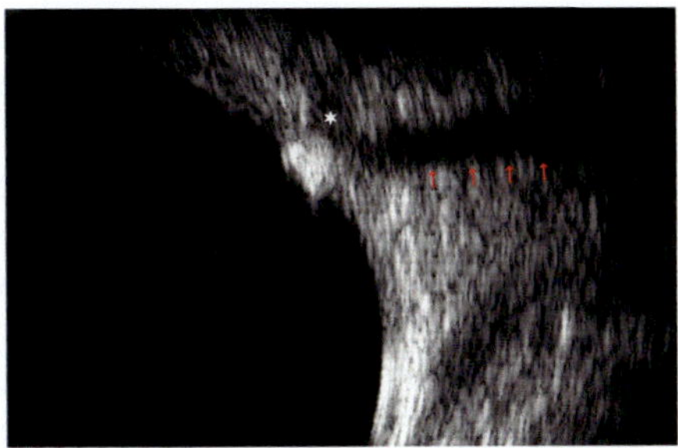

**Fig. 19.10 Calcified optic disc drusen of the left eye**. Section of the 3 o'clock meridian while asking the patient to look to the left; While in primary gaze, the posterior shadowing cone due to the calcifications of the drusen is projected over the shadow of the optic nerve (see Fig. 19.9); by moving the eyes, it is readily distinguishable (→ red arrows) from the optic nerve (✶ white star), which is entirely normal

When not calcified, a moderately echogenic nodule can be discerned, located under the optic disc, often on the nasal side. Buried drusen are difficult to see by ophthalmoscopy but are readily visualized on ultrasound.

Drusen can be uni- or bilateral and have asymmetrical morphological characteristics. In color Doppler imaging, calcified drusen result in a "twinkling artifact" [19]. This artifact can interfere with the collection and recording of the spectral Doppler signal from the central retinal vessels. The probe then needs to be positioned at the medial canthus (Fig. 19.11), or the signal collected from the central retinal artery "further away", well behind the optic disc, which often provides lower maximum systolic velocity values. For these data to be of any value, the hemodynamic measurements of the contralateral central retinal artery must be performed identically.

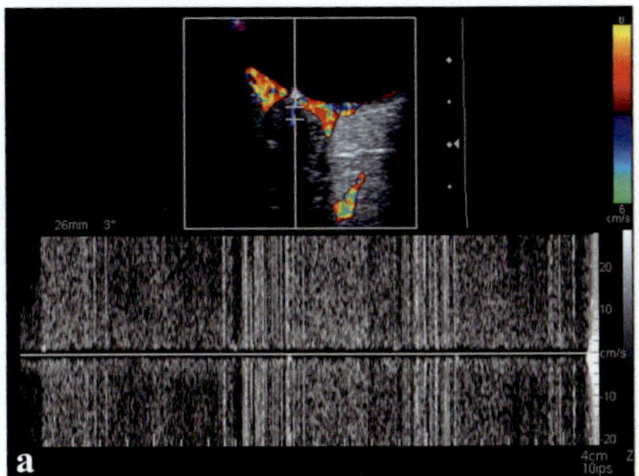
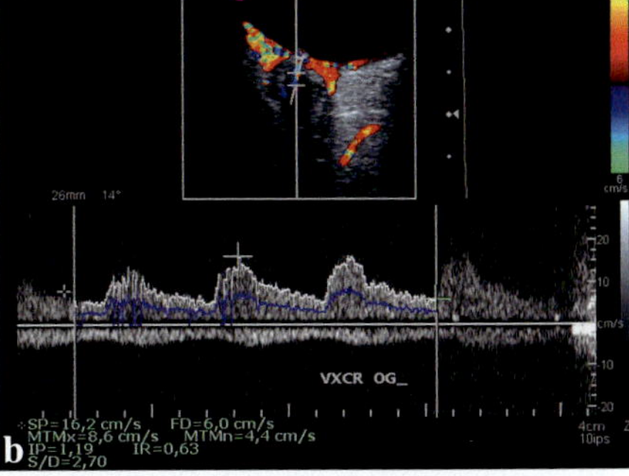

**Fig. 19.11 Optic disc drusen of the left eye**. CDI, color and spectral modes. By positioning the probe and the Doppler gate in the usual manner (**a**), the calcification of the voluminous drusen results in a **twinkling artifact** that prevents analysis of the flows of the central retinal vessels. By moving the Doppler gate back slightly (**b**), the flows can be recorded, which are entirely normal: PSV = 16.2 cm/s and RI = 0.63

The progression is usually marked by a significant increase in the volume of the drusen over several decades as well as moderate alterations of the visual field that are often asymptomatic.

Optic disc drusen can also, rarely, cause visual manifestations such as decreased visual acuity or symptomatic deficits of the visual field. These changes are linked to a mechanism close to that of AION, the drusen acting as a mechanical obstacle to blood flow at the optic nerve head. In one study [18], the authors reported that among 92 eyes with drusen, 55% were symptomatic (including 63% with reduced vision and 49% with visual field defects). Buried drusen, diagnosed by ultrasound, probably because of their smaller volume, are less frequently responsible for visual field deficits or visual disturbances.

In our experience, fortuitous discovery of optic disc drusen is not uncommon. Moreover, in the absence of vascular factors, in case of an AION-type of decrease in visual acuity, there is a high probability to discover optic disc drusen associated with AION-type hemodynamic alterations. In addition, these patients often have short eyes with an axial length < 21 mm and often the clinician tells us that ophthalmoscopy reveals a small crowded optic disc.

These drusen must be distinguished from peripapillary hyperreflective ovoid mass-like structures (PHOMS): relatively frequent, small, peripheral to the optic disc, easily diagnosed by Enhanced Depth Imaging Optical Coherence Tomography as hyperechoic nodules without posterior shadowing [20]. Yet their origin or their progression are not well known, in particular their impact on the visual field. They are also more frequently associated with myopia [21].

## 19.5  Stasis Papilledema

Papilledema related to CSF stasis around the optic nerve fibers and threatening visual function can be seen in intracranial hypertension. This situation is the result of an intracranial space-occupying lesion or in the context of idiopathic intracranial hypertension (IICH).

Ultrasound reveals elevation of the optic disc, with a dome protruding toward the vitreous, of variable echogenicity, more hypoechoic in chronically evolving and severe edemas. Ultrasound allows for rapid elimination of pseudopapilledema related to the presence of drusen (calcified hyaline deposits). Ultrasound reveals enlargement of the optic nerve sheath diameter (ONSD), with a diameter of the optical complex well above the threshold value of 5.7 mm in adults. The measurement is performed with a longitudinal section or, even better, a coronal section (using a transocular approach, the probe being placed on the lateral canthus or on the inferior lid). This B-mode measurement is reproducible and reliable. In standardized A-mode, the 30° test allows for differentiating a fluid-filled enlargement of the OSND from a "tumorous" enlargement of the optic nerve itself (see above).

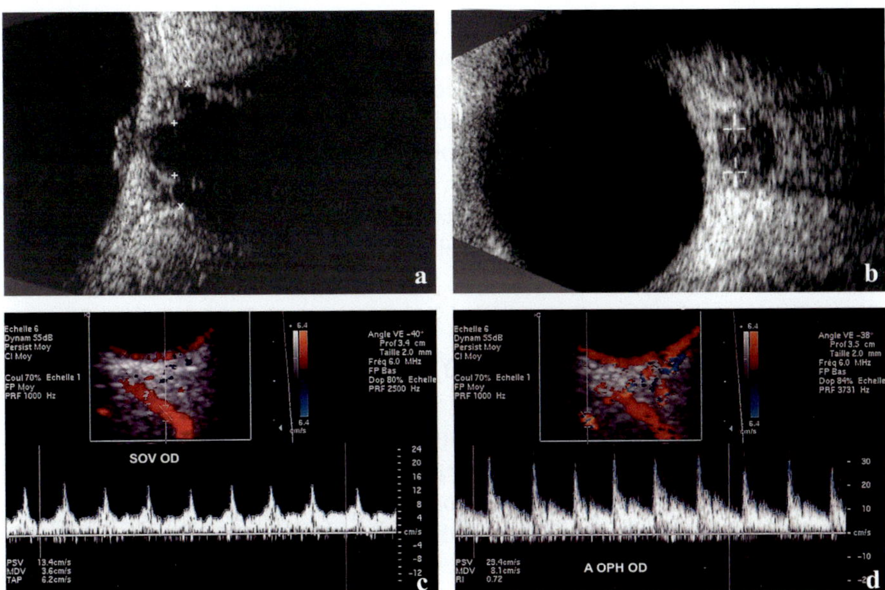

**Fig. 19.12   Stasis papilledema due to idiopathic intracranial hypertension (IICH). a:** 10 MHz B-mode: parasagittal section of the optic nerve head; **b:** 10 MHz B-mode, coronal section of the optic nerve; **c:** CDI, color and spectral modes of the right superior ophthalmic vein; **d:** CDI, color and spectral modes of the right ophthalmic artery. Major protrusion of the optic disc (**a**), which has retained its inverted omega shape, with a normal diameter of the optic nerve fibers, measured at 3.4 mm, and significant enlargement of the optic nerve, measured at 7.1 mm, by dilation of the subarachnoid space (**a** and **b**). Slight dilation of the superior ophthalmic vein, with a considerably pulsed flow corresponding to the pulsation of the cerebrospinal fluid (**c**), which is very different from the normal flow of the ophthalmic artery (**d**) that runs between the vein and the medial orbital wall

In case of suspected stasis papilledema, neuroimaging (ideally an MRI) should be performed without delay. With a negative MRI result (absence of tumor, meningoencephalitis, thrombophlebitis), the diagnosis of IICH, is suspected and based on the modified Dandy criteria [22]. In practice, the individual is typically female, overweight, and young, with all or part of the following symptoms: headache, tinnitus, and abducens cranial nerve palsy. Fundoscopy reveals typical papilledema, most often bilateral, ***which can be asymmetrical***. MRI reveals ptosis of the cerebellar tonsils, intrasellar arachnoidocele, thin ventricles, enlargement of the optic nerve subarachnoid space, flattening of the sclera around the optic disc by increased pressure of the CSF, and uni- or bilateral stenosis of the transverse venous sinuses with endoluminal protrusion of abundant Pacchioni granulations.

The initial diagnosis is based on measurement of the CSF opening pressure during a lumbar puncture performed in the supine position. (CSF pressure greater than 25 mmH$_2$O if an obese patient).

On ultrasound and Doppler, in addition to optic disc elevation and enlargement of the subarachnoid space, a clear enlargement of the superior ophthalmic vein (SOV) is seen, with a reverse flow, coded in red in color mode and with a positive spectrum in spectral mode, corresponding to the pulsation of the CSF transmitted to the SOV by the cavernous sinus through the superior orbital fissure (Fig. 19.12); the appearance differs greatly from what is observed with a fistula (see Figs. 20.23–20.25) and also (mirror image) from the flow of the ophthalmic artery. In addition, there is a loss of the undulated nature of the spectrum in relation to the breathing rythm.

## 19.6  Glaucomatous Neuropathy

Glaucoma is a progressive optic neuropathy that combines characteristic morphological changes in the optic nerve and disc (excavation), the death of retinal ganglion cells and their axons, and associated visual field loss. The visual field deficits are variable but are generally distributed in the arciform area of Bjerrum (superior or inferior), starting from the blind spot and extending to the horizontal axis, bypassing the central fixation point (although paracentral damage is common).

**The impairments are asymmetrical with regard to the horizontal axis, and they respect this axis.**

**However, these impairments never respect the vertical meridian; such a respect should prompt a search for another pathology, such as a compressive pathology.**

Intraocular pressure, which is the main risk factor for glaucoma, is regulated by the trabecular meshwork, through which the aqueous humor is evacuated out of the eye. A classification that is essential for the treatment distinguishes angle-closure glaucoma, in which the iris overlaps the trabeculum and obstructs it (see Chaps. 4 and 11), versus open-angle glaucoma, in which the trabeculum becomes less permeable. A second classification distinguishes glaucoma secondary to another condition and primary glaucoma. Finally, within primary open-angle glaucoma, which is by far the most common condition in the Western world, the distinction is between those with high pressure versus glaucoma with normal (or low) pressure, despite the existence of a continuum between these two entities.

The starting point of the axonal degeneration constituting glaucoma is the lamina cribrosa, a stack of lamellae riddled with holes that allow the axons of the retinal ganglion cells making up the optic nerve to exit the eye. At the level of this structure, axonal and vascular mechanical stress promoted by intraocular hypertension and certain biomechanical abnormalities appear to be the starting point of this axonal degeneration, through a cascade of events leading to their apoptosis [23].

The disappearance of nerve fibers widens the central area devoid of fibers. In addition, there is an almost pathognomonic anatomical modification: bulging of the lamina cribrosa. Depending on the stage of progression, when performed, B-mode ultrasound reveals various aspects of the optic disc: from a flat optic disc to the stage of major bean-pot optic disc cupping (Fig. 19.13).

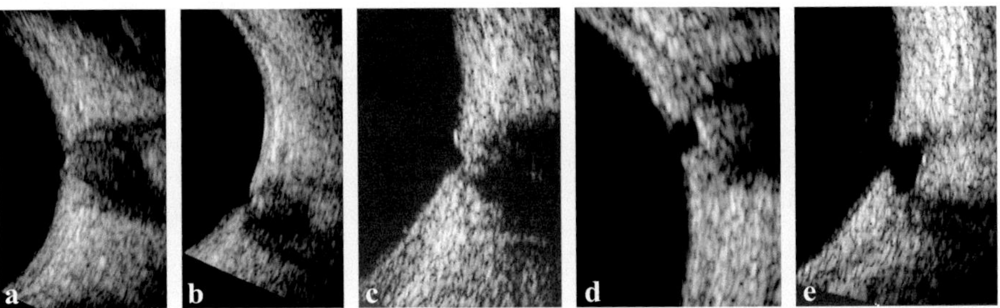

**Fig. 19.13 Optic disc excavation—different stages. a**: Minimal excavation: the optic disc having a "flat" appearance; **b**: small excavation; **c**: fairly large excavation, graded 0.9 clinically; **d**: large excavation; **e**: very large excavation, bean-pot optic disc cupping

The diameter of the optic nerve must be measured 3 mm behind the sclera on a coronal view. The normal diameter of optic nerve fibers is between 3 and 3.4 mm. Atrophy (< 2.9 mm) is not evident in the early stages of progression (Fig. 19.14).

Substantial excavation is easily detectable by ultrasound, which can be an essential contribution to the diagnosis when media are not clear, preventing access to the fundus, in particular, to help determine the indication for surgery (e.g. a corneal graft). Physiological autoregulation maintains a constant blood flow to the optic disc despite variations in ocular perfusion pressure. Dysfunction of this regulation has been demonstrated in primary open-angle glaucoma and particularly in normal-tension glaucoma [24, 25].

Color Doppler imaging (CDI) allows for analysis of circulatory flows of the large retinal vessels (central retinal artery and vein) and retrobulbar ones (short posterior ciliary arteries and ophthalmic artery). In open-angle glaucoma, there is a decrease in the circulatory velocities and an increase in the resistive index (RI) of the cilioretinal

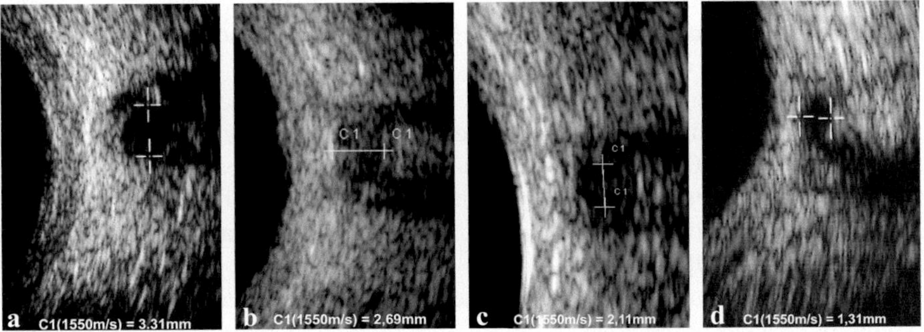

**Fig. 19.14 Optical atrophy: different stages. a**: Low-tension glaucoma, with a fairly large optic disc excavation (see Fig. 19.13c), and a normal-sized optic nerve (diameter = 3.31 mm); **b**: discrete optical atrophy (diameter = 2.69 mm) in association with advanced glaucoma; **c**: significant atrophy of the optic nerve (diameter = 2.11 mm) in connection with advanced-stage glaucoma and a bean-pot optic disc cupping. **d**: severe atrophy of the optic nerve (diameter = 1.31 mm)

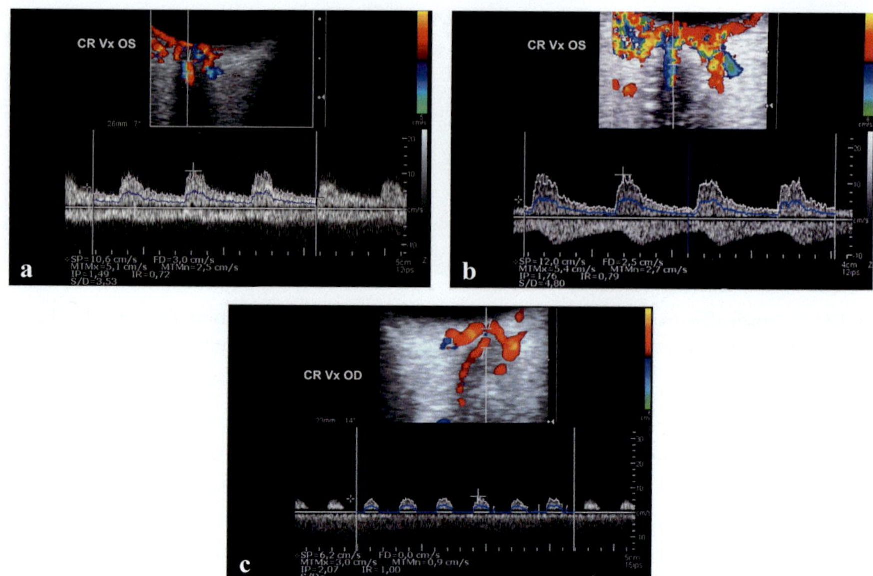

Fig. 19.15 **Velocimetric alterations of glaucomatous neuropathy - different stages. a:** Slight: PSV = 10.6 cm/s (value at the lower limit of normal) and RI = 0.72 (only slightly higher than normal) in a case of low-tension glaucoma with a large optic disc excavation but without significant optical atrophy (see Figs. 19.13**c** and 19.14**a**). **b:** moderate: PSV = 12 cm/s (normal value) and RI = 0.79 (moderately, but frankly high). **c:** severe, with a very low PSV = 6.2 cm/s and a very high RI at 1.00 by abolition of diastolic flow

arteries [3, 26, 27], in varying proportions, depending on the stage of the disease and the therapeutic response (Fig. 19.15).

However, CDI of the cilioretinal arteries, and the ophthalmic artery, is not a diagnostic test [28] because the sensitivity of detection of cilio-retinal hemodynamic alterations, in a population of untreated normal pressure glaucoma suspects, for a specificity of 90% is only 48%.

However, this examination can be useful for follow-up [3, 26], after an initial baseline examination has been completed, as corroborated by our experience. An increase in the RI (> 0.75) of retrobulbar blood flow and a decrease in its velocity are risk factors for conversion to primary open-angle glaucoma [29]. A lack of decrease in the RI of the ophthalmic artery under treatment (< 0.78) would constitute a poor prognostic factor [30].

In addition to monitoring changes in arterial flows under treatment, it is also useful to monitor changes in the flows of the superior ophthalmic vein.

## 19.7 Conclusion

CDI, by allowing assessment of the large retinal and orbital vessels, participates in the evaluation of the blood flow of the optic nerve head. It has led to great interest and hope for better diagnostic and therapeutic management. Over the years, with the experience gained in the field and the comparison of the experiences of different teams, this tool has naturally found its place in the diagnostic arsenal. The constant progress of ultrasound equipment, the refinement of the signal collection of low velocity flows, and improvement in inter-operator reproducibility with standardization of protocols [31] suggest an even better level of understanding of the vascularization of the optic nerve head in the future.

## References


1. Gans MS, Byme SF, Glaser JS. Standardized A-scan echography in optic nerve disease. Arch Ophthalmol. 1987;105(9):1232–6.
2. Dees C, Buimer R, Dick AD Atta HR. Ultrasonographic investigation of optic neuritis. Eye (Lond).1995;9(Pt4):488–94.
3. Tranquart F, Berges O, Koskas P, Pourcelot L, et al. Color Doppler imaging of orbital vessels: personal experience and literature review. J Clin Ultrasound. 2003;31(5):258–73.
4. Gerling J, Fanknecht P, Hansen LL, Kommerell G. Diameter of the optic nerve in idiopathic optic neuritis and in anterior ischemic optic neuropathy. Int Ophthalmol. 1997;21(3):131–5.
5. Elvin A, Andersson T, Sôderstrôm M. Optic neuritis. Doppler ultrasonograpy compared with MR and correlated with Visual evoked potential assessments. Acta Radiol. 1998;39(3):243–8.
6. Karaali K, Senol U, Aydin H, Cevikol C, et al. Optic neuritis: evaluation with orbital Doppler sonography. Radiology. 2003;226(2):355–8.
7. Akarsu C, Tan FU, Kendi T. Color Doppler imaging in optic neuritis with multiple sclerosis. Graefes Arch Clin Exp Ophthalmol. 2004;242(12):990–4.
8. Schmidt D, Hetzel A, Reinhard M, Auw-Haedrich C. Comparison between color duplex ultrasonography and histology of the temporal artery in cranial arteritis (giant cell arteritis). Eur J Med Res. 2003;8(1):1–7.
9. Arnold AC. Pathogenesis of nonarteritic anterior ischemic optic neuropathy. J Neuroophthalmol. 2003;23(2):157–63.
10. Foroozan R, Savino PJ, Sergott RC. Embolic central retinal artery occlusion detected by orbital color Doppler imaging. Ophthalmology. 2002;109(4):744–7; discussion 747–8.
11. Nedelmann M, Graef M, Weinand F, Wassill KH, et al. Retrobulbar spot sign predicts thrombolytic treatment effects and etiology in central retinal artery occlusion. Stroke. 2015;46(8):2322–4.
12. Keyser BJ, Flaharty PM, Sergott RC, Brown GC, et al. Color Doppler imaging of arterial blood flow in central retinal vein occlusion. Ophthalmology. 1994;101(8):1357–61.
13. WilliamsonTH BaxterGM. Central retinal vein occlusion, an investigation by color Doppler imaging. Blood velocity characteristics and prediction of iris neovascularization. Ophthalmology. 1994;101(8):1362–72.
14. Tranquart F, Arsene S, Aubert-Urena AS, Desbois I, et al. Doppler assessment of hemodynamic changes after hemodilution in retinal vein occlusion. J Clin Ultrasound. 1998;26(3):119–24.
15. Khonsari RH, Wegener M, Cochereau I, Milea D, et al. Drusen de la tête du nerf optique ou œdème papillaire? Rev Neurol. 2010;166(1):32–8.

16. Skougaard M, Heegaard S, Malmqvist L, Hamann S. Prevalence and histopathological signatures of optic disc drusen based on microscopy of 1713 enucleated eyes. Acta Ophthalmol. 2020;98(2):195–200.
17. Boldt HC, Byrne SF, DiBernardo C. Echographic evaluation of optic disc drusen. J Clin Neuroophthalmol. 1991;11(2):85–91.
18. Wilkins JM, Pomeranz HD. Visual manifestations of visible and buried optic disc drusen. J Neuroophthalmol. 2004;24(2):125–9.
19. Rahmouni A, Bargoin R, Herment A, Bargoin N, et al. Color Doppler twinkling artifact in hyperechoic regions. Radiology. 1996;199(1):269–71.
20. Mezad-Koursh D, Klein A, Rosenblatt A, Neudorfer M, Zur D, et al. Peripapillary hyper-reflective ovoid mass-like structures-a novel entity as frequent cause of pseudopapilloedema in children. Eye (Lond). 2021;35(4):1228–34.
21. Lyu IJ, Park KA, Oh SY. Association between myopia and peripapillary hyperreflective ovoid mass-like structures in children. Sci Rep. 2020;10(1):2238.
22. Friedman DI. Jacobson DM diagnostic criteria for idiopathic intracranial hypertension. Neurology. 2002;59(10):1492–5.
23. Denoyer A. Dégénérescence neurorétinienne glaucomateuse in Rapport SFO 2014: Glaucome Primitif à Angle Ouvert, Renard JP, Sellem E, editors. Elsevier-Masson, Paris, 2014. p. 79–88.
24. Mendrinos E, Pournaras CJ, Bouzas EA. Pathologie liée à l'ischémie artérielle in Rapport SFO 2008: Pathologies vasculaires oculaires. In: Pournaras CJ, editor. Elsevier-Masson, Paris; 2008. p. 574–75.
25. Chiquet C, Mottet B, Aptel F, Geiser M, Romanet JP. Facteurs vasculaires de la neuropathie optique glaucomateuse. In: Rapport SFO 2014: Glaucome Primitif à Angle Ouvert, Renard JP, Sellem E, editors, Elsevier-Masson, Paris; 2014, p. 95–100.
26. Gherghel D, Flammer J. Relationship between ocular perfusion pressure and retrobulbar blood flow in patients with glaucoma with progressive damage. Am J ophtalm. 2000;130(5):597–605.
27. Zeitz O, Galambos P, Wagenfeld L, Wiermann A, et al. Glaucoma progression is associated with decreased blood flow velocities in the short posterior ciliary artery. Br J Ophthalmol. 2006;90(10):1245–8.
28. Plange N, Kaup M, Harris A, Arend KO, et al. Performance of colour Doppler imaging discriminating normal tension glaucoma from healthy eyes. Eye (Lond). 2009;23(1):164–70.
29. Calvo P, Ferreras A, Polo V, Güerri N, et al. Predictive value of retrobulbar blood flow velocities in glaucoma suspects. Invest Ophthalmol Vis Sci. 2012;53(7):3875–84.
30. Galassi F, Sodi A, Ucci F, Renieri G, et al. Ocular hemodynamics and glaucoma prognosis: a color Doppler imaging study. Arch Ophthalmol. 2003;121(12):1711–5.
31. Barbosa Breda J, Van Eijgen J, Stalmans I. Advanced vascular examinations of the retina and optic nerve head in glaucoma. Prog Brain Res. 2020;257:77–83.

# Chapter 20
# Vascular Lesions

Patricia Koskas, François Lafitte, Elisabeth Nau, Mario de La Torre, and Olivier Bergès

**Abstract** The different lesions presented in this chapter are classified according to their hemodynamic characteristics: "Excluded" lesions are the lymphangiomas. Lesions with a predominant venous component are the orbital varicose veins (varices). Vascular lesions with arterial flow include cavernous hemangiomas, with characteristic diagnostic signs in A- and B-modes: hyperreflective, attenuating, with a usually homogeneous structure, and no spontaneous flow on color Doppler imaging (CDI) but with capillary arterial micro flows after injection of ultrasound contrast medium, their differential diagnosis being represented by hemangiopericytomas (= solitary fibrous tumor), fibrous tumors, and tumors of nerve sheath origin (neurofibroma and schwannoma); infantile hemangiomas (capillary hemangioma), arteriovenous fistulas and malformations, intravascular papillary endothelial hyperplasia (vegetative hemangioendothelioma or Masson's tumor), and arterial aneurysms. Vascular pathologies of the cavernous sinus impacting the orbit include direct carotid-cavernous fistulas, cavernous sinus dural arteriovenous fistulas, and intracavernous carotid aneurysm. Finally, orbital hematomas are discussed: often secondary to trauma or to the rupture of a pre-existing lesion (varicose vein+++, meningioma, cavernous hemangioma, lymphangioma, etc.) but which can also be spontaneous.

## 20.1 Classification

Vascular lesions account for a significant proportion of all orbital pathologies, around 10% [1]. The classification of these anomalies is sometimes difficult, especially if it aims to be exhaustive [2]; several terms cover the same histological entity. Conversely,

P. Koskas · F. Lafitte · E. Nau · O. Bergès (✉)
Rothschild Foundation Hospital, Paris, France
e-mail: oberges@for.paris

M. de La Torre
Universidad Nacional Mayor de San Marcos, Lima, Perú

© The Author(s), under exclusive license to Springer Nature Switzerland AG 2024     421
O. Bergès (ed.), *Echography of the Eye and Orbit*,
https://doi.org/10.1007/978-3-031-41467-1_20

some terms, such as hemangioma, are misused to refer to entities for which the clinical characteristics, progression, and histology are very different.

To clarify practices and treatments, the classification we retain is that of the Orbital Society [1], distinguishing three types of lesions:

- Type I, corresponding to lesions without flow, hemodynamically excluded: these are lymphangiomas.
- Type II, presenting a venous type of flow, corresponding to orbital varicose veins.
- Type III, characterized by the presence of arterial flows [3], such as high-flow arteriovenous malformations or cavernous hemangiomas. In this section, one can discern extra-orbital vascular lesions with intraorbital repercussions, such as aneurysms or carotid-cavernous and dural arteriovenous fistulas.

The special case of isolated orbital hematoma will be treated separately.


## 20.2 "Excluded" Vascular Lesions: Lymphangiomas

Lymphangiomas account for 1% of all orbital tumors, and 12% of all vascular tumors. These are lymphatic and/or venous malformations, occurring frequently in areas of the head and neck, especially in the orbit. These lesions do not have a capsule, which explains their tendency to extend into both the intra- and extraconal spaces and makes their completely surgical excision difficult. Within this meshwork of lymphatic ducts, there are thin septa containing capillaries responsible for spontaneous intraluminal lymphorrhagia.

They are discovered when the first complications arise, mainly before 10 years of age. They are revealed by the appearance of progressive or acute exophthalmos, a deviation of the eyeball, or more rarely by ptosis or palpebral telangiectasias. There can be an associated superficial lymphangioma, infiltrating the cheek, frontal region, or palate. The growth of this type of malformation is caused by repeated hemorrhage and not by cell growth.

B-mode ultrasound reveals a poorly delineated hypoechoic mass, with numerous microcysts (Fig. 20.1) or macrocysts with thick partitions (Fig. 20.2).

Similar to varicose veins, these lesions can increase in volume in procubitus or after Valsalva maneuver. Intralesional hemorrhages may occur giving these cysts a fine echogenic appearance. Color Doppler imaging can reveal Brownian motion within these hemorrhagic cysts (see Chap. 23) and demonstrates the vascularization of the active portion of lymphangioma (Fig. 20.3).

CT, and especially MRI, are better than ultrasound in showing the exact extension of the lesion, especially when it is voluminous, poorly defined, and infiltrating. Similarly, in case of sudden exophthalmos in connection with a massive hemorrhage, they are better for visualizing the stretching of the optic nerve, resulting in a characteristic triangular appearance of the eye; color Doppler imaging (CDI) can confirm vascular disorders of the optic nerve head requiring an emergency surgical procedure. They are also better than ultrasound for analyzing the extra-orbital lesional extension (deep

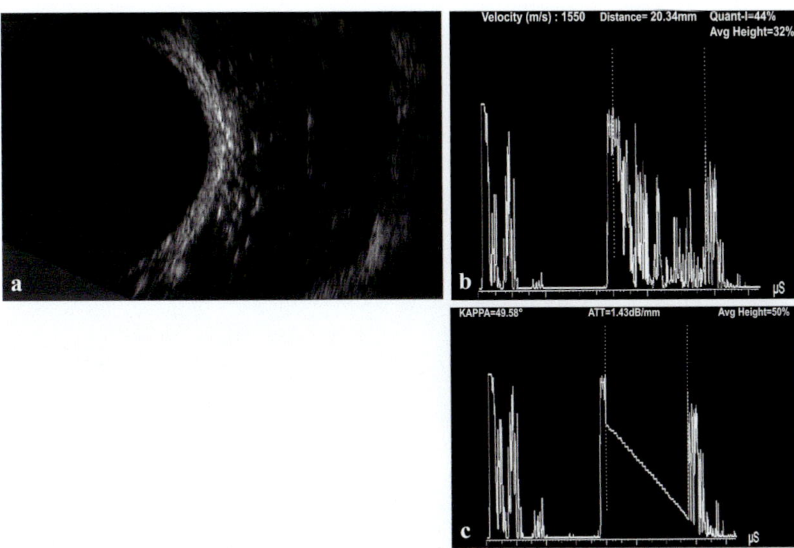

Fig. 20.1 **Microcystic lymphangioma**. **a**: 10 MHz B-mode section of the nasal quadrant of the right eye; **b**: standardized A-mode at tissue sensitivity (T = 76.3 dB), to assess the reflectivity: **c**: standardized A-mode at T+5.4 dB, with an average peak height equal to 50%, to assess the attenuation. B-mode reveals the micropolycystic structure of this voluminous intraconal mass. The echogenicity (**a**) and reflectivity (**b**) are less than for a cavernous hemangioma, and the honeycomb appearance is not obvious. However, the attenuation is not discriminating (*compare with* Fig. 20.9)

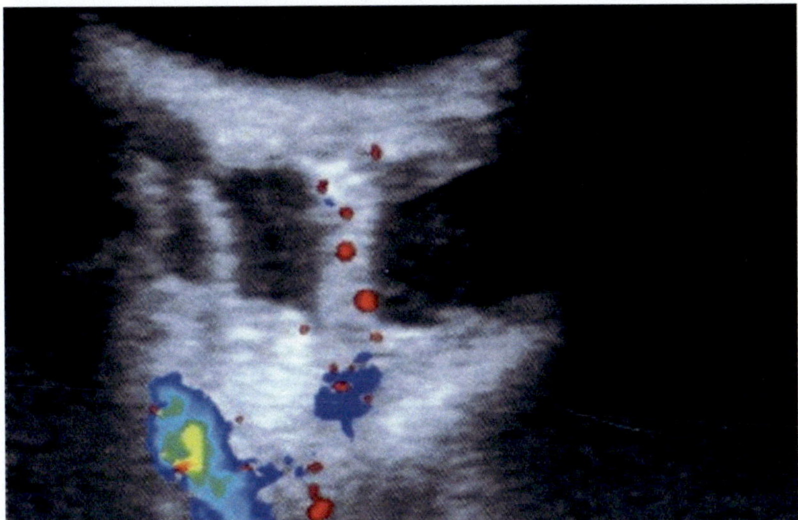

Fig. 20.2 **Macrocystic lymphangioma**. Color Doppler imaging (CDI) color mode. Voluminous intraconal mass with macrocysts, thick walls and some flows at the deep part of the lesion and at the level of the septa

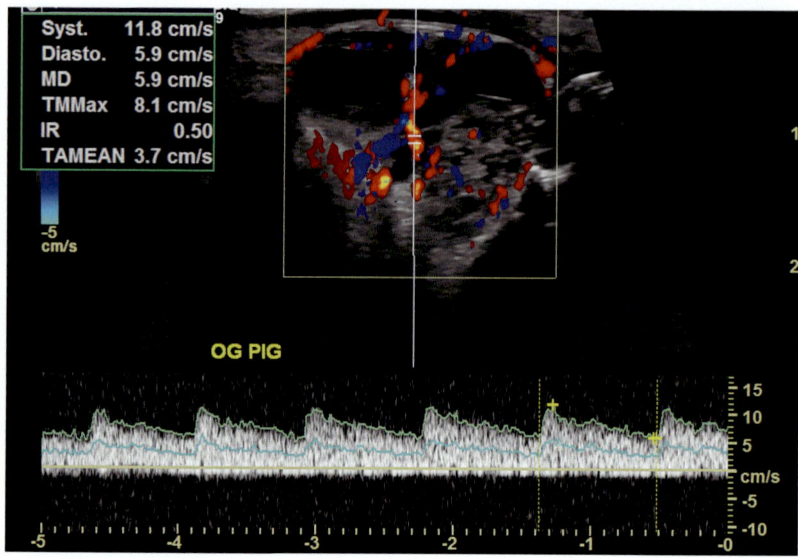


**Fig. 20.3** **Orbito-palpebral lymphangioma**. CDI, color and spectral modes. Flow is present in the deep, orbital part of the lesion and the thick septum separating two macrocysts. The resistive index (RI) is low: 0.50, in the main vessel

spaces of the face, endocranium), which is essential information for the therapeutic choice.

Their management is difficult: Currently, a non-aggressive surgical attitude prevails, with indications reserved mainly for the treatment of acute forms that jeopardize optic nerve function. In forms with excessive extension, an indication for an exenteration is sometimes required (for a benign lesion!!!).

## 20.3 Vascular Lesions with a Predominant Venous Component: Orbital Varicose Veins (orbital varix)

Orbital varices are congenital venous malformations, characterized by the proliferation of venous elements associated with major dilation of one of the orbital veins. They can be congenital, idiopathic, post-traumatic, associated with a hemangioma, or secondary to an arteriovenous fistula.

The symptoms related to orbital varicose veins consist of intermittent exophthalmos, dependent on the systemic venous pressure [4]. The exophthalmos fluctuates and occurs mainly when the patient leans forward or during a Valsalva maneuver [5]. At rest, a paradoxical enophthalmos can be seen. Occasionnaly they are suddenly revealed, when the malformation thromboses [6] or is complicated by a hematoma.

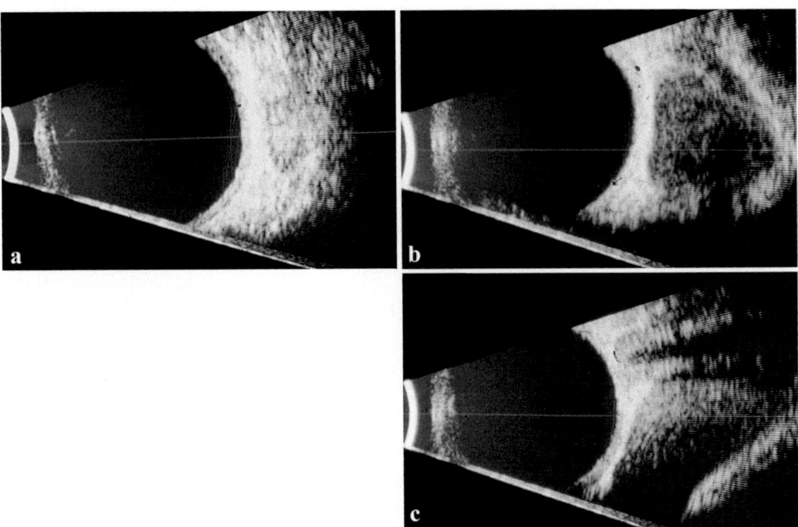

**Fig. 20.4  Orbital varix: effect of the Valsalva maneuver. a**: 10 MHz B-mode transverse view of the inferior quadrant in supine position at rest; **b**: the same view of the inferior quadrant after Valsalva maneuver; **c**: section of the 6 o'clock meridian after Valsalva maneuver. At rest, the appearance is strictly normal, and the malformation is not visible. After the Valsalva maneuver, the volume of the malformation is substantial, in width, and it occupies the entire inferior intraconal space, from the eyelid to the orbital apex

Ultrasound allows for a positive diagnosis by revealing an anechoic mass that is soft and depressible, with a volume that fluctuates according to the positions and maneuvers performed (Fig. 20.4).

In the supine position, the varicose malformation, when collapsed, may result in only a few small poorly delineated anechoic spaces relative to the orbital fat. Sometimes it can even be undetectable. Therefore, one must obtain imaging during a Valsalva maneuver or, with ultrasound in hyperdecubitus, for the head to be fully tilted back (= Hirtz's radiographic incidence), because although it is indeed not too difficult to perform CT or MRI sections in procubitus, performing an ultrasound in procubitus is unrealistic. In such cases, the appearance of a multilobed mass, more or less well delineated, both intra- and extraconal, then confirms the diagnosis of varix. Calcifications (phleboliths) are suggestive ans found in around 60% of the cases. These are hyperechoic nodules with posterior shadowing or comet-tail resonance artifacts, best seen when the malformation is filled, after a Valsalva maneuver (Fig. 20.5).

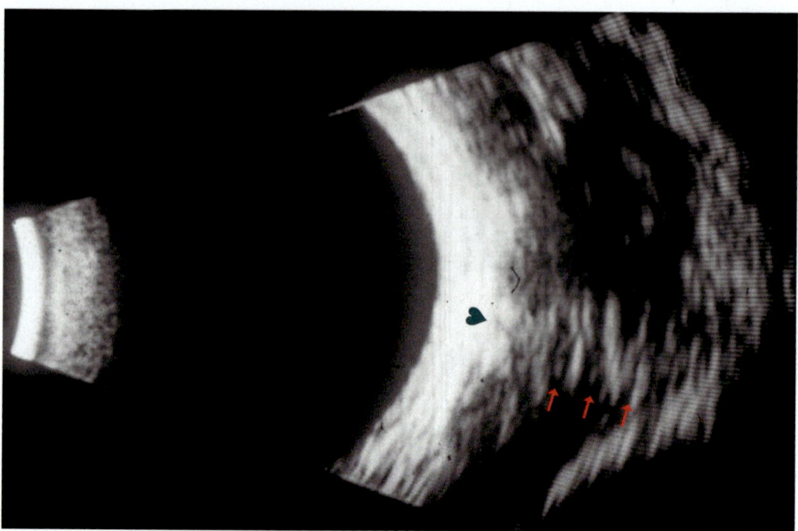

**Fig. 20.5  Orbital varix: presence of a phlebolith**. The phlebolith (♥) can barely be discerned because the small hyperechoic nodule is at the junction of the intraconal fat, which is also hyperechoic. However, the procession of posterior reverberation comet tail artifacts (→ red arrows) can readily be seen behind this calcification, particularly visible because the section was performed after a Valsalva maneuver

In color Doppler and power mode imaging, filling and emptying of the malformation can sometimes be seen with a venous type of flow (Fig. 20.6) in spectral Doppler.

However, this sign is variable because there are probably valves that limit these back-and-forth movements. A hematoma within the malformation results in an echogenic area, surrounded by a hypoechoic border, and the size changes are less obvious (Fig. 20.7).

The site of the lesion determines the prognosis and treatment. A purely palpebral localization, without posterior extension, supports undertaking surgical treatment. A retrobulbar localization contraindicates this surgery due to the almost constant recurrence of the malformation. A CT scan, MRI, or complement orbital phlebography should be considered.

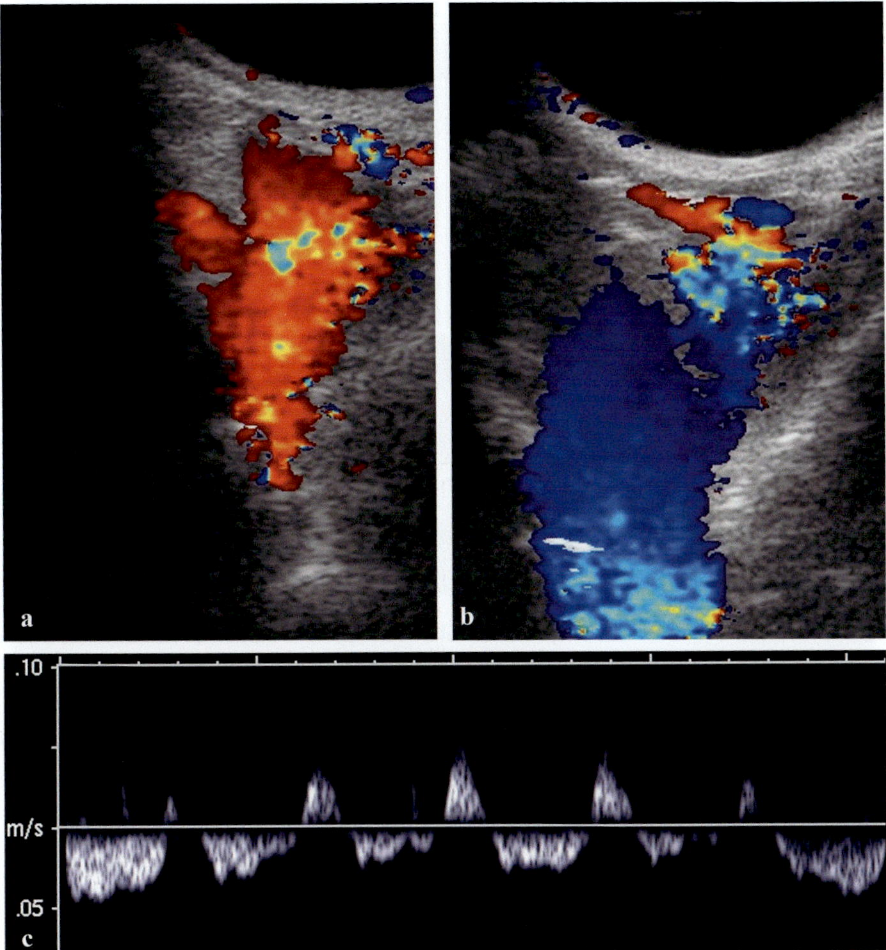

Fig. 20.6  **Orbital varix: CDI, color and spectral modes**. **a**: Color mode, filling phase; **b**: color mode, emptying phase; **c**: spectral mode. The malformation extends to the posterior orbit while filling and emptying freely at the level of the superior orbital fissure. Spectral mode shows that the malformation fills up quickly and empties over a longer period of time

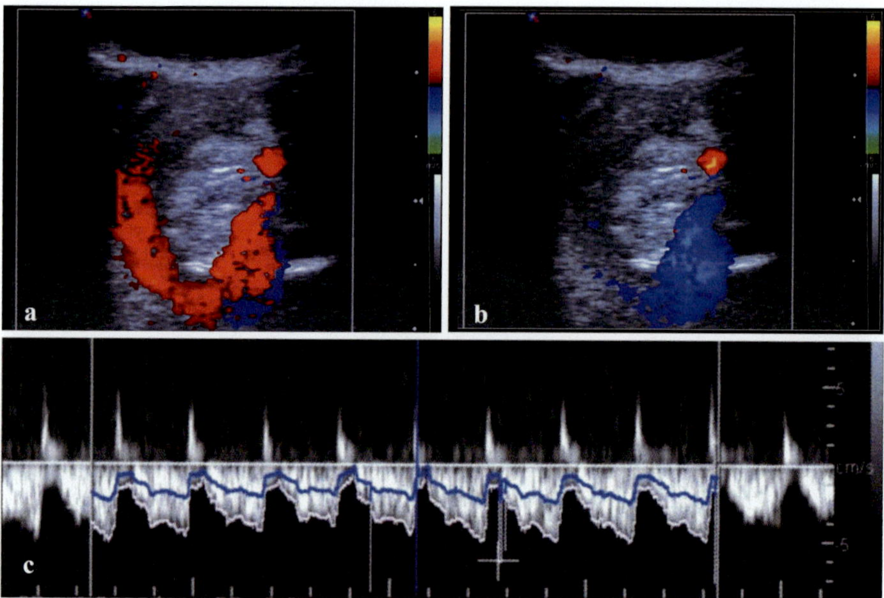

**Fig. 20.7 Thrombosed orbital varix: CDI, color and spectral modes. a**: Color mode, filling phase; **b**: color mode, emptying phase; **c**: spectral mode. The malformation is mainly occupied by a large echogenic clot, but a space that fills and then empties persists around it. Spectral mode shows that the filling is very brief, during the systole, and that the emptying is long, during the diastole, the cycle being synchronous to the pulsation of the cerebrospinal fluid, transmitted to the orbital malformation through the superior orbital fissure

## 20.4 Vascular Lesions with Arterial Flow

### 20.4.1 Cavernous Hemangioma

#### 20.4.1.1 Positive Diagnosis

It is the most common benign tumor in young individuals. The median age at discovery is 42 years, ranging from 18 to 67 years, with a preponderance in women, at 70% [7].

Of debatable etiopathogenesis, for some authors it corresponds to a congenital hemodynamically excluded venous malformation composed of blood lacunae, most often localized in the intraconal space, but in rare instances it can also develop in the extraconal and even the extra-orbital space [8]. Some can extend to the endocranium through the superior orbital fissure; others, very rarely, toward the eyelids, compressing the lacrimal ducts.

At the macroscopic level, it is an oval-shaped lesion, with regular contours, polycyclic, plum-colored, surrounded by a ± complete fibrous capsule; in rare instances they can be multiple. Histologically, cavernous hemangioma has large dilated vascular spaces, from 500 μm to 1 mm in diameter, limited by a layer of flattened endothelial cells, encapsulated in 1–5 layers of smooth muscle cells [9]. A variant of cavernous hemangioma is venous angioma, less well encapsulated, with more risk of intraoperative bleeding due to direct arterial intake, and a variant of venous angioma in the eyelids is the glomus tumor [10]. This benign tumor has no tendency to undergo spontaneous regression.

The clinical presentation, in most cases, is a slowly progressing exophthalmos over 4–5 years, axial in case of intraconal localization and lateral in case of extraconal localization, and non-pulsatile [7]. Although it is in contact with the optic nerve, or even repress it, visual field disorders are rare and transient amaurosis exceptional. This lesion is well tolerated, and corneal surface problems are extremely rare.

In B-mode, a cavernous hemangioma is visible in the form of a homogeneous mass, well delineated, round or oval, quite echogenic, and attenuating the ultrasound beam (Fig. 20.8a). Calcifications and hemorrhagic areas are sometimes found but less frequently than in varicose veins. The compression of the ocular wall by the mass, responsible for characteristic choroidal folds, is clearly visible in ultrasound (Figs. 20.8a and 20.9).

In standardized A-mode, in addition to the high reflectivity of the lesion, there is a typical "honeycomb" appearance, with an alternation of high peaks, corresponding to the fibrous tracts, and peaks of low intensity, corresponding to the blood circulating at very low velocity in the blood lacunae. The slope of decay of the echoes (angle κ) is approximately 45° (Fig. 20.8).

There is no spontaneous flow detectable in color Doppler imaging. However, after injection of ultrasound contrast medium, capillary arterial flows are readily visualized (Fig. 20.10).

MRI is only useful to complete the locoregional assessment for possible intervention (relation with the optic nerve and vessels and position of the lesion at the orbital apex).

Treatment is systematic beyond 25 mm in diameter because of the mass effect on nearby structures, including the optic nerve: Surgical excision uses different approaches depending on the location of the lesion.

If a cavernous hemangioma is discovered by chance (on a CT scan performed for another reason, exploration of the sinuses, for example) without exophthalmos and without any clinical signs and is small in size, the current attitude is simple monitoring, performed clinically and ultrasonographically (see Fig. 15.2).

### 20.4.1.2 Differential Diagnosis

(a) **Hemangiopericytoma**, despite its name, is no longer considered a vascular tumor but a **mesenchymal lesion** with pericyte differentiation; it has a suggestive immunohistochemical profile, with many of the cells expressing high levels of CD34 (90–95%) and CD99 (70%) with limited BCL-2 expression (35%). Mesenchyme is found throughout the orbit: striated extraocular muscles, connective tissue fibroblasts at the septa, adipocytes, smooth muscle cells of the

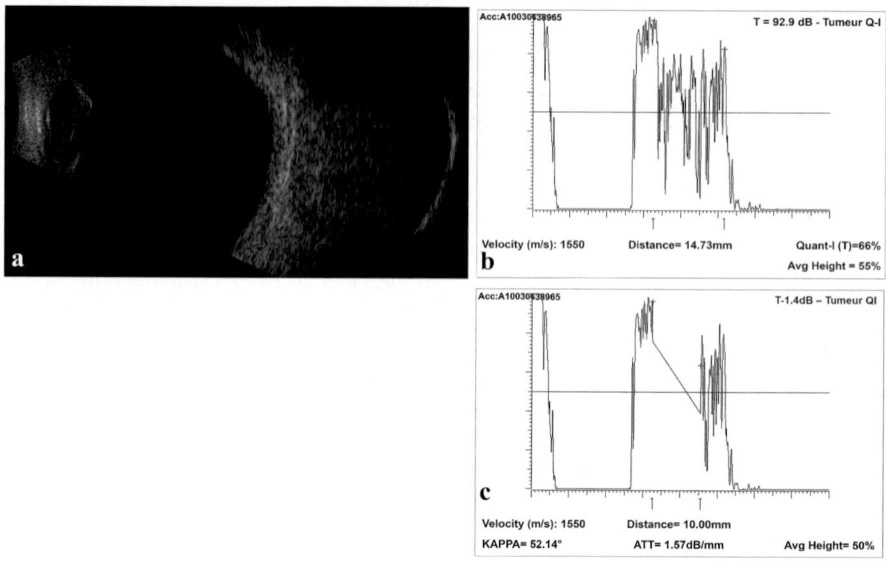

**Fig. 20.8 Cavernous hemangioma, characteristic echotexture. a**: 10 MHz B-mode section; **b**: standardized A-mode at tissue sensitivity (T = 92.9 dB), to assess the reflectivity, over the entire mass (17.73 mm); **c**: standardized A-mode at T = − 1.4 dB, so that the height of the peaks is equal to 50%, to assess the attenuation, on the first centimeter of the lesion. First, one can note the excellent concordance between B-mode and A-mode: the lesion is homogeneous, with an even appearance, and attenuating. At tissue sensitivity, the honeycomb appearance is particularly obvious and characteristic: with high peaks corresponding to fibrous septa and lower echoes corresponding to blood spaces. On the screen, echoes within these blood spaces are mobile, whereas those of the peaks are relatively stable. The reflectivity is high. The significant attenuation (kappa angle = 52°) is particularly characteristic when the first centimeter is evaluated

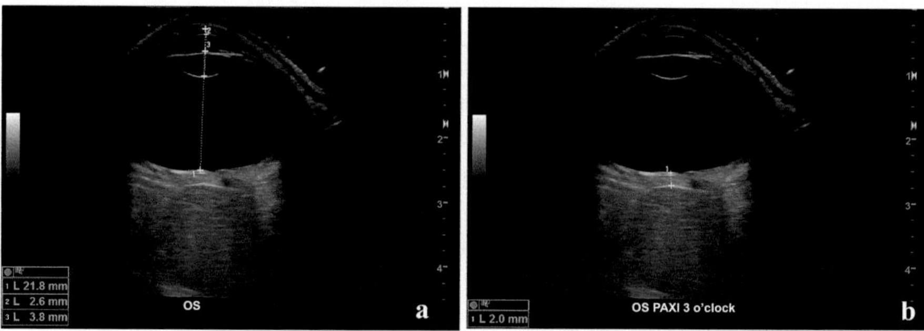

**Fig. 20.9 Cavernous hemangioma, impact on the posterior pole**. The lesion is located behind the posterior pole of the left eye and compresses it, resulting in recent hyperopia with a decreased axial length (21.8 mm vs. 23.4 mm OD) (**a**). There is also localized parietal thickening (2 mm vs. 1.2 mm OD) with an epimacular membrane (**b**)

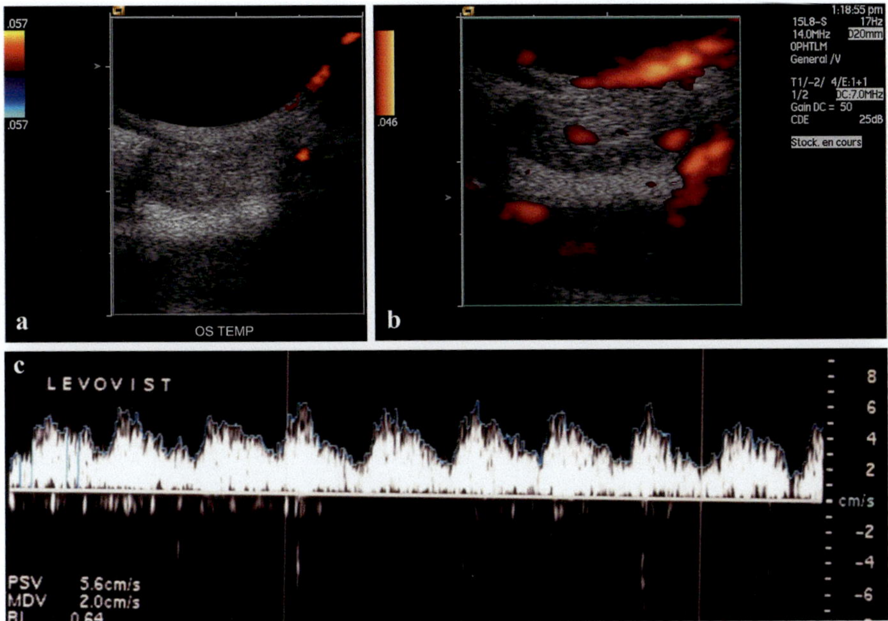

Fig. 20.10 **Temporal extraconal cavernous hemangioma**. CDI. Spontaneously (**a**), in color mode, absence of individualizable flow within the mass; in power mode, and after injection of ultrasound contrast medium providing an enhancement greater than 20 dB of the Doppler signal (**b**), the ocular parietal circulation and the two flows within this cavernous hemangioma can be seen and are highly characteristic of this diagnosis. In spectral mode (**c**), the capillary-arterial flows is slow

vascular walls (arteries and veins) but also Muller's muscle (superior eyelid) and connective septa covering the inferior orbital fissure and cartilage cells of the trochlea for the reflection of the superior oblique muscle. This mesenchyme in the orbit is responsible for 5–8% of orbital tumors. The WHO classification of soft tissue tumors has also removed hemangiopericytoma from its list (in extracranial localizations); the tissue forms being added to **solitary fibrous tumors**, and perivascular forms to smooth muscle tumors. This lesion is uncommon in the orbit but observed more frequently in the pleura. The lesion is most often benign, with slowly progressive exophthalmos, without inflammatory signs. Unlike cavernous hemangioma, the progression is faster with, in one third of patients, associated pain. The lesion is less often intraconal, sometimes palpebral or in the lacrimal fossa (Fig. 20.11) (see Fig. 21.9).

When the lesion is retrobulbar, in B-mode and A-mode, the lesion can resemble a cavernous hemangioma: echogenic, even texture, and attenuating, but in CDI, there are flows that can be low or abundant (Fig. 20.12).

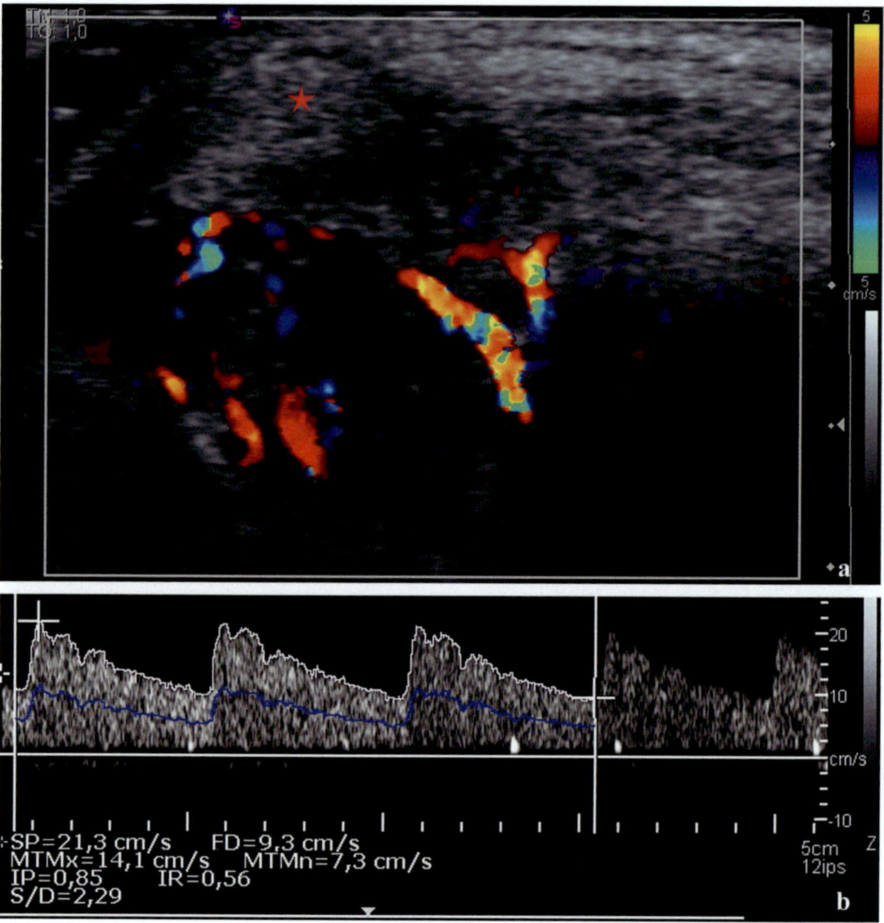

**Fig. 20.11 Solitary fibrous tumor of the lacrimal fossa**. CDI, paraocular approach. **a**: Color mode; **b**: spectral mode. CDI discloses a mass, hypoechoic and heterogenous, highly vascularized, with a relatively low RI (0.56). In retrospect, there is the impression of individualizing the more echogenic normal lacrimal gland (★ red star), repressed by the mass

Confirmation of the diagnosis can be achieved by MRI, which reveals a characteristic low signal on T2-weighted sequences and intralesional heterogeneous enhancement. These lesions are quite aggressive, with local invasive potential, even metastases, and a tendency to recur if the excision is not complete, sometimes long afterward. Some authors even propose life-long monitoring by imaging [11]. A biopsy is contraindicated because of the risks of bleeding and dissemination. Surgical resection should be as complete as possible respecting the capsule, possibly combined with radiotherapy/interferon α treatment.

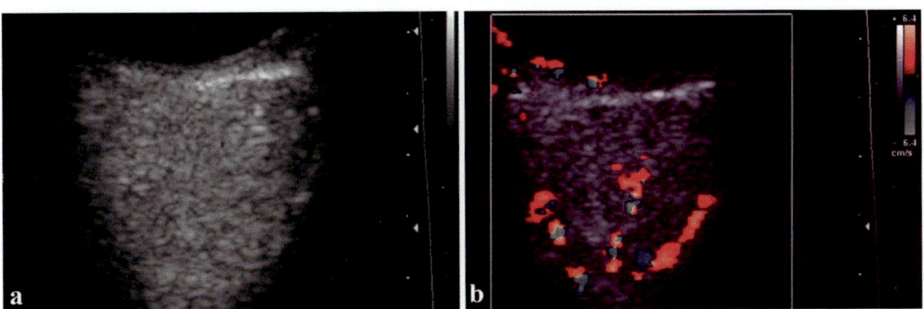

**Fig. 20.12  Retrobulbar solitary fibrous tumor**. In B-mode with an 8–12 MHz probe (**a**), the mass is moderately echogenic and very homogeneous but less attenuating than a typical cavernous hemangioma; and above all, weakly resistive flows are highlighted in CDI (**b**), incompatible with the diagnosis of a cavernous hemangioma

## (b)  Fibrous Tumors

There is a broad range of orbital fibrous tumors, both clinically and in terms of imaging, ranging from entirely benign lesions to locally aggressive lesions or even highly invasive malignant tumors [12]. Among the benign tumors, other than solitary fibrous tumors (see above), there are mainly fibrous histiocytoma, angiofibroma, nodular fasciitis/cellular fibromatosis, and leiomyoma. Diagnosis of these fibrous tumors is often difficult, based on optical microscopy, immunohistochemistry, and electron microscopy. Here, we analyze only purely benign lesions, which are limited, and we discuss the ultrasound signs that enables differential diagnosis with a cavernous hemangioma. As with solitary fibrous tumors, by revealing a hypointense lesion or with hypointense septa in T2-weighted imaging, MRI makes the diagnosis easier. They can be ubiquitous, intra- or extraconal, or palpebral. These lesions are less echogenic, often heterogeneous, and very attenuating, and in Doppler, some flows are frequently seen, with a rather low resistive index (RI) (Fig. 20.13).

The excision must be complete to avoid recurrence. Diagnosis with nerve tumors is sometimes difficult, both in terms of imaging and pathology.

## (c)  Tumors of Nerve Sheath Origin

Neurofibromas and schwannomas are the most common types [10].

- Orbito-palpebral plexiform **neurofibromas** are characteristic of von Recklinghausen's neurofibromatosis (NF1). The clinical aspect is already suggestive, with a feeling of a package of noodles on palpation. The purpose of imaging is to assess for extension, and therefore, MRI is the best for visualization of posterior extension of this lesion, according to the trigeminal branches, possibly associated with spheno-orbital dysplasia. Hence, ultrasound has little relevance in this indication. As for more localized forms outside neurofibromatosis type 1 (NF1), it can reveal a poorly echogenic, heterogeneous lesion, whose boundaries cannot always be precisely defined. In Doppler, some flows can be seen (Fig. 20.14).

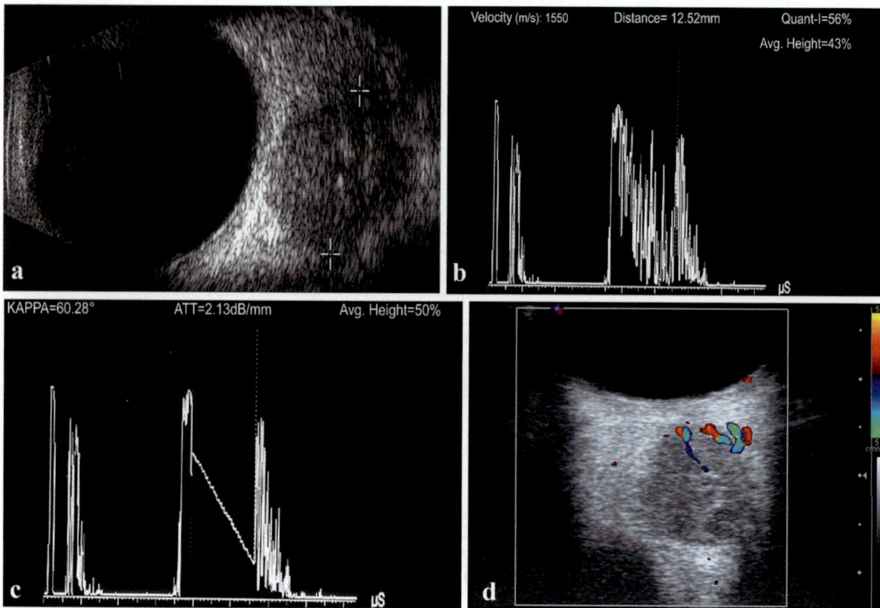

**Fig. 20.13** **Fibrous histiocytoma. a**: 10 MHz B-mode section; **b**: standardized A-mode at tissue sensitivity (T = 76.3 dB), to assess the reflectivity; **c**: standardized A-mode at T+1.9 dB with an average peak height of 50%, to assess the attenuation; **d**: CDI, color mode. The mass is more heterogeneous than a cavernous hemangioma, less reflective, and more attenuating. In addition, there is a centripetal flow to the center of the lesion

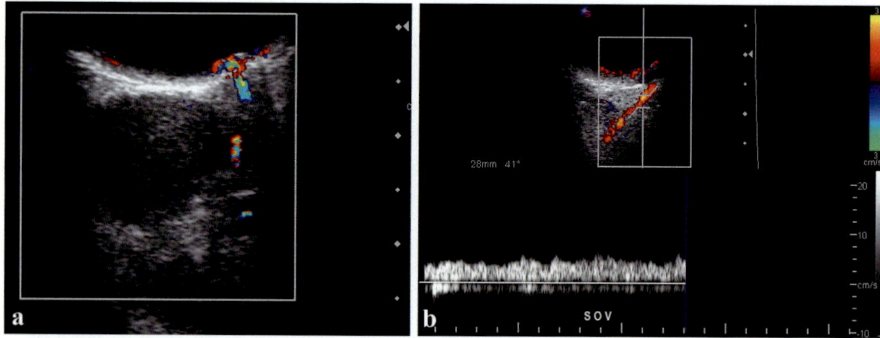

**Fig. 20.14** **Neurofibroma. a**: CDI, sagittal section; **b**: CDI, color and spectral modes of the superior ophthalmic vein. The mass is voluminous, very contoured, hypoechoic, with only a few detectable vascular flows; it is mainly localized in the inferior quadrant, but it has a posterior extension to the endocranium through the superior orbital fissure, resulting in reverse flow in the superior ophthalmic vein, coded in red in color mode and with positive venous flow in spectral mode

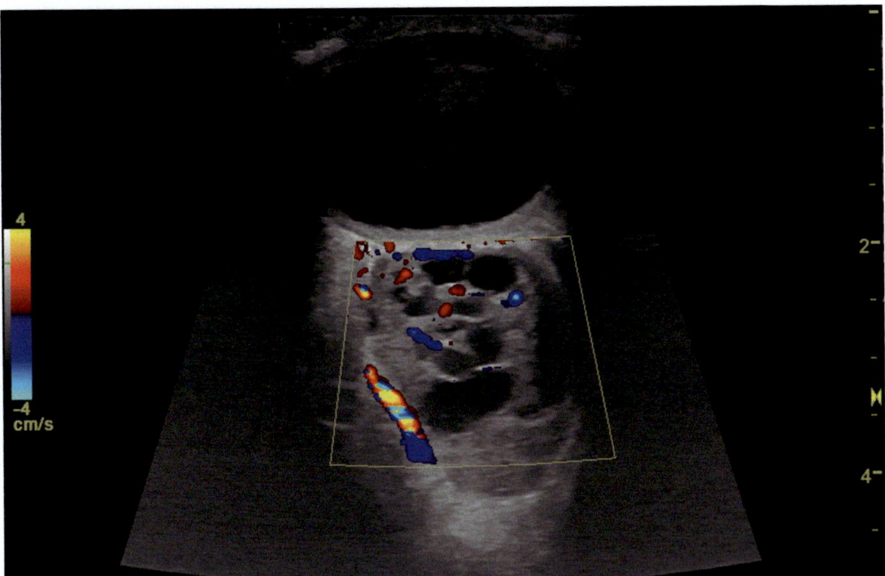

**Fig. 20.15  Schwannoma**. CDI, superior para-axial section. The mass is voluminous, extending to the posterior orbit, bordered by the ophthalmic artery. Numerous pseudocysts can be seen within the mass, corresponding to Antoni B spaces, and several vessels cross it from one edge to the other, especially at the level of the more echogenic (Antoni A) spaces

- **Schwannomas**, also called neurilemomas, are usually well limited, but they can extend outside the orbit (through the superior orbital fissure). They are also not very echogenic and heterogeneous, alternating dense cell zones = Antoni A and looser, pseudocystic areas = Antoni B (Fig. 20.15).

## 20.4.2   *Infantile Hemangioma*

This term replaces the name capillary hemangioma that was previously assigned to it. It is almost point by point the opposite of cavernous hemangioma. Moreover, the absolute difference in age of occurrence between infantile hemangioma and cavernous hemangioma supports the hypothesis that they are two different entities. It is a benign tumor, consisting of well-differentiated vessels, bordered by a single layer of endothelial cells. For some, more than a tumor, it is the result of anarchic postnatal vasculogenesis. At the histological level, it is a benign hemangioendothelioma, with benign proliferation of capillary-sized vessels with a flattened endothelium. The lesion consists of several very discrete nodules, each nodule supplied by a single arteriole. These nodules can be multiple in the form of hemangioma in tufts. There

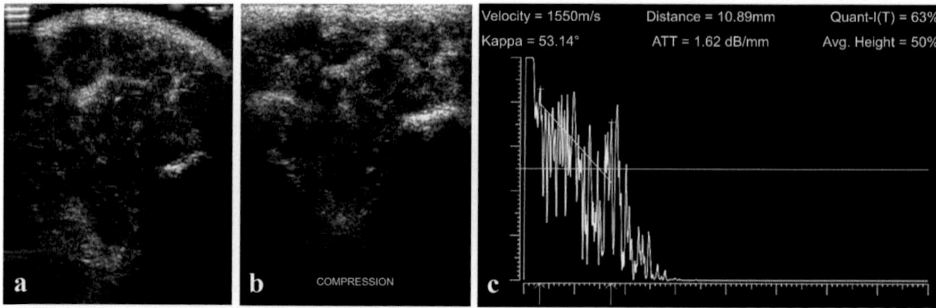



**Fig. 20.16 Infantile hemangioma of the inferior eyelid. a**: B-mode, horizontal section; **b**: the same section after gentle pressure on the mass by the probe; **c**: standardized A-mode with an average peak height of 50% to assess the attenuation. The lesion is moderately echogenic with an even echotexture; it is attenuating (angle kappa = 53°); after compression, the mass spreads under the probe, with a decrease in its anteroposterior axis

is never cellular atypia, but the endothelial cells can have noticeable mitotic activity. Discovered during the first year of life, with a disease-free interval from birth, its growth is rapid during the first 6 months after birth [13]. In 95% of cases, spontaneous regression can be observed, starting from the twelfth month to the sixth year. It more often affects girls (sex ratio 5 to 1) and often premature babies. Its diagnosis is clinical: a bluish elevation, or a depressible red spot, of the eyelids, which can reach the conjunctiva, associated with exophthalmos when there is retrobulbar extension. It is sometimes associated with neighboring skin abnormalities, and they can sometimes be part of a Sturge–Weber syndrome [14]. Ultrasound allows for easy differentiation between purely palpebral and orbitopalpebral forms; the mass appears hypoechoic, sometimes with echogenic areas related to endothelial proliferation. It is small and readily compressible (Fig. 20.16).

In standardized A-mode, it is even and attenuating. Doppler reveals the signs described for infantile hemangiomas of the soft parts [15] of the face and neck, and CDI results are highly characteristic, even **specific** in an infant: the hemangioma is an **extremely vascularized** lesion overall, resulting in a mosaic appearance with, albeit, very often small areas without vessels (especially in the process of progression) and in spectral mode, immature-type capillary-venous flows (with a low RI of $< 0.60$, equal to 0.49, on average, although it can be greater than 0.50 in one third of the cases) (Fig. 20.17).

In voluminous orbito-palpebral hemangiomas, there is frequently a low RI within the ophthalmic artery because it participates in the vascularization of this mass and an increase in size as compared with the contralateral side, of the superior ophthalmic vein. Cross-sectional imaging (CT and especially MRI) is only necessary in the rare cases in which it is entirely retrobulbar ($< 10\%$ of the cases) or when it extends broadly to the face. Its treatment, indicated in case of voluminous forms masking the visual axis or when there is an amblyogenic risk due to astigmatism, now involves beta-blockers systemically [16] or locally [17, 18].

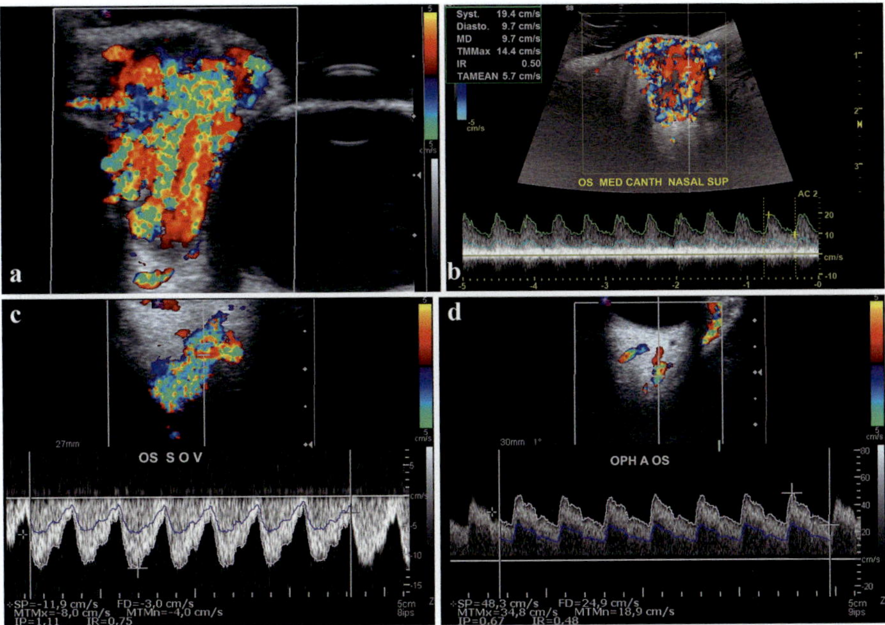

**Fig. 20.17** **Infantile hemangiomas.** CDI, four different cases. **a**: Color mode; **b**: color and spectral modes; **c**: superior ophthalmic vein; **d**: ophthalmic artery. The hypervascular appearance is obvious (**a**, **b**), characteristic, and, even specific when coupled to a low RI, $\leq 0.50$ (**b**). The peak systolic velocity (PSV) is between 11 and 20 cm/s. On the side of the hemangioma, the vein is dilated, with slightly elevated velocities: maximum velocity = 12 cm/s and mean velocity = 6 cm/s; and the artery exhibits little resistive flow (RI = 0.48), but this is usually equal to 0.70 for this vessel at this age

At this age, capillary hemangioma is the only existing Doppler hypervascularized mass. In adulthood, such hypervascularization can also be seen in arteriovenous malformations, intravascular papillary endothelial hyperplasia or Masson's tumor, and aneurysms (for these three diagnoses, see below), and even Merkel cell carcinomas. However, in the latter case, the clinical assessment and the imaging differ greatly, apart from this hypervascularization in Doppler.

## 20.4.3 Orbital Arteriovenous Fistulas and Malformations

These rare malformations connect arteries and veins without interposition of capillaries. They can be congenital or more often post-traumatic. The clinical picture resembles that of a carotid-cavernous fistula [19]. Palpation detects a quiver and

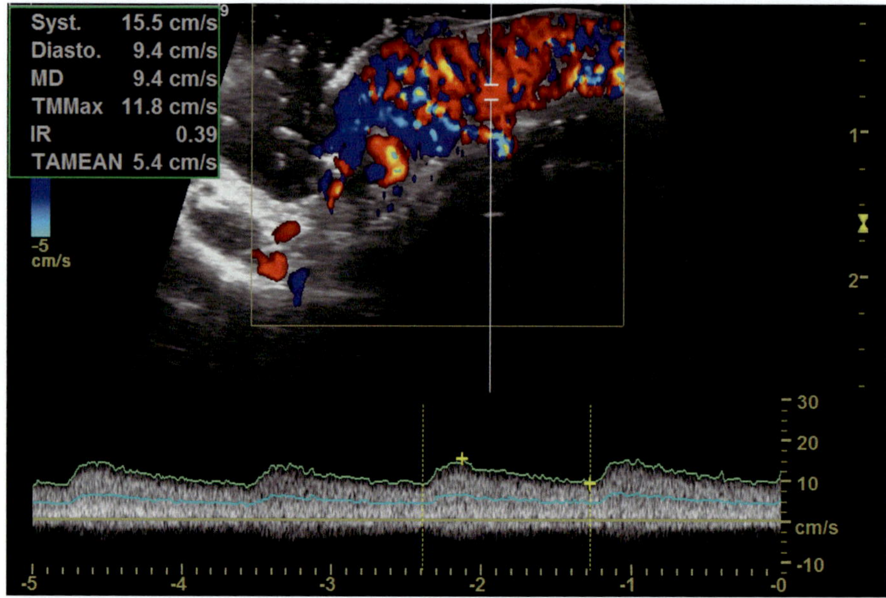

Fig. 20.18 **Orbito-palpebral arteriovenous malformation**. CDI, color and spectral modes. The malformation, having recurred despite several embolization sessions, occupies the entire width of the eyelid in a 24-year-old man. Absence of an avascular zone on color mode and very low RI = 0.39 on the spectral mode

auscultation a murmur that usually lead to carotid arteriography to undertake a diagnostic assessment of the lesions and consider the therapeutic possibilities (embolization). They mainly affect the eyelids, more frequently in men and young adults. In B-mode, the mass is moderately to quite echogenic and heterogeneous and appears hypervascularized in Doppler without a vessel-free area, as is frequently seen in infantile hemangiomas. In spectral mode, both the peak systolic velocity (PSV) and the resistive index (RI) are slightly lower than those of infantile hemangiomas (Fig. 20.18), RI ranging from 0.34 to 0.44, with an average of 0.41. They can recur after surgery or embolization.

### 20.4.4 Intravascular Papillary Endothelial Hyperplasia (Vegetative Hemangioendothelioma) or Masson's Tumor

The appearance differs greatly from an infantile hemangioma or an arteriovenous malformation: a mass is seen that is not very echogenic and very heterogeneous, more or less highly vascularized, with very high velocities, greater than 70 cm/s and low RIs of less than 0.50 (Fig. 20.19). It is difficult to differentiate from an

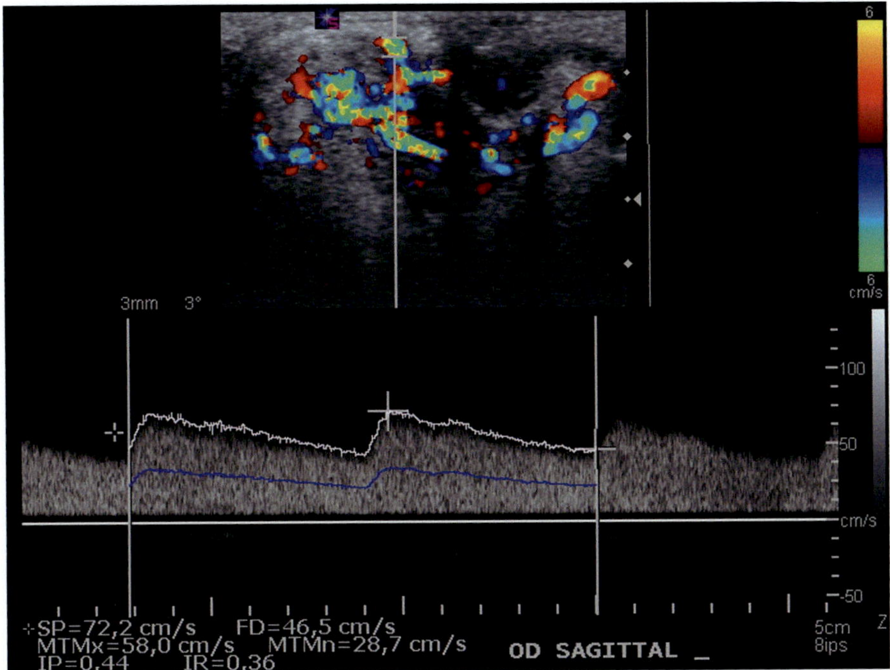

**Fig. 20.19 Intravascular papillary endothelial hyperplasia**. CDI, color and spectral modes. Hypoechoic and very heterogeneous mass, highly vascularized, with a very high PSV, 72.2 cm/s, and a very low RI, 0.36

angiosarcoma, except by histology, more periorbital than intraorbital; Histologically, this benign hyperplasia is associated with thrombi, without atypia or necrosis. On immunohistochemistry, there is elevated expression of CD31 and CD34 [20]. The outlook is favorable after excision.

### 20.4.5  Orbital Arterial Aneurysms

Very rare at the orbital level, they are located on the ophthalmic artery or lacrimal artery. The symptomatology is variable, the exophthalmos inconstant, and some aneurysms are revealed by a rapid and permanent decrease in visual acuity. Ultrasound reveals a mass with variable echotexture, anechoic or not very echogenic if the aneurysm is circulating or more echogenic if it is thrombosed. When the aneurysm is circulating, a hypervascular flow in the lesion can be seen on Doppler imaging (Fig. 20.20).

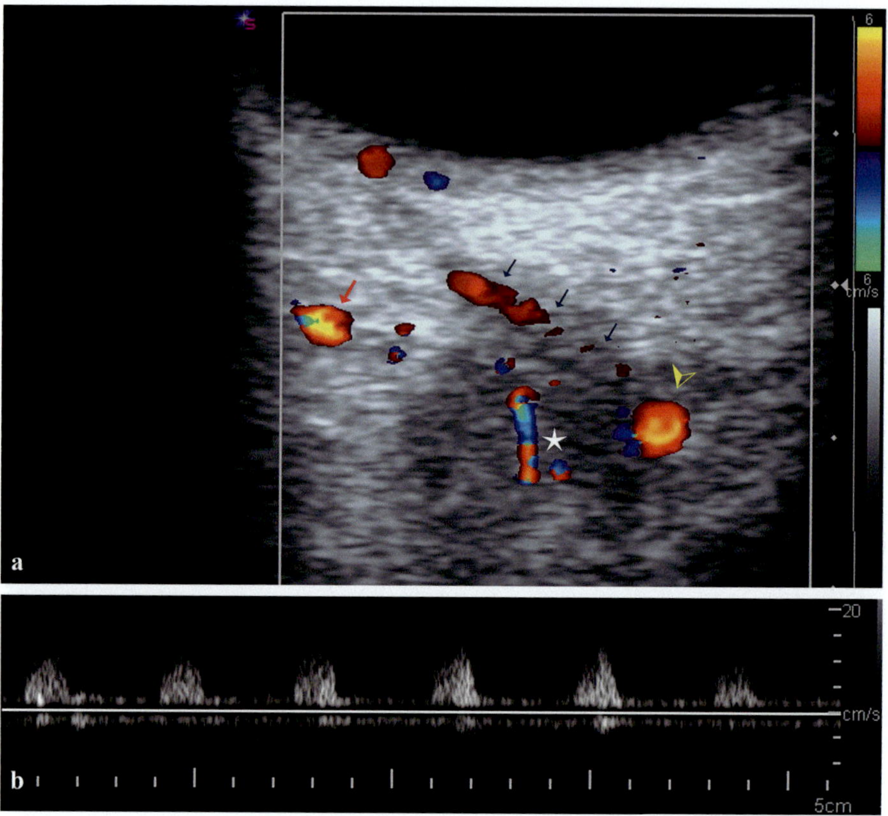

**Fig. 20.20 Ophthalmic artery aneurysm**. CDI. **a**: Color mode, superior para-axial section; **b**: spectral mode. The small aneurysmal dilation (▷ yellow arrowhead) is clearly visible outside the ophthalmic artery (→ red arrow) and the superior ophthalmic vein (→ dark blue arrows) and just below the outer part of the superior rectus muscle (⋆ white star), with its vessels in the center. In spectral mode, there is a blurred spectral envelope and a high RI, very different from the usual characteristics of the ophthalmic artery

Carotid arteriography confirms the lesion, its site, and the eventual options for embolization or surgical ligation of the nourishing pedicle. They can also be post-traumatic in the superior eyelid (Fig. 20.21), with turbulence in the aneurysmal sac.

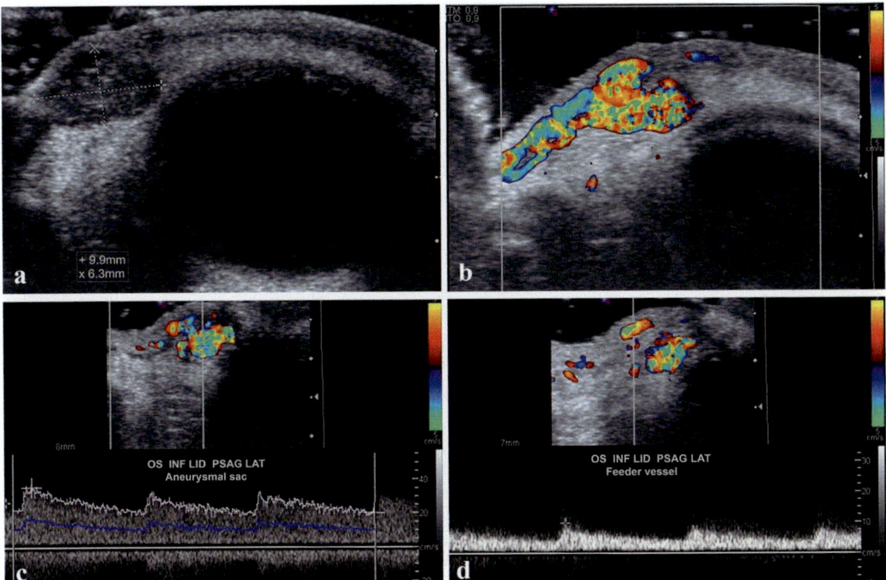

Fig. 20.21  **Post-traumatic aneurysm of the superior eyelid in a 24-year-old man. Assessment before surgery**. In B-mode, (**a**), the sac, well delineated, is poorly echogenic and heterogeneous, not calcified. In color mode (**b**), the appearance is shiny, reflecting turbulence, which is seen in spectral mode, both at the level of the aneurysmal sac (**c**), with a fringed envelope, and at the level of the feeder vessel (**d**), where the envelope is blurred and double. However, the PSV is not very fast, probably because it is a very distal vessel

## 20.5  Vascular Pathologies of the Cavernous Sinus Affecting the Orbit

### 20.5.1  Direct Carotid-Cavernous Fistula

This consists of a direct connection between the carotid siphon and the cavernous sinus. Most often post-traumatic, its constitution can also follow the rupture of an aneurysm of the intracavernous internal carotid artery, more often than a spontaneous rupture (Marfan, Ehlers–Danlos) [21].

The clinical presentation is obvious [22]. There is pulsatile exophthalmos associated with chemosis, conjunctival hyperemia, more rarely ophthalmoplegia, or even a decrease in visual acuity.

Venous drainage can be anterior or posterior and allow for hemodynamic adaptation, so the clinical presentation is less obvious.

B-mode ultrasound can provide the diagnosis in case of the occurrence of a very substantial dilation of the superior ophthalmic vein (SOV) (Fig. 20.22) and sometimes of the inferior ophthalmic vein, at times also associated with dilation of the angular vein or even facial veins.

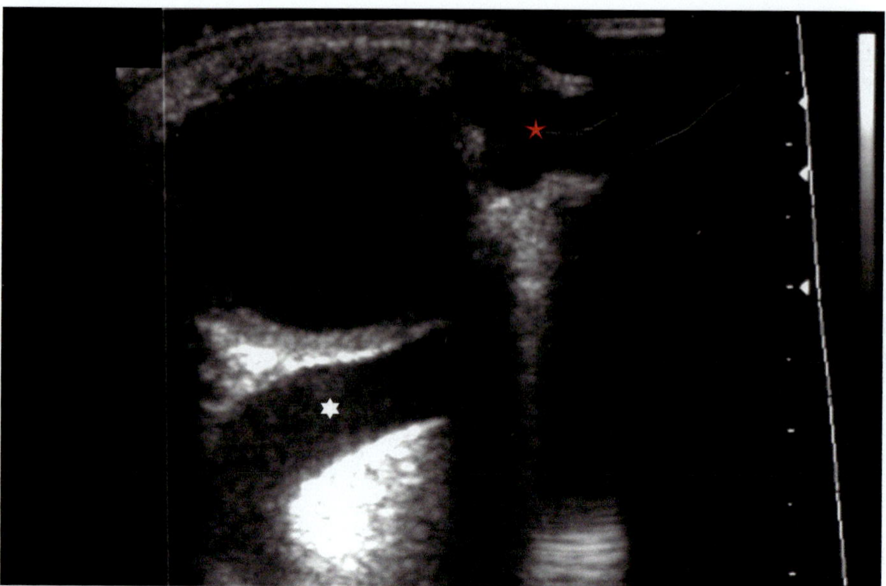

**Fig. 20.22 Direct carotid-cavernous fistula**. B-mode. Dilation of the superior ophthalmic vein (✳ white star), with its readily recognizable characteristic shape. Fluid mass of the internal canthus corresponding to an expansion of the angular vein (★ red star), with a posterior enhancement artifact

**Color Doppler imaging** (Fig. 20.23) **confirms the diagnosis**, the flow in this SOV is reversed (it appears red in color mode, with a positive spectrum in spectral mode). At the usual settings, the velocity of the flow leads to an aliasing phenomenon (inversion of the color by spectral ambiguity (see Chap. 6) in the center of the vessel. The flow is no longer venous, but it is arterialized, with a systolic peak in spectral mode; the PSV is high (50 cm/s), and the RI is low (< 0.50). In the absence of Doppler, A-mode can be useful. It shows an oscillating appearance of the peaks inside the dilated SOV, and the average height of the peaks at tissue sensitivity is less than 40% (see Fig. 25.9d) [23]. Venous involvement also affects the angular vein or even the facial veins. The extraocular muscles are often increased in volume. The existence of retroclival anastomoses can in some cases lead to a discrete increase in the contralateral SOV.

A high-resolution scanner is useful for assessing skull base fractures. Arteriography is essential, not so much to confirm the diagnosis but for therapeutic management.

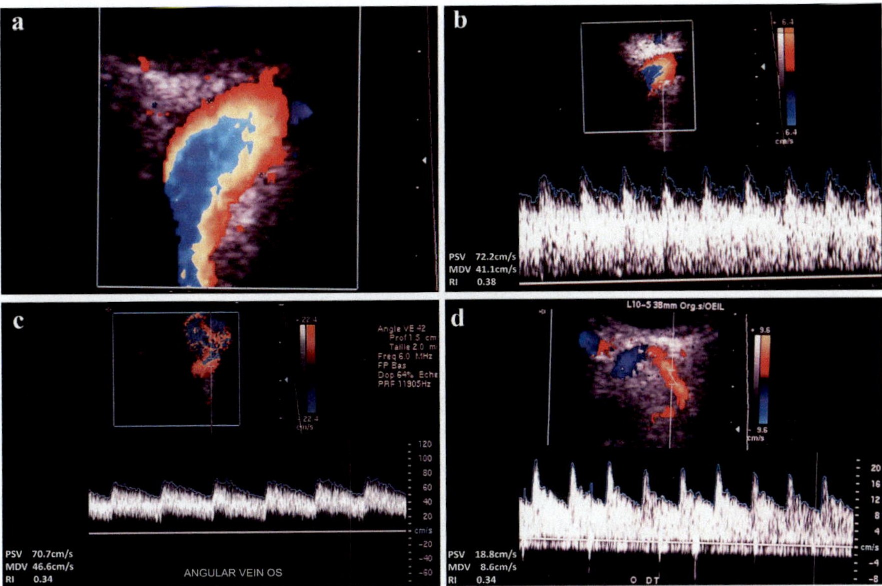

Fig. 20.23 **Direct carotid cavernous fistula**. CDI. Significant dilation of the superior ophthalmic vein in color mode (**a**), which should not be measured in color Doppler because of a blooming artifact (see Chaps. 3 and 6). The vein appears red, with a clear aliasing artifact indicative of very fast flow. In spectral mode (**b**), this very fast flow is confirmed, with PSV = 72.2 cm/s and very low RI, at 0.38. There are turbulences with similar values at the level of the angular vein (**c**) and a lesser dilation, with reverse flow and arterialization of the contralateral vein (**d**) due to retroclival anastomoses but circulating much slower, so without aliasing. At its level, the PSV is 18.8 cm/s and the RI is always very low, at 0.34

## 20.5.2 *Dural Fistula of the Cavernous Sinus*

Cavernous sinus dural arteriovenous fistulas are spontaneous and their initial description dates from 1966 [24]. They are often referred to as indirect/low-flow arteriovenous fistulas (AVFs) as opposed to direct/high-flow AVFs of traumatic origin that occur between the cavernous segment of the internal carotid artery and the homolateral cavernous sinus. Dural fistulas of the cavernous sinus are arteriovenous connections that develop in the dura mater between the arterial branches intended for meningeal purposes and the cavernous sinus.

Currently, most authors report that they are most often acquired [25], secondary to damage to the sinus wall (cerebral thrombophlebitis, nearby infection, trauma). They are frequently found in women between 60 and 80 years of age.

The most common clinical signs are unilateral exophthalmos, redness and congestion of the eye owing to dilation and tortuosity of the epibulbar venous plexus (the caput medusae sign) and inferior chemosis or even chronic glaucoma that does not respond to the usual eye drops. Given the atypical clinical picture, and the slow and often silent progression, a delay in diagnosis is frequent, even when CT scan or even MRI have been performed.

B-mode ultrasound reveals moderate pulsatile dilation of the SOV in the shape of an arciform structure with internal concavity on a para-axial section located above the plane of the optic nerve, or in cross-section, as an anechoic circle on a sagittal section; this dilation is less than in direct /high-flow AVFs (6 mm vs. 20 mm on average). **CDI confirms the diagnosis** by revealing reversal and arterialization of the flow in the dilated SOV.

Increase in volume of the left superior ophthalmic vein, arterialisation and flow inversion involves, the particularly visible medial root, with an anterolateral convexity, but also, frequently, the lateral root.

Peak systolic velocity is lower than in direct carotid-cavernous fistulas (10–15 cm/s vs. 50–70 cm/s). However, for both direct and dural fistulas, the RI is low, less than 0.50 (Fig. 20.24). In case of direct or dural AVFs of the cavernous sinus, dilation of the inferior ophthalmic vein can also be seen (Fig. 20.25).

As with direct carotid-cavernous fistulas, in the absence of Doppler, A-mode can be useful, with the average height of the peaks in standardized A-mode at tissue sensitivity greater than 40% (see Fig. 25.10d) [23]. Finally, very rarely, these dural fistulas

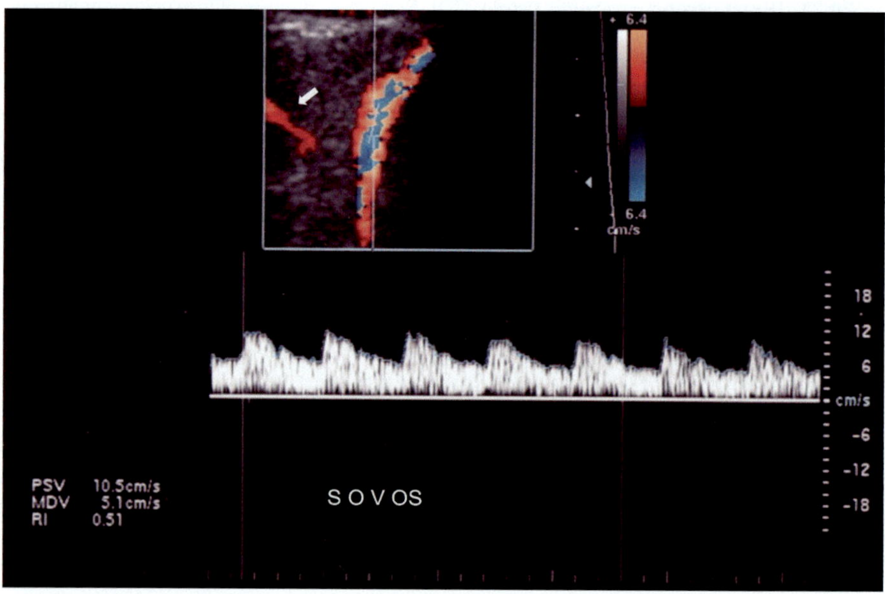



**Fig. 20.24 Dural fistula of the cavernous sinus** in a 63-year-old woman suffering from conjunctival hyperemia for 18 months with diagnostic wandering. Color and spectral Doppler imaging of the superior ophthalmic vein (SOV); Increase in volume of the left superior ophthalmic vein, with a particularly clear view of the medial root, with an anterolateral convexity, inverted and arterialized, and an aliasing phenomenon, whereas the recorded PSV is only 10.5 cm/s. However, the reverse flow in the superior ophthalmic venous system also involves the lateral root (→ white arrow), albeit thinner, and with a slower flow (without aliasing)

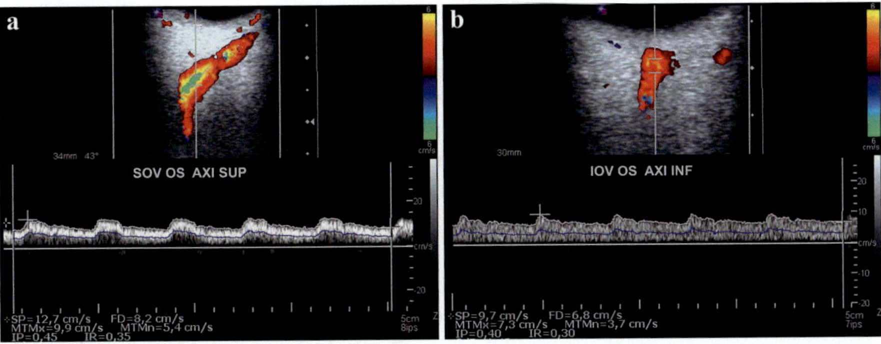

**Fig. 20.25** **Dural fistula of the cavernous sinus** in a 48-year-old man who consulted for diplopia with chemosis and conjunctival hyperemia. Color and spectral Doppler imaging. Increase in volume of the SOV (**a**) and the inferior ophthalmic vein (IOV) (**b**), the flows of which are reversed, coded in red in color mode and positive in spectral mode (in an adult without anesthesia; it is rare to be able to highlight the IOV), with a very low RI, 0.35 for the SOV and 0.30 for the IOV. Note the aliasing artifact within the SOV, whereas the PSV is only 12.7 cm/s but much higher than the velocity scale, set at 5 cm/s

can even occur in very small children, without obvious triggering circumstances (see Fig. 26.12).

The progression is variable. Most commonly, partial or total spontaneous stability or improvement (related to spontaneous occlusion) is observed in just under half of cases [21, 26].

Arteriography is only indicated if a therapeutic procedure is to be undertaken. It allows for mapping of arterial afferences and venous drainage, which is essential to the therapeutic strategy.

Venous embolization (coils) of a cavernous sinus affected by malformation remains the only permanent therapeutic solution.

This endovascular treatment should be carried out only in case of complications involving visual function, with disabling diplopia, chronic glaucoma, ophthalmoplegia, or significant esthetic discomfort.

### 20.5.3 Intracavernous Internal Carotid Aneurysm

This most often presents as a mass on the posterior part of the orbital apex, which can be responsible for visual field disorders, and/or ophthalmoplegia. The diagnosis is most often fortuitous, on CT scan, and Doppler ultrasound has no indication. Arteriography is an essential prerequisite for endovascular treatment.

## 20.6    Orbital Hematomas

They manifest as sudden onset painful exophthalmos, and they tend to regress in the days or weeks that follow. They are often secondary to trauma or to the rupture of a pre-existing lesion (varix+++, meningioma, cavernous hemangioma, lymphangioma, etc.) but can also be spontaneous. Such a pre-existing causal lesion should be sought at a distance from the acute episode.

From a topographical point of view, they can be intraconal, surrounding or repressing the optic nerve, extraconal, or straddle these two spaces [27].

In B-mode, they are in the form of a round or multilobed mass, the echotexture of which varies according to the stage of the hematoma. At the acute phase, there is a hard mass, homogeneous in appearance, with medium reflectivity and low attenuation. Liquid levels can sometimes be seen within the mass (Fig. 20.26).

The diagnosis can be difficult with a tumorous lesion. In fact, it is mainly the context of the occurrence (sudden onset, trauma, or pre-existing varicose vein)

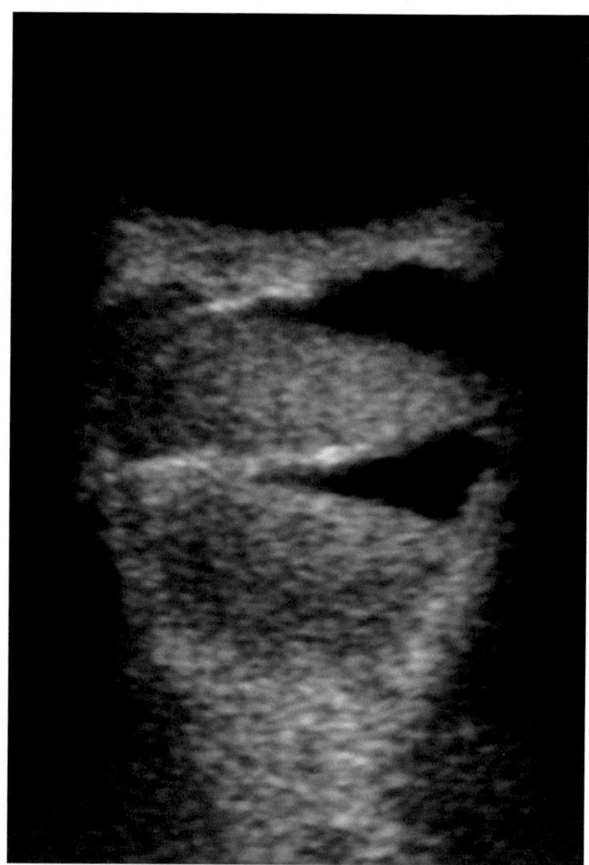

**Fig. 20.26  Post-traumatic orbital hematoma in the acute stage**. The hematoma is large, retrobulbar, with several cavities and liquid/liquid levels

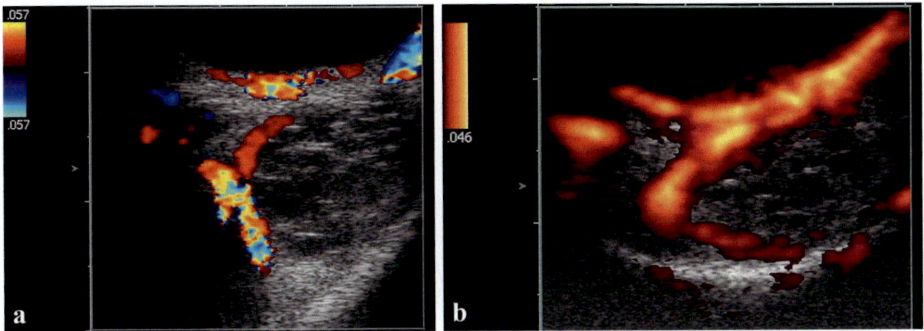

**Fig. 20.27 Superior temporal orbital hematoma complicating varicose veins**. **a**: CDI color mode, temporal parasagittal section; **b**: CDI, power mode after injection of ultrasound contrast medium, superior para-axial section. The superior temporal mass is moderately echogenic, with little or no attenuation, with a regular echotexture and laminated appearance, without detectable flow in Doppler, neither spontaneously nor after injection of ultrasound contrast medium (*compare with* Fig. 20.10)

and progression (progressive regression) that makes the difference. Color Doppler imaging, which reveals the absence of vascularization in the context of a simple hematoma, can be used, unlike with most tumors (except cavernous hemangioma) (Fig. 20.27).

In case of persistent doubt, a CT scan (spontaneously hyperdense mass) or MRI (hypersignal T1 and T2 mass after a few days) can confirm the diagnosis. After a few weeks, the hematoma becomes discretely hypoechoic, in connection with fibrinolysis, and a capsule with a varying degree of echogenicity appears. Eventually, it can disappear entirely.

Subperiosteal hematomas should be individualized because of their topography: it presents as a hypoechoic lenticular mass most often against the superior wall of the orbit, repressing the superior rectus muscle, and non-vascularized in Doppler.

These hematomas are most often post-traumatic, but they can sometimes correspond to hemorrhage in a cholesterol granuloma of the orbital roof, especially in case of recurrence [28]. Here again, a CT scan and especially MRI are useful to confirm the diagnosis. Spontaneous regression is common.

# References

1. Rootman J. Vascular malformations of the orbit: hemodynamic concepts. Orbit. 2003;22(2):103–20.
2. ISSVA classification for vascular anomalies © (Approved at the 20th ISSVA Workshop, Melbourne, April 2014, last revision May 2018). https://www.issva.org/classification.
3. Garzon MCEO, Frieden IJ. Vascular tumors and vascular malformations: evidence for an association. J Am Acad Dermatol. 2000;42(2 Pt 1):275–9.

4. Ramli N, Sachet M, Bao C, Lasjaunias P. Cerebrofacial venous metameric syndrome (CVMS) 3: Sturge-Weber syndrome with bilateral lymphatic/venous malformations of the mandible. Neuroradiology. 2003;45:687–90.

5. Cohen JACD, Norman D. Bilateral orbital varices associated with habitual bending. Arch Ophthalmol. 1995;113(11):1360–2.

6. Bullock JDGS, Connelly PJ. Orbital varix thrombosis. Trans Am Ophthalmol Soc. 1989;87:463–84; discussion 484–6.

7. Harris GJ, Jakobiec F. Cavernous hemangioma of the orbit. J Neurosurg. 1979;51(2):219–28.

8. D'hermies FCN, Hurbli T, Berges O, et al. Localisation inhabituelle préseptale d'un hémangiome caverneux orbitaire. J Fr Ophtalmol. 2000;23(6):631–4.

9. Ruchman MC, Flanagan J. Cavernous hemangiomas of the orbit. Ophthalmology. 1983;90(11):1328–36.

10. Jakobiec FA, Font RL. Orbit in ophthalmic pathology, an atlas and textbook. In: Spencer, 3rd ed. W.B. Saunders Company Philadelphia. 1986; p. 2459–2860.

11. Rice CDKR, Mrak RE. An orbital hemangiopericytoma recurrent after 33 years. Arch Ophthalmol. 1989;107(4):552–6.

12. Dalley RW. Fibrous histiocytoma and fibrous tissue tumors of the orbit Radiol. Clin North Am. 1999;37(1):185–94.

13. Boyd MJ, Collin JR. Capillary haemangiomas: an approach to their management. Br J Ophthalmol. 1991;75(5):298–300.

14. Dobyns WB, Michels VV, Groover RV, Mokri B, et al. Familial cavernous malformations of the central nervous system and retina. Ann Neurol. 1987;21(6):578–83.

15. Dubois J, Patriquin HB, Garel L, Powell J, et al. Soft-tissue hemangiomas in infants and children: diagnosis using Doppler sonography. AJR Am J Roentgenol. 1998;171(1):247–52.

16. Thoumazet F, Léauté-Labrèze C, Colin J, Mortemousque B. Efficacy of systemic propranolol for severe infantile hemangioma of the orbit and eyelid. A case study of eight patients. Br J Ophthalmol 14 Jun 2011.

17. Chambers CB, Katowitz WR, Katowitz JA, Binenbaum G. A controlled study of topical 0.25% timolol maleate gel for the treatment of cutaneous infantile capillary hemangiomas. Ophthalmic Plast Reconstr Surg. 2012;28(2):103–6.

18. Léauté-Labrèze C. Hémangiomes infantiles, actualités dans le traitement. Arch Pediatr. 2013;20(5):517–22.

19. Kupersmith MJBA, Choi IS, Warren F, Flamm E. Management of nontraumatic vascular shunts involving the cavernous sinus. Ophthalmology. 1988;95(1):121–30.

20. Dryden SC, Marsili S, Meador AG, et al. Intravascular papillary endothelial hyperplasia of the orbit: a case of Masson's tumor. Cureus. 2019;11(12):e6266.

21. Barrow DLSR, Braun IF, Landman JA, Tindall SC, Tindall GT. Classification and treatment of spontaneous carotid-cavernous sinus fistulas. J Neurosurg. 1985;62(2):248–56.

22. Henderson AD, Miller NR. Carotid-cavernous fistula: current concepts in aetiology, investigation, and management Eye (Lond). 2018;32(2):164–72.

23. Spector RH. Echography in Carotid-Cavernous Fistulas. In: Ophthalmic ultrasonography: proceedings of the 9th SIDUO Congress, Leeds, U.K. July 20–23, 1982, Hillman JS, Le May MM, editors. Springer Science & Business Media; 2012. p. 399–405.

24. Castaigne P, Blancard P, Laplane D, Djindjan R, Sorato M. Communications spontanées entre la carotide externe et le sinus caverneux. Bull Soc Ophtalmol Fr. 1966;66(1):47–9.

25. Chaudhary MYSV, Cho SH, Weitzner I Jr, et al. Dural arteriovenous malformation of the major venous sinuses: an acquired lesion. AJNR Am J Neuroradiol. 1982;3(1):13–9.

26. Phelps CDTH, Ossoinig KC. The diagnosis and prognosis of atypical carotid-cavernous fistula (red-eyed shunt syndrome). Am J Ophthalmol. 1982;93(4):423–36.

27. Bergès O, Torrent M. Echographie de l'œil et de l'orbite. Paris: Vigot; 1986.

28. Wiot JG, Pleatman GW. chronic hematic cysts of the orbit. AJNR Am J Neuroradiol. 1989;10:537–9.

# Chapter 21
# Masses of the Lacrimal Fossa

François Lafitte, Patricia Koskas, Augustin Lecler, Mario de La Torre, and Olivier Bergès

**Abstract**  Any tumor, regardless of its histology, can be located in the lacrimal fossa, but in this chapter, we focus on the ultrasound diagnosis of lesions of the lacrimal gland itself. The tumors of the lacrimal gland predominate in the deep lobe of the gland. Because the lacrimal gland is superficial, it is examined first with paraocular sections, but when the lesion is large, the deep (posterior) part must also be examined by transocular sections. Dacryops are cysts of the lacrimal gland, imaged only when bothersome. Color Doppler imaging has a key role in the diagnosis of tumors of the lacrimal gland because the resistive index (RI) guides the diagnostic perspective: a low RI, < 0.70, suggests a lymphoid lesion and indicates biopsy, whereas an RI > 0.70 suggests an epithelial tumor and indicates surgical excision, without effraction of the capsule. Epithelial tumors represent 11.5% of all primary orbital tumors. They include pleomorphic adenoma or benign mixed tumor, pleomorphic adenocarcinoma or malignant mixed tumor, and adenoid cystic carcinoma. But at the end of the chapter, lymphoid lesions are briefly examined along with other lesions such as solitary fibrous tumor, whose localization in the lacrimal fossa is not an anecdotal situation.

Masses of the lacrimal fossa, even more so than other orbital masses and tumors, are particularly amenable to ultrasound assessment. Careful clinical examination is often informative as the lesion is located anteriorly and easily accessible. The date of onset of the clinical symtoms must be precisely noted, and particular attention should be paid to pain and associated inflammatory signs which are important orientation signs. Any tumor, regardless of its histology, can be located in the lacrimal fossa. However, lesions of the lacrimal gland are naturally by far the most common. However, vascular masses and dermoid cysts can also be encountered. The ultrasound semiology of these latter lesions is identical regardless of the location, and we refer the reader to the corresponding chapters (see Chaps. 20 and 26).

F. Lafitte · P. Koskas · A. Lecler · O. Bergès (✉)
Rothschild Foundation Hospital, Paris, France
e-mail: oberges@for.paris

M. de La Torre
Nacional Mayor de San Marcos, Lima, Perú

© The Author(s), under exclusive license to Springer Nature Switzerland AG 2024
O. Bergès (ed.), *Echography of the Eye and Orbit*,
https://doi.org/10.1007/978-3-031-41467-1_21

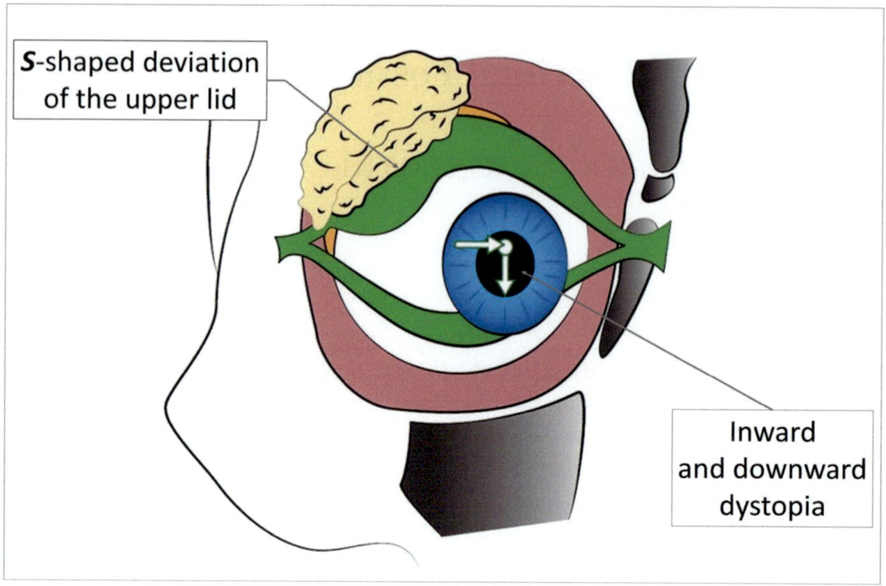



**Fig. 21.1  Clinical syndrome of the lacrimal fossa**. It combines an *S*-shaped deviation of the upper eyelid and an inward and downward dystopia. *Redrawn, with permission from an original drawing kindly provided by Dr. P.-V. Jacomet, Rothschild Foundation Hospital, Paris, France*

Tumor lesions of the lacrimal gland account for 6% of all orbital tumors [1]. They predominate in the deep lobe of the gland, while the superficial part is rarely affected [2]. They are most often suspected in case of a swelling of the upper part of the lateral canthus, exophthalmos with an S-shaped deviation of the upper eyelid associated with a displacement of the eyeball downward and inward (Fig. 21.1); these signs are very strongly suggestive of lacrimal fossa syndrome. Ptosis or pain can sometimes be encountered too [3].

The clinical examination is often already completed by CT scan or MRI. Nevertheless, although these examinations allow for confirming the existence of a lesion of the lacrimal fossa, specification of its volume, searching for calcifications, analysis of its extension, and etiological diagnosis of a tumor of the lacrimal gland are often difficult, with the exception of a few special cases (a fat lesion or entirely cystic).

However, the therapeutic management varies depending on whether it is an inflammatory lesion, a lymphoma, or an epithelial tumor. A biopsy is indicated for inflammatory lesions and lymphomas because the treatment in these cases is medical, whereas an epithelial lesion formally rules out biopsy and must be treated by complete surgical excision without rupture of the capsule to avoid the risk of recurrence in benign and even sometimes malignant forms [2].

## 21.1 Technique

The lacrimal gland is superficial. Therefore, it can be studied with paraocular sections, the probe placed over the lateral part of the upper eyelid with horizontal (transverse) and vertical (parasagittal) sections. A substantial amount of gel must be placed to be able to assess the anterior (superficial) part of the lesion (and not be impeded by the Fresnel zone). When the lesion is large, one can (one must) also examine its deep (posterior) part by transocular sections, placing the probe at the medial and lower part of the eye and orienting it toward the superior lateral quadrant. The examination must be completed with standardized A-mode. Tissue sensitivity setting (or reduced sensitivity setting in B-mode) is used first. Then the appearance can be analyzed with a high sensitivity setting (T + 9 dB) and a low sensitivity setting (T − 9 dB).

## 21.2 Dacryops

These are cysts of the lacrimal gland or cystic dilation of lacrimal canaliculi (canaliculops). In the countries concerned, trachoma is certainly the most common etiology. Elsewhere, they are relatively rare, sometimes occurring after cicatricial pemphigoid or chemical trauma. Their physiology is still debated. They can be associated with genuine tumors of the lacrimal gland.

Imaging is requested only when they are bulky or if patients find them bothersome. They are not painful and are not accompanied by inflammatory signs [4]. Small in size (accidental discovery), they appear intraglandular (Fig. 21.2).

When more voluminous, they can be eccentric and hence difficult to differentiate from conjunctival cysts. They are anechoic, entirely liquid, and very confined (Fig. 21.3).

There is, of course, no detectable flow upon color Doppler imaging, and the lacrimal artery flows are strictly normal.

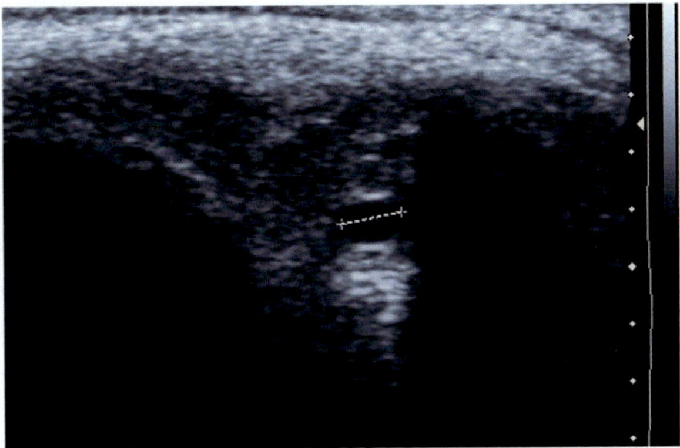

**Fig. 21.2 Small dacryops.** B-mode, horizontal section. The small cyst is deeply situated within the gland, measuring 2.1 mm in diameter. Both lobes of the lacrimal gland have a normal size and echotexture. Note the small posterior enhancement behind the cyst

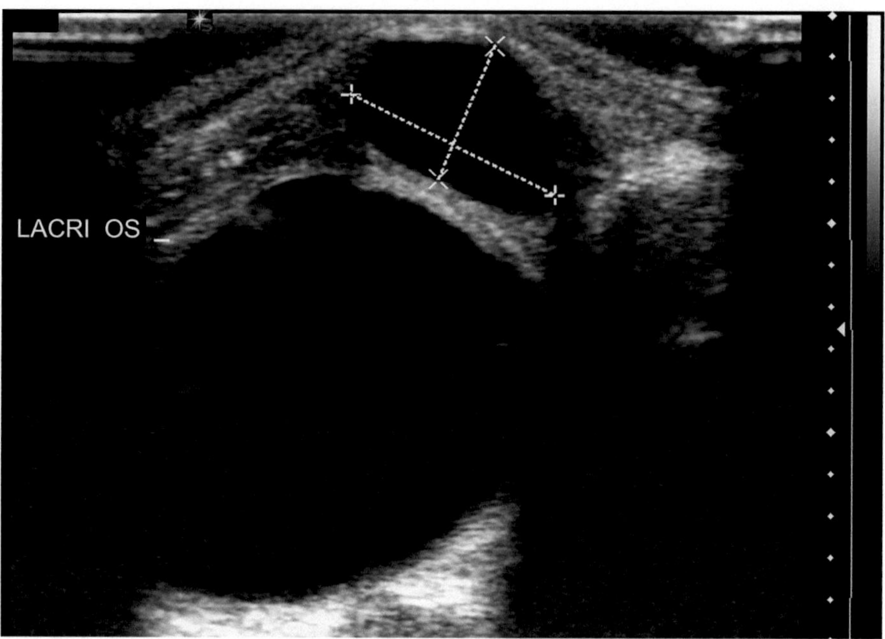



**Fig. 21.3** **Large superficial dacryops**. B-mode, horizontal section of the lacrimal gland. Developed at the superficial lobe of the lacrimal gland, it measures 14 mm × 11 mm in diameter × 7 mm thick

> Ultrasound and especially color Doppler imaging are the key to the diagnosis of tumors of the lacrimal gland because the resistive index (RI) guides the diagnostic perspective: a low RI, < 0.70, suggests a lymphoid lesion and indicates biopsy, whereas an RI > 0.70 suggests an epithelial tumor and indicates surgical excision, without effraction of the capsule [5].

## 21.3 Epithelial Tumors

Epithelial tumors of the orbit are essentially tumors of the lacrimal gland. They represent 11.5% of all primary orbital tumors according to the Mayo Clinic series [6]. The ratio of males to females is 1.5 to 1. The tumor most often concerns only the orbital portion of the gland and only rarely reaches the palpebral portion. The mass is firm on palpation, and when voluminous, it can extend quite far back, affecting the curvature of the eye wall. Patients often report pain, discomfort, and a feeling of pressure or tension, regardless of the type of tumor. There is no specific differential clinical sign between benign and malignant tumors. However, generally, malignant tumors most often have a shorter duration of symptom evolution (less than 1 year), they are often painful, and they can present intralesional calcifications and lysis of the adjacent bone wall. Therefore, the histology of the excision specimen is the key to diagnosis, even though ultrasound provides pertinent and useful information. For epithelial tumors, a biopsy without complete excision is contraindicated because it tends to promote recurrences and malignant transformations.

### *21.3.1  Pleomorphic Adenoma or Benign Mixed Tumor*

The older term "mixed tumor" dates back to when it was thought that these tumors consisted of epithelial and mesodermal contingents. The term pleomorphic adenoma proposed by the WHO is preferred nowadays. Most pleomorphic adenomas occur in young adults, between the 2nd and 5th decade. The typical clinical presentation combines a firm palpable mass without inflammatory signs and slowly progressive exophthalmos with dystopia, displacement of the globe downward and inward, which can be accompanied by oculomotor disorders in upward and outward gaze.

On ultrasound (Fig. 21.4), the lesion is well-limited, echogenic, > 70%, over the first centimeter of the lesion, and ≈ 50%, over the whole tumor in standardized A-mode, attenuating, with a kappa angle close to 45°. Oval, sometimes multilobed with round edges, it has an echotexture that is most often homogeneous and even, although sometimes irregular central clusters of myxoid or chondroid degeneration can be seen that have a varying degree of echogenicity and heterogeneity.

However, one cannot formally eliminate microfoci of malignant degeneration, sometimes only found on histological examination of the surgical specimen, and modifying, of course, the prognosis. A characteristic but inconsistent sign is a diffuse microcystic appearance of the lesion [7]. The posterior part of the tumor is best assessed transocularly because the lesion is indeed often voluminous at the time of diagnosis, measuring more than 2 cm along the main axis, extending toward the posterior part of the orbit. On color Doppler imaging, there are few vessels within the mass, and these have a very high RI (≥ 0.90), which differs greatly from that of lymphoid lesions (Fig. 21.5).

MRI, which would reveal a hyperintense T2 weighted lesion, is not useful. However, CT scan with bone windows in high resolution can be used to assess bone deformation (expansion) in contact with this voluminous and slowly progressing lesion; the bone can be very thin or often even exhibit contact osteolysis.

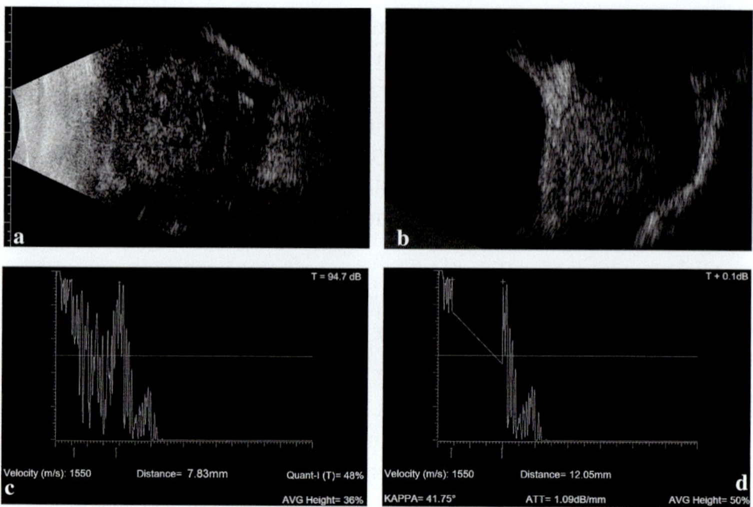

**Fig. 21.4 Pleomorphic adenoma. a**: B-mode, paraocular approach; **b**: B-mode, transocular approach of the posterior part of the large tumor; **c**: standardized A-mode at tissue sensitivity (T = 94.7 dB), to assess the reflectivity; **d**: standardized A-mode at T + 0.1 dB, so that the height of the peaks is 50%, to assess the attenuation. The lesion is moderately echogenic (48% in Quantification I in standardized A-mode), quite attenuating (kappa angle = 41.75°), and has an even echotexture; it is voluminous, and can be visualized both paraocularly and transocularly (for its posterior part)

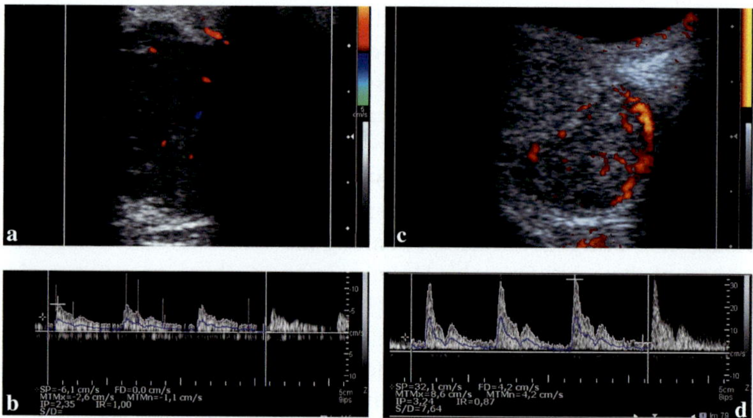

**Fig. 21.5 Pleomorphic adenoma.** Color Doppler imaging (CDI). **a**: CDI, color mode, paraocular approach; **b**: CDI, spectral mode of one of the small vessels in the center of the tumor; **c**: CDI, power mode, transocular approach of the posterior part of the large tumor; **d**: CDI, spectral mode of the most obvious vessel, under the innermost part of the tumor. In Doppler, there are few vessels, and all have a very high resistive index (RI), both those recorded paraocularly (RI = 1.00) and the most obvious vessel, recorded transocularly (RI = 0.87)

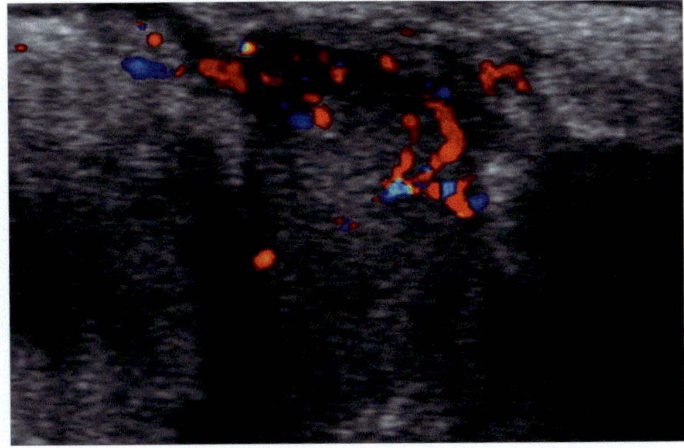

**Fig. 21.6 Pleomorphic adenocarcinoma**. Color Doppler imaging, paraocular section. The mass is heterogeneous, poorly to moderately echogenic, and poorly delineated, with many flows recorded in Doppler

## 21.3.2 Pleomorphic Adenocarcinoma or Malignant Mixed Tumor

In half of all cases, it is a recurrence of a pleomorphic adenoma that has previously undergone surgery. In other cases, it can be a malignant transformation of a tumor of the lacrimal gland that has been ignored for a long time (sometimes several decades) by the patient or cases that are clearly malignant from the outset. The two benign and malignant tumor contingents are readily distinguished by histology. Different histological subtypes can be encountered.

On ultrasound (Fig. 21.6), these are masses that are poorly delineated, with a hypoechoic, heterogenous, and uneven and attenuating echotexture, with anarchic vessels on color Doppler imaging, with a high RI (0.80–0.85).

CT scan frequently shows ($\geq 75\%$) malignant bone erosions or the appearance of permeation of the adjacent orbital walls.

The tumors present therapeutic problems in terms of both surgical technique and associated therapeuty, and their prognosis remains poor.

## 21.3.3 Adenoid Cystic Carcinoma

This is the most common epithelial tumor of the lacrimal gland after pleomorphic adenoma, occurring at any age but mainly in the 5th and 6th decade. Highly malignant, it is characterized by a high rate of recurrence and a survival rate at 5 years of almost zero, thus leading to the indication of early exenteration [8].

The tumor is often large (Fig. 21.7) and can be well defined but without an authentic capsule; it has a mainly posterior development. The echotexture is heterogeneous, of intermediate reflectivity, and attenuating. In CDI, there are anarchic vessels with a high RI ($\approx 0.80$).

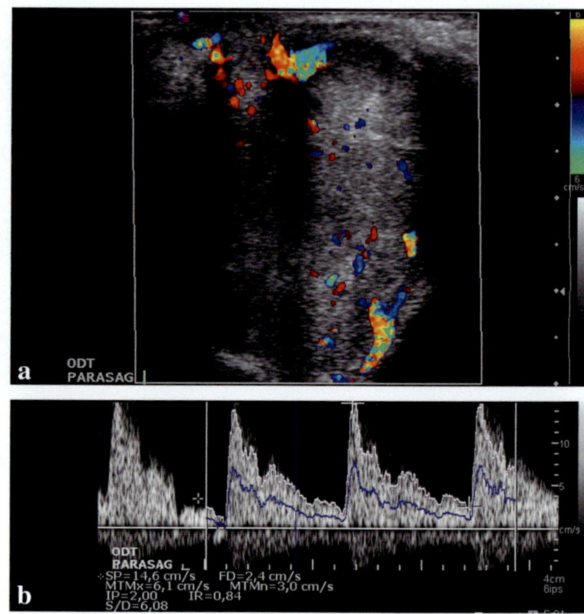

**Fig. 21.7 Adenoid cystic carcinoma:** CDI. **a**: CDI, color mode, paraocular, parasagittal section; **b**: CDI, spectral mode. The mass is voluminous, moderately echogenic, and heterogeneous. Doppler reveals many small vessels circulating rapidly with a high RI (= 0.84)

For these malignant tumors, the imaging assessment should be compared with a CT scan, to assess the bone walls and the extension [8].

At the histological level, oncocytomas, which are rare benign tumors, and other rare malignant tumors also warrant mention: de novo monomorphic adenocarcinomas, acinic cell carcinomas, myoepithelial carcinomas, squamous epitheliomas, and mucoepidermoid carcinomas.

## 21.4 Lymphomas and Pseudolymphomas

They undergo slow and progressive changes and are not very inflammatory, occurring in people of approximately 60 years of age. Palpation does not reveal a firm mass as in epithelial tumors, but it gives the impression of a certain degree of firmness.

The ultrasound appearance of lymphoma, pseudolymphoma, and lymphoid hyperplasia are identical: they are distinctly hypoechoic lesions ($\leq$ 40% in Quantification I in standardized A-mode) and yet attenuating, with an even echotexture, often crossed by fibro-conjunctival vascular septa that are discreetly more echogenic. They affect the entire gland, palpebral and orbital, and they become molded to adjacent structures and bone walls. Nevertheless, their anterior edge in relation to the eyelid is often multilobed. On color Doppler imaging, there is a multitude of characteristic arborescent vessels with a low RI of < 0.70 (Fig. 21.8).

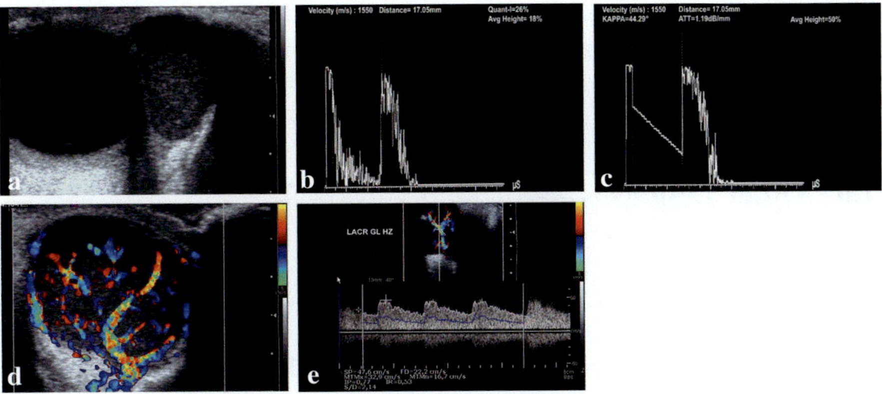

**Fig. 21.8 Lymphoma (MALT) of the lacrimal gland. a**: B-mode, paraocular section; **b**: standardized A-mode at tissue sensitivity (T = 84.3 dB), to assess the reflectivity; **c**: standardized A-mode at T + 6.4 dB, so that the height of the peaks is 50%, to assess the attenuation; **d**: CDI, color mode, paraocular, parasagittal section; **e**: CDI, spectral mode of one of the fast vessels within the tumor. In B-mode, the mass was only visible via the paraocular approach, being not very echogenic and homogeneous. In standardized A-mode it is low reflective (20% in Quantification I). The solid nature of the mass is reflected in the attenuation and vascularization; the attenuation is only appreciable in standardized A-mode at T + 6.4 dB (angle kappa = 44.29°); color mode shows vascular tree pattern, and spectral mode reveals their non-resistive nature (RI = 0.54)

## 21.5 Inflammations (Dacryoadenitis) (See Chap. 17)

### 21.5.1 Infectious Acute Dacryoadenitis

The diagnosis is purely clinical and does not usually require imaging. An ultrasound can reveal hypoechoic and relatively homogeneous dacryomegaly (see Fig. 17.2).

### 21.5.2 Chronic Dacryoadenitis and Chronic Orbital Inflammation

Exophthalmos and palpation of a mass are less common than in epithelial tumors, although local inflammatory signs are often present. There is never dystopia.

The lacrimal gland is the primary localization of chronic orbital inflammations, although they can be associated with other localizations (myositis, episcleritis, optic perineuritis, etc.). They may be idiopathic or specific (first and foremost sarcoidosis and tuberculosis).

On ultrasound, an increase in volume of the gland is seen, which is hypoechoic and heterogeneous, most often gently sloping with the adjacent orbital walls. The lesions are more echogenic than lymphomas (Quantification I = 20–50% in standardized

A-mode) and very attenuating (see Fig. 17.3). On color Doppler imaging, the lesion is even more hypervascularized than a lymphoma with, as for lymphomas, a low RI, $\leq 0.60$ (see Fig. 17.9).

## 21.6   Other Lesions

Finally, in the lacrimal fossa, but independent of the gland, we should mention dermoid cysts (see Fig. 26.9) and solitary fibrous tumors/hemangiopericytomas (Fig. 21.9 and see Fig. 20.11), for which the lacrimal fossa is far from being an anecdotal situation. In both cases, both on ultrasound and MRI, individualizing the lacrimal gland from the lesion is often difficult because the lesion volume can compress and/or repress the lacrimal gland.

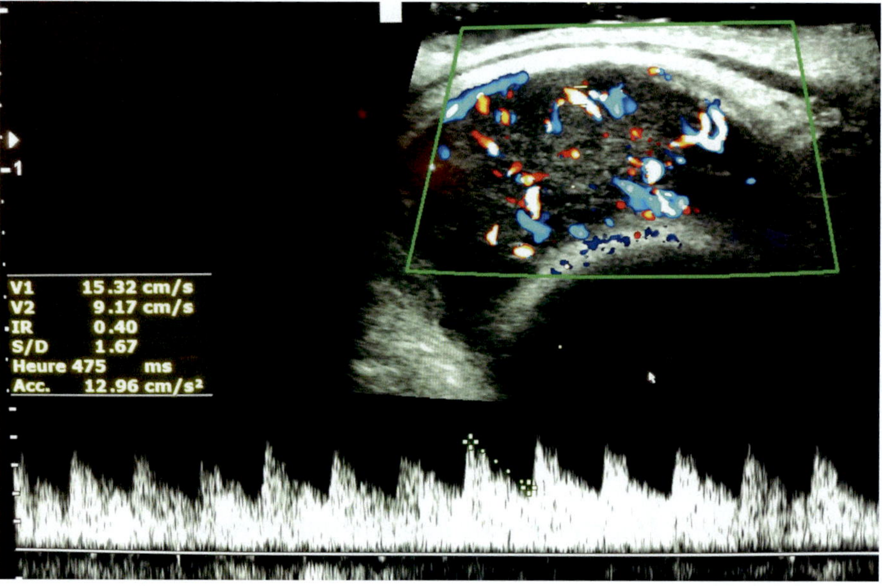


**Fig. 21.9 Solitary fibrous tumor of the right lacrimal fossa.** CDI. Color and spectral modes. Disclosing a voluminous mass measuring 3 mm × 1.8 mm, moderately echogenic with a discreetly uneven echotexture, well delineated and highly vascularized with low resistive flows (RI = 0.40). *Figure kindly provided by Dr. G. Braux, University Hospital of Caen, France*

## References


1. Levecq L, De Potter P, Guagnini AP. [Epidemiology of ocular and orbital lesions referred to an ocular oncology center] [Article in French] Épidémiologie des lésions oculaires et orbitaires adressées à un centre d'oncologie oculaire. J Fr Ophtalmol. 2005;28(8):840–4.
2. Auran J, Jakobiec FA, Krebs W. Benign mixed tumor of the palpebral lobe of the gland. Clinical diagnosis and appropriate surgical management. Ophtalmology. 1988;95(1):90–9.
3. Adenis JP, Saint-Blancat P. Tumeurs de la glande lacrymale. In: Adenis JP, Morax S, editors. Pathologie orbito-palpébrale, Rapport de la Société Française d'Ophtalmologie. Masson, Paris; 1998. p. 550–62.
4. Ozgonul C, Uysal Y, Ayyildiz O, Kucukevcilioglu M. Clinical features and management of dacryops. Orbit. 2018;37(4):262–5.
5. Lecler A, Lafitte F, Koskas P, Bergès O, et al. Usefulness of color Doppler flow imaging in the management of lacrimal gland lesions. Eur Radiol. 2017;27(2):779–89.
6. Henderson JW. Orbital tumors. 3rd ed. New York: Raven Press; 1994.
7. Till P, Steinkogler FJ. The importance of preoperative standardized echography for surgery in the temporal upper orbit. Orbit. 1987;6:129–33.
8. Han J, Kim YD, Woo KI, Sobti D. Long-term outcomes of eye-sparing surgery for adenoid cystic carcinoma of lacrimal gland ophthalmic. Plast Reconstr Surg. 2018;34(1):74–8.

# Chapter 22
# Pathologies of the Extraocular Muscles

François Lafitte, Mario de La Torre, and Olivier Bergès

**Abstract** This chapter presents muscle lesions other than those observed in dysthyroid orbitopathy and purely inflammatory lesions. Multiple and diffuse muscle hypertrophy can be related to systemic diseases: amyloidosis, porphyria, or orbital infiltration in neurofibromatosis type 1 or to a direct (post-traumatic) carotid-cavernous fistula or an (indirect) cavernous sinus dural arteriovenous fistula. When one deals with the presence of single or multiple muscle masses, one must first consider a tumor origin: in adults, metastases, and in children, rhabdomyosarcoma or more rarely metastases of neuroblastoma or localizations of leukemia or histiocytosis. Miscellaneous lesions may also be encountered: an invasion by contiguity of a bony lesion (spheno-orbital meningioma, metastasis), an infectious lesion, a parasitic localization (cysticercosis), a vascular localization (arteriovenous malformation), or giant cell myositis (sarcoidosis or myasthenia gravis). Finally, in case of muscle atrophy, one should think of sequelae of Graves' disease, or certain mitochondriopathies if several muscles are involved, and to post-traumatic fibrosis, or post-therapeutic rearrangements if atrophy affects a single muscle.

In most cases, muscle damage is related to dysthyroid orbitopathy (see Chap. 16) or with inflammatory involvement (see Chap. 17). But other diagnoses should be considered: tumors (especially metastases) as well as vascular, infectious, or metabolic lesions [1]. The clinical warning signs are most often non-specific: waves of orbital "pain", diplopia, palpebral edema, conjunctival redness, and lacrimation.

Most often, the affected muscle(s) appear hypertrophied and hypoechoic. However, the echotexture of the abnormal muscle rarely helps to identify the origin. Naturally, before considering a large muscle, especially when the increase in volume is minor, one must rule out a muscle that appears large simply because it is visualized in contraction. This is especially a pitfall for cross-sectional imaging, CT or MRI

F. Lafitte · O. Bergès (✉)
Rothschild Foundation Hospital, Paris, France
e-mail: oberges@for.paris

M. de La Torre
Universidad Nacional Mayor de San Marcos, Lima, Perú



O. Bergès (ed.), *Echography of the Eye and Orbit*,
https://doi.org/10.1007/978-3-031-41467-1_22

more so than for ultrasound, which is a dynamic examination. Schematically, one can distinguish thickening of a single muscle, several muscles in a uni- or bilateral manner, and muscle abnormalities associated with other orbital damage.

## 22.1 Multiple and Diffuse Muscle Hypertrophy

### 22.1.1 Systemic Diseases

Global and bilateral hypertrophy of the extraocular muscles, sometimes associated with infiltration of the orbital fat, has been described, albeit rarely [1, 2], during certain systemic diseases such as amyloidosis, with the orbital localization remaining isolated or associated with systemic manifestations, justifying an extensive assessment. One must determine the histological form because the prognosis differs greatly, the AA (Amyloid A protein, secondary) form being associated with a chronic inflammatory pathology and the AL (amyloid light chain, primary) form associated with myeloma and Waldenström's disease. Even more rarely, the cause of infiltration is porphyria (deposits of specific material and inflammation) or is associated with acromegaly. The clinical-biological context is quite important.

### 22.1.2 Neurofibromatosis Type 1

With neurofibromatosis type 1 (NF1), orbital infiltration by neurofibromas can be pronounced and affect all of the elements of the orbit, including the muscles [3].

### 22.1.3 Fistulas

A direct (post-traumatic) carotid-cavernous fistula or an (indirect) dural cavernous sinus arteriovenous fistula may be responsible for muscle hypertrophy, which, in this case, is usually unilateral. The increase in muscle volume, moderate and of average echogenicity, takes a back seat to flow inversion and arterialization in the superior ophthalmic vein in Doppler (see Fig. 26.12).

## 22.2   Presence of Single or Multiple Muscle Masses

### *22.2.1   Tumor Origin: This Is the Etiology to Be Considered First*

- In adults, metastases are the first thing that comes to mind. They can present a necrotic part (Fig. 22.1), resulting in a V-shaped appearance in A-mode and for certain origins (e.g., primary digestive cancer or bronchial neuroendocrine), calcifications [2] (Fig. 22.2). The possibility of hemopathy (lymphoma, leukemia, myeloma) is also a consideration, whose imaging (especially in case of lymphoma) is quite characteristic: a hypoechoic mass (Fig. 22.3) with quite echogenic spans that are typically hypervascularized on color Doppler imaging (with a low resistive index), although sometimes, the appearance is similar to that of inflammatory myositis (Fig. 22.4), especially because the spans are less obvious than in a larger bulky lesion, but in the case of lymphoma, the tendon is not thickened [4]
- In children, a muscle mass in principle must suggest rhabdomyosarcoma or more rarely, metastases of neuroblastoma or localizations of leukemia or histiocytosis (see Chap. 26), but in these cases, the lesions are not entirely localized to one muscle but are more extensive, often encompassing several muscles.

Especially in children, one must also consider the rare possibility of rhabdomyoma, which is a benign lesion for which a fetal form and an adult form (very differentiated) can be distinguished [5], with a muscle that has increased in volume, moderately echogenic, and with an uneven appearance.

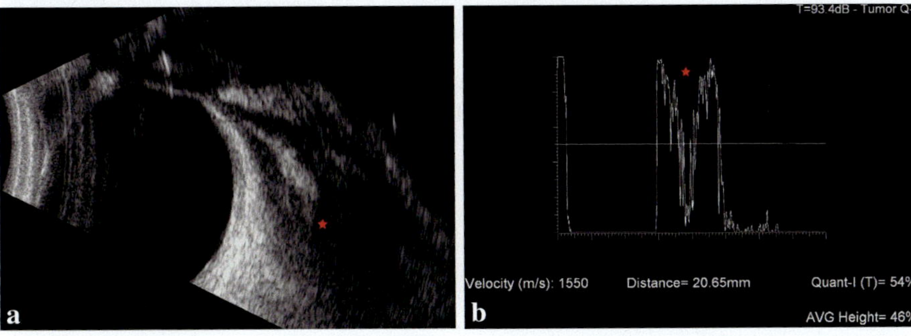


**Fig. 22.1  Breast cancer metastasis affecting the superior rectus muscle. a**: B-mode longitudinal section; **b**: standardized A-mode at tissue sensitivity setting, T = 93.4 dB. Substantial increase in volume of the muscle, overall not very echogenic, but heterogeneous, with a central hypoechoic area, necrotic (★ red star), resulting in a V-shaped appearance in A-mode, which was not obvious in B-mode

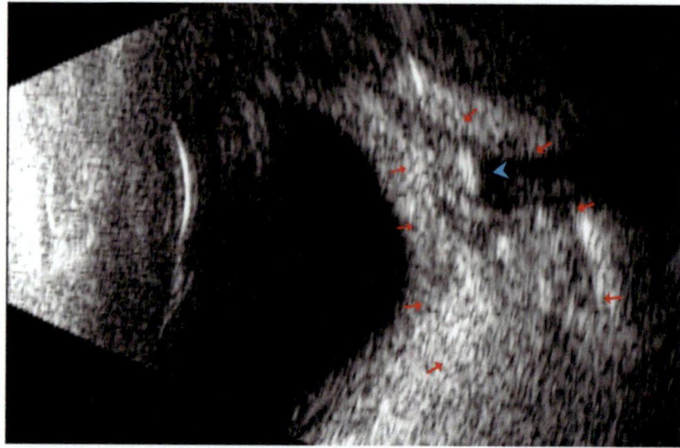

**Fig. 22.2 Stomach cancer metastasis affecting the left lateral rectus muscle**. B-mode. The muscle is voluminous (→ red arrows), echogenic, and heterogeneous, with several hyperechoic nodules, the largest resulting in a posterior shadowing (▶ blue arrowhead), suggesting calcifications

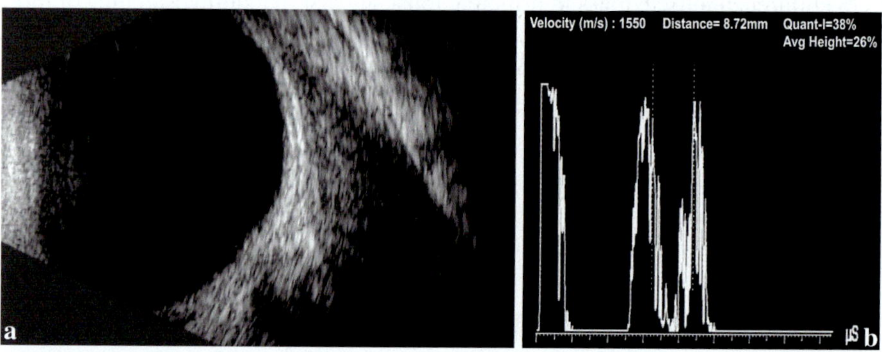



**Fig. 22.3 Lymphoma of the medial rectus muscle. a**: B-mode; **b**: standardized A-mode at tissue sensitivity (T = 93.4 dB) to study the reflectivity. The muscle is large, 8.7 mm thick, and hypoechoic (38% in standardized A-mode), as in myositis (see Fig. 17.1), but the tendon has a normal appearance

## 22.2.2 Traumatism

(See Fig. 25.16).

## 22.3 Miscellaneous Lesions

- A bone lesion (spheno-orbital meningioma, metastasis) can invade a muscle by contiguity.

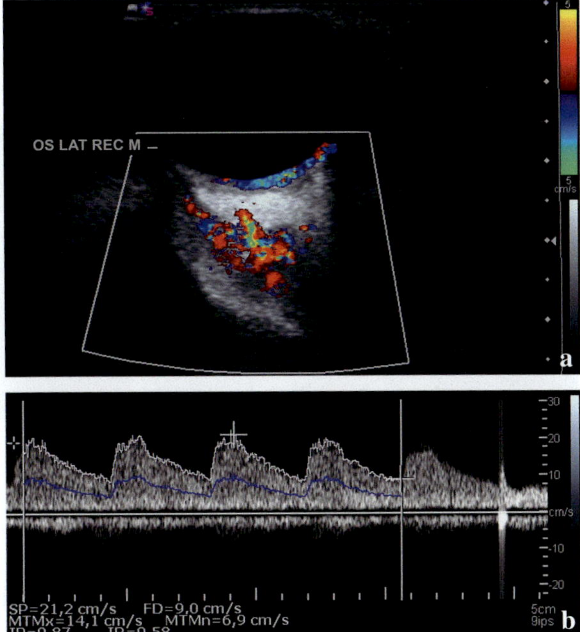


**Fig. 22.4 Lymphoma of the left lateral rectus muscle.** Color Doppler imaging. **a**: Color mode; **b**: spectral mode. The voluminous hypoechoic muscle is highly vascularized, with low resistive flows (resistive index = 0.58)

- An infectious lesion should be considered in an infectious context: myositis (diffuse and homogeneous involvement) or a pyogenic abscess, with a central pseudoliquid zone, and peripheral hypervascularization can be observed on color Doppler imaging.
- A parasitic localization is to be considered in case of oculomotor disorders and inflammatory signs, not only in endemic areas, but also outside such countries. The most common is cysticercosis (see Fig. 23.4), a cystic lesion in which scolex, hyperechoic, and sometimes an associated intravitreal lesion can be seen. In the absence of treatment, a chronic, heterogeneous lesion, sometimes with calcifications, is seen [6]. Rare cases of muscle-localized hydatidosis have also been described [7].
- A vascular localization. Angiomas are rare within a muscle; however, arteriovenous malformations can be encountered (Fig. 22.5). Their treatment is naturally very complex.
- Giant cell myositis, which is rare, can be associated with sarcoidosis or myasthenia gravis.

## 22.4 Muscle Atrophy

The muscles are small, sometimes hyperechoic in case of fatty infiltration, and there is no hypervascularization on color Doppler imaging.

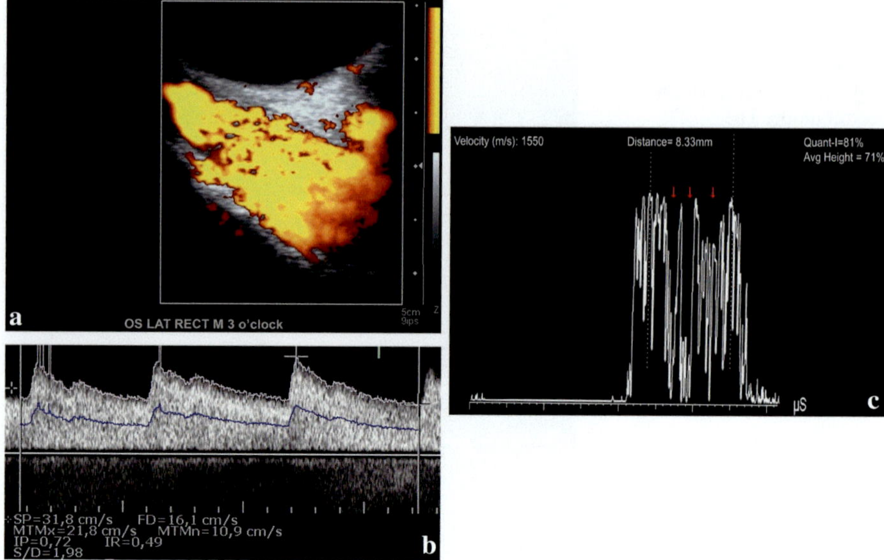



**Fig. 22.5** **Arteriovenous malformation affecting the left lateral rectus muscle in a 35-year-old woman**. **a**: Doppler imaging, power mode; **b**: spectral mode; **c**: standardized A-mode at tissue sensitivity. The hypervascular malformation, with a low RI, = 0.49, occupies the entire muscle and is large. It is very reflective (81% in Quantification I in standardized A-mode), non-attenuating (kappa angle = 30°), and has vascular spaces filled with weak echoes circulating rapidly (→ red arrows) separated by hyperreflective septa

- If several muscles are involved, it may be the sequellar phase of Graves' disease, myopathy, or certain mitochondriopathies (Kearns–Sayre syndrome) [8].
- Atrophy of a single muscle can be seen following post-traumatic fibrosis or post-therapeutic rearrangements.

# References


1. Lacey B, Chang W, Rootman J (1999) Nonthyroid causes of extraocular muscle disease. Surv Ophthalmol. 1999;44(3):187–213.
2. Ossoinig KC. The diagnosis and differential diagnosis of neoplastic lesions of the extraocular muscles with Standardized Echography. In: Thijssen JM, Fledelius HC, Tane S, editors. Ultrasonography in ophthalmology14 proceedings of the 14th SIDUO congress, 1992. Documenta Ophthalmologica Proceedings Series, vol. 58. Tokyo, Japan: Springer Science + Business Media Dordrechl; 1995. p. xxxiii–lvi.
3. Shah VS, Cavuoto KM, Dubovy SR, Schatz NJ, et al. Systemic amyloidosis and Extraocular muscle deposition. J Neuro Ophthalmol. 2016;36(2):167–73.
4. Mombaerts I, Rose GE, Verity DH. Diagnosis of enlarged extraocular muscles: when and how to biopsy. Curr Opin Ophthalmol. 2017;28(5):514–21.

5. Knowles DM 2nd, Jakobiec FA. Rhabdomyoma of the orbit. Am J Ophthalmol. 1975;80(6):1011–8.
6. Salim S, Alam MS, Backiavathy V, Raichura ND, Mukherjee B. Orbital cysticercosis: clinical features and management outcomes. Orbit. 2020;27:1–7.
7. Rajabi MT, Berijani S, Asadi Amoli F, Mohammadi SS. Hydatid cyst of inferior rectus. Ophthalmic Plast Reconstr Surg. 2021;37(3S):S168.
8. Lee SJ, Na JH, Han J, Lee YM. Ophthalmoplegia in mitochondrial disease. Yonsei Med J. 2018;59(10):1190–1196.

# Chapter 23
# Orbital Cysts and Cystic Lesions

**François Lafitte, Mario de La Torre, and Olivier Bergès**

**Abstract** Cysts are anechoic if their content is pure liquid, or they may be hypoechoic to a certain extent but always associated with a posterior enhancement artifact. Their etiologies are varied, and schematically, one can distinguish malformative orbital cysts, acquired orbital cysts, superficial cysts, cysts from adjacent structures, epithelial inclusion cysts, and cystic tumors. Superficial cysts include dermoid cysts and palpebral cysts: chalazion, stye, hidrocystoma, and pilomatrixoma, and dacryops. Abscesses, bacterial or fungal, correspond to one or more collection areas within a patch of cellulitis or within a pre-existing lesion (tumor, granuloma following foreign body injury). Parasitic cysts are mostly related to hydatidosis or cysticercosis. Cystic granulomas are usually secondary to penetration of a foreign body into the orbit. Hematomas are characteristic of hemolymphangiomas but can occur within other benign vascular lesions such as cavernous hemangiomas and varices, or within all malignant tumors. Cystic tumors, rare, are mainly observed in children. Congenital malformative colobomatous cysts can be encountered under the optic nerve. Cystic lesions extending to the orbit from adjacent spaces include mucoceles, dacryoceles (or dacryocystoceles), and cephaloceles. Finally, epithelial inclusion cysts can be seen after any eye or orbital surgery but are particularly observed after placement of a prosthesis.

Semiologically speaking, cysts always appear as hypoechoic entities, well delineated, with distinct walls, and without intrinsic vessels on color Doppler imaging. Their content is anechoic if it is pure liquid, or hypoechoic to a certain extent depending on its content. As for the eyeball, which is a pure liquid cyst, the anterior and posterior walls are clearly visualized, but the side walls are less clear, and a posterior enhancement artifact can be seen.

F. Lafitte · O. Bergès (✉)
Rothschild Foundation Hospital, Paris, France
e-mail: oberges@for.paris; oberges@wanadoo.fr

M. de La Torre
Universidad Nacional Mayor de San Marcos, Lima, Perú

© The Author(s), under exclusive license to Springer Nature Switzerland AG 2024
O. Bergès (ed.), *Echography of the Eye and Orbit*,
https://doi.org/10.1007/978-3-031-41467-1_23

**Table 23.1** Etiologies of orbital cysts

- **Malformative orbital cysts**
  - Choristoma (epidermoid, dermoid, dermolipoma)
  - Teratomas
  - Congenital cystic eye
  - Colobomatous cysts
- **Acquired orbital cysts**
  - Cystic lesions of vascular origin
      Lymphangioma
      Hematomas ("chocolate" cyst) / encysted
  - Epithelial cysts (chalazion, hidrocystoma, pilomatrixoma, etc.)
  - Aneurysmal bone cyst
  - Cystic myositis
  - Orbital abscess
  - Parasitic cysts
      Hydatidosis
      Cysticercosis
- **Superficial cysts**
  - Eyelid cysts
  - Conjunctival cysts
  - Dacryops
- **Cysts from adjacent structures**
  - Mucoceles and mucopyoceles
  - Meningoceles and meningoencephaloceles
  - Dacryoceles
  - Exogenous cysts
  - Cysts of dental orgin
- **Epithelial inclusion cysts**
- **Cystic tumors**

Their etiologies are varied and considering a classification may be useful. Schematically, one can distinguish the following: malformative cysts, acquired cysts, superficial cysts, cysts from adjacent structures, epithelial inclusion cysts, and cystic tumors (Table 23.1).

In children, Kaufman [1] proposed another classification, which is in fact complementary (Table 23.2).

## 23.1 Superficial Cysts

### 23.1.1 Dermoid cysts

These are mainly observed in children, and they will be dealt with in Chap. 26 (see Fig. 26.9).

**Table 23.2** Etiologies of orbital cysts in children, from Kaufman LM, Villablanca JP, and Mafee MF [1]

- **Malformative orbital cysts**
  - Choristoma (epidermoid, dermoid, dermolipoma)
  - Teratomas
  - Congenital cystic eye
  - Colobomatous cysts

- **Acquired orbital cysts**
  - Cystic lesions of vascular origin
      - Lymphangioma
      - Orbital varicose vein
      - Blood cyst ("chocolate" cyst)
  - Epithelial cysts (chalazion, hidrocystoma, pilomatrixoma, etc.)
  - Epithelial inclusion cyst
  - Peri-optic meningocele
  - Aneurysmal bone cyst
  - Cystic myositis
  - Orbital abscess
  - Parasitic cysts (hydatid, cysticercus cellulosae)

- **Cyst fom adjacent structures**
  - Mucoceles and mucopyoceles
  - Dacryops
  - Meningoceles and meningoencephaloceles
  - Enterogenous cysts
  - Cysts of dental origin

## *23.1.2   Eyelid Cysts*

A distinction is made between chalazion, stye, hidrocystoma, and pilomatrixoma. Their diagnosis is clinical, and the use of ultrasound is rare: only when voluminous. Also, their clinical appearance is not characteristic or raises fears of a complication, such as encystment. In this case, an anatomopathological examination after excision surgery is useful.

**A chalazion** is a benign cyst caused by inflammation of one or more sebaceous glands. These so-called Meibomian glands produce sebum, an oily substance that is used in the composition of tears (Fig. 23.1). A stye is a bacterial infection; centered on a pilosebaceous follicle of the eyelash. **A hidrocystoma** produces small translucent, shiny, single or multiple cysts that form(s) at the expense of the eccrine or apocrine sweat glands (Fig. 23.2). **A pilomatrixoma**, preferably "pilomatricoma", formerly called a calcifying (or sometimes mummified) epithelioma of Malherbe (an improper term), observed most often during the first two decades of life, is a rare benign adnexal skin tumor, developed from the cells of the hair matrix.

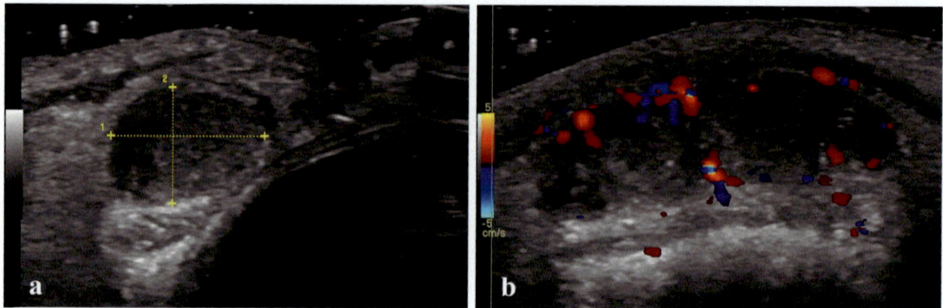

**Fig. 23.1** **Voluminous encysted chalazion**. **a**: B-mode, sagittal section; **b**: Color Doppler imaging (CDI), axial section. The lesion, measuring 16.3 mm × 7.4 mm in diameter × 5.7 mm thick, has progressed for more than 1 month, despite treatment, although possibly not well monitored. It is poorly to moderately echogenic, heterogeneous with septa in formation; it is rather poorly delineated with posterior enhancement and rather blurred boundaries, vascularized on Doppler, and inflammatory

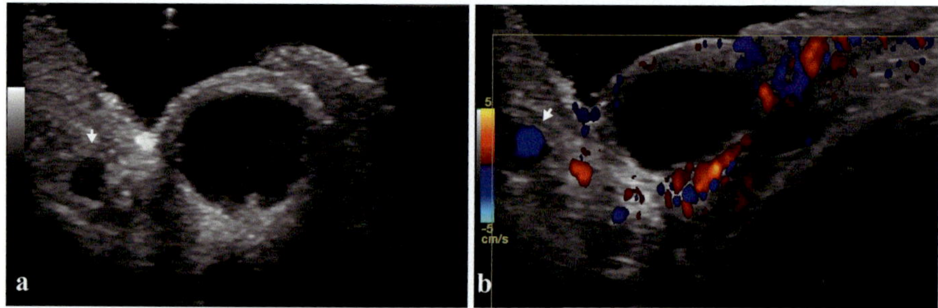

**Fig. 23.2** **Small hidrocystoma of the upper right eyelid at the medial canthus**. **a**: B-mode; **b**: CDI, axial section. Small cystic cavity, with clear posterior enhancement, measuring 7.5 mm × 6 mm in diameter × 5.8 mm thick, very hypoechoic, at a distance from the angular vessels (➡ white arrows). Histologically, the lesion was bordered by a cubic epithelium and contained eosinophilic serosity

### 23.1.3 *Lacrimal Gland Cysts: Dacryops*

These are dealt with in Chap. 21 (see Figs. 21.2 and 21.3).

## 23.2 Abscesses

These correspond to one or more collection areas within a patch of cellulitis or within a pre-existing lesion (tumor, granuloma following a foreign body). They are most often secondary to bacterial infections but sometimes also to fungal infections (mucormycosis, aspergillosis), especially in diabetic or immunocompromised patients. They take the form of a rounded mass with a varying degree of fluid content: if the abscess is purulent, the fluid may be frankly echogenic, with possibly a level (which appears sloping, changing during lateral decubitus). As they progress, the liquid becomes poorly echogenic, and a thick wall can be seen, corresponding to a genuine shell. In all cases, there is clear posterior enhancement. On color Doppler, the vascularization is minimal and only peripheral. The topography of the abscess often provides an indication of its origin (ethmoid, preseptal region, lacrimal sac, etc.) (see Figs. 26.13, 25.7 and 25.8).

Peripheral abscesses are more flattened: subperiosteal abscesses, like hematomas, have a biconvex lens shape.

A CT scan with injection confirms the diagnosis, completes the locoregional assessment, and helps monitor the therapeutic indications (surgery) [2].

The basic rules of asepsis are to be followed before and after the exam.

## 23.3  Parasitic Cysts

These are rare, but they should be considered when the patient is from or is returning from a country where these diseases are endemic.

**23.3.1 Hydatidosis** [3] occurs mainly around the Mediterranean basin (North Africa, Turkey, etc.). Orbital hydatid cysts account for less than 1% of hydatidosis localizations, and they most often result in progressive exophthalmos. On ultrasound, there is a single lesion (rarely multiple), with regular contours, hypo- or anechoic, limited by a thick capsule, without objectifiable vascularization on Doppler (Fig. 23.3).

The diagnosis is confirmed if necessary by serology.

The treatment is surgical (total excision avoiding rupture).

**23.3.2 Cysticercosis** is mainly found in southern Europe (Portugal ++), Reunion, India, and Latin America. Lesional diffusion is performed by hematogenous spread. These are generally young patients, more frequently men, who complain of pain and oculomotor disorders. Orbital involvement, rarer than ocular involvement, most often concerns an extraocular muscle at the origin of an intramuscular cystic lesion, 10 mm in diameter, on average [4, 5], which on ultrasound results in an overall anechoic nodule containing a hyperechoic area corresponding to the scolex (Fig. 23.4).

Medical treatment reduces the volume of the cyst, which disappears in 6 months.

**23.3.3** Other parasitic lesions (toxoplasmosis etc.) only rarely result in intraorbital locations [6].

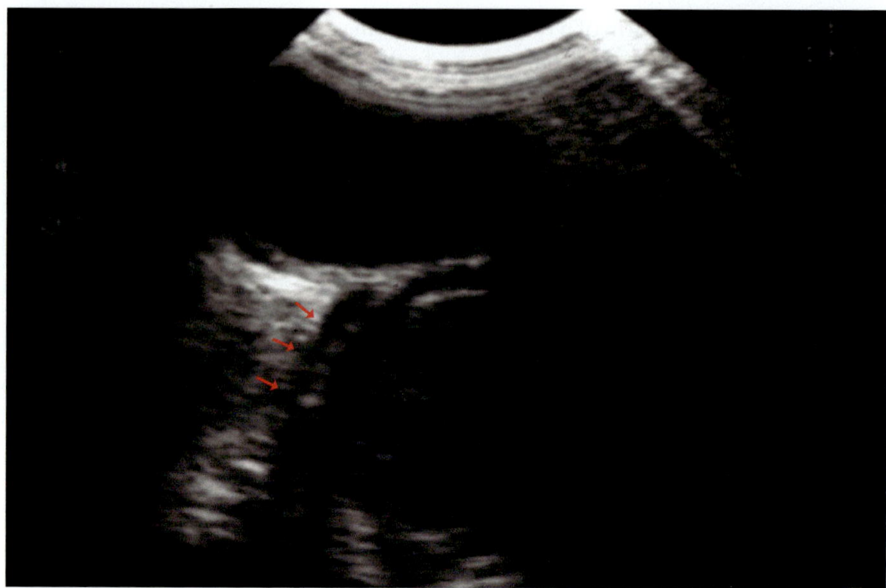

**Fig. 23.3** **Retrobulbar intraconal hydatid cyst**. B-mode para-axial section. The large cyst, with a thick wall, represses the optic nerve (→ red arrows)

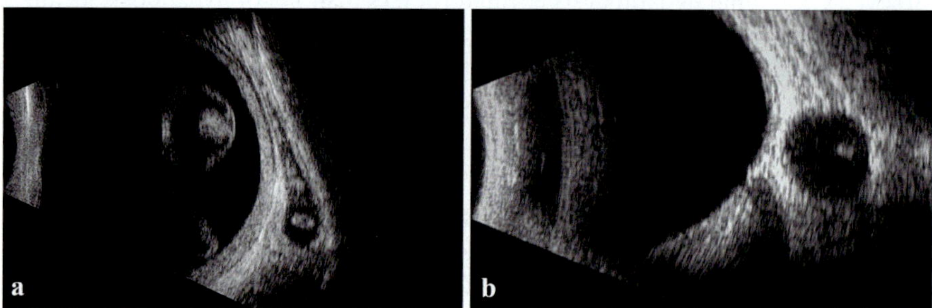

**Fig. 23.4** **Ocular and orbital cisticercosis. a**: 20 MHz annular probe B-mode section of the temporal quadrant in a 24-year-old man; **b**: 15 MHz B-mode section along the 9 o'clock meridian of the left eye in another 26-year-old patient. In **a**, an intraocular lesion and another lesion centered on the lateral rectus muscle is highlighted. In **b**, the lesion is centered on the belly of the medial rectus muscle. All lesions are cystic and anechoic, with a small echogenic bell-shape material corresponding to the scolex

## 23.4 Cystic Granulomas

These lesions are usually secondary to penetration of a foreign body into the orbit, and they can occur several months after the trauma [7]. They are a reaction to a foreign body that results in cystic changes (anechoic or heterogeneous in case of superinfection). A foreign body should be considered in case of a more echogenic intracystic image, with often resonance artifacts or a posterior shadowing. The nature of the foreign body is diverse: metal, glass, and sometimes plant debris in case of trauma from a stem or a tree branch.

## 23.5  Hematomas

Chocolate cysts are characteristic of hemolymphangiomas (Fig. 23.5), but they can also complicate a varicose vein.

Cystic transformation of a hematoma occurs after a few weeks, in connection with fibrinolysis, and a capsule of varying echogenicity appears. Eventually, it can disappear, sometimes even completely. The same progression can be seen for subperiosteal hematomas, which present as peripheral lenticular lesions. If the hematoma is not already known, one relies on the clinical context, Doppler (avascular lesion,

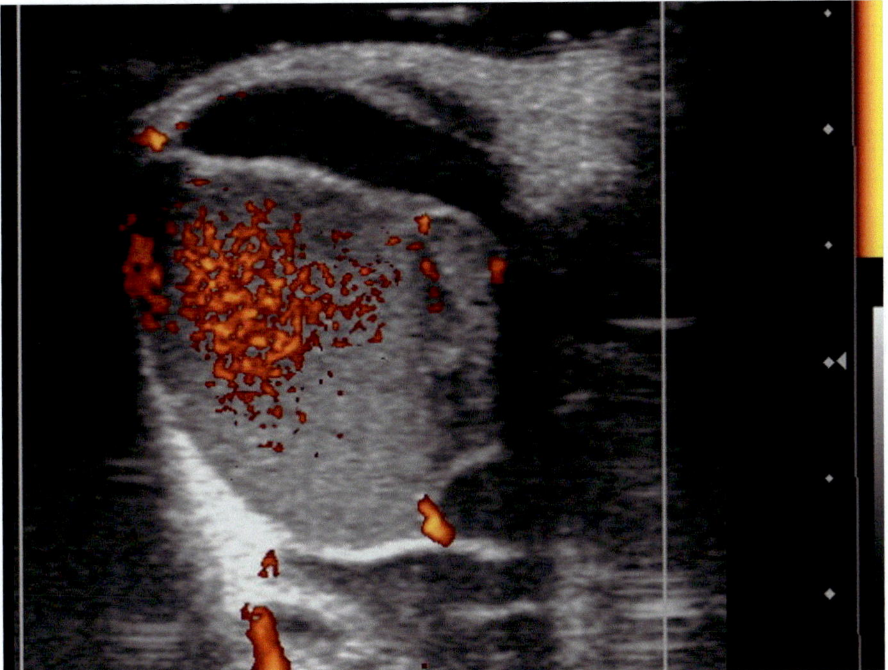

**Fig. 23.5 Chocolate cyst complicating hemolymphangioma**. CDI, power mode. The mass, paraocular, is echogenic, with a liquid/liquid level. Small colored dots can be seen within the echogenic part, corresponding to sedimentation of the red blood cells. This section is centered (focused) on the hematoma, but some posterior cystic cavities are seen, characteristic of the causal lesion

                                                                                    

possible associated varicose vein, etc.), and especially the progression, which will be toward progressive regression.

Aside from hemolymphangiomas, hematomas can occur within other benign vascular lesions such as cavernous hemangiomas and varices or within all malignant tumors.

These hematomas should not be mistaken for the giant dilatations of the superior ophthalmic vein observed in varicose veins and in arteriovenous fistulas that present as tubular cystic images, displaying a colored flow on Doppler (see Chap. 20).

## 23.6 Cystic Tumors

These are rare, observed mainly in children (teratomas, choristomas, dermoid, and/ or epidermoid cysts) (see Chap. 26), the tissue portion of tumors generally being predominant. However, some schwannomas (see Fig. 20.15) can appear as almost entirely cystic lesions; the tissue periphery of the lesion is hypervascularized on Doppler [8]. Rare cases of melanoma and cystic intraorbital myxomas [9] have been reported.

## 23.7 Cystic Dilatations of the Posterior Pole of the Globe and the Optic Nerve

Coloboma is a congenital malformation related to non-closure of the fetal choroidal fissure [2], with the set of abnormalities thus located in the inferior nasal quadrant. They can affect the eye, to varying degrees, associating the iris, the choroid and retina, and the optic disc (see Chap. 14). However, orbital colobomatous cysts can also be encountered, located under the optic nerve, and they are always associated with microphthalmia, hence the often-valid aphorism that microphthalmia without enophthalmos indicates the existence of an associated colobomatous cyst, until proven otherwise (see Figs. 18.17 and 26.1).

This anomaly can be bilateral and associated with other malformations (see Fig. 14.30).

In addition, the subarachnoid spaces surrounding the optic nerve can be dilated under different circumstances, presenting as an anechoic circular image surrounding the optical fibers. This dilation is observed in case of an obstacle: extrinsic compression by a tumor such as a glioma (see Fig. 18.3), an infection, such as cysticercosis [10]), or intracranial hypertension (bilateral and usually moderate, sometimes asymmetrical dilation) (see Fig. 19.12). In such cases, brain MRI is indicated.

## 23.8  Cystic Lesions Extending to the Orbit from Adjacent Structures

### *23.8.1  Mucoceles*

They are slowly progressive cystic lesions that straddle a sinus (or an ethmoid cell) and the orbit, with more often a superonasal localization [11]. They are caused by an accumulation of mucus, usually the result from sinus ostium obstruction by inflammation, infection, fibrosis, trauma, surgery or by tumors.

On ultrasound, a well-limited extraconal lesion is found, with little or no compressibility. This lesion is anechoic or hypoechoic, in connection with the mucous content of the mucocele. Sometimes a small hypoechoic bell-shaped entity is seen within the anechoic cyst related to thicker, denser mucus (Fig. 23.6), sometimes with a horizontal sloping level, mobile with the patient's position; it is of course avascular. Erosion of bony walls is a characteristic sign (Fig. 23.7). In case of superinfection, the content appears more echogenic and heterogeneous (Fig. 23.8).

The assessment is completed by CT (very thinned and expansive appearance of the cortical bone) and/or by MRI (assessment of cerebral impact in frontal mucoceles). The treatment is surgical.

### *23.8.2  Dacryoceles (or Dacrocystoceles)*

They represent a particular form in infants [12], corresponding mainly to a pseudo-cystic dilation of the lacrimal sac and the nasolacrimal duct due to an obstruction at the level of the Hassner valve, which is the lower ostium of the canal at the level of the

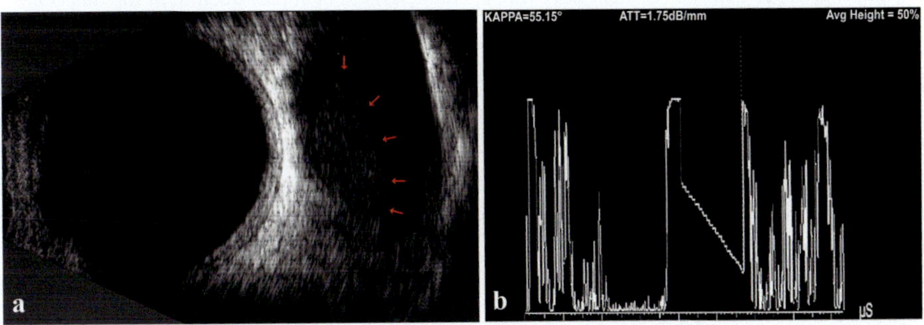


**Fig. 23.6  Hypoechoic bell-shaped mucus within an anechoic mucocele. a:** B-mode; **b:** standardized A-mode, the height of the peaks at 50% to assess the attenuation. In B-mode, the small, slightly denser bell-shaped mucus (→ red arrows) is clearly visible within the anechoic mucocele. In standardized A-mode, this small anechoic bell-shaped entity is attenuating (kappa angle = 55°) the ultrasound beam

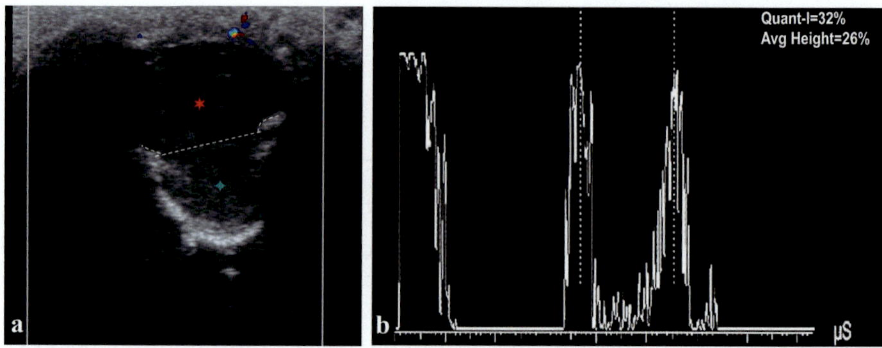

**Fig. 23.7** **Frontal mucocele with lysis of orbital roof**. **a**: B-mode; **b**: standardized A-mode, at tissue sensitivity (T = 76.3 dB), to assess the reflectivity. The bone lysis, indicated by the pale gray dotted line, is clearly visible and creates a wide-open connection between the sinus part (green star) and the orbital part (red star) of the mucocele

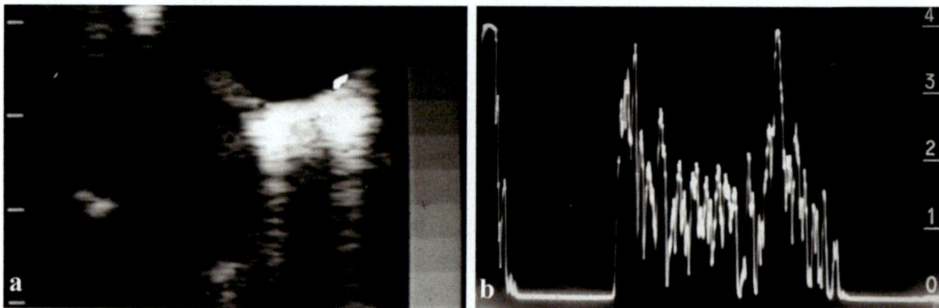

**Fig. 23.8** **Ethmoid mucopyocele**. **a**: B-mode; **b**: standardized A-mode, at tissue sensitivity (T = 81.4 dB), to assess the reflectivity. In B-mode, assessing the echotexture of such an extraconal lesion is sometimes difficult when one cannot be perpendicular to it. However, the moderately reflective and heterogeneous nature is evident in A-mode, characteristic of superinfection of the mucocele

nasal cavity behind the head of the inferior nasal concha (turbinate). They are treated by probing from the third month, with a 90% cure rate, and by probing with silicone intubation in case of failure, impossibility of restraint, or in children over 1 year of age, with a 99% success rate. However, the impermeability of the lacrimal ducts can also be due to lacrimal, facial, or nasal malformations of a complex, congenital, or acquired nature.

They are centered on the medial canthus (Fig. 23.9). Even when atypical, they can be easily differentiated from abscesses, dermoid or epidermoid cysts, choristomas, or cephaloceles. The role of ultrasound is mainly to measure them and evaluate their extension.

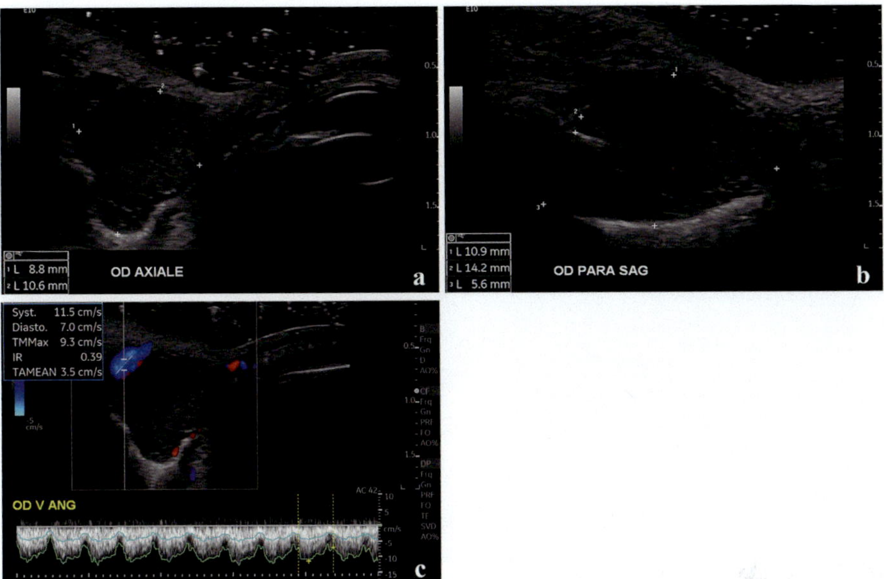



**Fig. 23.9 Dacryocele**, in a 2-week-old infant. Sections focused on the lacrimal sac. **a**: B-mode axial section; **b**: B-mode, sagittal section; **c**: CDI, color and spectral Doppler with recording of the angular vein flow. Significant expansion of the lacrimal sac measuring 8.8 mm × 14.2 mm × 10.9 mm but buried at the level of the medial canthus and not protruding under the skin; the content is hypoechoic and homogeneous and of course without flow. The nasolacrimal duct is dilated, measuring 5.6 mm in diameter, but it cannot be followed very far because of its bony walls. The lacrimal sac represses the angular vein, which nethertheless has a normal flow (**c**)

## 23.8.3 Cephaloceles

These are hernias of a part of the encephalic content, often dysplastic, through bone dehiscence that is mainly post-traumatic or post-surgical and rarely congenital [13]. They are uncommon. Their classification is based on their content and location [14]. There is not much of a role for ultrasound, and the diagnosis is mainly based on MRI (± CT) [15].

## 23.9 Epithelial Inclusion Cysts

Observed particularly after placement of a prosthesis, they can be seen after any eye or orbital surgery (Fig. 23.10) [16]. In case of an ocular prosthesis, the fluid collection is trapped between the prosthesis and the scleral shell, which was closed during the procedure. On ultrasound, an anechoic nodule is seen, often anterior and adjacent to the prosthesis. The assessment is often completed by CT scan or MRI, in particular, to determine the relation between the cyst and the attachments of the prosthesis.

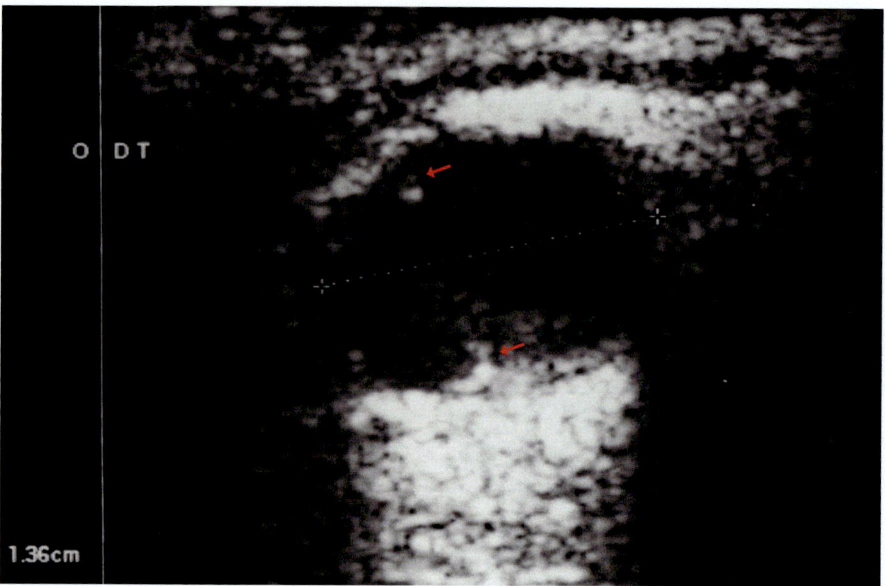

**Fig. 23.10 Epithelial inclusion cyst,** secondary to strabismus surgery. B-mode with a 7–12 MHz probe. The cyst is in fact molded to the medial wall of the eyeball within and below the tendon of the medial rectus muscle. Measuring 13.6 mm in its largest diameter, it is hypoechoic and one guess a septum in formation (→ red arrows), on its anterior and especially posterior surfaces. Note the poor visualization of the side walls and the clear posterior enhancement

# References


1. Kaufman LM, Villablanca JP, Mafee MF. Diagnostic imaging of cystic lesions in the child's orbit. Radiol Clin North Am. 1998;36(6):1149–63.
2. Bourjat P. In: Bourjat P, Veillon F, editors. Imagerie radiologique tête et cou. Vigot Paris; 1995.
3. Turgut AT, Turgut M, Kosar U. Hydatidosis of the orbit in Turkey: results from review of the literature 1963–2001. Int Ophthalmol. 2004;25(4):193–200.
4. Dhiman R, Devi S, Duraipandi K, Sen S, et al. Cysticercosis of the eye. Int J Ophthalmol. 2017;10(8):1319–24.
5. Salim S, Alam MS, Backiavathy V, Raichura ND, Mukherjee B. Orbital cysticercosis: clinical features and management outcomes. Orbit. 2020;27:1–7.
6. Lee MW, Fong KS, Hsu LY, Lim WK. Optic nerve toxoplasmosis and orbital inflammation as initial presentation of AIDS. Graefes Arch Clin Exp Ophthalmol. 2006;244(11):1542–4.
7. Yazdanfard Y, Heegaard S, Fledelius HC, Prau JU. Foreign body orbital cyst. Acta Ophthalmol Scand. 2001;79(1):97–9.
8. Byrne BM, van Heuven WA, Lawton AW. Echographic charasteristics of benign orbital schwannomas. Am J Ophthalmol. 1988;106(2):194–8.
9. Lieb We, Goebel HH, Wallenfang T. Myxoma of the orbit: a clinopathologic report. Graefes Arch Clin Exp Ophthalmol. 1990;228(1):28–32.
10. Gulliani BP, Dadeya S, Malik KPS, Jain DC. Bilateral cysticercosis of the optic nerve. J Neuro-Ophthalmol. 2001;21(3):217–8.
11. Rochels R, Geyer G, Bleier R. Echographic diagnosis in orbital mucoceles. Laryngol Rhinol Otol (Stuttg). 1985;64(4):181–4.

12. Allali J. Pathologie lacrymale du nourrisson et de l'enfant. Arch Pediatr. 2010;17(11):1609–16.
13. Koch B, Ball W Jr. Congenital malformations causing skull base changes. Neuroimag Clin North Am. 1994;4:479–98.
14. Barkovich AJ, Vandermarck P, Edwards MS, Cogen PH. Congenital nasal masses : CT and MR imaging features in 16 cases. AJNR Am J Neuroradiol. 1991;12:105–16.
15. Levy R, Wald S, Aitken P, et al. bilateral intraorbital meningoencephaloceles and associated midline craniofacial anomalies: MR and three-dimensional CT imaging. AJNR Am J Neuroradiol. 1989;10:1272–4.
16. Al-Shehah A, Khan AO. Subconjunctival epithelial inclusion cyst complicating strabismus surgery: early excision is better Saudi. J Ophthalmol. 2010;24(1):27–30.

# Chapter 24
# Malignant Neoplasms

Olivier Bergès

**Abstract** These various and rare lesions are often hypoechoic, attenuating and heterogeneous, with possible hemorrhagic rearrangements, and firm, with blurred or ill-defined contours and bumpy boundaries. On Doppler, they are often fairly to very vascularized with usually a high resistive index > 0.70 except for lymphoid lesions, for which the resistive index is low, < 0.70.

Malignant tumors are varied but rare. In Table 24.1, we propose a classification based on the key reference works [1, 2] for orbital pathologies.

In addition, ultrasound is rarely used first for the diagnosis of malignant tumors of the orbit but often follows MRI (and/or CT scan) and is not as clearly useful for characterizing such tumors as for the other already discussed lesions. Histological diagnosis is crucial, as is the eventual search for a primary lesion and assessment of extension, best provided by MRI and a high-resolution CT scan for assessing orbital walls.

We refer the reader to the corresponding chapters for vascular malignant tumors (Chap. 20), tumors of the lacrimal gland (Chap. 21), and tumors in children (Chap. 26) as well as muscle metastases (Chap. 22). Nonetheless, it seems useful to point out their common ultrasound signs: a hypoechoic and heterogeneous lesion, with quite blurred and ill-defined contours, often firm, all signs encountered in a case of primary malignant melanoma of the orbit (Fig. 24.1), diagnosed because the patient had a nevus of Ota, promoting the occurrence of ocular and orbital melanomas. Sometimes the lesion is distinctly hypoechoic (Fig. 24.2). In contrast, sometimes the heterogeneous nature of the echotexture predominates (Fig. 24.3). The hypercellularity of these lesions means that even though they are not very echogenic, the attenuation is evident in standardized A-mode (Fig. 24.4). All these malignant lesions can be complicated, like vascular lesions, by hemorrhagic rearrangements, which alter their ultrasound appearances (Fig. 24.5).

O. Bergès (✉)
Rothschild Foundation Hospital, Paris, France
e-mail: oberges@for.paris


O. Bergès (ed.), *Echography of the Eye and Orbit*,
https://doi.org/10.1007/978-3-031-41467-1_24

**Table 24.1** Malignant orbital tumors from Henderson [1] and Jakobiec [2]

- **Malignant vascular tumors**
  - Angiosarcoma (malignant hemangioendothelioma): highly anaplastic = malignant hemangiopericytoma, Kaposi's sarcoma, malignant lymphangiosarcoma, etc., *extremely rare, very aggressive*

- **Malignant fibrous tumors**
  - Primary fibrosarcomas: very rare
  - Fibrosarcomas extending to the orbit (from the nasal cavities)

- **Bone tumors of the walls of the orbit**
  - Osteosarcoma
  - Ewing's tumor
  - Chondrosarcoma

- **Malignant mesenchymal tumors**
  - Rhabdomyosarcoma
  - Liposarcoma: *difficult to define; the rarest of orbital tumors*
  - Leiomyosarcoma
  - Malignant hemangiopericytoma

- **Malignant tumors of the peripheral nerves (e.g. malignant triton tumor)**

- **Neuroblastoma and ganglioneuroblastoma/esthesioneuroblastoma**

- **Primary orbital melanomas**

- **Hematopoietic tumors**
  - Non-Hodgkin lymphomas / Burkitt lymphomas
  - Multiple myeloma and plasmacytoma
  - Chloroma = extramedullary form of myeloid leukemia
  - Leukemias (leukemic infiltration/hematoma)
  - Hodgkin: controversial for some time, but possible

- **Primary epithelial tumors**
  - Mixed malignant tumor / Pleomorphic adenocarcinoma
  - Adenoid cystic carcinoma
  - Adenocarcinoma
  - Malignant oncocytoma
  - Myoepithelial carcinoma (lacrimal gland)
  - Squamous cell carcinoma (to be distinguished from malignant mixed tumors)
  - Mucoepidermoid carcinoma

- **Propagated epithelial tumors**
  sinus +++: maxilla > ethmoid > frontal
  skin of the ocular appendages (eyelids, eyebrow, nose, temple, face)
  lacrimal and conjunctival epibulbar sac
  nasal cavity and nasopharynx
  - Squamous cell carcinoma
  - Adenoid cystic K and malignant Adéno K (sinus)
  - Melanoma (sinus → orbit)
  - Mesenchymal tumors: osteosarcoma, chondrosarcoma, fibrosarcoma, embryonal rhabdomyosarcoma (sinus → orbit)
  - Transitional cell carcinoma (transformation of an inverted papilloma)
  - Ameloblastoma (teeth → sinus → orbit)
  - Basal cell carcinomas/sclerodermiform/squamous cell carcinoma
  - Sebaceous carcinoma
  - Melanoma (conjunctival)
  - Mucoepidermoid carcinoma
  - Sweat gland carcinoma
  - Pharyngeal or hypopharyngeal squamous cell carcinoma (lymphoepithelioma)
  - Esthesioneuroblastoma

(continued)

**Table 24.1**  (continued)

• **Metastases**

In children

— neuroblastoma (often bilateral, the + often associated with a primitive adrenal. If thoracic or cervical (Horner syndrome)

— Ewing's sarcoma

— medulloblastoma

— Wilms tumor

In adults

*Less common (1/10) than choroidal metastases*

— Breast (infiltrating mass versus malignant)—adenocarcinoma

— Pulmonary (bronchial)—adenok/epidermoid/undifferentiated/small cells

*Metastasis can precede and be indicative*

— Prostate—adenok

— Kidney—adenok (hypernephroma): highly vascularized

• **Various tumors**

— Alveolar soft tissue sarcoma = malignant paraganglioma, granular cell myoblastoma = malignant angiocarcinoma

— Carcinoids

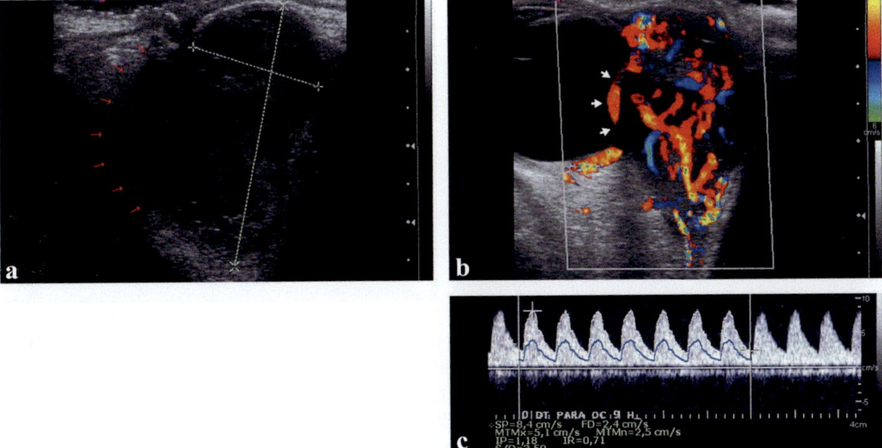

**Fig. 24.1  Primary malignant melanoma of the orbit. a**: B-mode paraocular section of the temporal quadrant of the right orbit; **b**: Color Doppler imaging (CDI), color mode, paraocular section along the 9 o'clock meridian of the right orbit; **c**: CDI, spectral mode. Exophthalmos and rapidly progressing palpable mass in a patient with a nevus of Ota. It is clearly a malignant tumor, the voluminous mass (35 mm × 18 mm) being poorly echogenic and heterogeneous with blurred contours, poorly delineated (→ red arrows) and with very hard consistency, indenting the lateral wall of the eyeball (⇨ white arrows). On Doppler, the mass is very vascularized, with relatively slow flow (PSV < 10 cm/s) with high resistivity (RI > 0.70)

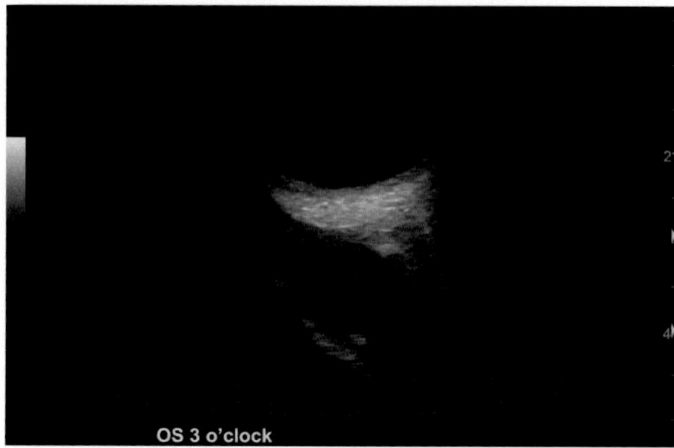



**Fig. 24.2 Liposarcoma of the left lateral rectus muscle**. B-mode. The size of the muscle is greatly increased, measuring 18 mm thick; it is higly hypoechoic, with two moderately echogenic micronodules, and it has slightly bumpy boundaries. Even though these signs suggest a malignant tumor, histology is mandatory

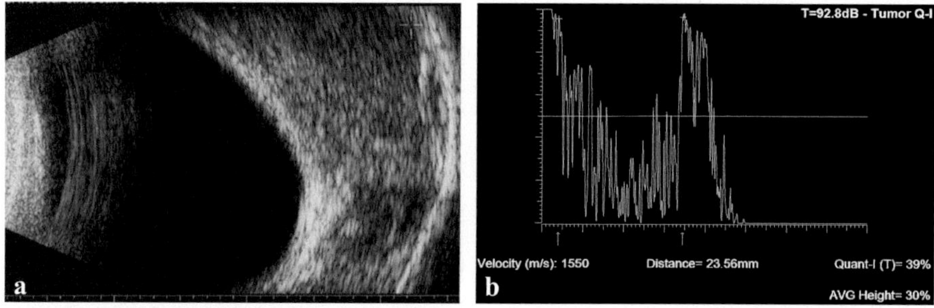



**Fig. 24.3 Rhabdomyosarcoma in a 5-year-old child. a**: B-mode transocular section of the inferolateral quadrant of the left orbit; **b**: standardized A-mode at tissue sensitivity (T = 92.8 dB) by a paraocular approach; The voluminous mass deforms the eye wall; it is moderately echogenic in B-mode and slightly low reflective in A-mode (39% in Quantification-I). A-mode also shows the heterogeneity of the lesion better than B-mode, with peaks of very uneven height

On Doppler, malignant lesions tend to be fairly to highly vascularized (Fig. 24.1b), but this is not always the case, and they present, as for the solid masses of the lacrimal gland, a high resistive index > 0.70 (Fig. 24.1c), except for lymphoid lesions, for which the resistive index is low, < 0.70 (see Figs. 21.8 and 22.4) [3].

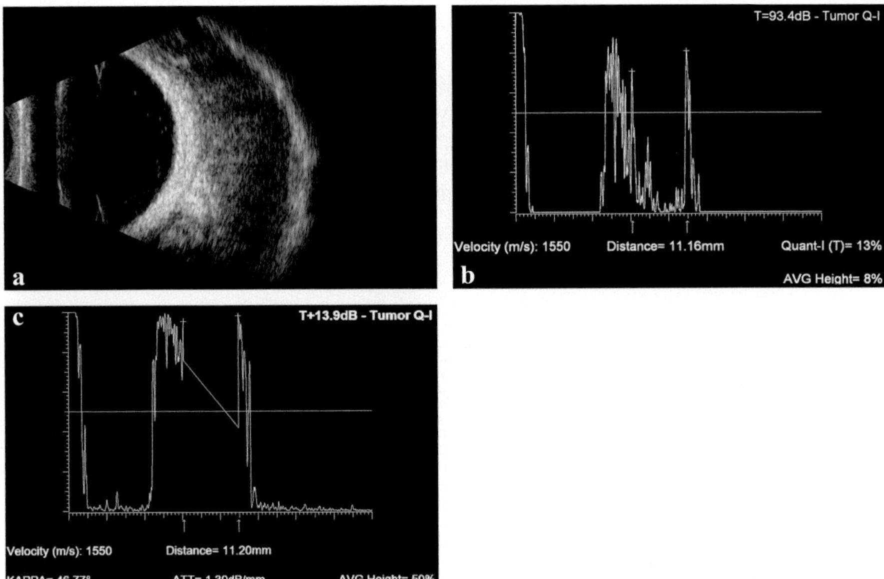



**Fig. 24.4  Superior extraconal lymphoma. a**: 10 MHz B-mode transocular section of the left orbit; **b**: standardized A-mode at tissue sensitivity (T = 93.4 dB) for assessing the reflectivity; **c**: standardized A-mode at T + 13.9 dB so that the average height of the peaks is 50%, to quantify the attenuation. The lesion is very low reflective (13% in Quantification-I), homogeneous, and strongly attenuating (kappa angle = 46.77°); in A-mode, attenuation is perceptible despite the low reflectivity of the lesion

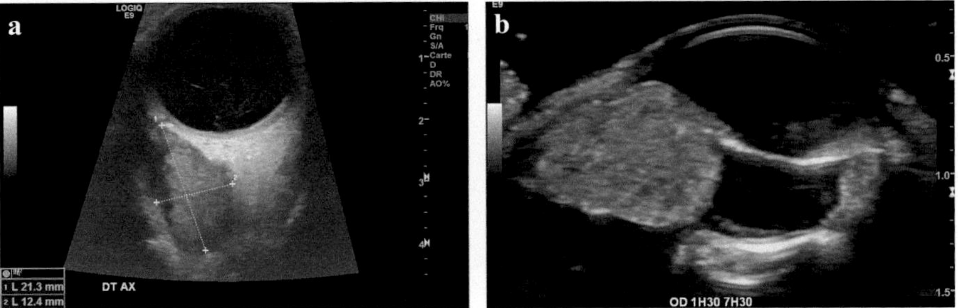



**Fig. 24.5  Metastases of breast cancer, to the lateral rectus muscle and to the ciliary body. a**: B-mode transocular section of the left orbit with an 8–18-MHz probe; **b**: Immersion B-mode centered on the temporal ciliary body of the left eye at 18 MHz. The muscle is hypoechoic and significantly increased in size, measuring 12 mm in diameter, and slightly bumpy, and there is a broad moderately echogenic span with scalloped edges, corresponding to a voluminous hemorrhage. In contrast to the anterior chamber and vitreous, the ciliary body lesion appears as echogenic as the muscle lesion, even though it is hemorrhage-free and perfectly homogeneous

# References


1. Henderson JW. Orbital tumors, 3rd ed. New York: Raven Press; 1994.
2. Jakobiec FA, Font RL. Orbit. In: Spencer WH, editor. Ophthalmic pathology, an atlas and textbook. Philadelphia: Saunders Co; 1986. p. 2459–860.
3. Lecler A, Lafitte F, Koskas P, Bergès O, et al. Usefulness of Color Doppler Flow Imaging in the management of lacrimal gland lesions. Eur Radiol. 2017;27(2):779–89.

# Chapter 25
# Orbital Traumatic Pathologies

Mario de La Torre

**Abstract** Ultrasound is useful for exploring traumas; after suture of an open wound, without any pression and in a sterile environment. Evaluation of motility is crucial. Orbital cellulitis may be pre-septal (grade 1) or orbital, retroseptal (grade 2) or correspond to a subperiosteal abscess (grade 3). Grade 4 corresponds to the orbital abscess. In post-traumatic carotid cavernous fistula, B-mode shows a significant dilation of the superior ophthalmic vein with an average height of the peaks less than 40% at tissue sensitivity (T) in standardized A-mode. Doppler confirms the diagnosis by showing a high peak systolic velocity, between 50 and 70 cm/s, with a low resistive index, less than 0.60. Retrobulbar hematoma is rare. Ultrasound can be performed as an emergency procedure and can reveal a small lesion at the very beginning. A-mode allows for more precise analysis of the echotexture. One of its real contributions, in addition to diagnosis, is to allow evacuation of the hematoma under ultrasound guidance. Terson syndrome associates an intraocular hemorrhage, related to a subarachnoid hemorrhage. Before vitrectomy, ultrasound reveals a retro equatorial hemorrhage, and must look for retinal detachment, choroidal thickening and maculopathy. A-mode may note a slight increase in the size of the optic nerve, persistent in abduction. For muscle trauma (incarceration, disintegration, or laceration), ultrasound is useful, combining B- and A-modes. It may show an abnormality of volume or echotexture, particularly revealing a hematoma. For the optic nerve, ultrasound is useful for traumatic optic neuropathy and for avulsion of the optic nerve head.

## 25.1 Introduction

Even more so than for other indications, traumatic, orbital, and ocular lesions require extremely rigorous performance and semiological analysis. Additional examinations are often necessary because the clinical examination is frequently disappointing, difficult, or impossible because of the opacity of the media or the affected structure

M. de La Torre (✉)
Universidad Nacional Mayor de San Marcos, Lima, Perú
e-mail: mariodlt@gmail.com



O. Bergès (ed.), *Echography of the Eye and Orbit*,
https://doi.org/10.1007/978-3-031-41467-1_25

is buried and hence difficult to access; clinical signs must be searched for with finesse and interpreted with great precision.

Severe orbital trauma frequently involves all or part of the eyeball. The contribution of ultrasound in eye trauma has been discussed in Chaps. 11 and 12, and we focus mainly on orbital lesions in this chapter.

For these severe traumas, CT scan is considered the "gold standard" for additional examinations, with recent helical scanners and their ultra-thin multiplanar reconstructions. The main advantage of CT scan is that it allows for simultaneous and exhaustive assessment of the eyeball, the orbit, and other structures of the face as well as the brain and skull; the patient's life is often at stake, and this must remain a priority.

MRI is sometimes difficult to perform in an emergency, and it remains contraindicated in case of a suspected ferromagnetic metallic foreign body, and, moreover, it provides a poor analysis of bone lesions. Indications for plain radiographs have become limited, mainly when other techniques are not available.

The development of ultrasound techniques at very high resolution, such as evaluation of the anterior segment at 25 or 50 MHz (very-high-frequency ultrasound or ultrasound biomicroscopy), analysis of the posterior pole and the retro equatorial wall at 20 MHz with a long focal length or at 20 MHz with an annular probe and standardized A-ultrasound allow for assessing small structures with very high resolution and is even far superior to other medical imaging techniques.

Probably unnecessary reminders: ultrasound is a non-aggressive, non-ionizing, and inexpensive technique. Both B-mode and A-mode, which are complementary, are relatively easy to perform; a clinical analysis of the anterior segment should first rule out an open wound before considering an ultrasound.

However, an open wound is only a relative contraindication. Nonetheless, an initial suture of the wound is recommended before any ultrasound, and even then, one must undertake the examination with the utmost care and minimum pressure to avoid contamination of the wound and aggravation of the traumatic lesions already present.

In rare instances, ultrasound may be indicated before the wound is sutured, in this case with particular caution and especially after having considered the risk/benefit of the information to be obtained. However, being cautious remains a good rule to follow.

In any case, when an examination is performed shortly after trauma has occurred, working in a sterile environment is a priority: with dedicated sterile areas and after having covered the probe, after decontamination, with a sterile protection without talc identical to what is used for intraoperative ultrasounds. In addition, nitrile gloves are preferrable to latex gloves because the latter may contain talc powder, which can act as very small foreign bodies (Fig. 25.1). In A-mode, the small end of the probe is placed on the conjunctiva, but it remains at a distance from the wound (Fig. 25.2).

In B-mode, the probe can certainly be placed on closed, uncontracted eyelids coupled with a thick layer of methylcellulose gel or carbomer. That said, the eyelids often strongly attenuate and disrupt the ultrasound beam, especially when they are the site of a hematoma: the images obtained are often poor, even when the gain is

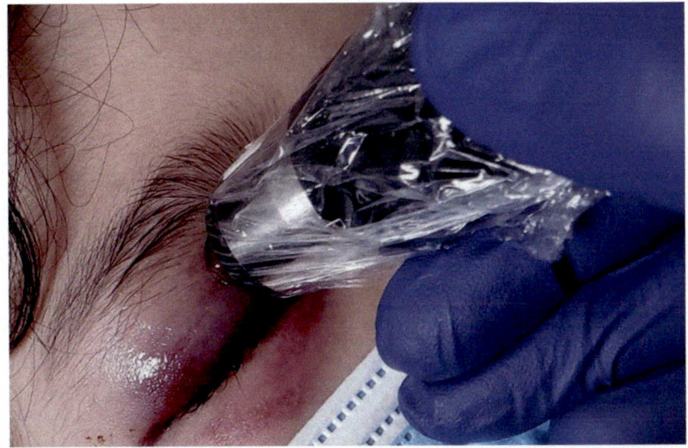

**Fig. 25.1  In B-mode**, physical barriers should be used to avoid contamination: sterile plastic protection around the probe; in addition, nitrile gloves that do not contain talc are preferable

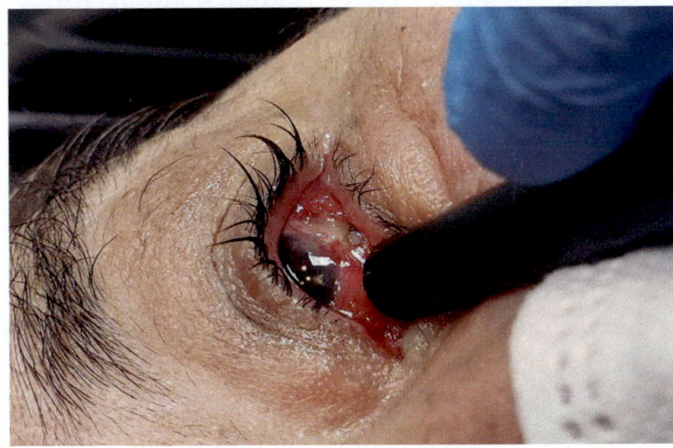

**Fig. 25.2  Examination of a traumatized eye in A-mode.** A small A-probe is placed on the conjunctiva, at a certain distance from the wound

increased, which does not allow to obtain images with a sufficient resolution and penetration. A transconjunctival approach is preferrable, if possible, remaining as atraumatic as possible, using the vitreous as an acoustic window and allowing for images of retrobulbar structures that are of much better quality.

A periocular approach is sometimes useful for assessing the anterior periocular structures. Even with all these precautions, assessing the posterior and apical part of the orbit is nonetheless difficult, except in certain circumstances when there is retrobulbar fluid collection.

Even when there is a degree of opacity of the media, ultrasound remains a contributory examination. In addition, to avoid iatrogenic complications, the examination should not be postponed or prolonged unnecessarily.

One of the advantages of ultrasound is that it requires somewhat less cooperation from the patient and a lesser degree of immobility. Another is the resolution, which is often higher than with CT scan and sometimes MRI, depending on the sequences performed (except for detailed assessment of the optic nerve), especially for high- and very-high-frequency probes. However, the main advantage of ultrasound is its dynamic nature, in real-time, allowing assessment of the mobility (muscle function, fistulas) and the compressibility/firmness of a lesion (hematoma, cystic lesion), which is different (and much better) than what can be obtained with other imaging techniques.

In contrast, in addition to the lack of resolution at the orbital apex, a notorious disadvantage of ultrasound is the absence of an image, or the presence of images with artifacts due to the presence of air in the orbit (e.g., orbital emphysema after a fracture).

Because ultrasound images taken quickly after trauma are often difficult to interpret, it is frequently useful to repeat the examination, sometimes several times, and to take into account the changes in the images to make a decision based on detailed information.

In orbital traumatic pathology, ultrasound is useful for the following: **assessment of ocular motility, orbital cellulitis, subperiosteal abscess, carotid-cavernous fistula, a foreign body, hemorrhage/hematoma, muscle trauma, the optic nerve, and subcutaneous emphysema**.

## 25.2 Evaluation of Ocular Motility

In case of orbital trauma, this test is very important and is easy to perform by ultrasound. It rules out edema, bleeding as well as disinsertion or muscle incarceration. Direct trauma affecting only the muscles or the optic nerve is rare, and ophthalmoplegia not explained by orbital or adnexal injury may be of central origin. Such an etiology must be searched for and ruled out.

The probe is placed on the eyelid, or on the conjunctiva after topical anesthesia; the patient is asked to look in different directions. Cross-sections of the muscular body (Fig. 25.3) provide an idea of the morphology and the thickness of the muscle, from its tendon to the orbital apex, and the longitudinal sections of the muscle (Fig. 25.4) show the insertion of the muscle on the globe. In addition, the position and attachment of the optic nerve (Fig. 25.5) should be noted. This eye motility test is a simple dynamic examination that can detect abnormalities in muscle movements but also any interior alteration in the volume of the orbit. However, because of the patient's pain and/ or lack of cooperation after the trauma, this test may not be feasible; similarly, with significant palpebral edema or orbital hematoma, results may be difficult to interpret. The existence of paralysis or muscular paresis after fracture of a wall of the orbit is an indication to operate without delay. There is merit in performing a forced reduction test, in the ward and under General Anesthesia, just before the repair of bone dehiscence to differentiate between muscle incarceration and an innervation problem, and to repeat it immediately afterward to verify that there is no conflict between the implant and the muscle.

**Fig. 25.3 Cross-section of a muscle**. Scanning the probe from the front to the back allows for assessing the entire muscle, from its tendon to its most posterior part near the orbital apex, providing an indication of the morphology and the thickness of the muscle (see Fig. 7.6). It is best to analyze the changes and displacements of the muscle during eye movements

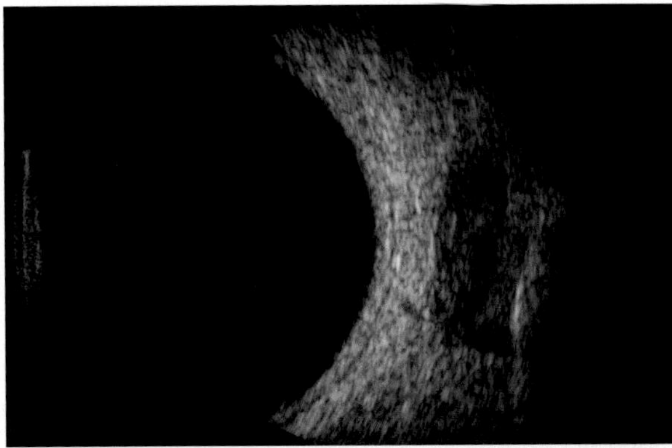

**Fig. 25.4 Longitudinal section of a muscle**. This section clearly shows the insertion of the tendon on the globe. During eye movements, the traction it exerts on the eyeball can be evaluated

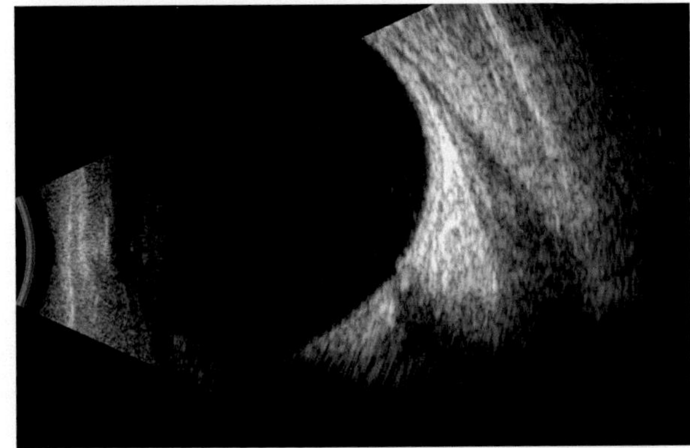

**Fig. 25.5 Position and insertion of the optic nerve**. Parasagittal section. Normal situation and appearance of the optic disc and the immediately retrobulbar optic nerve

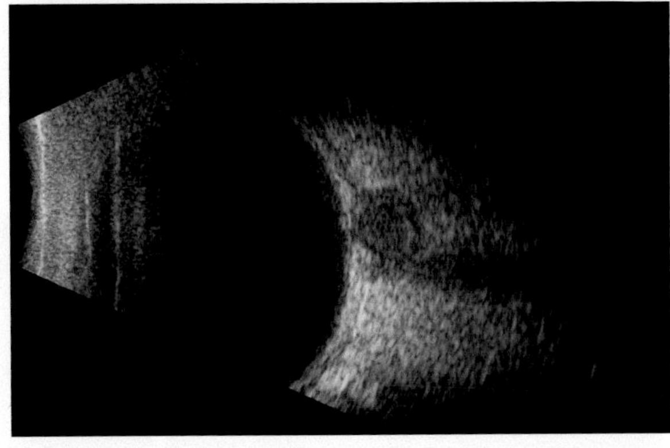

## 25.3 Orbital Cellulitis

Preseptal cellulitis and orbital cellulitis are generally distinguished according to Chandler's classification [1]:

- Preseptal (grade 1): this follows infections secondary to facial or palpebral trauma, from insect stings or animal bites.
- Orbital, retroseptal (grade 2): this is secondary to the extension of an infection of an adjacent sinus after a fracture.

In both cases, the most common microbial entities involved are *Streptococcus pneumoniae* and *Staphylococcus aureus*, to which anaerobic microorganisms must be added in children [2, 3].

- In grade 1 preseptal forms, the patient experiences relatively little pain, complaining mainly of tension of the subcutaneous tissues. There is inflammatory edema of the eyelids, which are red and tense. By slit lamp, chemosis is rare. There are no disorders of oculomotricity nor a decrease in visual acuity. In 30% of cases, there is moderate exophthalmos due to inflammatory edema of the orbit.
- In orbital forms, the patient experiences pain and has edema and redness of the eyelids and conjunctiva (chemosis) as well as pronounced exophthalmos and abnormalities in regard to ocular motility. Infiltration of tissues by microorganisms and inflammatory cells is seen in the sub-Tenon episcleral space as well as in the extraocular muscles (Fig. 25.6). In standardized A-mode, there is a decrease in the reflectivity of the orbital fat in the infiltrated area, and the ultrasound absorption is low.
- Subperiosteal abscess:

This corresponds to grade 3 of the Chandler classification. The collection of pus is located between the bone and the periorbit, with localized edema around the abscess. They can also be encountered after trauma. Clinically, there is non-axial exophthalmos (displacement opposite to the abscess) and limitation of oculomotricity.

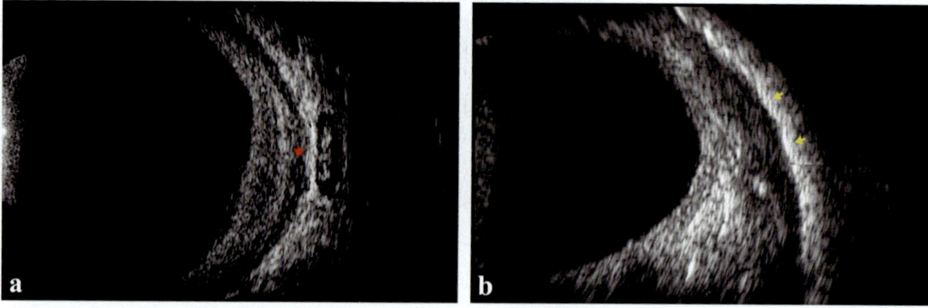

**Fig. 25.6 Orbital cellulitis. a**: B-mode, vertical section of the lateral quadrant; **b**: B-mode, sagittal section along the 12:00 o'clock meridian. Thickening of all ocular parietal tunics and inflammatory heterogeneous hypoechoic enlargement of the sub-Tenon episcleral space (★ red star). In addition, extraconal inflammation masks the confines of the superior rectus muscle (➡ yellow arrows)

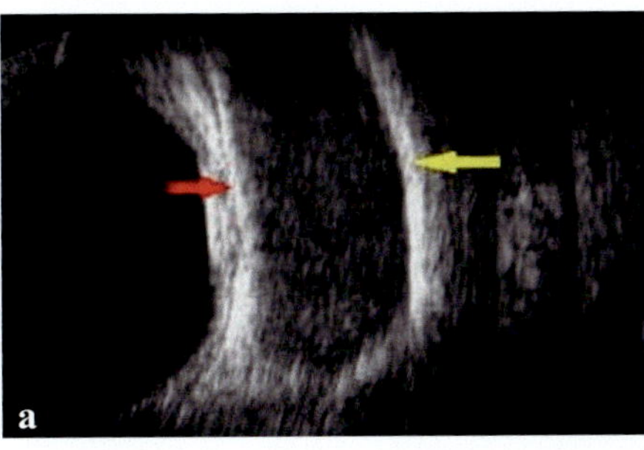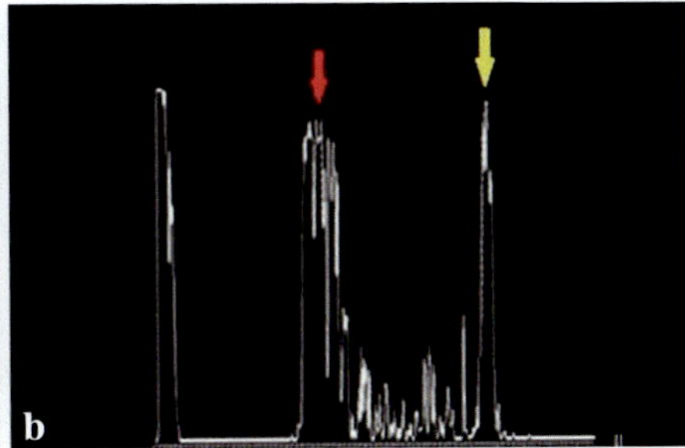

**Fig. 25.7 Subperiosteal abscess. a**: B-mode; **b**: standardized A-mode at tissue sensitivity. The mass is well delineated, with a double peak toward the orbit, corresponding to detachment of the peri-orbit (red arrow), better seen in A-mode. The posterior boundary corresponds to the orbital wall (yellow arrow); the purulent content is very hypoechoic and homogeneous

Generally, there is no decrease in visual acuity, unless the abscess is large and leads to compression of the optic nerve. The orbital pain varies. Anterior orbital palpation can reveal exquisite pain or even a mass. Figure 25.7 provides a clear summary of the ultrasound signs: the good delineation of the process, with a double peak in A-mode due to the detachment of the periorbit and a very hypoechoic and homogeneous content due to purulent nature, and of course, there is no deformation of the lesion after pressure of the probe.

– Grade 4 corresponds to an orbital abscess. At this stage, the chemosis is pronounced and there is generally exophthalmos. There may be complete ophthalmoplegia and often a decrease in visual acuity. At the ocular fundus, papilledema with venous dilation can be noted. The pain is very strong. On ultrasound, the outline is clear, unlike phlegmon, which is more diffuse. In the abscess, poorly echoic areas, corresponding to edema or pus, alternate with brighter areas (dotted images) corresponding to infiltration by inflammatory cells. Palpebral abscesses may also be observed in front of the septum (Fig. 25.8).

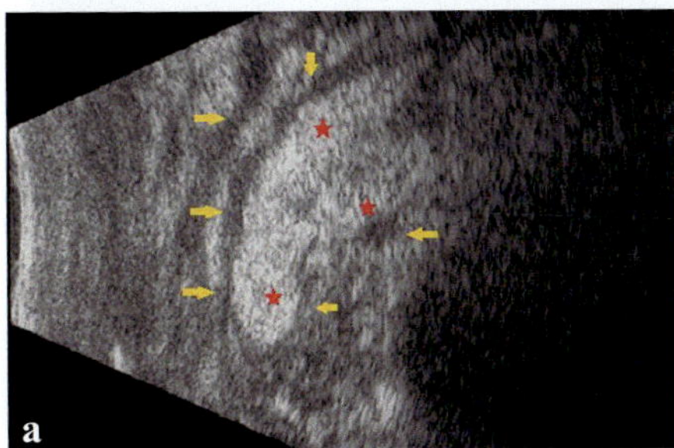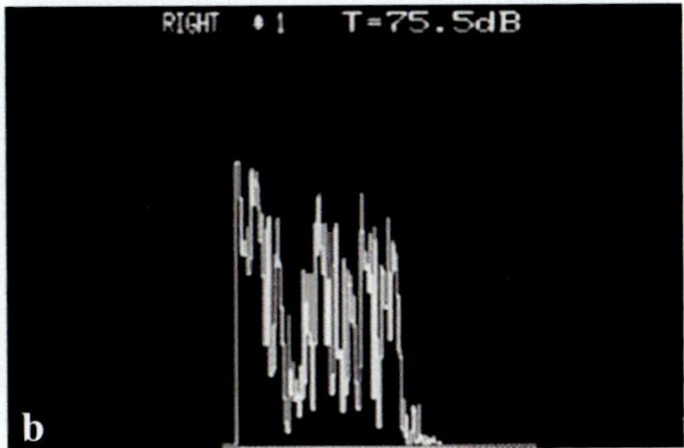

**Fig. 25.8 Preseptal abscess. a**: B-mode; **b**: standardized A-mode at tissue sensitivity (T = 75.5 dB). The lesion is well delineated. Curved areas of very low echogenicity (yellow arrows), corresponding to the hyporeflective areas in A-mode which represent edema or pus alternate with brighter areas (red stars) with "dotted" images corresponding to the moderately reflective areas in A-mode which represent infiltration of the fat by inflammatory cells

The kinetic criteria have only a secondary role: however, in case of massive infiltration of the orbital fat, there is a soft consistency, with also a certain resistance to the pressure of the probe.

These different forms must be differentiated quickly to consider an appropriate treatment without delay, depending mainly on the clinical signs: oral antibiotic therapy for preseptal forms, intravenous double antibiotic therapy for retroseptal forms, and surgical drainage indicated in case of abscesses [2, 4]. This allows for a generally favorable outcome, without reaching grade 5: thrombosis of the cavernous sinus.

## 25.4 Post-traumatic Carotid Cavernous Fistula

These are secondary to any type of craniofacial trauma, with or without fracture of the base of the skull. The clinical diagnosis is usually obvious (see Chap. 20), especially because in most cases, there is evidence of recent trauma. Ultrasound should confirm the diagnosis, showing significant dilation of the superior ophthalmic vein (SOV) (Fig. 25.9, see Figs. 20.22 and 20.23). Doppler affirms the diagnosis by showing a

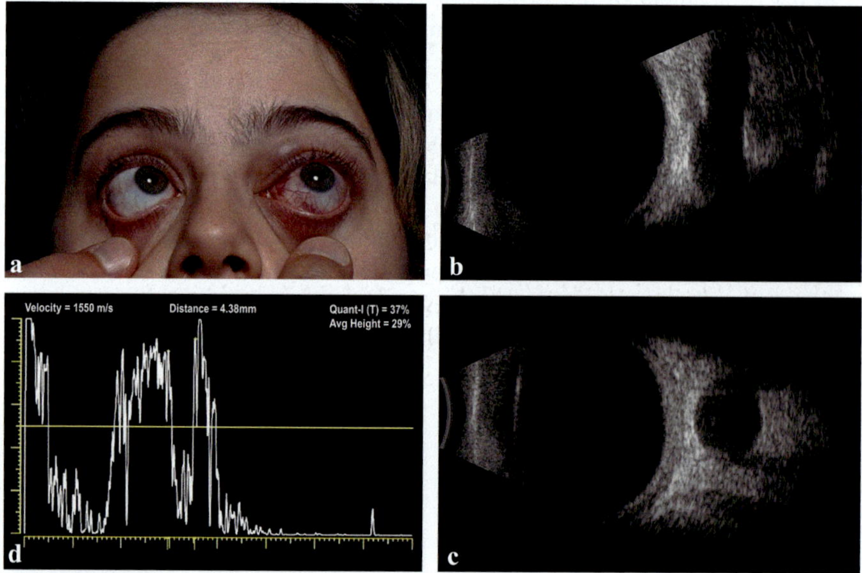


**Fig. 25.9  High-flow post-traumatic carotid-cavernous fistula. a**: Clinical presentation; **b**: B-mode superior para-axial section; **c**: B-mode parasagittal section; **d**: standardized A-mode at tissue sensitivity (T = 85.8 dB). Small left exophthalmos and conjunctival dilation (**a**) in a 34-year-old woman, 10 days after a car accident without a skull fracture, are very suggestive of the diagnosis. The dilation of the superior ophthalmic vein is readily highlighted in B-mode by its morphology, convex forward and temporal, above the optic nerve (**b**) and as a hypoechoic circle above the optic nerve (**c**). In dynamic mode, faint small punctiform echoes can be seen, corresponding to the red blood cells, going from back to front. When the flow is fast (**d**), the average height of the peaks in standardized A-mode is less than 40%

high peak systolic velocity (PSV), at 50–70 cm/s, and a low resistive index (RI), less than 0.60 in the dilated SOV, with an inverted and arterialized flow, often with aliasing artifact in the center of the vessel. In the absence of Doppler, A-mode can be of value: it shows an oscillating appearance of the peaks inside the dilated SOV, with the average peaks height at tissue sensitivity (T) being less than 40% [5].

In contrast, in cavernous sinus dural fistulas (Fig. 25.10, see Figs. 20.24, 20.25, and 26.12), the SOV is generally less dilated, the PSV is 10–25 cm/s, the RI always low, less than 0.60, and in standardized A-mode at tissue sensitivity (T), the average height of the peaks is greater than 40% [5]. These slow-flowi fistulas are responsible for vascular congestion, giving rise to the classic jellyfish sign image with conjunctival edema (chemosis), thickening of the extraocular muscles or even the optic nerve, and ocular hypertension with sometimes choroidal detachment.

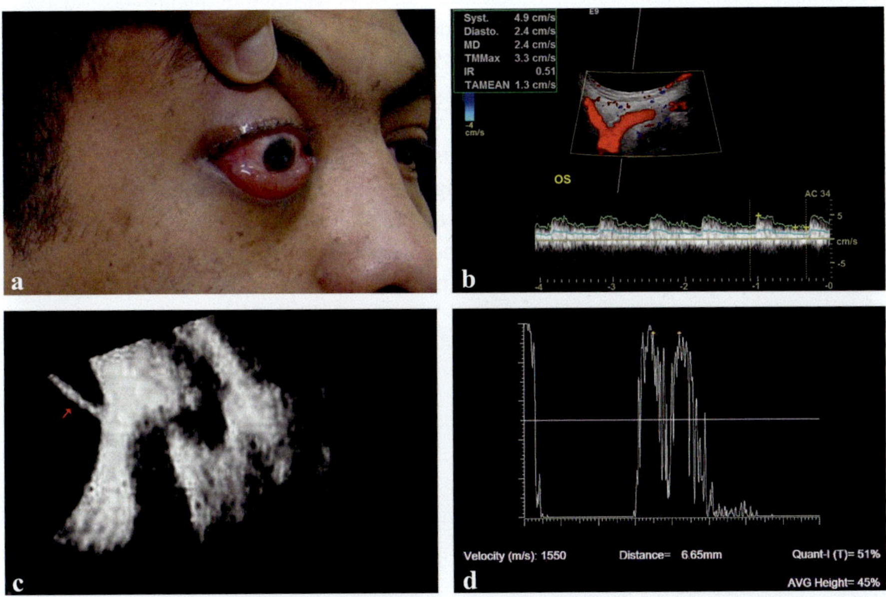


**Fig. 25.10  Dural fistula of the cavernous sinus. a**: Clinical presentation; **b**: Color Doppler imaging (CDI), color and spectral modes, superior para-axial section; **c**: B-mode, superior cross-section; **d**: standardized A-mode at tissue sensitivity (T = 94.7 dB). The clinical picture (**a**) is also very suggestive: diffuse conjunctival redness and because of gravity, pronounced inferior conjunctival chemosis in this 50-year-old woman with no history of trauma. Moderate dilation of the two roots of the superior ophthalmic vein (SOV) (**b, c**); in CDI, the flow is reversed, coded in red in color mode. Spectral mode shows an arterialized flow with a slow peak systolic velocity (PSV), at 4.9 cm/s, and a low resistive index (RI), at 0.51. Note in **c** the choroidal detachment (→ red arrow) in connection with ocular hypertension associated with the fistula. In standardized A-mode (**d**) the average peak height is greater than 40%

## 25.5   Hemorrhage

### *25.5.1   Hematoma*

Retrobulbar hematoma is a rare complication of traumatic brain injuries but can, when large, lead to permanent vision loss. Whether intraconal, extraconal, or subperiosteal [6], bleeding can lead to a senstion of tension (which may result in dizziness), exophthalmos, sometimes painful, and have an impact on the vessels of the optic nerve head, mainly the ciliary arteries, which can eventually progress to ischemic optic neuropathy and retinal ischemia. Attention should be paid to subconjunctival hemorrhage (Fig. 25.11), optic disc papilledema or pallor, decreased vision, restriction of ocular motility, and ocular hypertension. In cases of multiple trauma and to avoid irreversible visual disturbances, ultrasound can be performed in the emergency room or even while the patient waits for CT scan or MRI. The ophthalmological clinical examination is sometimes difficult to perform because of disorders of consciousness or periorbital edema, and under these conditions, ultrasound may reveal a small lesion at the very beginning, compatible with a small hematoma in its early stage (Fig. 25.11). A-mode allows for more precise analysis of the echotexture (Fig. 25.12): very low reflective, uneven, and attenuating. When the lesion is larger, one may need to assess the relationships with adjacent structures and in particular the optic nerve (Fig. 25.13). However, in addition to diagnosis, one of the real contributions of ultrasound is to allow evacuation of the hematoma under ultrasound guidance (Fig. 25.14) [7].

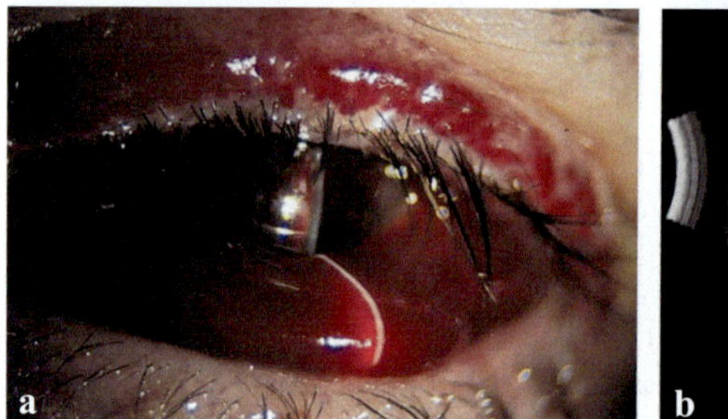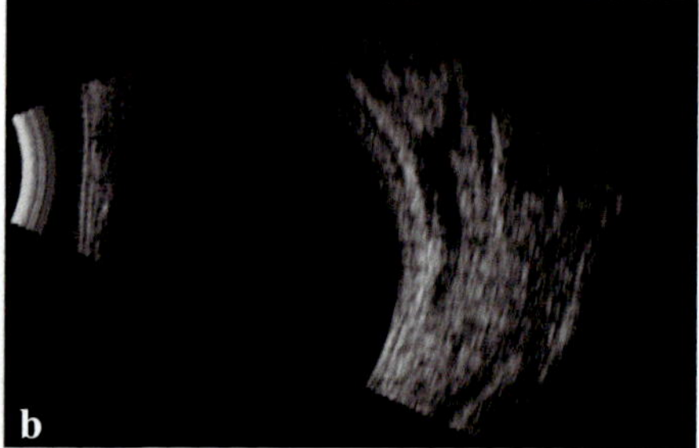

**Fig. 25.11 Massive subconjunctival hemorrhage associated with a small retrobulbar hematoma** at the early stage, after blunt trauma in a 36-year-old man. **a:** Clinical presentation; **b:** B-mode, inferior para-axial section. Discrete retrobulbar fluid collection with irregular contours, infiltrating the orbital fat

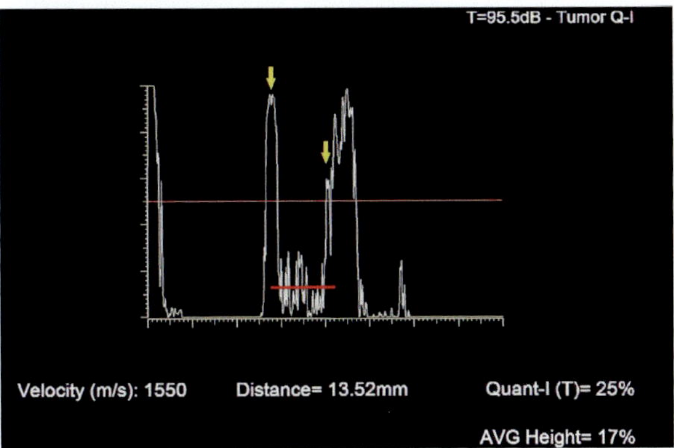


**Fig. 25.12 Retrobulbar hematoma**. standardized A-mode at tissue sensitivity (T = 95.5 dB). The lesion, which is 13.5 mm thick, is well delineated (→ yellow arrows). It exhibits little reflectivity (red line), with an average peak height of 17% and an uneven and attenuating echotexture

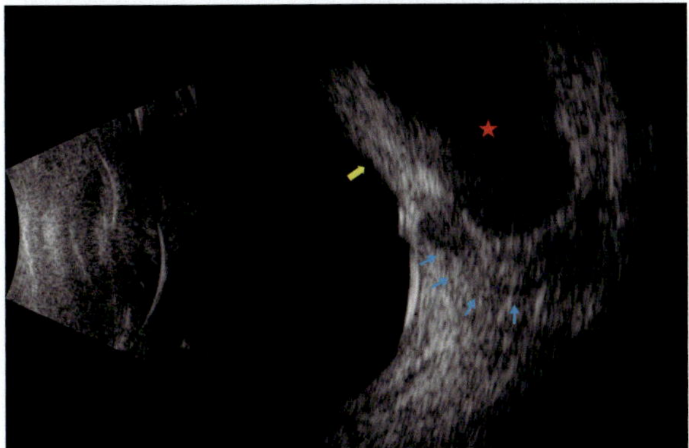

**Fig. 25.13 Large intraconal hematoma**. B-mode, parasagittal section. Fairly large hypoechoic oval retrobulbar mass (★ red star) deforming the ocular wall (➡ yellow arrow), compressing the optic nerve (→ blue arrows) and pushing it downward

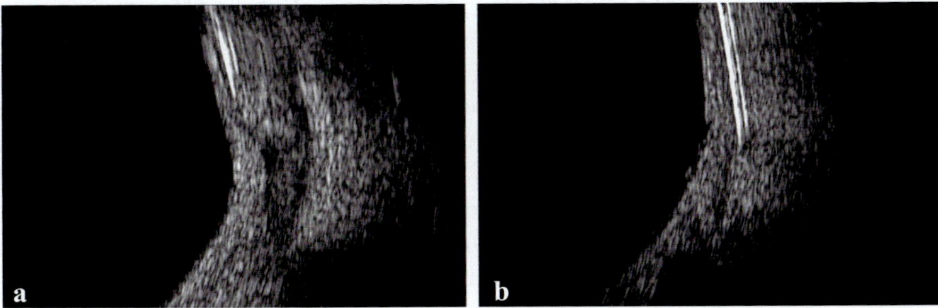


**Fig. 25.14 Puncture/evacuation of a hematoma under ultrasound guidance. a**: At the beginning of the procedure; **b**: at the end of the evacuation

### *25.5.2 Terson Syndrome*

This associates an intraocular hemorrhage, associated with a subarachnoid hemorrhage, related to an intracranial hemorrhage, by rupture of an aneurysm, head trauma, etc. The pathophysiology is controversial. One of the hypotheses is the sudden increase in pressure in the cerebrospinal fluid hindering the venous return, thus causing rupture of the internal blood–retinal barrier. Hemorrhage may be present in the vitreous, the retrohyaloid space, under the internal limiting membrane, under the retina, and in the subarachnoid spaces surrounding the orbital optic nerve fibers.

There can be spontaneous slow favorable progression, but persistence of the blood can lead to various complications (hemosiderosis, cataracts, epiretinal membranes and other macular abnormalities, retinal detachment, etc.) that, with certain excessively slow resorptions, are considered reasons to justify a vitrectomy [8], without knowing whether it is better to operate early on or more than 3 months after the accident [9]. On ultrasound, hemorrhage, whether intraocular, intravitreal, or subretinal, tends to be located behind the equator (Fig. 25.15), in relation to gravity, with patients being in a recumbent position during their hospitalization (see Chap. 12). A slight increase in the size of the optic nerve is noted, more readily in A-mode, that is persistent in abduction. Choroidal thickening may also be noted in connection with venous stasis. Ultrasound is strongly indicated for assessment before vitrectomy [10] and to detect maculopathies behind the intraocular hemorrhage [11].

## 25.6 Muscle Trauma

Trauma can lead to muscle incarceration, disintegration, or laceration. In addition to the mechanisms already described, there can also be a hematoma that increases the ischemia of an already traumatized/incarcerated muscle. After a fracture, the muscles most often affected are the inferior rectus and the medial rectus. Clinical examination is crucial (Fig. 25.16), in particular the characteristics of diplopia and examination of oculomotricity, notably a Lancaster test, as well as analysis by CT scan, in search of lesion of a wall, incarceration of soft tissues at the fracture site: pinching of the orbital fascia and fat, exceptionally of the muscle [12]. Ultrasound is complementary, useful in case of persistent diplopia with a slightly displaced fracture, without obvious incarceration. In B-mode, one immediately sees, on both longitudinal and cross sections, the abnormalities of the affected muscle: increase volume, abnormal echotexture, visualization of a sinus, in relation to hematic content, which is not visible when normally aerated (Fig. 25.17a). However, A-mode is also crucial, first of all for measurement in its thickest point and comparison with its contralateral counterpart but also for assessment of its echotexture, revealing a hematoma, of medium or high reflectivity, without obvious attenuation but with an even and homogeneous echotexture (Fig. 25.17b).

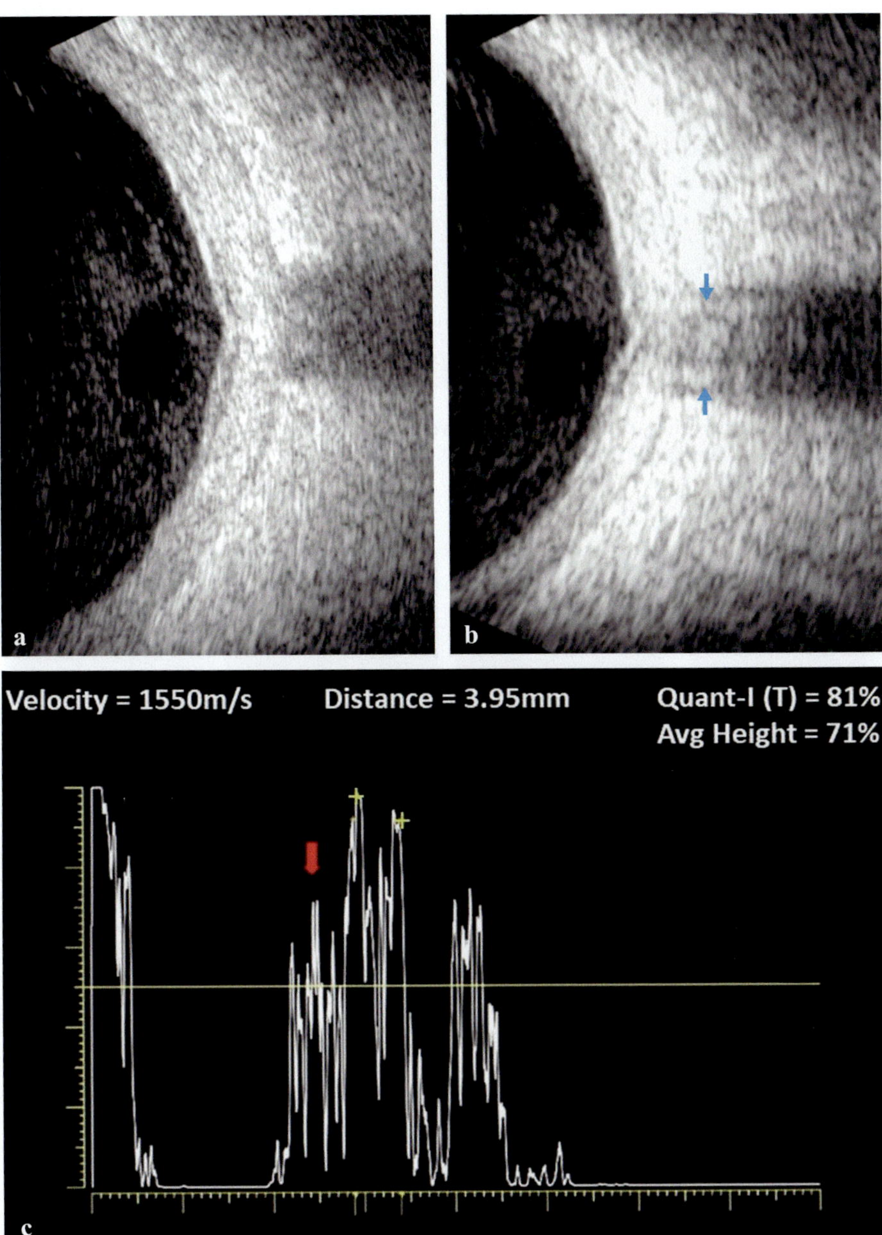

**Fig. 25.15 Terson syndrome. a**: B-mode with a 20 MHz annular probe, retina program; **b**: B-mode with a 15 MHz probe, orbit program; **c**: standardized A-mode, at tissue sensitivity (T = 86.2 dB). Posterior intravitreal hemorrhage, not very mobile after ocular movement (red arrow ➡), associated with slight choroidal thickening (**a**). Slight increase in the size of the optic nerve, with a very echogenic appearance of the hemorrhagic subarachnoid spaces (→ blue arrows) (**b**), more evident in A-mode, where it is measured 3.95 mm (small yellow crosses +) (**c**)

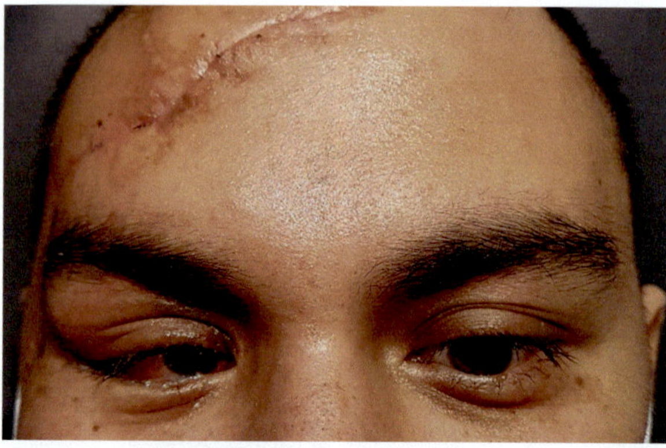

**Fig. 25.16 Incarceration of the right medial rectus muscle** in a fracture of the medial orbital wall after severe craniofacial trauma. It is responsible for esotropia, the incarcerated muscle being entirely immobile

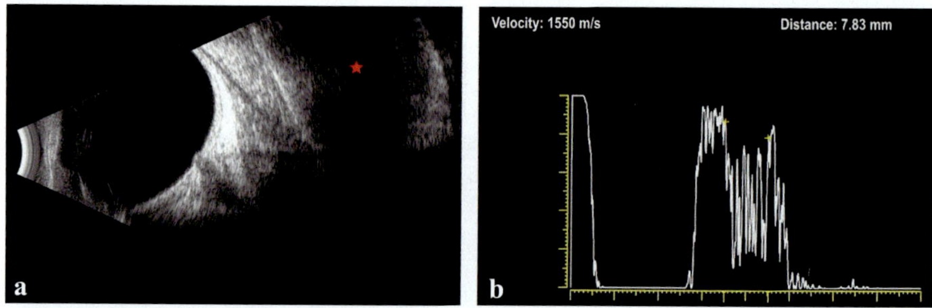



**Fig. 25.17 Incarceration and hematoma of the right medial rectus muscle. a**: B-mode; **b**: standardized A-mode, at tissue sensitivity (T = 86.2 dB). The thickening of the muscle predominates at its belly, measured as 7.83 mm in standardized A-mode (between the yellow crosses +). The hematic muscle has a higher reflectivity than an inflammatory muscle (see Fig. 17.1). Discontinuity of the wall of the orbit can also be seen as well as the ethmoid cell next to it (★ red star), in relation to the hematic content of the sinus

## 25.7 Optic Nerve Trauma

### 25.7.1 Traumatic Optic Neuropathy

Although this is probably underrated, it is one of the most common neurological complications of head injuries [13]. It can result in a loss of visual function, be it partial or total, as well as temporary or permanent. It can be a direct or indirect trauma (the most frequent); direct traumas comprise a wound (by a knife or a projectile), a bone fracture (of the optical canal), or an avulsion or sectioning. Indirect traumas comprise craniofacial contusions, especially frontal, with transmission of force through the bone to the optic canal whereby the shearing effect leads to edema

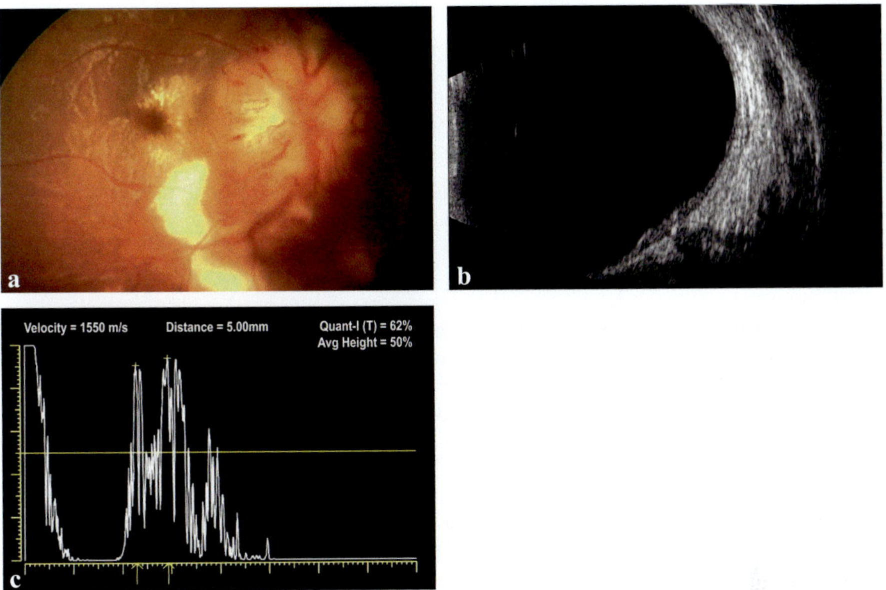

**Fig. 25.18  Post-traumatic neuroretinitis. a**: Appearance of the fundus; **b**: B-mode of the posterior pole; **c**: standardized A-mode of the optic nerve at tissue sensitivity (T = 85.8 dB). Protrusion of the optic disc relatively moderate, but extensive (**b**), compact and homogeneous appearance and distinct widening of the optic nerve, measured at 5 mm (between the yellow crosses +) (**c**) with moderate and homogeneous reflectivity, without attenuation, and with clear delineation in relation to infiltration by inflammatory cells

and hemorrhage. Finally, it can be due to compression, by a hematoma or a subarachnoid hemorrhage (see Figs. 25.13 and 25.15). On ultrasound, measurement of the optic nerve in A-mode indirectly translates to measurement of the intracranial pressure as well as assessment of the superior ophthalmic vein in color Doppler imaging. This correlation is particularly the case and useful in acute situations such as head injuries. However, trauma to the optic nerve can also lead to neuroretinitis, whereby at the level of the nerve itself, there is an enlargement of the nerve of average reflectivity by infiltration of inflammatory cells as well as a papillary protrusion (Fig. 25.18). Unfortunately, consensus is lacking regarding the treatment of such patients [14].

## 25.7.2   Avulsion of the Optic Nerve Head

Avulsion means to tear away by force. It is a rare but serious condition. Secondary to violent trauma, it consists of a sectioning of all or part of the ganglion fibers at the level of the lamina cribosa, responsible for its retraction into the intact dural sheath of the optic nerve. Its pathogenesis is not fully known but probably involves the following mechanism: the usually blunt traumatic agent penetrates the orbit between

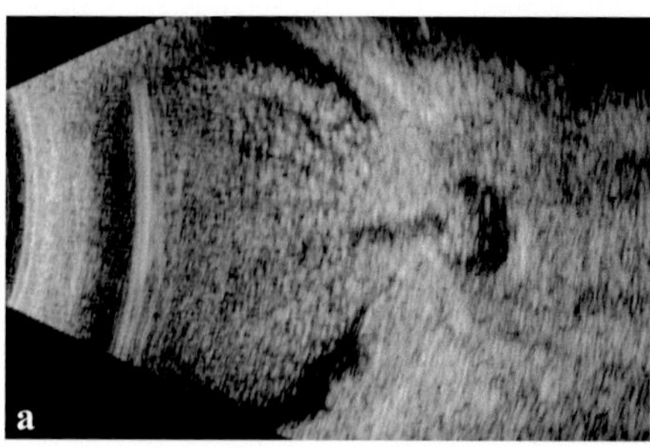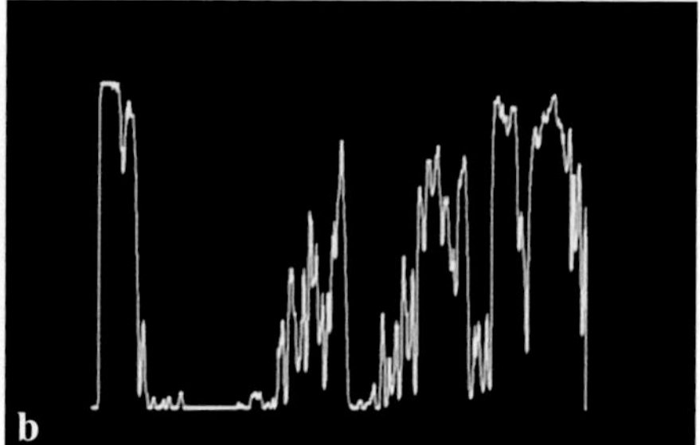

**Fig. 25.19  Avulsion of the optic nerve head**. **a**: B-mode, parasagittal section; **b**: standardized A-mode. In B-mode (**a**), significant intravitreal and parietal hemorrhage with choroidal thickening. The optic disc is disinserted, replaced by an anechoic hole with some echoes inside. In A-mode (**b**), the posterior wall is seen with the sclera, but behind this, the absent optic nerve is replaced by an empty space

the orbital rim and the eyeball, inducing an extreme and forced rotation of the latter, which leads to stretching and tearing of the optic nerve at its emergence from the globe, where the optical fiber support tissue is the least abundant. The diagnosis is easy when the ocular fundus is accessible: the optic disc is then replaced by a hole surrounded by a hemorrhage. Ultrasound is useful (Fig. 25.19) when the hemorrhage is denser [15–17], and color Doppler imaging is also useful for studying the vessels of the optic nerve head [18].

However, the avulsion can also be partial, with an almost normal ultrasound appearance (Fig. 25.20).

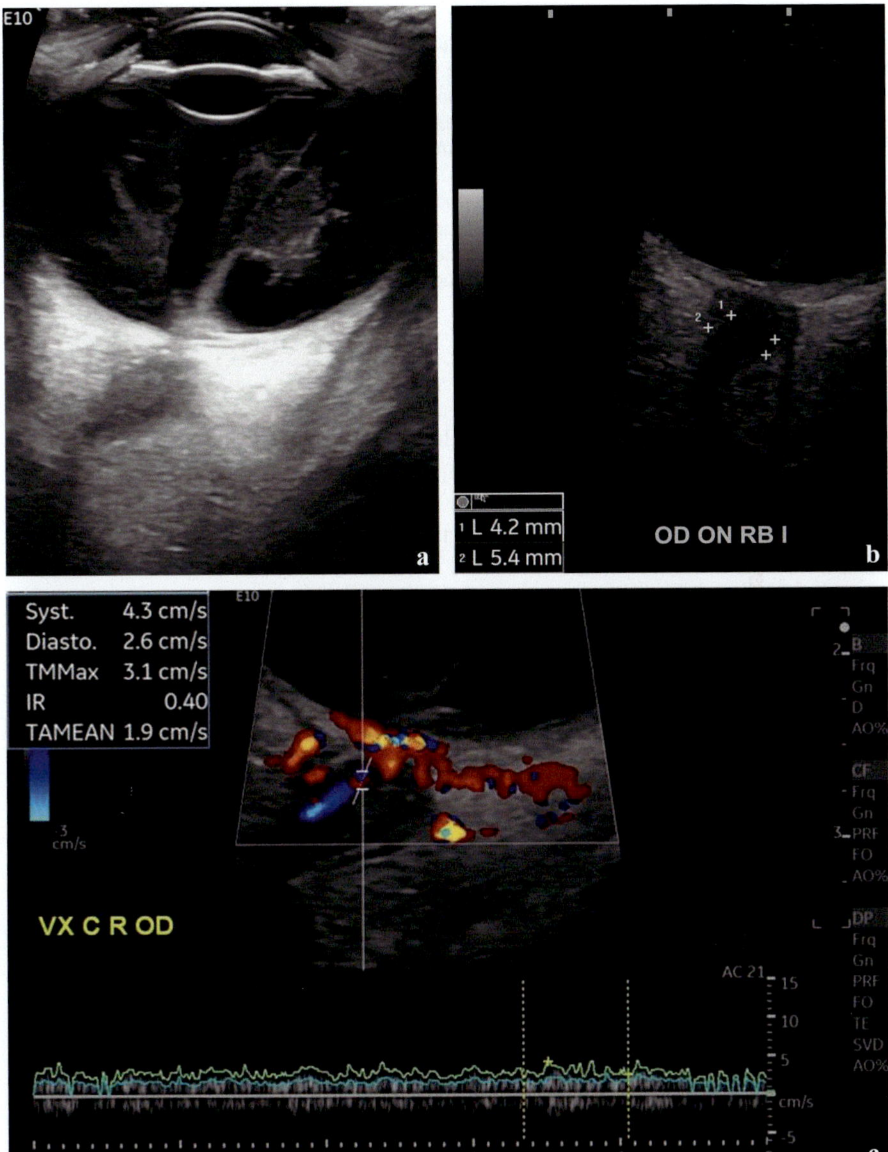
E10
1 L 4.2 mm
2 L 5.4 mm
OD ON RB I
Syst.      4.3 cm/s
Diasto.   2.6 cm/s
TMMax   3.1 cm/s
IR            0.40
TAMEAN 1.9 cm/s
.3
cm/s
VX C R OD
AC 21
a
b
c

◄**Fig. 25.20 Partial avulsion of the optic nerve head of the right eye** after an eye contusion with a wooden spoon in a 2½-year-old child. **a**: B-mode with a multipurpose ultrasound unit and an 8–18 MHz probe at high sensitivity setting; **b**: B-mode of the posterior pole with a reduced sensitivity setting; **c**: CDI, color and spectral modes of the central retinal vessels. A dense and organized intravitreal hemorrhage prevents access to the ocular fundus. Ultrasound detects an inter-maculopapular hematoma. At both high and reduced sensitivity settings, the optic nerve head remains at a distance from the parietal curvature, without individualizable papillary elevation, with normal diameters of the optic nerve behind the lamina cribosa. Finally, severe velocimetric disorders of the central retinal vessels, with a very slow flow even for the age of the child: PSV = 4.3 cm/s (left PSV = 6.9 cm/s) and entirely demodulated, RI = 0.40 (left, RI = 0.57)

## 25.8 Orbital Emphysema

Any fracture of the orbit that connects to the sinus or the nasal cavity can be complicated by pneumo orbit or intraorbital emphysema. This emphysema is most often moderate. When pronounced, it can be the cause of optic neuropathy or occlusion of the central retinal artery, requiring emergency surgical decompression [19]. Usually, it follows the trauma, but it can occur at a later time, after blowing one's nose or by Valsalva maneuver. It can be entirely orbito-palpebral but it is rarely entirely palpebral. When it reaches the eyelids, one can feel a subcutaneous crackling (Fig. 25.21). In the orbit, the air stopping ultrasound results in posterior shadow artifacts (see Figs. 6.6 and 6.15). Unlike the eye, where one can make an air bubble move, the air in the orbit is motionless and, therefore, one cannot explore the orbit in case of pneumo orbit or even adequately estimate its volume.

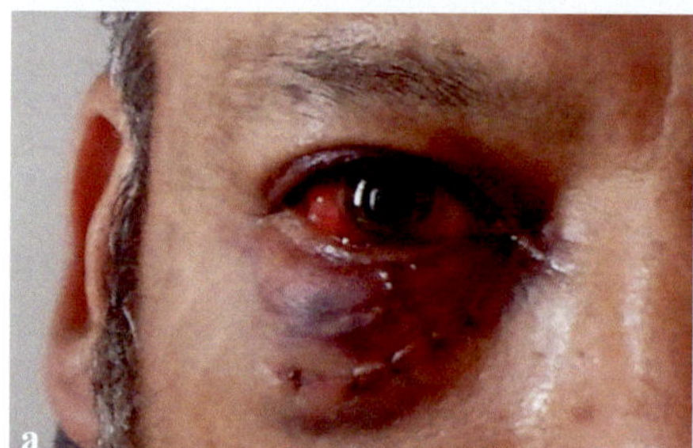
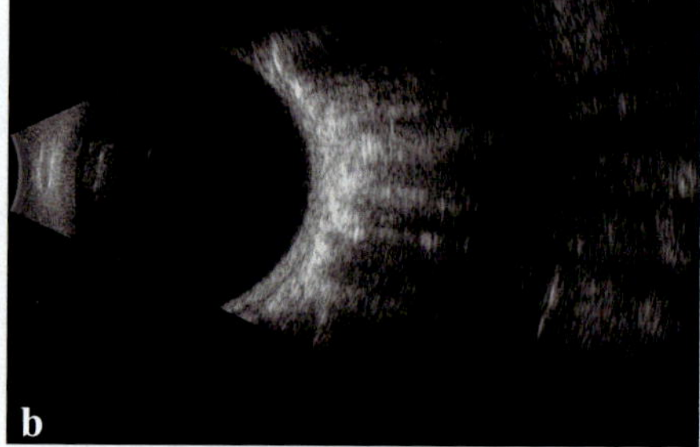

**Fig. 25.21 Orbito-palpebral emphysema**. **a**: Clinical presentation; **b**: B-mode exploring the retrobulbar space. Patient with a sutured facial trauma and fracture of the medial wall of the orbit. Palpable subcutaneous emphysema in the inferior eyelid and around the scar (**a**). The numerous air bubbles result in multiple posterior shadowing cones completely preventing assessment of the orbit

# References


1. Chandler JR, Langenbrunner DJ, Stevens ER. The pathogenesis of orbital complications in acute sinusitis Laryngoscope. 1970;80(9):1414–28.
2. Mouriaux F, Rysanek B, Babin E, Cattoir V. Cellulite orbitaire. J Fr Ophtalmol. 2012;35(1):52–7.
3. Haas H, Lorrot M, Hentgen V, Cohen R, Grimprel E. Antibiothérapie des infections ORL sévères du nourrisson et de l'enfant: sinusites aiguës compliquées Arch Pediatr. 2013;20 Suppl 3:e5–9.
4. Van der Veer EG, van der Poel NA, de Win MML, Kloos RJ, et al. True abscess formation is rare in bacterial orbital cellulitis; consequences for treatment Am J Otolaryngol. 2017;38(2):130–4.
5. Spector RH. Echography in carotid-cavernous fistulas. In: Hillman JS, Le May MM, editors. Ophthalmic ultrasonography: proceedings of the 9th SIDUO Congress, Leeds, U.K. July 20–23, 1982. Springer Science & Business Media; 2012, pp. 399–405
6. Kondoff M, Georges Nassrallah G, Ross M, Deschênes J. Incidence and outcomes of retrobulbar hematoma diagnosed by computed tomography in cases of orbital fracture. Can J Ophthalmol. 2019;54(5):606–10.
7. Orlandi D, Sconfienza LM, Lacelli F, Bertolotto M, et al. Ultrasound-guided core-needle biopsy of extra-ocular orbital lesions Eur Radiol. 2013;23(7):1919–24.
8. Kuhn F, Morris R, Witherspoon CD, Mester V. Terson syndrome. Results of vitrectomy and the significance of vitreous hemorrhage in patients with subarachnoid hemorrhage. Ophthalmology. 1998;105(3):472–7.
9. Nazarali S, Kherani I, Hurley B, Williams G, et al. Outcome of vitrectomy in Terson syndrome: a multicenter Canadian perspective. Retina. 2020;40(7):1325–30.
10. Czorlich P, Burkhardt T, Knospe V, Richard R, et al. Ocular ultrasound as an easy applicable tool for detection of Terson's syndrome after aneurysmal subarachnoid hemorrhage. PLoS One 2014;9(12):e114907.
11. Weingeist TA, Goldman EJ, Folk JC, Packer AJ, Ossoinig KC. Terson's syndrome. Clinico-pathologic correlations Ophthalmol. 1986;93(11):1435–42.
12. Adenis JP, Morax S. Pathologie orbito-palpébrale. Rapport de la Société Française d'Ophtalmologie. Paris: Masson; 1998.
13. Le Guern A, Marks-Delesalle C, Vasseur V, Defoort-Dhelemmes S, et al. Neuropathies optiques post-traumatiques: à propos de 8 cas et revue de la littérature. J Fr Ophtalmol. 2016;39(7):603–8.
14. Steinsapir KD, Goldberg RA. Traumatic optic neuropathy: an evolving understanding. Am J Ophthalmol. 2011;151(6):928–33.e2.
15. Talwar D, Kumar A, Verma L, Tewari HK, Khosla PK. Ultrasonography in optic nerve head avulsion. Acta Ophthalmol (Copenh). 1991;69(1):121–3.
16. Espaillat A, To K. Optic nerve avulsion. Arch Ophthalmol. 1998;116:540–1.
17. El Kettani A, Benhaddou M, Hamdani M, Amraoui A, Zaghloul K. L'avulsion du nerf optique. J Fr Ophtalmol. 2005;28(8):872.e1–4.
18. Foster BS, March GA, Lucarelli MJ, Samiy N, Lesselle S. Optic nerve avulsion. Arch Ophthalmol. 1997;115:623–30.
19. Gloaguen Y, Cochard-Marianowski C, Potard G, Rogez F, Meriot P, Cochener B. Emphysème orbitaire post-traumatique: à propos d'un cas. J Fr Ophtalmol. 2006;29(8):942.e1–4.

# Chapter 26
# Orbital Masses in Children

Monique Elmaleh-Bergès and Olivier Bergès

**Abstract** Orbital masses in children have different etiologies than in adults. In newborns and infants, when the eye is abnormal, one must consider a colobomatous cyst of the optic nerve or a teratoma, and if the eye is normal, cysts arising from adjacent structures, such as dacryo(cysto)celes and meningocencephaloceles, or vascular lesions, such as infantile hemangioma (benign hemangioendothelioma/ capillary angioma) and lymphangioma, or venous-lymphatic malformations. In older children, malignant tumors are more common, for which ultrasound is less relevant: rhabdomyosarcoma, lymphoproliferative lesions (various forms of histiocytosis, orbital involvement of leukemias, lymphomas), and neuroblastoma metastases. However, one should not forget the possibility of dermoid and epidermoid cysts, nerve tumors (gliomas of the optic nerve, neurofibromas and schwannomas) and vascular lesions (lymphangiomas or venous-lymphatic malformations, vascular malformations). Finally, inflammatory exophthalmos requires first ruling out rhabdomyosarcoma. In case of acute ethmoiditis, ultrasound when performed first, may detect a retroseptal extension.

## 26.1 Introduction

The etiologies of orbital masses in children differ from those in adults [1]. The frequency of malignant/benign lesions varies according to age:

- in newborns and infants, mainly "vascular" tumors and malformative pathologies are observed.
- in older children, malignant tumors are more common.

M. Elmaleh-Bergès
Robert Debré University Hospital, Paris, France

O. Bergès (✉)
Rothschild Foundation Hospital, Paris, France
e-mail: oberges@for.paris



O. Bergès (ed.), *Echography of the Eye and Orbit*,
https://doi.org/10.1007/978-3-031-41467-1_26

The most common clinical sign is exophthalmos, which occurs more rapidly than in adults because of a smaller space between the globe and the bone orbit [2]. Imaging has an important role in diagnosis and therapeutic management.

Of course, ultrasound appears to be the "ideal" technique in children, as it is non-irradiating, and most often does not require sedation. But it readily reaches its limitations in orbital pathology: Indeed, it does not allow for assessing the orbital bone framework (such as CT scan) or retrobulbar, facial, or intracranial extension assessment of voluminous lesions (such as MRI). Nevertheless, its contribution is undeniable and often even sufficient in the diagnosis of small orbital and periorbital lesions, in particular with the assessment of vascularization by color Doppler imaging (CDI) [3–6].

## 26.2 Technique

Sedation is less frequently necessary for orbital ultrasound, than for assessment of the eye, but is still required before 5 years of age if CDI with detailed analysis of vascular velocimetric constants is to be performed [7]. General anesthesia is rarely performed for ultrasound alone, but this can be coupled with a clinical examination and/or MRI. Unlike for adults, for children, topical corneal anesthesia is not useful, but it is advisable to use lukewarm contact gel (at body temperature), the same as for adults: 0.2% carbomer ophthalmic gel (Lacrygel® Europhta, or Lacrynorm® Chauvin).

The examination must always be bilateral and comparative and begin with biometry: B-mode guided, easy to perform, through the eyelids and not with simplified immersion, certainly a little less precise, but nonetheless useful and reliable.

The orbit is first studied at a reduced sensitivity setting, but there is also merit in assessing poorly echogenic lesions with a high sensitivity setting (and to compare them to the vitreous). This helps separate hypoechoic from anechoic lesions. CDI is always useful, either to show the absence of flows within a process, or to study these if the process is vascularized and, in all cases, to assess the impact of the mass on the oculo-orbital vascularization.

## 26.3 Lesions

Most of the lesions presented in this chapter have largely been discussed previously, particularly in the chapters on vascular tumors, optic and peri-optic nerve masses, cysts and malignant tumors. Table 26.1 proposes a classification of orbit tumors [2], but the clinical aspects and the relevance of ultrasound for diagnosis have guided us in the layout of this chapter, by separating the lesions in newborns and infants from those in older children.

**Table 26.1**  Childhood orbital tumors from Ben Hadj Hamida and Morax [2]

| **Primary orbital tumors** |
| --- |

**Mesenchymal (muscular) tumors**
- Rhabdomyosarcoma

**Bone lesions**
- Fibrous dysplasia
- Fibrous dysplasia + precocious puberty, + café-au-lait skin pigmentation: McCune-Albright syndrome
- Ossifying fibroma
- Aneurysmal bone cyst
- Osteoblastoma
- Osteosarcoma
- Ewing's sarcoma

**Lymphoproliferative lesions** (orbital localizations of a systemic disease or hemopathy)
- Histiocytosis X
      Eosinophilic granuloma
      Hand-Schüller-Christian disease
      Letterer-Siwe disease
- Rarer histiocytic and granulomatous lesions
      Sinus histiocytosis
      Juvenile xanthogranuloma
      Erdheim-Chester disease
      Sarcoidosis
      Fibrous histiocytoma
- Leukemias (chlorhoma)
- Lymphomas

**Nerve tumors**
- Optic nerve glioma
- Tumor of peripheral nerves (neurofibromas, schwannomas)

**Vascular lesions**
- Vascular tumors
      Lymphangiomas
      Capillary/infantile hemangioma
- Vascular malformations
      Varix
      Fistulas

**Cystic tumors and et ectopias**
- Dermoid and epidermoid cysts
- Colobomatous cyst
- Meningoencephalocele
- Teratoma
- Hydatid cyst
- Orbital mucocele
- Orbital hematoma

**Rare tumors**
- Liposarcoma, fibrosarcoma
- Primary orbital melanoma

(continued)

**Table 26.1** (continued)

| Orbital inflammations |
| --- |

| **Metastatic tumors** |
| --- |
| – Neuroblastoma |
| – Ganglioneuromas |

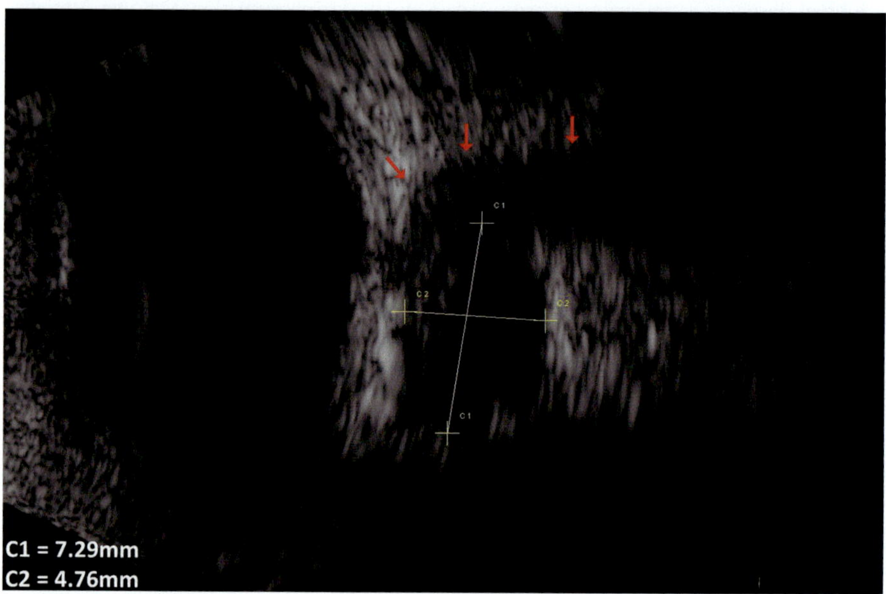


**Fig. 26.1 Small colobomatous cyst of the left optic nerve associated with severe microphthalmia**. B-mode parasagittal section according to the 7:30 o'clock meridian. The eye is microphthalmic: AL OS = 12.2 mm versus AL OD = 18.9 mm. The cyst is located under the optic nerve in the nasal inferior quadrant, measures 7.3 mm high × 4.2 mm deep, and pushes the optic nerve (→ red arrows) slightly upward

## 26.3.1 In Newborns and Infants

### 26.3.1.1 With an Abnormal Eye Examination

Colobomatous Cyst

(See Chaps. 14, 18 and 23).

These are most often located at the infero-nasal part of the orbit, in contact with the optic nerve (Fig. 26.1), the eye being more or less severely microphthalmic [8].

These elements are clearly seen in ultrasound (see Fig. 14.30). Sometimes large, the cyst can collapse the septum and manifest clinically as a bluish mass of the lower eyelid that can be incorrectly interpreted as a vascular mass (see Fig. 18.17). On imaging, it appears as a cystic, non-vascularized mass. A CT scan helps to set the indications of the surgical procedure and to specify the technique, in order to preserve the growth of the orbital cavity. The indication is mainly aesthetic, as visual acuity is usually always very poor [9], **MRI looks for associated intracranial abnormalities, including midline malformations.**

These orbital malformative cysts of childhood must be differentiated from acquired cysts (vascular, epithelial, infectious, and parasitic) and cysts from adjacent periorbital structures, mainly mucoceles and meningoceles (see Chap. 23) [10].


Teratoma

Teratomas [11], also called dysembryomas or dysembryoplastic tumors, are tumors that develop from primary germ cells. They are a rare type of congenital tumor, for which the diagnosis can sometimes be made antenatally. Depending on the stage of differentiation of the tumor, the diagnosis can be:

- **immature teratomas,** also called teratocarcinomas, which are solid, malignant tumors;
- **mature teratomas**, which are benign and cystic tumors;
- **mixed teratomas**.

The imaging assessment uses MRI and CT scan. However, ultrasound can reveal a moderately to mildly echogenic lesion, with calcifications and cystic areas. These lesions can be diagnosed at an early age (Fig. 26.2). Treatment consists of complete surgical excision, which sometimes requires exenteration. For mature forms, the long-term prognosis is good.


### 26.3.1.2  With a Normal Eye Examination

**26.3.1.2.1 Cysts**. These have been discussed in Chap. 23.

- dacryo(cysto)celes: these can be discovered antenatally; they manifest after birth as a mass of the medial canthus, inferior to the lacrimal puncta, and can clinically suggest hemangioma. They are rounded usually large lesions, protruding to a certain degree (Fig. 26.3), cystic, with a hypoechoic content that is most often homogeneous but that may contain moderately echogenic debris due to mucus stasis and without Doppler flow (see Fig. 23.9).
- meningoencephalocele: unlike dacryocystocele, it appears as a mass of the upper part of the medial canthus. It is a cystic or mixed fluid–solid mass. Due to the ill-defined posterior boundary on ultrasound, a complementary MRI is required.

**26.3.1.2.2 Vascular lesions**. These have been discussed in Chap. 20. In newborns and infants, we can consider:

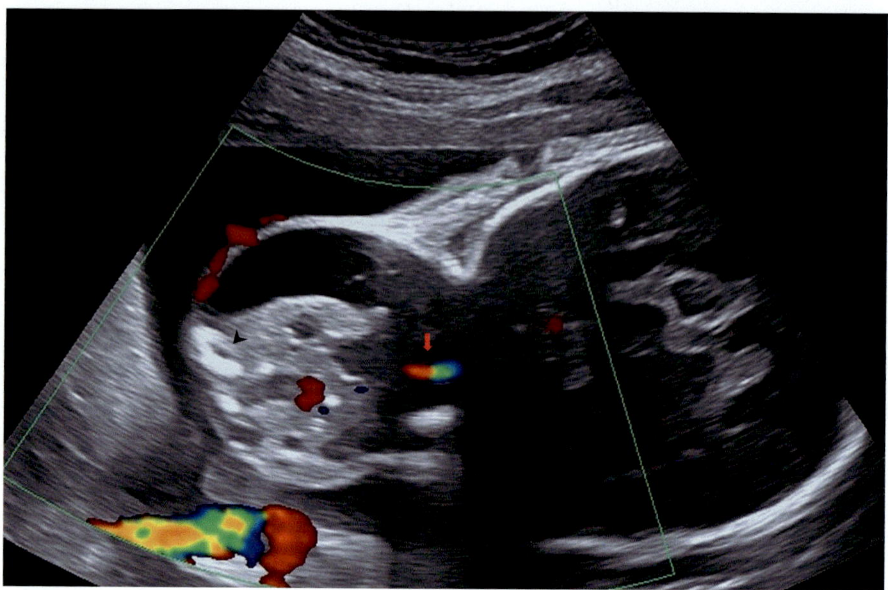

**Fig. 26.2** **Left orbital teratoma**. Fetal ultrasound. Very large mass, measuring 77 mm × 72 mm, occupying the entire orbit, and protruding widely from the face, very heterogeneous, with cystic areas and solid portions (with vessels [→ red arrow] and calcifications[arrowhead])

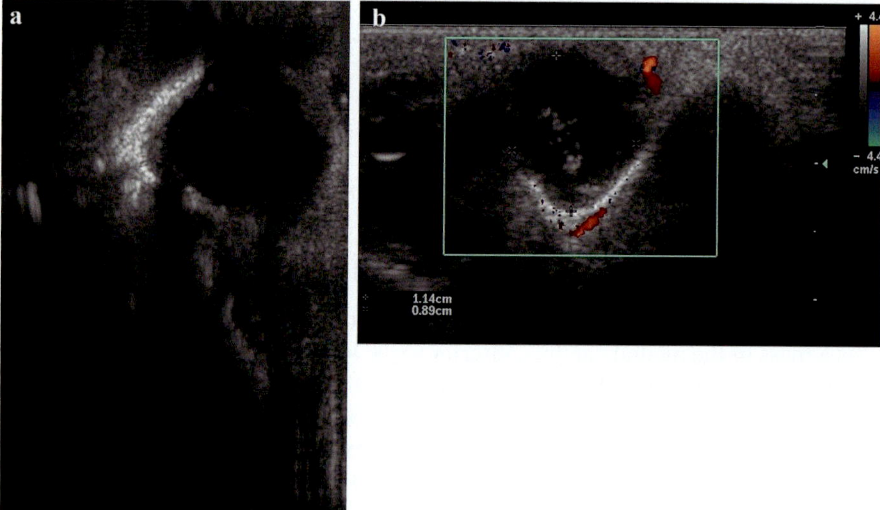

**Fig. 26.3** **Voluminous dacryocystocele in a 10-day-old newborn**. **a**: B-mode parasagittal section; **b**: CDI, axial section of the dilated lacrimal sac. Significant expansion of the lacrimal sac, measuring approximately 10 mm in diameter. This sac is hypoechoic, with the presence of some moderately echogenic debris due to mucus and/or superinfection. Absence of intrinsic flow. Slight dilation of the nasolacrimal duct, which cannot be followed over a long distance due to the bony wall

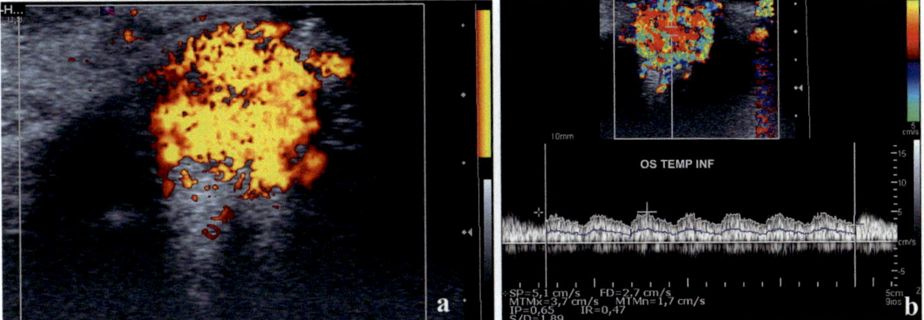

**Fig. 26.4 Small infantile hemangioma of the lower eyelid. a**: CDI, power mode; **b**: CDI, color and spectral modes. The mass, measuring 7 mm × 10 mm × 13 mm, is hypervascular with low resistive flows: RI = 0.47

- infantile hemangioma, also called benign infant hemangioendothelioma, and capillary angioma. CDI reveals a hypervascular lesion, with a low RI affirming the diagnosis (Fig. 26.4); this presentation is characteristic at this age and is sufficient to indicate beta-blocker treatment depending on the clinical findings (see Fig. 20.17)
- lymphangioma, or venous-lymphatic malformation. Their appearance is identical in infants and older children (see below).

## 26.3.2   In Older Children

### 26.3.2.1   Rhabdomyosarcoma (RMS)

This is a malignant tumor of mesenchymal origin whose cells reproduce, in an anarchic manner, the different stages of muscle differentiation [2, 11]. These are rare tumors, but RMS is the most common malignant mesenchymal tumor in children and adolescents. The average age of occurrence is 7 to 8 years of age. The progression is rapid, with often an inflammatory exophthalmos. This is a therapeutic **emergency**, and, therefore, ultrasound is rarely performed. MRI ± CT scan must be performed without delay to properly assess the lesion, especially to probe for parameningeal extension or at the level of the nasal cavity (which darkens the prognosis).

When performed, ultrasound reveals a hypoechoic (Fig. 26.5) and firm lesion that can deform the ocular wall and is heterogeneous; this heterogeneous nature is even more evident in A-mode (see Fig. 24.3).

On Doppler, the lesion is highly vascularized with fairly resistive flows, with an RI > 0.70 (Fig. 26.6).

A biopsy must also be urgently performed: the most common form is embryonic rhabdomyosarcoma, which has a better prognosis than the alveolar form. Recent

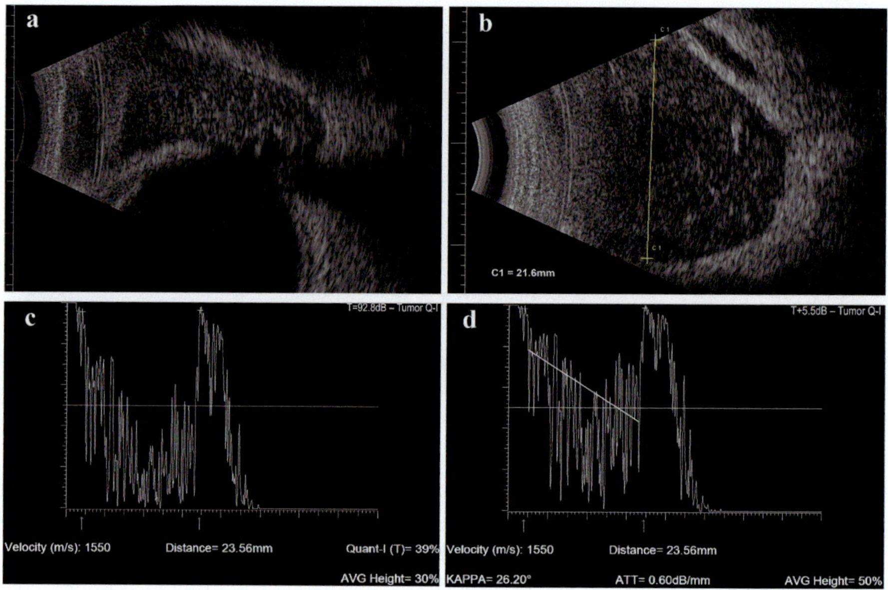



**Fig. 26.5 Superior orbito-palpebral rhabdomyosarcoma. a**: B-mode, paraocular sagittal section; **b**: B-mode, paraocular axial section; **c**: standardized A-mode at tissue sensitivity, T = 92.8 dB, for assessing the reflectivity; **d**: standardized A-mode, with average peak height at 50% for assessing the attenuation. Voluminous hypoechoic mass (39% in Quantification-I) and heterogeneous, (high variability in the height of peaks) of the upper eyelid and the superior extraconal space, measuring 24.8 mm × 21.6 mm in diameter × 9 mm in height

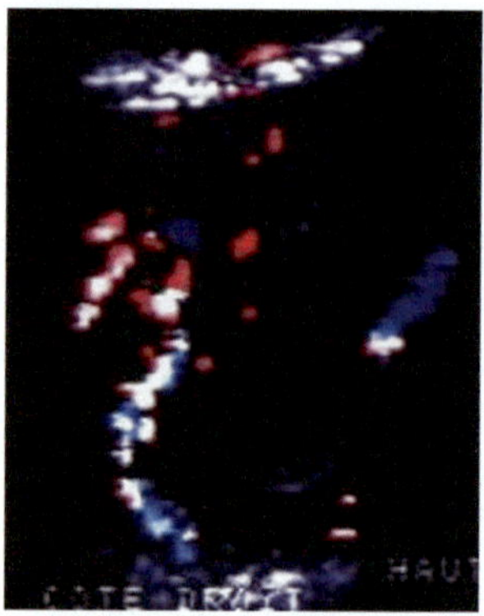

**Fig. 26.6 Rhabdomyosarcoma**. CDI: highly vascularized, hypoechoic mass

treatments, combining chemotherapy ± orbital radiotherapy allow for 90% survival [12, 13].

**Finally, one must systematically consider rhabdomyosarcoma with any inflammatory orbital mass in a child.**

### 26.3.2.2   Lymphoproliferative Lesions

These are the orbital localizations of a systemic disease or hemopathy. For all these conditions, ultrasound is of little use and rarely performed. These lesions can include the following:

- a form of histiocytosis X [14]: eosinophilic granuloma, Hand–Schuller–Christian disease or Apt–Letterer–Siwe disease.
- rarer histiocytic and granulomatous lesions: sinus histiocytosis with massive lymphadenopathy (Rosai–Dorfman) [15]; juvenile xanthogranulomatoma (already discussed in Chap. 13 for its anterior uveal form), which can have orbital localizations [16]; and finally sarcoidosis (see Chap. 17).

Orbital Involvement During Leukemia

These represent a non-exceptional cause of exophthalmos. They are more common in acute than chronic forms and in myeloid than lymphoblastic forms. *Myeloid sarcoma* (sometimes called granulocytic sarcoma or chloroma) is a greenish, solid malignant tumor of myeloid cells and is localized outside the bone marrow; it is frequently located in the orbit.

Clinical signs include exophthalmos, eyelid edema, chemosis, and pain. The condition can be uni- or bilateral. Exophtalmos can be related to the presence of a mass consisting of leukemia cells or to orbital hemorrhage. Orbital involvement is often present in the terminal phase of the disease but can sometimes be the telling sign [17]. Ultrasound reveals a voluminous hypoechoic mass, often extra- and intraconal, quite heterogeneous, poorly delineated, with visible vessels on Doppler. MRI is essential to analyze the extent of the lesion.

Lymphomas

Lymphoproliferative diseases are rare in children. Childhood lymphomas are mostly diagnosed after 5 years of age. Ultrasound is not sufficient for the diagnosis; it is rarely performed, but may reveal a mass with low echogenicity, often homogeneous, with visible vessels on Doppler. MRI allows for assessing the lesion and its extension and for reaching the indication of biopsy for histological evaluation with immunohistochemical typing.

In children, Burkitt lymphoma is the most common (Fig. 26.7); lymphoblastic lymphoma and anaplastic large-cell lymphoma are rarer. These are three aggressive,

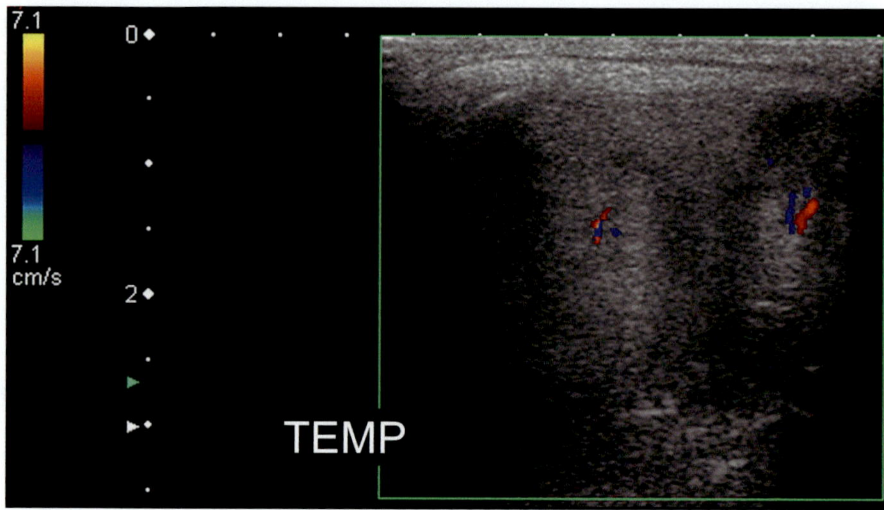


**Fig. 26.7 Burkitt lymphoma**. CDI: poorly delineated, hypoechoic, orbito-palpebral mass with some vessels

rapidly progressing non-Hodgkin lymphomas. Endemic Burkitt lymphoma occurs mainly in Africa. It is almost always associated with Epstein-Barr virus infection.

### 26.3.2.3 Neuroblastoma Metastases

In children, the most common malignant lesions are secondary locations (leukemias, metastatic neuroblastoma) [11]. In 90% of cases, neuroblastoma is diagnosed before 5 years of age. The primary tumor is most often diagnosed before the onset of orbital metastasis, but metastasis is revealing in 10% of cases. Clinically, rapidly progressing bilateral exophthalmos associated with bilateral periorbital ecchymosis (raccoon eyes) indicates Hutchinson syndrome. Neuroblastoma is a malignant tumor of the sympathetic nervous system. The primary tumor can be located in the adrenal glands or other retroperitoneal structures but also in the lymphatic system of the neck, mediastinum, and pelvis. Abdominal ultrasound can be used to search for adrenal lesions and hepatic localization (Pepper syndrome). When the orbital ultrasound reveals a hypoechoic and vascularized lesion (Fig. 26.8), in a child, a hematological localization or metastatic neuroblastoma must be considered and an abdominal ultrasound should be performed. Assessment of the extension is based on MRI and/or CT scan.

Ewing's sarcoma, less common, can also cause orbital metastases.

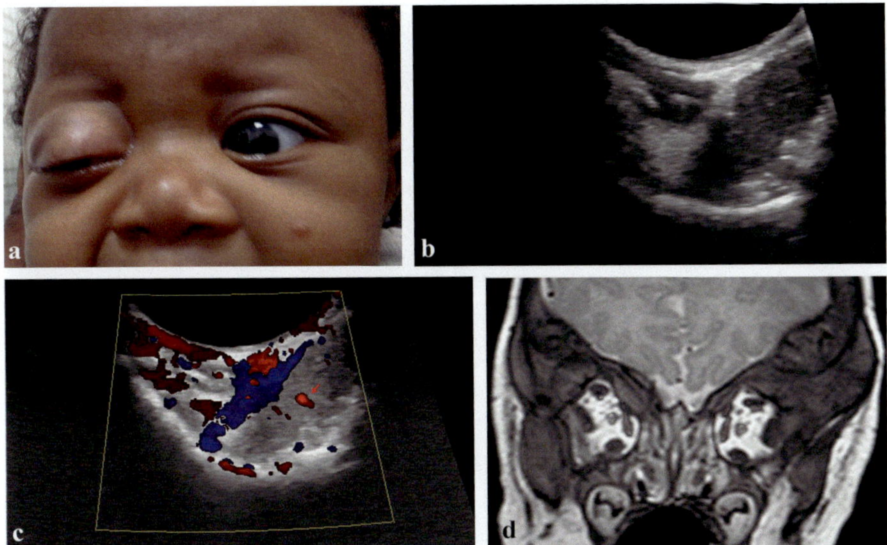

**Fig. 26.8  Metastasis of neuroblastoma. a**: clinical aspect: voluminous right exophthalmos with ptosis and hemorrhage in the superior eyelid, equating Hutchinson syndrome; **b**: B-mode: large, hypoechoic, poorly delineated mass in the superior temporal region; **c**: CDI; despite numerous motion-related artifacts, there is at least one obvious vessel (→ red arrow) within the hypoechoic mass; **d**: MRI, T2 weighted coronal section: clearly showing the impressive extent of the bone involvement of the orbital walls and the skull base, naturally not visualized on ultrasound

### 26.3.2.4   Cystic Lesions

Dermoid cysts are the most common type of cystic lesion in children [18], so we chose to present examples in this chapter rather than in the one devoted to cystic lesions (Chap. 24).

### Dermoid and Epidermoid Cysts

These are congenital choristomas (normal tissue formation with abnormal localization) discovered most often before 10 years of age that tend to develop in the superolateral quadrant of the orbit or at the tail of the eyebrow. Histologically, they are surrounded by epithelium and contain sebaceous glands, hair follicles, keratin, and cholesterol [19]. Ultrasound should be performed before considering surgical removal of the lesion to ensure no bone damage or posterior intraorbital or intracranial extension. This ultrasound reveals a lesion of variable echotexture, anechoic or moderately echogenic, sometimes heterogeneous with anechoic portions, but in any case, with no Doppler-detectable intrinsic flow, but with sometimes visibility of normal vessels around the cyst (Fig. 26.9).

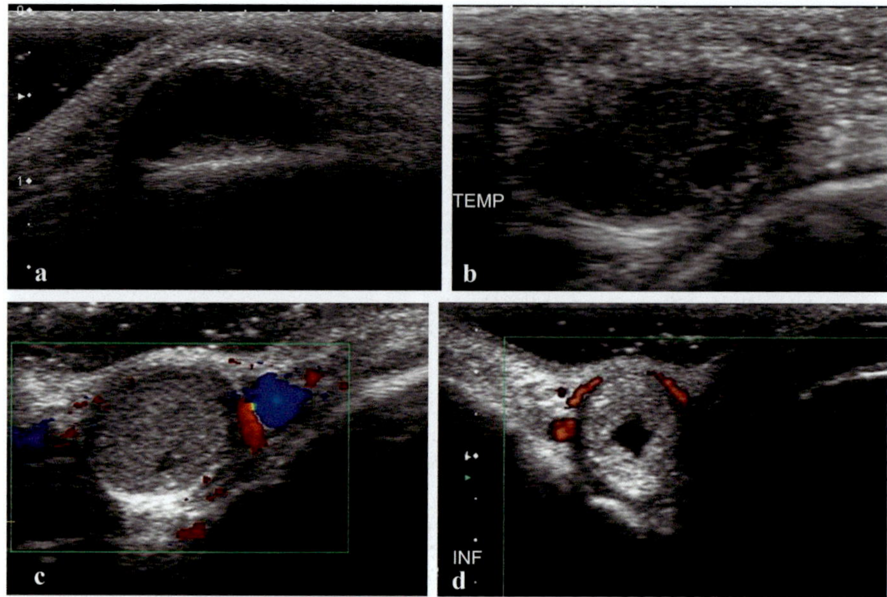



**Fig. 26.9** **Small periorbital dermoid cysts. a**, **b** (B-mode) and **c** (color Doppler imaging), cysts located at the tail of the eyebrow; **d**: CDI, power mode of a cyst located at the medial canthus. The echotexture is hypoechoic (**a**) or moderately echogenic with a small hypoechoic nodule in the center (**b**, **c** and **d**). On Doppler (**c** and **d**), flows at the periphery of the cyst can be seen

If the lesion is not clinically mobile, if its limits are poorly defined, or if it is located in the medial canthus or retrobulbar space (Fig. 26.10), complementation of the ultrasound with MRI ± CT scan is indicated [20]. The excision should be complete and the cyst removed as a whole because intraoperative rupture of the cyst could be responsible for a secondary inflammatory reaction.

The other cysts, meningoencephalocele, parasitic cysts, mucocele and orbital hematoma, have been discussed in Chap. 23.

### 26.3.2.5　Nerve Tumors

These can be gliomas of the optic nerve (see Chap. 18) or tumors of peripheral nerves, neurofibromas and schwannomas (see Chap. 20). For all these lesions, ultrasound is rarely performed, with MRI preferred.

### 26.3.2.6　Vascular Lesions

- **26.3.2.6.1 Tumors (Lymphangiomas or Venous-Lymphatic Malformations)**

These have been discussed in Chap. 20. They can be discovered in the antenatal

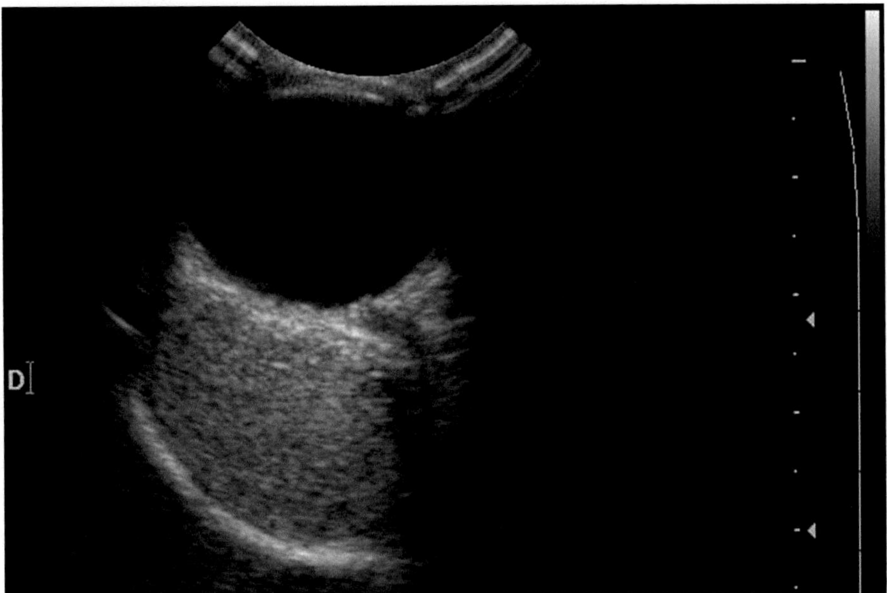

**Fig. 26.10 Large retrobulbar dermoid cyst**. The highly echogenic nature already indicated a fatty content, and there was no intrinsic flow in Doppler, and a preoperative MRI confirmed this hypothesis

or perinatal period, but they occur most often in older children at the time of the first complications. These are infiltrating tumors consisting of ducts surrounded by an endothelium, the appearance of which is similar to that of the lymphatic ducts. Progressive flares of exophthalmos can be observed with nasopharyngeal infection. There is often enlargement of the orbit. Because of the poorly systematized nature of the lesion, ultrasound has great difficulties in seeing the entire lesion (Fig. 26.11) and assessing its extension.

The appearance in imaging is often multicystic, and the solid part of the mass only sometimes exhibits flows on CDI (see Figs. 20.2 and 20.3). However, ultrasound can reveal intracystic hemorrhages (chocolate cysts) that frequently complicate this lesion (see Fig. 23.5). The problem is both esthetic and functional. Surgical removal of the tumor is difficult because of its infiltrative nature.

- **26.3.2.6.2 Vascular malformations**

These are the same as in adults (see Chap. 20).

- varicose vein
- fistula; post-traumatic fistulas can occur naturally in older children; dural fistulas are rare in children (Fig. 26.12). However, diagnosis should be considered in case of suggestive clinical and ultrasound signs.

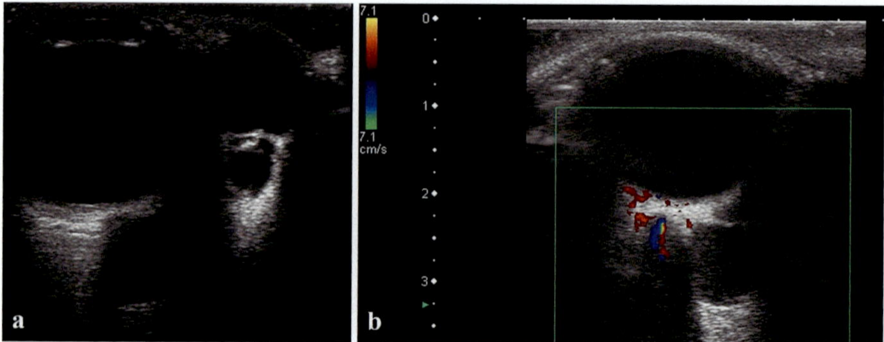

**Fig. 26.11 Left orbital lymphangioma in a 7½-year-old child**. **a**: B-mode axial section, revealing two liquid periocular extraconal lesions and one intraconal lesion; **b**: CDI axial section of the optic nerve head and the intraconal lesion, which is poorly echogenic and non-anechoic because of a hemorrhagic rearrangement and does not present any intrinsic flow

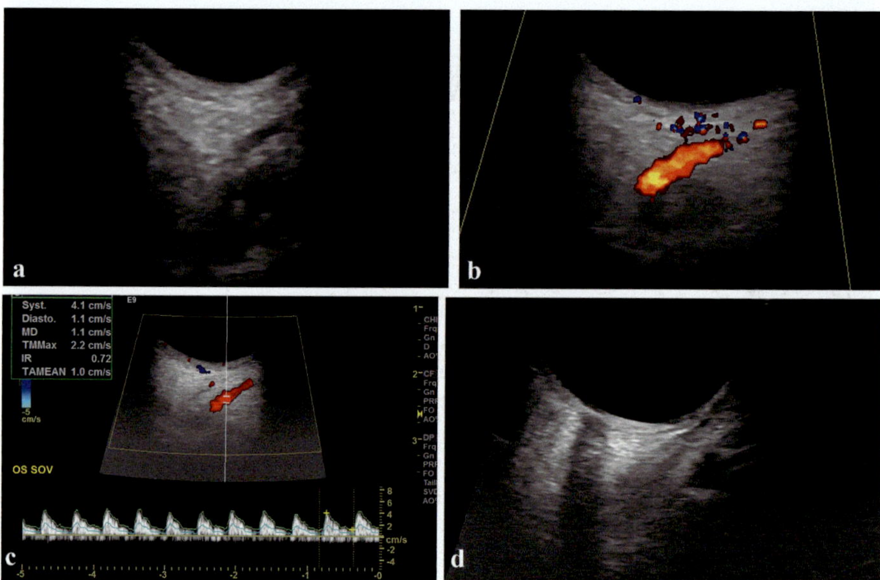

**Fig. 26.12 Cavernous sinus dural fistula** in a 1-year-old child with small left exophthalmos, discrete conjunctival hyperemia, and orbital pain. **a**: B-mode, para-axial section superior to the optic nerve; **b**: CDI, color mode, same incidence; **c**: CDI, color and spectral modes of the superior ophthalmic vein: slight increase in volume of the superior ophthalmic vein, circulating in the opposite direction, anterograde, coded in red in color mode and arterialized with a rather low PSV (4.1 cm/s) and a rather high RI (0.72) compared to the fistulas observed in adulthood (compare with Figs. 20.24 and 20.25); **d**: B-mode, 9 o'clock meridian OS: clear increase in volume of the medial rectus muscle (and other extraocular muscles), measuring 4.7 mm for the largest diameter, the muscle is more echogenic than normal in relation to the blood stasis caused by the fistula

### 26.3.2.7  Inflammations

The same causes are found as in adults (see Chap. 17). However, again, any rapidly progressing inflammatory exophthalmos requires ruling out rhabdomyosarcoma.

### 26.3.2.8  Cellulitis and Abscesses

These can occur after trauma (see Chap. 25), but they are mainly complications of sinusitis [21]. Acute ethmoiditis is suspected with febrile unilateral periorbital edema. When the infiltration is pre-septal, the prognosis is most often good with medical treatment. However, with retroseptal collection, there is a functional and life-threatening risk, requiring management in a surgical setting depending on the size of the lesion. If the clinical signs of retroseptal involvement (proptosis, decrease in visual acuity, oculomotor palsy) are not obvious, ultrasound may help for affirming or refuting retroseptal, extension especially in infants (Fig. 26.13).

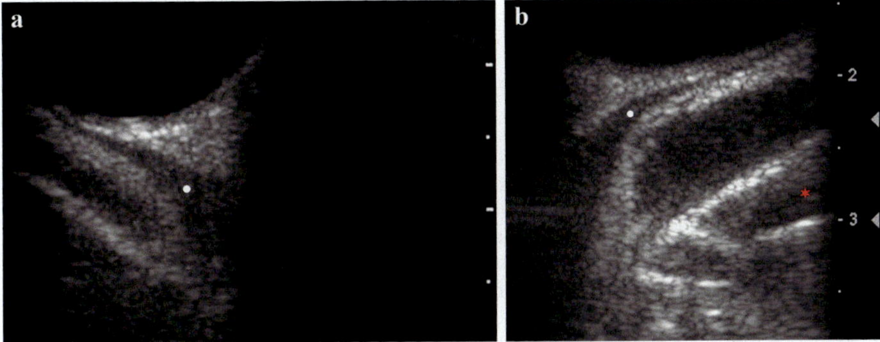

**Fig. 26.13  Two cases of orbital cellulitis with subperiosteal abscess. a:** The abscess is small in volume, 7 mm thick, likely to be monitored under medical treatment; **b:** voluminous abscess, 17 mm thick, with visualization of infected ethmoid cells (⋆ red star), requiring CT scan before surgical drainage. In both cases, the medial rectus muscle (● small white circle) is repressed, at a distance from the medial wall of the orbit

If the retroseptal extension is substantial, then CT scan with contrast is necessary, which allows for assessing the intra-orbital process: cellulitis, or subperiosteal abscess to be drained surgically, accurate measurement of the exophthalmos (overestimated by edema), visualization of the sinus walls and cavities, and to search for complications (thrombosis of the superior ophthalmic vein and/or the cavernous sinus, or intracranial complications [abscess, empyema]).

Finally, orbital cellulitis can be secondary to a tumor process evolving in an inflammatory setting: mucocele, dermoid cyst, retinoblastoma, rhabdomyosarcoma, etc.

# References


1. Henderson JW. Orbital tumors, 3rd ed. New York: Raven Press; 1994.
2. Ben Hadj Hamida F, Morax S. Tumeurs orbitaires de l'enfant chapitre 15.I. In: Adenis JP, Morax S, editors. Pathologie Orbito-Palpébrale rapport de la Société Française d'Ophtalmologie 1998. Paris: Masson; 1998. p. 495–501.
3. Glasier CM, Brodsky MC, Leithiser RE Jr, Williamson SL, et al. High resolution ultrasound with Doppler: a diagnostic adjunct in orbital and ocular lesions in children. Pediatr Radiol. 1992;22(3):174–8.
4. Ramji FG, Slovis TL. Baker JD Orbital sonography in children. Pediatr Radiol. 1996;26(4):245–58.
5. Arndt C, Bergès O, Elmaleh-Bergès O, Meunier, I, Bernard JA. Examens complémentaires. In: Meux P, editor. Ophtalmologie pédiatrique DeLaage de, chap. 2. Paris: Masson; 2003. p. 36–68.
6. Gorospe L, Royo A, Berrocal T, García-Raya P, et al. Imaging of orbital disorders in pediatric patients. Eur Radiol. 2003;13(8):2012–26.
7. Elmaleh-Bergès M, Bergès O. Pathologie opphtalmologique. In: Adamsbaum C, editor. Imagerie pédiatrique et fœtale. Paris: Médecine-Sciences Flammarion; 2007. p. 174–186.
8. Onwochei BC, Simon JW, Bateman JB et al. Ocular colobomata. Surv Ophthalmol. 2000;45(3):175–94.
9. Hornby S, Gilbert C. Orbital cyst and bilateral colobomatous microphthalmos. Br J Ophthalmol. 2008;92(11):1568–9.
10. Kaufman LM, Villablanca JP, Mafee MF. Diagnostic imaging of cystic lesions in the child's orbit. Radiol Clin North Am. 1998;36(6):1149–63, xi.
11. Desjardins L. Les tumeurs en ophtalmo-pédiatrie. J Fr Ophtalmol. 2000;23(9):926–39.
12. Ducrey N, Nenadov-Beck M, Spahn B. La thérapie actuelle du rhabdomyosarcome orbitaire de l'enfant. J Fr Ophtalmol. 2002;25(3):298–302.
13. Pontes FS, de Oliveira JI, de Souza LL, de Almeida OP, et al. Clinicopathological analysis of head and neck rhabdomyosarcoma: a series of 10 cases and literature review. Med Oral Patol Oral Cir Bucal. 2018;23(2):e188–97.
14. Koka K, Alam MS, Subramanian N, Mukherjee B, et al. Clinical spectrum and management outcomes of Langerhans cell histiocytosis of the orbit. Indian J Ophthalmol. 2020;68(8):1604–8.
15. McAlister WH, Herman T, Dehner LP. Sinus histiocytosis with massive lymphadenopathy (Rosai-Dorfman disease). Pediatr Radiol. 1990;20(6):425–32.
16. Hidayat AA, Mafee MF, Laver NV, Noujaim S. Langerhans' cell histiocytosis and juvenile xanthogranuloma of the orbit. Clinicopathologic, CT, and MR imaging features. Radiol Clin North Am. 1998;36(6):1229–40, xii.
17. Schwyzer R, Sherman GG, Cohn RJ, et al. Granulocytic sarcoma in children with acute myeloblastic leukemia and t(8;21). Med Pediatr Oncol. 1998;31(3):144–9.

18. Rao AA, Naheedy JH, Ramkumar HL, et al. A clinical update and radiologic review of pediatric orbital and ocular tumors. J Oncol. 2013;2013: 975908.
19. Shields JA, Kaden IH, Shields CL et al. Orbital dermoid cysts: clinicopathologic correlations, classification, and management. The 1997 Josephine E. Schueler Lecture. Ophthalmic Plast Reconstr Surg. 1997;13(4):265–76.
20. Kumar R, Vyas K, Kundu J, et al. Deep orbital dermoid cyst bulging into the superior orbital fissure: clinical presentation and management. J Ophthalmic Vis Res. 2017;12(1):110–2.
21. Mouriaux F, Rysanek B, Babin E, Cattoir V. Les cellulites orbitaires. J Fr Ophtalmol. 2012;35(1):52–7.

# Index

Page numbers suffixed with 'f' and 't' refer to index terms in figures and tables, respectively.